Rave reviews for

PREEMIES:

THE ESSENTIAL GUIDE FOR PARENTS OF PREMATURE BABIES

"For families experiencing the emotional and complex journey of the NICU, *Preemies* is a practical and reassuring source of information on their premature baby's hospitalization, as well as the early years. A helpful resource for every NICU lending library!"

—Liza Cooper, LMSW, Director, NICU Family Support, March of Dimes Foundation

"*Preemies* is a wonderful book. It covers all the bases. During the panic and confusion of having and nurturing a premature baby, *Preemies* will become a parent's constant companion. As a clinical psychologist and father of a preemie, I deeply appreciate many aspects of *Preemies* and its new edition. Here are two. One is that *Preemies* is unique in that it provides additional information about what the doctors are thinking. Secondly, it conveys an understanding of what preemie parents are feeling, so we can realize that our fears and concerns are universal and normal."

—Michael T. Hynan, Ph.D., Chair, National Perinatal Association

"This second edition of *Preemies* is essential reading for parents of premature infants and equally for their caregivers. . . . This book is important."

—Peter A.M. Auld, M.D., Emeritus Professor of Pediatrics, Weill Cornell Medical College, New York

"*Preemies* is quite simply an extraordinary book. Its authors (they are parents who 'have been there,' and an empathetic neonatologist who 'has seen it all') have written a comprehensive manual which gives voice to the feelings and fears of parents in an easy-to-read question-and-answer format. . . . The book adopts a reassuring and comforting tone when dealing with the disappointment, the grief, the joy, and the roller-coaster ride that is the experience of many parents. . . . I cannot think of a topic that has not been addressed. This updated book is a comprehensive reference suitable for parents and health professionals alike. I learnt a lot from it and recommend it highly."

—Saroj Saigal, M.D., Professor Emerita, Department of Pediatrics; Director, Neonatal Follow-Up Clinic, McMaster University, Ontario, Canada

"The problem with most books about premature babies is that they tend to emphasize everything that can go wrong, no matter how rare. *Preemies: The Essential Guide for Parents of Premature Babies* is a reassuring yet realistic manual on caring for a preemie."

—*Parenting* magazine

"A must-have for parents and caregivers of premature infants. The authors have done a fantastic job of writing a guide that is both comprehensive and easily understandable. I recommend this book to all parents, caregivers and educators who work with infants born prematurely."
—Joelle Mast, Ph.D, M.D., Chief Medical Officer, Blythedale Children's Hospital, Valhalla, NY

"Parents will treasure this sensitively written guide that supplies the reader with valuable information, resources, and emotional support."
—Laura Kennedy, M.A., Director, Staten Island Early Childhood Direction Center, Staten Island University Hospital

"Complex medical and psychological information is imparted in a reassuring tone to parents coping with the rigors of premature birth and premature baby care. An extensive collaboration of a neonatologist and two experienced preemie parents . . . *Preemies* will make you a more informed parent—in the NICU and after."
—Allison Martin, Founder, Prematurity.org, Preemie Child, and ChildrensDisabilities.info

"The authors fulfill the need for information with remarkable clarity, offering answers to a multitude of questions [in] a personal, reassuring tone. . . . Since parents can't always plan ahead for the possibility of a preemie, this book provides a valuable crash course and serves as a useful tool for communicating with medical staff."
—*Publishers Weekly*

"This informative book reassures parents who have been thrust suddenly into the scary and unfamiliar world of the NICU. . . . I highly recommend purchasing a copy of this book if your little one has decided to be born too soon."
—Julie M. Snyder, Editor-in-Chief, Pregnancy.org, LLC

"An invaluable resource . . . a comprehensive, authoritative yet sensitive reference which explains a spectrum of issues in easy to understand language. . . . Whether read from cover to cover or used as reference text, parents of premature infants will be enlightened from the clinical wisdom provided by this book."
—Frank A. Chervenak, M.D., Given Foundation Professor and Chairman, Obstetrics and Gynecology, Weill Cornell Medical Center, New York

"Although one out of ten children born in this country is born prematurely, until now there has never been an authoritative, practical, and encouraging reference tool for their parents. This book . . . will prove to be a bible for parents of 'preemies' . . . and in fact is certain to be a blessing to them. Enthusiastically recommended."
—*Library Journal*

PREEMIES

The Essential Guide for Parents of Premature Babies

SECOND EDITION

Dana Wechsler Linden, Emma Trenti Paroli,
and Mia Wechsler Doron, M.D.

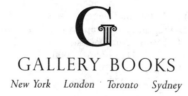

GALLERY BOOKS
New York   London   Toronto   Sydney

The ideas, procedures, and suggestions in this book are not intended as a substitute for the medical advice of your trained health professional. All matters regarding your health require medical supervision. Consult your physician before adopting the suggestions in this book, as well as about any condition that may require diagnosis or medical attention. The authors and publisher disclaim any liability arising directly or indirectly from the use of the book.

G

Gallery Books
A Division of Simon & Schuster, Inc.
1230 Avenue of the Americas
New York, NY 10020

Copyright © 2000, 2010 by Dana Wechsler Linden, Emma Trenti Paroli, and Mia Wechsler Doron, M.D.

Illustrations by Daniela Rossato and Sarah Wedge

All rights reserved, including the right to reproduce this book or portions thereof in any form whatsoever. For information address Pocket Books Subsidiary Rights Department, 1230 Avenue of the Americas, New York, NY 10020

This Gallery Books trade paperback edition November 2010

GALLERY BOOKS and colophon are trademarks of Simon & Schuster, Inc.

For information about special discounts for bulk purchases, please contact Simon & Schuster Special Sales at 1-866-506-1949 or business@simonandschuster.com.

The Simon & Schuster Speakers Bureau can bring authors to your live event. For more information or to book an event contact the Simon & Schuster Speakers Bureau at 1–866–248–3049 or visit our website at www.simonspeakers.com.

Designed by Ruth Lee-Mui

Manufactured in the United States of America

5   7   9   10   8   6   4

Library of Congress Cataloging-in-Publication Data
Linden, Dana Wechsler.
Preemies : the essential guide for parents of premature babies / Dana Wechsler Linden, Emma Trenti Paroli, Mia Wechsler Doron.
p.   cm.
1. Infants (Premature).   2. Infants (Premature)—Care.   3. Birth weight, Low—Complications.   4. Pregnancy—Complications.   I. Paroli, Emma Trenti.
II. Doron, Mia Wechsler.   III. Title.
RJ250.L56   2000
618.92'011—dc21   00-028554
ISBN 978-1-4165-7232-9

To our children,
and to all preemies

ACKNOWLEDGMENTS

We feel deeply grateful to our families, who all made sacrifices for this book, and especially can't find enough ways to thank Larry, Leonardo, Scott, Tess, Maya, Luigi, and Lily, whose support was precious and unending through it all; to a few, extraordinary doctors—Kathryn Crowley, Joelle Mast, Barney Softness, and Mark Souweidane—who took care of Dana's and Emma's babies with a rare combination of clinical skill and compassion; to the families of the preemies Mia has cared for, who shared their joys and fears and were examples of courage and strength; and to the experts who generously contributed their time and expertise to this book:

Heidelise Als of Harvard Medical School

Marie Anzalone of Columbia University

Ronald Ariagno of Stanford University School of Medicine

Diane Asbill of University of North Carolina Hospitals

Grace Baranek of University of North Carolina Hospitals

Jane Barlow of University of North Carolina Hospitals

Judy Bauman of University of North Carolina Hospitals

Patricia J. Becker of University of North Carolina Hospitals

Laraine Borman of Mothers' Milk Bank, Presbyterian St. Luke's Medical Center, Denver

R. V. Paul Chan of New York Presbyterian Hospital

Frank Chervenak of New York Presbyterian Hospital

Martha Collette of Massachusetts General Hospital

Myra Collins of University of North Carolina Hospitals

Liza Cooper of March of Dimes NICU Family Support

Rosalyn Benjamin Darling of Indiana University of Pennsylvania

Sharon K. Davis of New York, NY

Kathleen Donkin of New York, NY

Stacy Emack of Portland, Maine

Barry Fleisher of Stanford University School of Medicine

Sharon Freedman of Duke University Eye Center

Miriam Mazzoni Frigerio of Ospedale Sant'Anna, Como, Italy

Carol Gilmer of University of North Carolina Hospitals

Stanley Graven of University of South Florida College of Public Health

Victor Groza of Case Western Reserve University

Ruth Eckstein Grunau of British Columbia Children's Hospital, Canada

Wendy Hansen of University of Iowa Hospitals and Clinics

M. Ashley Hickman of University of North Carolina Hospitals

Carol Hubbard of University of North Carolina Hospitals

Thomas Ivester of University of North Carolina Hospitals

Melissa Johnson of WakeMed, Raleigh, North Carolina

Laura J. Kennedy of Staten Island University Hospital

Emily Pearl Kingsley of Children's Television Workshop

Laboratory Corporation of America, Burlington, North Carolina

Susan Shier Lowry of Governor Morehead School, Raleigh, North Carolina

Leah MacMillan of University of North Carolina Hospitals

Jane Madell of Beth Israel Medical Center, New York

Diane Marshall of University of North Carolina Hospitals

Joelle Mast of Blythedale Children's Hospital, Valhalla, NY

Joni McKeeman of University of North Carolina Hospitals

M. Kathryn Menard of University of North Carolina Hospitals

Florence Milch of New York Eye and Ear Infirmary

Management of PSA Healthcare

Molecular Genetics Laboratory of Mayo Clinic

Jennifer Rayburn of University of North Carolina Hospitals

Madeline D. Ribaudo of New York, NY

Jonathan Roth of Kaiser Permanente, Denver, Colorado

Barney Softness of West End Pediatrics, New York, NY

Lynn Spivak of North Shore/Long Island Jewish Health System

Judith Stadler of New York Presbyterian Hospital

Mark Steele of Pediatric Ophthalmic Consultants, New York, NY

Robert Strauss of University of North Carolina Hospitals

Stuart Teplin of University of North Carolina Hospitals

Mary Tully of Mothers' Milk Bank, WakeMed, Raleigh, North Carolina

Steven Wells of University of North Carolina Hospitals

Rhonda Weiss of Office of Special Education and Rehabilitation, U.S. Department of Education

Janice Wereszczak of University of North Carolina Hospitals

Randah Whitley of University of North Carolina Hospitals

Jason Williams of U.S. Army, Fort Bragg

Ida Wise of Blythedale Children's Hospital, Valhalla, NY

Karen Wood of University of North Carolina Hospitals

We also want to thank Tracy Berran of New York Presbyterian Hospital for reaching out to us and other parents of preemies; Lisa Gubernick for always pointing us in the right direction; the many other doctors and nurses at UNC Hospitals whose lessons fill the pages of this book, and especially Carl Bose for his unwavering support; Lisa Vogel for her cheerful, tireless typing efforts; Danielle Poiesz for moving mountains to get the manuscript in shape; our fabulous literary agent, Kris Dahl; and our phenomenal editors, Nancy Miller, who believed in this book from the first minute she heard about it; and Abby Zidle, who challenged us up to the last minute with her wit, intelligence, and patience to make the second edition the very best that it could be.

CONTENTS

Chapter 4. The First Week

PARENTS' STORIES: THE FIRST WEEK

THE DOCTOR'S PERSPECTIVE: THE FIRST WEEK

YOUNGEST PREEMIES TO OLDEST PREEMIES: WHAT YOUR BABY IS DOING AND SENSING

QUESTIONS AND ANSWERS

IN DEPTH

Chapter 5. Settling Down in the Hospital   237

Chapter 6. If Your Baby Needs Surgery   346

INTRODUCTION: IF YOUR BABY NEEDS SURGERY   346

QUESTIONS AND ANSWERS

KINDS OF SURGERY A PREEMIE MAY NEED   353

PART III: A LIFE TOGETHER

Chapter 9. When Parents Have Something Special to Worry About

INTRODUCTION: WHEN PARENTS HAVE SOMETHING
SPECIAL TO WORRY ABOUT

QUESTIONS AND ANSWERS

PART IV: OTHER CONSIDERATIONS

APPENDICES

INTRODUCTION TO
THE FIRST EDITION

Preemies was conceived a few years ago, when our lives took turns that we never could have predicted.

Dana and Mia were two sisters with professional lives that had never overlapped: Dana was a journalist writing for a business magazine in New York, and Mia a doctor who specialized in the care of premature and sick babies at the University of North Carolina at Chapel Hill. They hadn't met Emma, who lived a few miles from Dana and was also a journalist, writing about medical issues for the leading publications in Italy, where she grew up.

Dana and Emma were pregnant. Dana had a two-year-old daughter already, but this time she was expecting twins, so she had much to discover about the extraordinary experience of a multiple gestation. Emma was in her first pregnancy, the result of six years of infertility treatments. She was finally allowing herself to believe that, after all, she would become a mother.

It was for both expectant mothers a wonderful time in our lives. We expected our pregnancies to last nine months, of course, and felt safe as our favorite pregnancy books led us by the hand. But we never got to read the last chapters as we had pictured: lying on the sofa with swollen feet and giant bellies vibrating from vigorous baby kicks. Instead, Dana's water broke suddenly one night, and Emma developed an infection. We leaped over the last trimester of our pregnancies in a matter of days, delivering our babies almost three months before term.

Before we had even started to think about cribs and baby clothes, we were hurled under the glaring lights of the neonatal intensive care unit, where our children would spend the first months of their immature lives. We met in the nursery—in that high-tech world of frail, tiny babies, attached to machines that set off loud alarms whenever breathing or heart rate faltered for a few seconds, where our children were fighting for their lives.

And we were hardly alone. Our children had become part of a growing crowd—the one out of ten births in this country that are premature.

In the beginning, we didn't know anything about prematurity. We had to learn a great deal just to understand what was happening to our babies, and what it might mean for their futures. We asked questions of the medical staff. We called our friends' doctors for further explanations. Dana's sister Mia—how fortunate that she was a neonatologist!—left her family and job to be with Dana and Dana's husband during the most difficult days of their twin daughters' hospitalization.

But every day we needed more information, and the conversations with doctors and nurses were never enough. Sometimes the professionals taking care of our babies gave us conflicting answers to crucial questions. Sometimes they delivered news in callous or terrifying ways, adding unnecessary worries. There were many times when we were told things that we were simply too distressed to remember a few hours later.

Emma's son, Luigi, was diagnosed with a brain bleed and soon developed hydrocephalus, a buildup of fluid in the brain, which required surgery—how could he withstand it, at his tiny size, and what would this mean for his development? Dana's daughter Elena was breathing vigorously in the delivery room—did that mean she was out of danger? Why did Maya's ears fold over in a funny way? Were our babies as aware as they seemed? Were they in pain? We had hundreds of questions; some profound, others so seemingly trivial that we didn't dare ask.

As a neonatologist, Mia had counseled many parents about their premature babies over the years. She knew that even the most empathetic doctor, when charged with caring for dozens of tiny or critically ill babies in an intensive care nursery, doesn't have enough time in the day to give each parent all of the information he or she so desperately wants. She bought Dana and her husband, as a "birth-day" gift, a book about premature babies, the only guide she knew of for parents. But even though the time she spent with them, explaining and advising and comforting, was invaluable, the book terrified them, emphasizing all of the things that can go wrong in premature babies (but that most parents really don't have to worry about). At the hospital where Dana and Emma met, the doctors said regretfully that there was no book they could wholeheartedly recommend.

A few months later, memories from the NICU brought us together, and so, from our experiences, *Preemies* was born, as the book Dana and Emma wished they could have had, and Mia wished she could have given—a companion and resource, guide and teacher, realistic but reassuring. It is a book that parents can keep on their nightstand, or keep handy as they travel back and forth to the hospital, to consult briefly and frequently, as new questions and doubts arise almost every day. It is a book for all future parents, and those close to them, who will both suffer and rejoice in their children's premature births.

What happened to our preemies in the NICU and after is the personal legacy we carry into this book. Luigi had his surgery, came out of it stronger than ever, and went home a few days later. Maya had some serious ups and downs—including a sudden illness and rehospitalization just a few days after she got home—but grew gradually healthier, and came home for good before her due date. Elena, although she was slightly bigger than her twin sister at birth, suffered much more. She developed a tear in her lung, and a spiral of complications followed. She died in the hospital. Her parents miss her badly.

Our inspirations in writing *Preemies* have been Mia's little patients and their parents, whose bravery and openness she admires and finds constantly amazing, and Dana's and Emma's preemies: the memory of Elena Linden, and Maya Linden and Luigi Trenti Paroli, who are now normal, beautiful, thriving preschoolers, so happy to be alive.

POSTSCRIPT TO
THE SECOND EDITION

Already ten years have passed—bringing knowledge, medical advances, and changes in the care of premature babies—and it is time to revise this book. We look back at the years when we were first writing *Preemies* with wonder.

Dana and Emma were taking care of Maya and Luigi, their own high-risk children, and at the same time writing about all premature babies, trying to put themselves in other parents' shoes: What do they need to know at this time? What is the best way to convey the information to them? For Mia, the struggle was between being the doctor for each of her little patients in the hospital and then writing for a general audience of parents with the same degree of authority and compassion. The task was so demanding that our memories of that time are still fresh, as if it were yesterday. Now that Maya and Luigi are grown beyond belief and—we're happy to say still beautiful and thriving, we realize that our book has come a long way, too.

Preemies has been very successful. It has received outstanding reviews from medical experts and has become the companion book for a huge number of parents of premature babies. All of the grateful letters and comments that have come to us over the years are a constant reward and reminder that we met our goal: to write the informative yet hopeful book Dana and Emma wished they could have had and Mia wished she could have given when their babies were born.

Today, there are more premature births than ever: over half a million babies a year, or more than 12.5 percent of births in the United States alone. Not long after the publication of *Preemies*, we gained some extraordinary allies in our quest to help families of premature babies. Since 2003 the March of Dimes has devoted its tremendous resources to fighting prematurity and the toll it takes on families. Thanks to them and to the efforts of the Association of Maternal and Child Health Programs and the sponsorship of bipartisan representatives, a law known as the "PREEMIE" act was passed by Congress on December 22, 2006. This law supports medical research, surveys, education, and programs aimed to help lessen and limit the dangers and harms of premature birth.

Empowered by this positive energy, we and our publisher decided to update *Preemies*. While incorporating new findings in medical research and practice and other changes of recent years, we've tried to keep the book what we originally wanted it to be: a realistic but reassuring guide for all adults who love and care for a preemie, and a comprehensive but not overwhelming source of information, to be taken in a step at a time. We hope we have succeeded and that this second edition will be as appreciated as the first.

In these past ten years, while our book took on a life of its own as a guide for other parents, we watched—at first with trepidation—our own preemies grow. At this moment, Luigi and Maya are in middle school, poring over their homework and very serious about their studies. They are average height for their age, but while Maya is reedy, Luigi is big-boned like his maternal grandfather. They both adore dogs. Maya is training a puppy she's raising to become a guide dog for the blind, and with daily practice she has her doing amazing things. Luigi just likes to play and have fun with his dog. When it comes to playing the piano, though, he practices. He's a gifted young musician with eclectic tastes, from classical to rock to electronic music. We sometimes wonder whether this psychological trait or that physical attribute comes from their difficult start in life, but the truth is we've been so lucky with them that you'd never know they were preemies. When someone new learns that Maya was born at two pounds or Luigi at three pounds, six ounces (a big 29-weeker), there's usually a gasp of disbelief. The pain of missing Elly is less sharp now for Dana and her family, but her memory is just as important—beyond measure—to all of them, including Maya.

To all of our present and future readers: Our fervent wish is for you to enjoy all the good moments with your premature baby despite the hurdles. Your baby's first months and years are a precious gift you can experience only once. We wish we could go back and rejoice more often during our own experiences. We send you our loving thoughts, wishing you all the luck we have had with our own preemies and more.

A NOTE TO THE READER: HOW TO USE THIS BOOK

There are a few things you need to know, as a reader of *Preemies*. This book cannot and is not intended to replace conversations with your baby's doctors. Every baby is different, and each case has its own subtleties. In fact, we hope *Preemies* will encourage more meaningful conversations with your baby's doctors, by giving you background knowledge and helping you to know what questions to ask.

Very important: *Don't read all of this book!* We purposely wrote it in bite-sized pieces, with each question-and-answer or box addressing a separate topic, so that you can read about the specific issues that are relevant for you and your baby—and skip all of the rest. Every preemie's story is different, and if you read about the wide range of problems that occur in different children—most of which you'll never have to deal with—you'll develop a scary, highly distorted image of what to expect for your baby. Most babies who are born premature today grow into healthy, happy, normal children and encounter only a fraction of the hurdles you can read about here. So browse through each chapter or use the index to follow your baby's own unique experience.

Use the table of contents to find the questions or topics you may encounter during that period of your baby's life. Read *Parents' Stories* at the beginning of most chapters if you are interested in reflecting on your emotional reactions, and on how some other parents of premature babies respond to this experience. *The Doctor's Perspective* section gives you an insight into something we found mysterious and very much wanted to know: what your baby's doctor might be looking for and concerned about at each stage. This section also provides a good overview of the whole chapter's issues, if you want one. If you would like statistics on the outcomes and paths of premature babies in general, you can find them in *Youngest Preemies to Oldest Preemies: Survival and Long-Term Health* on page 55. Look under your baby's gestational age for the information that applies to him.

Keep in mind that different nurseries do things differently. Our descriptions cover some of the most common ways of doing things but not all, so if the medical staff at your hospital does things in ways that diverge from our descriptions, that doesn't mean they're wrong. That's also true for services that are available to preemies after they leave the hospital. State-run organizations in particular vary widely across the country.

Thankfully, neonatal care is changing and progressing all the time. We'll update this book periodically, but for information on the most recent research and developments, you should rely on your baby's doctors. For all of the general parenting issues that aren't unique to preemies and relate just as much to full-term babies (there are lots of things that are not different for a premature baby, and we'll be pointing many of these out to you), you should turn to the many excellent pregnancy and child-care guides in print.

We suggest you keep *Preemies* on hand throughout your baby's early childhood, since many parents continue to have occasional questions. Our hope is that it will be a reliable, reassuring companion for you, always there when you need it—and a good luck charm, too!

Part I

BEFORE THE BIRTH

CHAPTER 1

IN THE WOMB

Why Premature Birth Happens and What Can Be Done to Prevent It

. . . .

For parents trying to grasp the extent of their risk and what they can do to minimize it.
Also for parents looking back, trying to make sense of what happened.

. . . .

INTRODUCTION: IN THE WOMB

A normal pregnancy that leads nine months later to the birth of a healthy baby is a natural life experience in which doctors are mostly watchful bystanders until the time of delivery. But if you're at risk for a premature birth, your experience is going to be different. Some women will be aware of their risk before they conceive. For many others, suddenly becoming a patient comes as a shocking surprise.

If you're likely to have a preterm birth, you'll probably get assistance from an obstetrician who specializes in high-risk pregnancies (called a perinatologist). Your doctor's efforts will be directed at preventing a premature birth or postponing it as much as is possible and advisable.

Why prematurity happens is still a puzzle. In fact, experts believe that most preterm births result not from a single cause but from several risk factors that interact throughout the pregnancy. Doctors know many reasons for preterm birth (as you'll see from the list in Appendix 1 on page 575) and can identify many pregnancies at risk, but almost half of the expectant mothers who go into preterm labor have no known risks for it. If you've already given birth to a preemie and never suspected that it might happen to you, you're certainly not alone.

Perhaps even more frustrating is that many premature births cannot be prevented even when mothers are known to be at risk. Still, even if a premature delivery cannot be avoided, a lot can be done to delay it for at least a few days (and sometimes much longer), enough time to take some precautions that can greatly reduce the health risks for both you and your baby. For example, you may be admitted to a hospital where you and your baby can be monitored 24 hours a day, or transferred to a facility with more expertise in perinatology and newborn intensive care. If you have an infection, you'll be started on antibiotics to help prevent your baby from getting it, too. And you may be given steroids to help your baby's organs mature faster before birth.

Sometimes, your doctor may decide to purposely deliver your baby before term because he is not growing or doing well in the womb or because it has become too dangerous for your own health to continue the pregnancy. About 20 percent of all preterm births are such so-called elective, or medically indicated, preterm births. The rest occur spontaneously, about 30 percent after a woman's water breaks too early and about half after preterm labor.

As you read through the information in this chapter, remember that only an experienced obstetrician can evaluate your individual case. It's important for you to develop a good, trusting relationship with your obstetrician so that you can count on her for support as well as for state-of-the-art medical care as you travel the demanding road of a high-risk pregnancy.

QUESTIONS AND ANSWERS

Bed Rest

My doctor told me to go on bed rest, but I have so many things in my life I need to do. Will bed rest really help prevent an early birth?

Nobody knows for sure. Bed rest is probably the oldest prescription for a high-risk pregnancy. Yet despite its widespread use—one in every five pregnant women in the United States is put on bed rest—it has not been studied extensively. Although more research is needed before anyone can answer your question for sure, so far the few studies that have been done have produced no convincing evidence that bed rest helps reduce preterm births.

So why do almost all obstetricians prescribe it to women with preterm labor, premature rupture of membranes, preeclampsia, bleeding, or other pregnancy problems, and sometimes even as a preventive measure to women who are expecting multiples? Because even without proof, there are situations in which bed rest makes sense to doctors for some solid, scientific reasons.

For example, say your baby isn't growing as well as she should in the womb. Fetuses depend entirely on blood flowing through the placenta for their supply of nutrients and oxygen, and a mother's blood flow to the placenta is greatest when she is lying down. So it makes sense that your baby will have the best chance of growing better if you spend a few extra hours in bed each day.

Or say your water has broken early. It makes sense that you could maximize the amount of fluid remaining around your baby by spending more time off your feet, since increased blood flow to the baby leads to greater production of amniotic fluid. Also, the fluid is less likely to drip out when you're lying down.

Bed rest also makes sense when gravity may be dangerous for a pregnancy. For example, once a woman's membranes have ruptured, there is a risk that the umbilical cord could slip down through her cervix—an absolute emergency, because the cord could get caught there and squeezed, cutting off blood flow to the baby. Gravity also can be risky when a woman has a weak, or "insufficient," cervix, which could open if the fetus presses down on it too hard.

There is also good evidence that blood pressure is higher in women who are walking around. So it is assumed that bed rest is helpful to pregnant women with preeclampsia, a condition involving high blood pressure that when it's severe can necessitate a premature delivery. Although research hasn't demonstrated so far whether bed rest itself makes the difference, there has been a dramatic improvement in the outcomes of pregnancies with preeclampsia. It may partly have to do with the increasing use of hospitalization, which allows for both intensive monitoring and more bed rest than most women can get at home.

But if sometimes there is sound reasoning behind the prescription of bed rest, other times there is simply a mixture of observation and wishful thinking. Take preterm labor. Many doctors believe that women who remain active in the third trimester of pregnancy have more Braxton-Hicks contractions, the normal "false labor" contractions that don't lead to cervical change and delivery, and are of no concern. It's natural to assume that bed rest might reduce the risk of real labor, too. Nobody knows whether the initial observation about Braxton-Hicks contractions or its extension to real labor is valid.

(*Continued on page 7*)

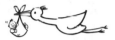

Bed Rest Survival Tips

OK. You've been put on bed rest, and you're understandably feeling miserable. How are you going to make it through the long weeks ahead? These survival tips may help:

* **Recognize that you are performing a job, one of the hardest you'll ever do.** If you are an active person with a tendency to ask, "What have I gotten done today?" it's easy to feel frustrated and inadequate while on bed rest—unless you give yourself credit for a daily achievement: an investment in your child's and family's future. Whenever you feel that you can't take it anymore or are about to give in to the many temptations to get up, remind yourself of the job you have to do and focus on your goal!

* **Make your physical comfort a priority.** Lying down for long stretches at a time can be very uncomfortable, and aches and pains are going to make your job far more difficult. You may have heard that you should lie on your left side because blood flow to the placenta will be greatest, but your right side is good for your baby, too. What's most important is simply to avoid lying flat on your back, because blood flow is reduced that way. Rest a pillow under one side of your tummy or back, so you're on a slight tilt. That's fine!

* **Do light exercises in bed.** To avoid muscle and bone loss, some obstetricians now arrange for a physical therapist to visit their patients on complete bed rest. If your doctor doesn't mention this, don't hesitate to ask. The therapist can teach you light isometric exercises you can do while lying down. Or you can try to make up your own very light exercise regime: no abdominal crunches (since they could stimu-

late your uterus), but point and flex your toes, rotate your ankles and hands, do head rolls, tense and relax the muscles of your arms and legs, and lift some light hand weights.

* **Stay clean and attractive.** It's amazing how this can affect your mood. Many hospitals have arrangements with hairdressers who will come to your room and expertly wash your hair without ever asking you to sit up. If you're at home, ask friends or the staff of your hair salon if they know of a hairdresser who makes house calls. Put on makeup every morning. Some women find that when they're feeling down, it lifts their mood to pamper themselves with manicures, pedicures, or facials.

* **Make your environment attractive, too.** It will just take a couple of minutes for a friend or your partner to tape up some family photos or artwork by your children. When you're feeling imprisoned, warm touches go a long way!

* **Don't expect the household to run as smoothly or cleanly as usual.** It's a fact of life: Women on bed rest don't have clean houses! If your family eats pizza for the seventh time in a week, you're not alone, either. The best thing is to lower your expectations, recognize that these things aren't a priority right now, and plan to fix them later when you're up and about.

* **Organize your space.** It's terrible to have to ask for every little thing you need. Instead, ask your partner to put a table next to your bed with the following items within easy reach: a telephone, books and magazines, grooming items, tissues and disposable cleansing wipes or liquid (to wash your hands), the remote control, an iPod or laptop, paper and pencil, things you need for your hobby, and a cooler with water and lunch that your partner sets out for you each morning. No matter how much your partner wants to help, it will minimize tension between you if he doesn't have to act as your constant gofer.

* **Be understanding that bed rest is hard on your partner and children, too.** Your partner's life is also disrupted. He may be as worried and distressed as you are, and he's probably picking up lots of extra tasks while holding down his usual responsibilities. Try not to be resentful of him for still being able to move around or for not being able to meet your every need. And give him as much time off as you can. It's important to keep supporting each other.

It's normal for your children to show some reaction, either behaving badly toward others or toward you. It's also normal for you to worry about them and to think how long this period feels to them. But believe us, they will forget about it soon afterward. In the meantime, encourage them to spend time with you by making your bedside into a play area with their toys and putting up a little table where they can eat some meals. Try to arrange special time for them with grandparents. Some mothers say it helped a lot for their child to be present when the doctor explained the need for bed rest; hearing it from an outside authority made the child understand better and even eager to cooperate.

* **If you were working, make sure to discuss financial arrangements with your employer.** Find out if you are eligible for disability payments and whether this time is being counted as part of your maternity leave or sick leave. Remember that the Family and Medical Leave Act requires employers with 50 or more employees to give up to 12 weeks of unpaid leave related to pregnancy problems or childbirth. You are eligible if you have been working for your employer for 12 months, have worked at least 1,250 hours during the last year, and work in a location where your company has at least 50 employees. (Companies are allowed to make exceptions for their highest-paid "key" employees.)

* **Get some easy things done from bed.** You haven't bought furniture or linens for the nursery yet? There are child care books you've wanted to read and don't have? Shop by catalog or computer. Or give your mother-in-law a list of all the layette items you need—she'll probably be thrilled to help, and it's like having a personal shopper! Now is also a good time to do those quiet things that haven't quite made it to the top of your to-do list because they aren't urgent and take hours, like organizing your files, photo albums, or recipe box, writing letters to the editor or to old friends, constructing a family tree, or trying out the craft ideas you've saved from magazines. Not only will the time pass more quickly, but you'll have the satisfied feeling that you made this period of inactivity into something even more productive than it would have been.

* **Don't be surprised if you get depressed or have ups and downs.** Many women say that some days their spirits are up and then suddenly they find themselves in tears. Irritability, lots of anxiety, anger, and inability to concentrate are all normal reactions. You can expect a few naïve comments from friends, like "I'd love to be on bed rest and catch up on my reading." But most people who have been on bed rest themselves will tell you that it's hard. When you think what you're doing it for, though, it's worth it.

Even though studies on pregnant women haven't found that bed rest decreases preterm labor, well-meaning obstetricians want to do *something* for women with preterm labor, so as long as there is a possibility that bed rest might help, many suggest it.

Some obstetricians also have observed that a prescription of bed rest can bring a helpful focus to a pregnancy. The thinking is that your pregnancy may have the best chance of succeeding if you, your family, and even your doctor focus more attention on your needs, concerns, and symptoms. Some women say this worked for them: that after trying to juggle a lot of things during the early part of their pregnancies, bed rest actually reduced their stress by allowing them to shift their emphasis away from their many other daily obligations.

Undoubtedly, obstetricians also prescribe bed rest partly as a holdover from past medical practice. As recently as two decades ago, nearly every woman with a pregnancy risk or problem was put immediately to bed and told to stay there 24 hours a day.

Today, however, on top of a lack of proof of bed rest's effectiveness, there's a growing awareness of its potential costs. Total bed rest quickly causes bone and muscle loss (much of which is regained after a woman becomes active again) and increases the chance of developing a blood clot in the legs. And for plenty of women, bed rest causes more stress not less. In fact, it can be really hard on an entire family, especially when there are older children or job and financial concerns. So more and more doctors are recommending reduced activity—lying down for a few hours each morning and a few hours each afternoon—rather than complete bed rest, except in a few situations, such as an already open cervix, ruptured membranes, or severe preeclampsia.

Thankfully, you'll rarely see the once-common Trendelenburg position, in which a woman lies with her feet raised higher than her head. There's no evidence that it makes a difference and a general consensus that no one can tolerate that position for long!

While you nestle in bed, try to stay as optimistic as possible (remember that medical treatments often work best when patients believe they will) and take a look at the practical tips in Appendix 1 on page 575 to make that experience more tolerable.

Predicting the Birth Date

My doctor says I'm at risk for having a premature baby. Is there any way of telling how long my pregnancy will last?

If pregnancy researchers had a Holy Grail, it would be the ability to predict whether an expectant mother would deliver her baby early and, if so, when. That crucial information would allow doctors to intervene early, when therapies are most likely to be effective, and treat only women who really need them.

The good news is that if you or your baby has a known medical complication, there are excellent tests of fetal well-being (see page 42) that can help your doctor determine how long your pregnancy can safely go on. But most methods adopted so far to help predict whether preterm labor or premature rupture of the membranes might cut short a pregnancy that is otherwise proceeding well—such as adding up and scoring a mother's risk factors or closely monitoring her uterine contractions—have had disappointing results. In recent years, researchers have been looking at a new set of tests, some more promising than others.

Many obstetricians have started using ultrasound to examine the cervix in addition to the cervical exam they've always done by hand. At each pregnancy visit, doctors traditionally feel a woman's cervix with their fingertips to see if it is starting to open (or dilate), but they can feel only the outermost part of the cervix. With ultrasound, they can do a more precise assessment, including observing its inner opening at the connection with the uterus, where dilation

sometimes begins, and measuring its length (since the cervix shortens before it dilates).

If you have an ultrasound exam of your cervix, it may be performed by your obstetrician in his office or by a specialist (a doctor or ultrasound technician) at a hospital. You'll lie in the usual position you're so accustomed to for obstetrics exams, with your legs apart and your feet on footrests, while an ultrasound probe with a sterile cover is inserted in your vagina. An image of the lower part of your uterus and cervix will appear on the monitor. You may feel some gentle pressure, but it doesn't hurt, and the exam is not dangerous to you or your baby.

Don't be concerned if your obstetrician doesn't recommend this test because doctors agree it shouldn't be used to screen all pregnant women. If your risk of delivering early is low, it's still imperfect and can lead to useless medical treatment and unnecessary scares. If you're at higher risk, though, it's more reliable: There is a strong relationship between a shortened or dilating cervix in the second trimester of pregnancy (when the cervix should still be long and closed) and delivery of a premature baby.

Deciding how to use this information once you have it is still a tough call. A great many high-risk women with a short cervix—about 25 percent—will nevertheless still go to term. And in any case, the ultrasound exam doesn't tell the doctor *why* a cervix is shortening or opening. If it is a sign of cervical weakness or "insufficiency," a cerclage (a surgical procedure to help the cervix stay shut) might be called for. If it's because of an infection, medication might be the answer. Or there could be inflammation from unknown causes, which doctors don't yet know how to treat effectively. So unfortunately, moving from finding a short or dilated cervix on an ultrasound to preventing a premature delivery is neither straightforward nor always possible.

What if a cervical ultrasound finds nothing wrong? Then it *is* helpful, telling you that a premature birth is not imminent. For instance, even though you're having some contractions, if your cervix isn't shortened and there are no signs of inner dilation, your contractions almost certainly won't progress to true preterm labor. What a relief to find that out! You might avoid an unnecessary hospitalization, surgery, or treatment with anti-labor drugs and proceed with your pregnancy feeling reassured.

Two other new tools for predicting prematurity are now available, thanks to research on the biomarkers of preterm labor, as scientists call the substances in a woman's body whose levels change when she's about to deliver her baby. The Food and Drug Administration has approved tests that measure the biomarkers fibronectin and salivary estriol.

Fibronectin is a protein that helps keep the placenta and the membranes well attached to the uterine lining. If high levels of it leak through the cervix into the vagina during the second trimester of pregnancy (your doctor can do a simple swab of your vagina to find out), it may indicate that the placenta and amniotic sac's membranes are loosening. Just like cervical ultrasound, this test isn't accurate in women whose risk of delivering prematurely is low. But if you have reasons to be concerned—say you have symptoms of preterm labor or are pregnant with twins and are getting ready to take a trip—then a normal test can be extremely reassuring, almost guaranteeing that you won't deliver within the next week or two. High levels of fibronectin aren't nearly as reliable a predictor as low levels, so don't let them worry you too much. Only about 15 percent to 25 percent of women with high levels end up delivering prematurely.

The other test measures a pregnant woman's saliva to see how much of the hormone estriol it contains. Estriol is a type of estrogen that helps prepare the uterus for labor and delivery. It gradually increases as pregnancy advances, but a steep surge can indicate that labor is likely to occur within two to three weeks. Unfortunately, salivary estriol is much more reliable in predicting a late premature birth (after 35 weeks of gestation) than an earlier one. Since babies born after 35 weeks are at low risk for medical complications, the clinical usefulness of this test is not great.

Your obstetrician will decide which tests to use in monitoring your pregnancy. None of them is the panacea we'd all like to have, and predicting a premature birth—hard as it is—is still easier than preventing one. But they can help your doctor decide what needs to be done, and if your test results are reassuring, you and your family can relax and sleep tighter at night.

Exercise and Preterm Labor

My mother thinks I went into preterm labor because I kept playing tennis while I was pregnant. Could that be true?

Actually, contrary to conventional wisdom, studies have found women who exercise regularly during pregnancy are less likely to give birth prematurely than women who don't.

True, part of the reason may be just that women who feel good throughout their pregnancy are more inclined to be physically active. But another reasonable explanation is that exercise reduces stress. Stress is being investigated as a possible trigger of preterm labor, because we now know that it can wear and tear our bodies' adaptive and immune systems over time, opening the door to illnesses and inflammation. It's possible that exercising helps lower the risk of prematurity by reducing stress—as long as exercising is not so excessive that it becomes a source of stress itself.

Interestingly, one study done in India found that practicing yoga and meditation during pregnancy went along with a lower risk of preterm birth. The study compared the effect of one hour of daily yoga postures, breathing, and meditation techniques to the effect of twice-daily 30-minute walks. Only 14 percent of the women who practiced yoga delivered prematurely compared with 29 percent of those who didn't. Now if you're a yoga fan, take this news with a grain of salt, since it's intriguing but by no means definitive. At this point, practice yoga only with your obstetrician's permission and avoid hot yoga (which aims to raise your core temperature and could potentially damage a developing baby) and extreme stretching postures, which could possibly reduce blood flow to your uterus or injure ligaments that are laxer as a result of pregnancy's hormonal changes.

If you haven't already asked your doctor why you went into labor early, it would be a good idea: Finding out what he suspects will be helpful if you are thinking about getting pregnant again. But for now, you can stop feeling guilty. If you felt comfortable running on a court and hitting a good forehand while you were pregnant, it's almost certain that this didn't cause your preterm labor.

Family History and Ethnicity

I'm African-American and have a sister who gave birth prematurely. Does prematurity run in families or ethnic groups?

The short answer is yes, but there are still lots of uncertainties about why. And of course, as with any trait, some members of a family or group may have it and others not.

After observing that women who have one preemie tend to deliver early again and that women who were born prematurely themselves often have their own preemies, particularly if they were born at 30 weeks of gestation or less, physicians long suspected that some women have an inherited predisposition to deliver prematurely. Many studies of twins and siblings, and close examination of family histories, support the existence of a genetic susceptibility to give birth early.

One reason genes may matter is that they make a difference in how, and how strongly, a woman's body reacts to trauma, toxins, and certain microorganisms, including the peaceful bacteria that live on the skin, mouth, or vagina without anyone knowing it. A pregnant woman who mounts a particularly vigorous inflammatory response (as doctors call the physical reaction to bodily insult or invasion) can find herself in premature labor, while one whose body is more tolerant may sail through her pregnancy. You and your sister are more likely to be similar to each other in these sorts of reactions than to a stranger who isn't related to you.

But prematurity can run in families for nongenetic reasons, too. Family members tend to be similar in their diet, living conditions, activities, and habits, and each of these can make a preterm birth more likely or less. The same is true for members of the same ethnic group, who also share cultural behaviors and practices, as well as some genes. And socioeconomic disadvantages, more common in some ethnic groups, go hand in hand with chronic stress and greater exposure to infection, which can increase inflammation throughout the body and lead to a premature birth.

Of course, your sister may have delivered prematurely for reasons having nothing to do with your shared genes and family history. She may smoke, for example, or have another of the risk factors described in Appendix 1 on page 575. If she does have one that you don't, you're less likely to have a preemie of your own.

(Continued on page 13)

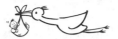

Lifestyle Choices and Preterm Birth

Exercise is one of the many lifestyle choices that have been thought—rightly or wrongly—to play a role in premature birth. Here are the latest findings on some others:

✴ **Sexual activity.** Interesting recent studies indicate that sex is not a cause of premature delivery and, despite popular belief, does not stimulate labor when pregnancy has reached full term. On the contrary, the statistics show that sexual activity and orgasm throughout pregnancy are strong predictors of a full-term delivery. So why do most obstetricians say to avoid sexual intercourse if you've had episodes of premature labor, rupture of membranes, or bleeding? Because, as with exercise, it's possible that self-selection is a factor. Women whose pregnancies are going well may feel more comfortable with intimacy. Sex can cause minor injury to your cervix and spread infection into your uterus, and substances in a man's semen, and a woman's sexual response, can stimulate uterine contractions. It could be that in normal pregnancies, when sex stirs up uterine contractions they die down before progressing to true labor. But if you're already at high risk for a premature delivery, your doctor may fear that the relatively minor effects of sexual intercourse just could be the straw that breaks the camel's back. (If your pregnancy is going well but you're nervous about a premature delivery anyway, you could consider using a condom, so you aren't exposed to semen.)

✴ **Physical exertion.** A physically demanding job was once believed to cause preterm labor, but new data show that standing for up to 30 hours a week, lifting heavy objects, or working long hours do not increase the risk of prematurity. Pregnant women who work at least 46 hours a week actually have a lower risk for preterm birth, probably because they feel healthy and capable of doing so (while women with pregnancy complications might choose or be advised to stop working). There's just one job situation—working night shifts—that seems to be associated with a higher risk for premature delivery, for reasons that aren't yet known.

✴ **Smoking.** Obstetricians recommend that a woman immediately quit smoking when she finds out she's expecting—or even better, before that—for the sake of her health as well as her child's. Cigarette smoke can stunt fetal growth and also cause preterm rupture of membranes, placental abruption, placenta previa, and premature birth. The more you smoke, the greater the risk. Ideally you should quit altogether right away, but every little bit helps, and even cutting back on cigarettes in the second half of your pregnancy can reduce your chance of having a small-for-gestational-age or premature baby. (You'll also really improve your baby's future health by not exposing him to secondhand smoke.)

✴ **Drinking coffee.** The final word is still out on the safety of drinking coffee during pregnancy. Some studies have found that more than one or two cups of coffee a day during pregnancy might lead to higher rates of miscarriage and low birthweight babies, but many doctors are still skeptical. In the meantime, moderation is probably best. Think about cutting back your coffee to no more than a cup a day or switching to decaf (caffeine is believed to be the culprit, although decaffeinated coffee hasn't been studied much). If you reduce your daily caffeine intake gradually, you will avoid unpleasant side effects like morning headaches or constipation.

* **Licorice.** In the United States, where white teeth are so prized, concentrated licorice candies—the black ones—aren't popular. But many people in other parts of the world do love their licorice. Heavy licorice consumption during pregnancy increases the risk of prematurity because of some still unknown effect of glycyrrhizin, the main extract of the licorice plant. Don't worry, there's no need to stop eating red licorice (which isn't really licorice at all) or delicious anise cookies (since anise flavoring doesn't come from the licorice plant, it's OK).

* **Drinking alcohol.** Drinking alcoholic beverages early in pregnancy increases the risk of birth defects. It has also been linked to a higher rate of preterm deliveries but only in women who have more than seven drinks a week during their pregnancy, compared with those who completely abstain. No increased risk of prematurity has been found in expectant mothers who have fewer than four drinks a week. Sound advice would be to avoid alcohol completely in the first few months of pregnancy and later to enjoy only an occasional cocktail or glass of wine.

* **Recreational drug use.** Cocaine or amphetamines during pregnancy can cause birth defects, poor fetal growth, placental abruption, and preterm birth. They may also lead to neurological and behavioral problems in the baby.

* **Environmental pollution.** Mothers who live in environments that are particularly full of everyday pollutants like automobile exhaust, cigarette smoke, and other chemicals (such as those contained in pesticides), have a higher risk of delivering babies who are small for their gestational age, have smaller heads, and are more likely to develop asthma and cognitive delays later in life.

  Environmental pollution tends to be worse in inner-city neighborhoods. Because most people can't completely change the environment in which they live or work, avoiding pollution is not a simple lifestyle choice you can make. But you should try to avoid contact with pesticides or toxic disinfectants and direct exposure to strong fumes, such as those of paint thinners, dry cleaning solution, or oven cleaners—when possible. (The safety of most common household cleansers during pregnancy hasn't been well researched. Most experts think they are OK in normal amounts but say it can't hurt to keep a window open when you're using them, just to be cautious.)

* **Diet and vitamin supplements.** There is some evidence that taking daily multivitamins before and during pregnancy may reduce the risk of preterm birth, particularly in women who don't have good nutrition. Your obstetrician will give you information about the optimal pregnancy diet and will recommend vitamin supplementation if he thinks you need it. The U.S. Public Health Service recommends that all women of childbearing age take 400 micrograms of folic acid a day to prevent birth defects. A pregnant woman might also need extra calcium, iron, and other supplements in her diet, but she should talk to her doctor, who will prescribe the quantities she needs.

In the United States, black women are twice as likely to have a preemie as white women of the same educational level and three times as likely to deliver a very young preemie—before 32 weeks—according to the latest data. Overall, black women have a prematurity rate of nearly 18 percent, compared with 12 percent for Hispanic women, 11.5 percent for white women, and 10.5 percent for Asian women. (Interestingly, the prematurity rate is higher for second-generation Hispanic women than for their immigrant mothers, even though they tend to be better off, possibly because the younger generation adopts some bad American habits like smoking or eating fast food.) Experts still can't fully explain why there are such big differences but suspect that stress related to racism or social status (which can lead, for example, to changes in the inflammatory response) in addition to genetic predisposition, behavior, and exposures in the environment may all be working together to cause a premature birth.

With the recent decoding of the human genome, researchers have new tools that might help them understand the connection between ethnicity and premature birth. For example, new studies show that black babies are three times more likely than white babies to have a genetic variation that makes their bodies produce less collagen, one of the building blocks of the amniotic sac. Lower levels of collagen may mean weaker amniotic membranes that are more likely to rupture prematurely and lead to premature birth. A future step could be experiments on treatments to boost production of collagen in early pregnancy and help a healthy, strong amniotic sac develop around the fetus.

Just as in other parts of our lives, we get good things from our families and bad. If there's a bright side, it's that sharing the hard things with people close to us can sometimes make them easier. When you think about it, why would something as basic as birth be any different?

If You Are Overweight

I needed to lose 35 pounds before conceiving, but here I'm pregnant with my first baby and overweight. Is this going to hurt my baby?

Probably not. An overweight mother who is healthy doesn't have a higher chance of delivering a preemie. There's even evidence that if you are healthy and overweight, you have a lower than average risk (whereas mothers who are too thin are more apt to deliver prematurely).

But you shouldn't throw caution to the wind and take this reassuring news as encouragement to "eat for two." A balanced, nutritious diet is very important for you and your baby. Your obstetrician will advise you on the amount and kind of calories you need for your baby to grow well without your accumulating too many more extra pounds.

That's important because even if you are fit and exercise regularly, being overweight means you have a greater chance of developing high blood pressure due to your pregnancy, or gestational diabetes. These diseases, which show up for the first time during pregnancy, are not only a problem for you but they can affect your baby's growth in the womb (high blood pressure can slow his growth and diabetes can make him grow too much) and can lead to a premature delivery. C-sections are more common in overweight mothers because of these complications. And being overweight makes it more likely that your breast milk will come in later than usual, more than three days after your baby is born. (If this happens, don't get discouraged or give up trying to breastfeed. You can trust that your breast milk will arrive soon, and your baby can be fed formula in the meantime if he needs it.)

The most important question is: Knowing this, is there anything you should do? First, don't start worrying unnecessarily. You can be proud of your womanly body and the new life you're nurturing in your womb. But do be vigilant about regular doctor's visits for prenatal care. You'll get physical exams, which together with blood and urine tests will catch any possible problem at the best time—early—when you can do something about it. Or even more likely, you'll be reassured that you and your baby are fine and everything is going well.

High Blood Pressure and Preeclampsia

I've always eaten right and exercised. But now in my pregnancy I suddenly have high blood pressure. I'm stunned.

Because high blood pressure is often associated with an "unhealthy" lifestyle, it can be a real shock for a health-conscious woman to be told she has it just when she's expecting. But there is a certain kind of high blood pressure that occurs only during pregnancy and can strike out of the blue. It's called—fittingly—pregnancy-induced hypertension (or PIH). Fortunately, the vast majority of women with PIH end up with healthy babies born at term, so you have every reason to be optimistic. Your doctor will help you keep your blood pressure under control so that it doesn't damage your placenta and your baby grows normally. By three months after delivery, your blood pressure should return to normal, although you may be at slightly increased risk of developing hypertension in the future.

When high blood pressure in pregnancy is accompanied by protein in the urine and sometimes other signs and symptoms, it's a more serious illness that doctors call preeclampsia. If you have it, a time may come before you've reached term when your doctor tells you it's best to de-

liver your baby as soon as possible. Luckily, the prognosis is usually very good, because most cases of preeclampsia are mild and occur late in pregnancy, when a baby is unlikely to have any complications from an earlier-than-expected birth. And because preeclampsia always goes away after delivery, the vast majority of mothers are back at their previous state of health within several weeks of their baby's birth.

Although most people haven't heard of it, preeclampsia is surprisingly common, affecting nearly 10 percent of pregnant women. Doctors have many theories, but the exact cause of this disease is still mysterious. Women at risk for it are those who are younger than 20 or older than 40; are pregnant with their first baby or multiples; are overweight or already have high blood pressure, kidney disease, or diabetes; or have a mother or sister who had it. If you had preeclampsia in a previous pregnancy, you're also more likely to get it again, especially if it came on early and was severe. For women who are at high risk, taking low-dose aspirin, calcium, or vitamins C and E early in pregnancy and possibly doing regular, gentle exercise may help prevent preeclampsia from developing. But nearly three-quarters of women who get preeclampsia have no risk factor for it at all, and these preventive measures don't seem to help women who are at low risk.

Most of the time, preeclampsia is an easy diagnosis for your obstetrician to make. He'll measure your blood pressure, check your weight, and do some simple urine and blood tests. Sometimes, though, it isn't clear whether a pregnant woman has preeclampsia or some other medical condition. It is important for your doctor to try to figure this out, because the cure for preeclampsia is delivery.

The reason preeclampsia can be dangerous is that it causes changes in the body that are the opposite of what should occur during pregnancy.

(Continued on page 16)

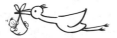

Diabetes and Premature Birth

If you have diabetes, it means you have trouble using the sugar that circulates in your blood as fuel. Blood sugar is the body's energy supply. It comes from food you've eaten or fat you've metabolized, but if you have diabetes, instead of passing into your body's cells where it can be turned into energy or stored for future use, it stays in your bloodstream, giving you the high blood sugar that is characteristic of the disease. If blood sugar remains high for too long, it can damage various organs. During pregnancy it can cause problems for the developing fetus.

What confuses many people is that there are three types of diabetes: type 1, type 2, and gestational. They are different in some ways but have similar health consequences when you're pregnant. In type 1 diabetes (also called juvenile diabetes), the body doesn't make insulin, the hormone that is responsible for getting blood sugar into the cells. In type 2 diabetes (often related to being overweight and not exercising), the body does make insulin but is resistant to its action so the insulin doesn't work well. Gestational diabetes is like type 2—it involves insulin resistance—but is triggered by pregnancy. It tends to be milder and goes away after delivery. (One thing to be aware of: Many cases of what seem to be gestational diabetes are in fact type 2 diabetes that weren't diagnosed before conception. Only time can tell for sure. If a mother's blood sugar levels remain too high after her baby is born, she has type 2 diabetes; if they go back to normal, she just had gestational diabetes.)

If you have any type of diabetes during your pregnancy, there are some potential problems your doctor will be sure to watch out for. For example, you're more likely to develop high blood pressure or preeclampsia. Both of these— especially preeclampsia—can lead to poor fetal growth and serious health complications in the mother, causing the doctor to recommend an elective premature delivery. Women who suffer from advanced type 1 diabetes with vascular disease, even without preeclampsia, are prone to have smaller than normal babies and health problems during pregnancy.

Diabetes can cause the opposite situation as well: a fetus that is too big. This happens when the mother's high blood sugar is transferred to her baby, who uses all that excess fuel to grow too much. A baby whose weight is above the ninetieth percentile for his gestational age is called large-for-gestational-age, or macrosomic. If you are carrying a large-for-gestational-age baby, the obstetrician may recommend an early elective delivery because macrosomic fetuses have a higher incidence of stillbirth and delivery complications.

Large-for-gestational-age babies often face some extra hurdles after birth, too, including hypoglycemia (blood sugar levels that are too low), respiratory distress, poor feeding, jaundice, and a higher incidence of SIDS (sudden infant death syndrome).

With type 1 and type 2 diabetes, if a woman's blood sugar is very high early in pregnancy, during the embryo's first stages of development, there's a small increased risk of birth defects. This isn't a problem with gestational diabetes, which arises later in pregnancy after a fetus's organs have already been formed.

To help prevent all of these complications, your doctor will counsel you on ways to keep your blood sugar in check and will prescribe insulin if it's necessary. Insulin is safe during pregnancy, but be sure to talk to your obstetrician about whether and how to safely stop any other medications you may already be on, because many of the oral drugs used to treat diabetes, and also some medications for high cholesterol and hypertension (common problems if you have diabetes), aren't safe during pregnancy. (If you happen to be planning a pregnancy, it's best to do this even before you conceive.) Fortunately, if you simply have gestational diabetes, you have a very good chance of being able to stabilize your blood sugar just with careful diet and regular exercise, which will be healthy for you and your baby in so many ways. Be sure to get close medical follow-up after you deliver, though, because women with gestational diabetes have a higher chance (estimates range from 20 percent to 50 percent) of developing type 2 diabetes in the decade after their pregnancy. Eating healthfully and exercising can greatly lower your risk.

Breastfeeding is good for all babies, and especially for preemies whose mothers are diabetic. Studies have found that preemies and children of women with diabetes are both more likely to develop insulin resistance later in life, and breastfeeding helps prevent that. So think of your breast milk as one of the best preventive medicines you can give your baby. What a great gift!

As you call on your willpower day after day to stick to your diet and exercise plans, don't get demoralized and stop trying if your blood sugar level isn't always perfect. It doesn't have to be! All it has to be is good enough. Most pregnant women with diabetes deliver healthy babies at full term. Chances are, you will be one of them.

Normally the amount of circulating blood in a woman's body increases to provide for both her and her fetus, and her blood vessels open wider to accommodate it. But when a mother has preeclampsia, her blood vessels tighten, and not as much blood can flow through them. Her blood pressure rises, and all of her organs, including her uterus, receive less blood.

That's not a big problem when preeclampsia is mild; the amount of blood flow is slightly reduced but still adequate. But when it's severe, a mother's vital organs may not get enough blood. Your doctor will watch you closely for kidney, liver, or intestinal problems (be sure to tell him if you have pain in your belly), fluid retention (which can show up as very rapid weight gain or a puffy face and hands—not the normal leg swelling that many pregnant women have), and symptoms like blurry vision and headaches, which could indicate that your eyes or brain are suffering. In a few women with preeclampsia (only about 5 percent), the symptoms progress to seizures (called eclampsia) or abnormalities of blood clotting with liver damage (called HELLP syndrome, for hemolysis—destruction of red blood cells—elevated liver enzymes, low platelets). Women with these most severe forms of preeclampsia occasionally have strokes, or even die—that's why your obstetrician takes it so seriously.

For a fetus, the main consequence of preeclampsia is receiving less blood flow through the placenta and therefore less oxygen and nutrients. For that reason, babies of mothers with preeclampsia are often small for their gestational age. If the restriction of blood flow becomes extreme or the placenta separates from the wall of the uterus (a complication called placental abruption, which is more common in pregnant women with high blood pressure), there's a risk of fetal death. But thanks to alert doctors and careful fetal monitoring, this is an uncommon tragedy today.

The simplest and most commonly prescribed treatment for preeclampsia is rest, which can lower your blood pressure and help your baby get more blood flow. Your doctor may recommend bed rest at home or admit you to the hospital. You may also be given medications to lower your blood pressure and to prevent seizures. The usual drug to prevent seizures is magnesium sulfate, which is safe for both mother and baby but can have some bothersome side effects, such as making you feel sick and possibly temporarily depressing a newborn baby's breathing. (Don't worry about that, though—if necessary, a ventilator can help your baby breathe until the magnesium wears off, usually within a day or two.) If it's early in your pregnancy, you'll also get steroid shots to help your baby's lungs and brain mature more quickly. Steroids often bring a nice bonus: The preeclampsia improves temporarily, giving you a little extra time.

The earlier that preeclampsia occurs during pregnancy and the more severe its symptoms, the more it can affect a mother's and fetus's health. While you're in the hospital, your obstetrician will closely observe you and your baby and make fine-tuned decisions day by day. She'll get crucial information from tests that monitor your medical status, your baby's growth and well-being, and the blood flow through the placenta. Fortunately, most women with mild preeclampsia can safely continue their pregnancies to term. But women with severe preeclampsia usually deliver within a couple of weeks of being hospitalized, often by C-section.

If it ever appears that your pregnancy is becoming too risky for you, your obstetrician will decide that your baby needs to be delivered. When you hear that, you might think: "I don't care about myself if it would help my baby to stay longer in my womb." It's heroic to be willing to take such risks for your child. But your family, including your baby, needs you. And when preeclampsia becomes that severe in a mother, her fetus usually begins to suffer severely, too, and is in real danger of dying in the womb. So it's better to look at your doctor's decision as the best chance for you *and* your baby. Once you put the dangers of preeclampsia behind you, you can focus on the positives: the excellent care your premature baby will receive in a neonatal intensive care unit and your imminent recovery.

Previous Premature Delivery

My first baby was a preemie, and now that I'm pregnant again I'm so anxious, fearing that it might happen again.

It's true that you have a higher risk of delivering prematurely once you've already had a premature baby. Studies put the recurrence rate at around 20 percent to 50 percent for mothers of preemies as a whole. But every case is different, and the scariest data might not reflect your own chances.

For example, if you gave birth early because of a problem with your placenta, such as a placenta previa, you really can be optimistic, since that rarely occurs again in a second pregnancy. If your last pregnancy resulted from infertility treatments and this one was spontaneous, you're less likely to deliver prematurely this time, because all assisted pregnancies carry a higher risk for premature birth. And if you had an older preemie last time, your chances of bringing this pregnancy to term may be higher than you think, because the later in pregnancy you delivered your previous baby, the lower your current risk.

On the other hand, if you're pregnant with multiples, your chance of delivering early is very high, 50 percent for twins and 90 percent for triplets. (Fortunately, most twins and triplets are born after 30 weeks of gestation when the consequences of prematurity don't tend to be severe.) So the trick is understanding your particular circumstances.

That's especially important because if your first baby's premature delivery was caused by something you or your obstetrician can do something about, you may be able to reduce your risk substantially. For example, if your doctor thinks you had a preemie partly because of smoking or drug use, being significantly underweight or overweight, or perhaps working the night shift, these are all things you might already have changed or can change as soon as possible to bring your risk down. Your doctor will be able to advise you on the best nutrition, lifestyle choices, and stress-control techniques, all with a view to promoting your well-being and helping you bring this pregnancy to a happy full term.

Your doctor may also suggest certain medical treatments or tests. For instance, if you gave birth early because you have cervical insufficiency (a weak cervix that tends to open before term), there's a good chance it can be treated by a cerclage, in which the cervix is stitched closed during pregnancy. Infections that might have caused your premature delivery (especially urinary tract infections or sexually transmitted diseases) can be detected with tests and treated with antibiotics; your doctor will certainly try to rule out any hidden infections this time. If you suffer from gum disease, you will be advised to see a dentist and undergo treatment, because—strange as it may seem to talk about flossing and childbirth in the same breath—research has shown that inflamed or infected gums may contribute to premature delivery. And if you have a chronic illness, such as diabetes or high blood pressure, closer medical surveillance may lengthen this pregnancy.

Finally, the most encouraging news is that you might benefit greatly from a promising new treatment: progesterone, a hormone that keeps the uterus from contracting during pregnancy. Recent studies show that, for women who have had one premature baby, weekly shots of progesterone between 16 and 20 weeks of pregnancy can significantly lower the risk of having another preemie.

What's really important for you now is to be followed by an experienced obstetrician who specializes in high-risk patients like you and is familiar with all of the choices you can make to minimize your risk of a second premature delivery. It's natural for you to feel nervous, considering what you've been through already. But by following your doctor's recommendations, you'll give yourself and your little growing baby the best possible chance.

Progesterone to Prevent Premature Delivery

Our first baby was born nine weeks early. Now that I'm pregnant again, my doctor is recommending that I take progesterone shots. Would this treatment really be helpful—and safe for my baby and me?

Since you've already had one premature baby, your doctor knows there's a good chance you could have another, even if you're healthy and get excellent prenatal care. The good news, though, is that there's a treatment that might help. A large study found that mothers like you who started getting weekly shots of progesterone between 16 and 20 weeks of pregnancy brought down their risk of another premature delivery by a third or more.

In the quest to find ways to prevent premature birth, progesterone stands out as the only success story in recent years. Doctors have known for a long time that this hormone keeps the uterus from contracting during pregnancy and that its levels usually drop just before labor begins. But so far attempts to use it as a treatment to postpone delivery have worked only for a specific group of women, those who went into spontaneous, preterm labor in a previous pregnancy and delivered a preemie. Your obstetrician is probably recommending progesterone treatment because you fall into this category.

Naturally, doctors are hoping that progesterone can help prevent premature birth in other groups of women, too, and research so far has turned up mixed results. One promising study found that progesterone reduced the rate of premature delivery in pregnant women who had a short cervix (a short cervix seen by ultrasound can presage a preterm birth), while another study found that it did not prevent preterm birth in women who were expecting multiples.

Most obstetricians have high expectations for progesterone but agree there are still many questions to be answered, such as how effective it is in other groups of women at risk for delivering early, what the right doses are, and how best to administer it. One thing that's tremendously encouraging is that progesterone treatment as yet hasn't caused any serious side effects in mothers or their babies (who've been followed for up to two years of age so far). But safety concerns can't be completely ruled out until these children are grown and many more women have been treated, a process that will take many years.

The American College of Obstetricians and Gynecologists already feels confident enough about progesterone to recommend it for patients like you who are at high risk for a second premature delivery. But keep in mind that in some ways progesterone treatment is still experimental and needs more research before its efficacy and safety are truly known. If you decide to ask another obstetrician for a second opinion on whether progesterone is appropriate for you, be assured that most doctors would not interpret this as a lack of trust in them; they might even welcome a colleague's participation.

One thing to keep in mind: If you are going to take progesterone, be sure to check whether your insurance carrier or state Medicaid program will pay for it, because the indications for this new therapy are still being established. Don't be discouraged if it isn't covered; your doctor might be able to enroll you in a research study, where the medication is provided for free.

Diagnosing and Treating Preterm Labor

Sometimes I feel some tightening in my stomach that I think is false labor. Or could it be something serious I should report to my doctor?

By all means if you're feeling frequent contractions—coming every 15 minutes or less—you should call your doctor, even outside of office hours, because she needs to decide whether you are in true labor or false. Some women just have unusually active uteruses, well before real labor starts. Still, it's not always easy to tell whether your contractions are the real McCoy—ones that will lead to cervical change and birth—or just harmless ones whose only consequence is to give you and your doctor a hefty dose of anxiety. Catching the early stages of real preterm labor is important, because that's when treatment has the very best chance of succeeding.

Harmless contractions (also called Braxton-Hicks contractions) can be regular, frequent, and painful, but they eventually stop by themselves, whereas contractions that herald true labor are accompanied, sooner or later, by shortening and opening of the cervix. There's always a mixture of science and art in the practice of medicine, but when it comes to treating preterm labor, the balance tilts solidly to art. Doctors want to avoid mak-

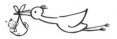

Are You in Preterm Labor?

Even if you are having contractions before term, you may not be in preterm labor. But it is very important to identify real labor early, because it can lead to thinning and opening of your cervix and progress to an early delivery.

What should you look for to know if you are in preterm labor? Be alert for any of the following signs, and call your doctor if their appearance represents a change for you:

* **Uterine contractions, painful or not, that occur more than four times an hour.** You may feel these as a tightening sensation in your belly. If you place your fingertips over your uterus when one is happening, it will feel firm. (If you think you are feeling some contractions, but they aren't that frequent yet, you can try drinking two or three large glasses of water and lying down for half an hour. Often, the contractions will gradually decrease in frequency.)
* **A dull ache or sharp pain in your lower back.**
* **Menstrual-like cramps, possibly with gas pains or diarrhea.**
* **Pressure in your pelvis.**

* **An increased or changed vaginal discharge.** A blood-tinged discharge could mean the loss of the mucus plug that's like a stopper for the uterus. A greater than usual leakage of clear fluid could be your water breaking.

If you think you have any of these symptoms or have any doubt, do not hesitate to call your doctor. Don't worry about being a pest. First of all, the people who worry about being pests rarely are. Also, you have obligations: to your doctor, who can't be with you all the time and who counts on you to call with your concerns, and to your baby, whose well-being is at stake and counts on you to represent him!

ing too hasty a diagnosis so that they don't expose a mother and her fetus to the side effects of anti-labor drugs and the stresses of hospitalization unnecessarily. But they also don't want to wait too long, because once labor becomes advanced, medications are unlikely to be successful. If anti-labor treatment is started early enough, it usually stops contractions and delays delivery for a week or longer. Even postponing delivery for a short time is valuable, because just a couple of more days in the womb can improve a very young preemie's outcome substantially.

If your doctor does suspect that you're having real preterm labor, here's what you can expect. Most likely you will be sent to the hospital, the safest place to be in case you do deliver. There your contractions will be monitored, and so will your baby's heartbeat, to make sure he is not sick or in distress. While your doctor tries to determine whether a treatable problem like dehydration or infection is causing your contractions, you'll be put on bed rest and given intravenous fluids (to enhance the flow of blood to your uterus).

(Continued on page 22)

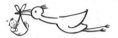

What Is Home Monitoring?

To detect preterm labor in women at high risk, an obstetrician will sometimes prescribe home uterine activity monitoring (HUAM). This involves two things: a device you strap over your belly to record your uterine contractions and a daily phone call from a nurse. You use the monitor for an hour twice a day; the nurse retrieves a record of your contractions by computer, examines it, and asks you whether you are having any other signs of labor. Depending on your symptoms and the number of contractions you have, the nurse can decide to contact your doctor or send you to the office, hospital, or emergency room to be evaluated. You also have access to a toll-free information line staffed by nurses seven days a week, 24 hours a day, so you can ask questions and get advice.

Whether home uterine monitoring works is controversial. Some studies found that it was effective in detecting labor at an early stage and prolonging pregnancy, whereas others found that it merely increased visits to doctors and hospitalizations without reducing premature birth.

Doctors who don't believe in home monitoring point out that the relationship between the frequency of uterine contractions and preterm delivery isn't straightforward. Some women have so-called "irritable" uteruses, meaning they contract a lot even though they're not in labor. And even if preterm labor is detected, it may not be possible to stop it. These doctors feel that home monitoring causes false alarms and anxiety without any better results than good, careful prenatal care.

On the other hand, believers in home monitoring argue that when it is done correctly—with the right equipment and only for women at high risk of delivering early, such as those who have had a previous episode of preterm labor or are carrying twins or triplets—it can help detect labor almost as soon as it starts, when anti-labor drugs are most effective. It's also possible that the daily personal involvement of a nurse who can reassure and guide an expectant mother and answer her questions—an integral part of HUAM—is as useful in preventing prematurity as the monitoring technology itself.

An expert review of the research on home monitoring is expected soon and will help doctors come to a consensus. In the meantime, in the absence of conclusive evidence that it works, some insurance companies will not pay for it. So if your obstetrician prescribes HUAM, be sure to inquire about the cost. If you really want to try it and your physician doesn't recommend it—or vice versa—be sure to ask lots of questions and don't be afraid to press your case. There's professional support on both sides. Whatever makes you feel more secure and in control of your pregnancy could be helpful.

About half the time, if you don't also have bleeding and your water hasn't broken, fluids and bed rest alone will be enough to stop it.

Let's say that bed rest and fluids don't do the trick, and you and your baby are doing well otherwise. Then your doctor will probably prescribe anti-labor drugs (which in medical parlance are called tocolytics) to relax your uterus and halt the contractions. If she doesn't, it may be that you haven't reached 20 weeks of gestation yet (because medication is unlikely to work long enough for your fetus to mature to the point when he could survive outside the womb), or that you've already reached 34 weeks of gestation (since preemies this old do very well, even if they enter the world a little early), or an amniotic fluid test has indicated that your baby's lungs are already mature (meaning that he'll probably avoid the serious complications of a preterm birth and the risks of anti-labor treatment therefore aren't worth taking). Your doctor also won't try to stop your labor if she thinks delivery now is safer for you or your baby.

There are several types of drugs a doctor can choose from. They work differently but all have the same effect of decreasing uterine contractions. Magnesium sulfate is the first choice of some obstetricians, especially when it's early in pregnancy, because some studies have shown that very young preemies whose mothers got magnesium had the best neurological outcomes. Magnesium is given intravenously. A downside is that it may not work as well as some other tocolytics, and many women feel horrendous while they're on it, with nausea, hot flashes, headaches, or weakness. There are also a few potentially dangerous complications your doctor will watch out for, such as breathing problems or low blood pressure, but they are rare. Babies whose mothers get high doses of magnesium are sometimes born a little floppy and lethargic, possibly even to the point of not breathing regularly or being able to eat, but don't worry. This problem will completely disappear in a day or two, and your baby's doctor will support him until it goes away.

Popular in the past but less commonly used now, in part because of their frequent unpleasant side effects, are terbutaline, ritodrine, and other so-called beta-mimetic drugs, which can be administered by injections, pills, or a tiny pump implanted under the skin. Some women tolerate them well, while others feel jittery or have heart palpitations, nausea, headaches, or muscle cramps. Women who have high blood pressure, heart disease, diabetes, or hyperthyroidism are more apt to have dangerous complications, so doctors generally don't prescribe these kinds of drugs for them.

Two other types of tocolytics are used more often these days: anti-inflammatory medications (such as indomethacin, which is similar to Motrin or Advil) and calcium channel blockers (such as nifedipine). Both can be given as pills or intravenously. One recent study found that anti-inflammatory medications were the most effective type of anti-labor drug, with very few side effects for pregnant women. But because they can cause some problems for the fetus if a mother takes them for too long, most doctors use them carefully and only briefly. Calcium channel blockers can cause low blood pressure and a fast heart rate, but fortunately these side effects are rarely severe enough to be dangerous.

As you can see, each of these medications—and any others that your obstetrician might use—has its own advantages and disadvantages; you can ask your doctor how she's deciding which one is best for you.

No matter how stiff an upper lip you keep, if you're lying in a hospital bed having to endure uncomfortable side effects from anti-labor medicine, you may well ask: Is it worth it? Most of the time the answer is, absolutely! These medications are usually given for 48 hours or less and can often put a quick stop to preterm labor that isn't far along. Even if your labor returns as soon as the anti-labor drugs are stopped, the couple of days gained can be long enough to allow you to get a course of prenatal steroids (see page 34), which can boost your preemie's maturity and give him the best chance of doing well after he's born. That alone can be a major benefit. Or better yet, you may be one of the many mothers for whom preterm labor passes, the medication is stopped, and your uterus is quiet and calm again. Sometimes the doctors never learn why preterm labor came and went—whether it was an infection that flared up fleetingly, dehydration, or some other cause.

It's hard to predict what will happen in the rest of your pregnancy after you've had an episode of preterm labor. Many women end up bringing their pregnancy happily to term without any more problems. For others, preterm labor returns in a few days or at some later date. Some doctors try to prevent a recurrence by having their patients continue taking anti-labor drugs for weeks or months at home. Most studies, though, have found that long-term tocolytic therapy doesn't help delay delivery.

If your preterm labor does start again, your doctor will readmit you to the hospital and reassess whether it is safe for you and your baby for the pregnancy to continue. If she thinks it is, she will try again to stop your contractions—and although you'll feel that you are back where you started, your pregnancy will be further along, your baby bigger, and a new treatment starting that may give you yet more precious time.

But there are times, upsetting as it is, when delivery is the better course. Doctors believe that the fetus often participates in the "decision" to initiate labor—and that the decision can be a wise one. For example, if your labor is due to an infection that has reached the amniotic sac, it's probably safer for your baby to get out of the womb before he gets infected, too. A healthy preemie tends to do better than a sick preemie,

even if he's born a few weeks earlier. Similarly, if preterm labor is accompanied by vaginal bleeding and fetal distress, you may have a placental abruption and your baby may not be getting enough blood flow.

So if your doctor can't stop your preterm labor, consider that your baby's rush to come into the world can be a self-protective move. Try to trust that when Mother Nature can't be overruled, she may be doing what's best, even if the outcome isn't what you would choose.

Cerclage

My last baby was born too early, and before that I had several miscarriages. Now I'm pregnant again and my doctor thinks a cerclage will help. What is it, and what will it do?

A cerclage is a minor surgical procedure, done by an obstetrician, in which the cervix—the opening at the base of your uterus through which your baby emerges—is temporarily sewn shut. Obstetricians recommend a cerclage when they conclude that a woman has a weak or, as doctors say, "insufficient" cervix. (You may also hear the old expression "incompetent cervix," which thankfully has largely been abandoned. As though a woman's cervix should get a performance rating!) This means that instead of staying tightly closed until labor begins the cervix tends to open earlier during pregnancy.

If your doctor says you have cervical insufficiency, it means not only that your cervix opened too early in your previous pregnancy but that it did so painlessly and without any driving force like an infection or preterm labor, which can cause even a perfectly "sufficient" cervix to loosen and open up. The reason an open cervix is a problem is that the membranes of the baby's amniotic sac are then exposed to bacteria and other substances in the vagina, which make them more likely to become infected or rupture, leading to a miscarriage or a preterm birth. If you have an insufficient cervix, it can be a relief to hear that a cerclage might help prolong your pregnancy until your baby, even if he's born before term, has a good chance of being fine.

Now you may be wondering why your cervix is insufficient. A common cause is an injury from a past obstetric or gynecological procedure. For example, any surgery on your cervix, tearing during a difficult vaginal delivery, or second trimester abortion you've had could have caused insufficiency. But often the reason remains unknown. Some experts suspect that there simply may be natural differences in how soft, loose, or long the cervix is (just like natural differences in hair color or texture), making a woman's cervix more or less resistant to pressure from the amniotic fluid and growing fetus.

While it can be hard to accept that your obstetrician didn't predict and prevent your last baby's early birth, the frustrating fact is that in most cases doctors can't diagnose cervical insufficiency in advance. Like you, most women are found to have a weak cervix only after it has already opened too early. Actually, even in hindsight cervical insufficiency can be difficult to diagnose; for example, a pregnant woman may have had silent preterm labor contractions or an infection that caused her cervix to open early without being aware of them.

And it's equally difficult to predict whether cervical insufficiency will happen again; just because you had it in one pregnancy doesn't mean you'll have it in another. As a result, it can be a hard call whether to put in a cerclage. So even with the best medical care, cerclages are given to some women who don't really need them and are not given to all women who do.

The good news is that for women who have had three or more miscarriages or premature deliveries, a cerclage almost always works: Nearly

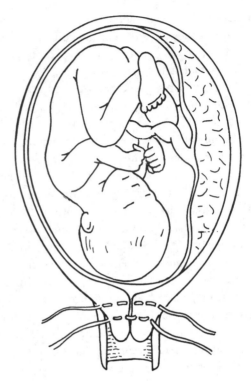

In a cerclage, sutures are sewn around the cervix to hold it closed.

90 percent of the time, it helps extend pregnancy to 34 weeks or longer, when most babies do very well. But when the diagnosis of cervical insufficiency is less certain, a cerclage may not be such a good idea. Research suggests that in women with just one or two losses, a cerclage may hurt more than it helps, causing complications (most commonly, injury to the cervix, infection, an increase in contractions because the stitches irritate the uterus, or premature rupture of the membranes) without lengthening the pregnancy.

Most doctors think the best time to do a cerclage is early in pregnancy when the cervix is still closed. They worry that if the procedure is done later, after the cervix has opened or an infection has set in, bacteria could be carried into the uterus or the obstetrician might damage the exposed membranes of the amniotic sac.

(Continued on page 26)

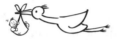

How a Cerclage Is Performed and Removed

There are two kinds of cerclage procedures. Your doctor will recommend the one that is right for you:

Transvaginal cerclage (through the vagina)

This is the most common procedure, with different variations depending on where on the cervix the cerclage is placed (toward the end or in the middle) and what kinds of stitches are used. In most cases, a transvaginal cerclage is a quick, safe procedure that allows a woman to be in and out of the hospital within a few hours. First you'll be given anesthesia (usually spinal) and light sedation. Then your obstetrician will reach through your vagina and sew several stitches around your cervix in a circle (in French, *cercle*), pulling them tight and knotting them to seal it shut.

If the cerclage is performed before your cervix has begun to open, other than relaxing for a day or two after the procedure, you probably won't be advised to do anything differently. If your cervix has already begun to open and your membranes are exposed, you may be given antibiotics and told to reduce your activity or remain in bed. You may also be advised not to have sexual intercourse in order to avoid stimulating the cervix and to reduce the risk of infection, which is higher than normal with a cerclage in place. (Instructions will vary, depending on your personal situation and your obstetrician.) Periodically, your obstetrician will examine you to look for any changes in your cervix and any signs of infection.

The cerclage will be removed in your doctor's office before you deliver your baby, generally at around 37 weeks. If you go into labor or develop an infection before then, the cerclage will be taken out earlier in the hospital.

Transabdominal cerclage (through the abdomen)

This is a more demanding type of surgery, requiring a longer hospitalization, and is usually performed only if a transvaginal cerclage hasn't worked or can't be done (in women who have serious cervical malformations, for example). It allows the obstetrician to place the stitches very high on the cervix where the tissue is stronger and to close it tighter. This surgery may be performed laparoscopically (through tiny incisions, the surgeon maneuvers surgical instruments from the outside, with the help of a video camera), shortening the recovery time and leaving just tiny scars.

A transabdominal cerclage can be placed even before you conceive or up to 14 weeks of pregnancy. Just as with a transvaginal cerclage, most women are advised to reduce their activity for a while and to abstain from sexual intercourse. You will be checked regularly for any signs of infection or cervical changes.

After a transabdominal cerclage, delivery is almost always performed by C-section because the cervix can't be reopened by removing the stitches through the vagina. After delivery, the cerclage is usually left in place, where it will do its good work during another pregnancy if you have one or will just become an invisible part of you.

Doctors also want to be sure not to wait until a woman has already gone into labor, when doing a cerclage would be too risky and no longer helpful.

But some doctors think that if a woman's risk of cervical insufficiency isn't too great—if she's had just one or possibly two preemies, for instance—it's wiser to adopt a wait-and-see approach. They carefully monitor her cervix with frequent ultrasound exams, which can pick up shortening and thinning of the inner part of the cervix—signs that it might be getting ready to open. Only when these changes, or a little dilation, take place do they give her a cerclage. Even though ultrasound testing, like most medical tests, is still not 100 percent reliable and small amounts of cervical dilation don't necessarily lead to preterm birth, it's a way to avoid unnecessary cerclages and their complications. Some small studies suggest that the wait-and-see approach is safe and works well, but the good results need to be confirmed by larger studies before anyone can say for sure.

What probably matters most to you now is to bring your baby closer to term. You can feel hopeful that a cerclage may help you reach that crucial goal.

Bleeding During Pregnancy

I've had some vaginal bleeding during my pregnancy. Am I at risk for a premature delivery?

Not necessarily. Vaginal bleeding during pregnancy is much more common than you might think: up to one in four expectant mothers have some. While it's definitely scary, bleeding can be harmless and have no consequences. For instance, if you've had just a single episode of light spotting during the second trimester and your placenta looks normal on an ultrasound, you have no greater risk of a preterm birth than usual. On the other hand, if your bleeding initially occurred during the first trimester, you've had several episodes, or your bleeding was heavy, your chance of

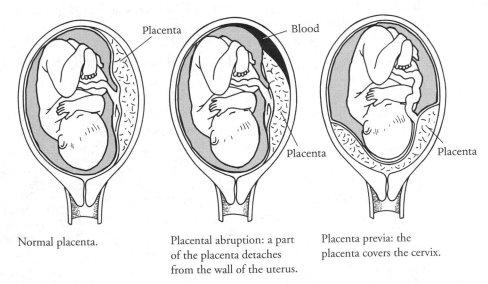

Normal placenta.

Placental abruption: a part of the placenta detaches from the wall of the uterus.

Placenta previa: the placenta covers the cervix.

Adapted with permission from *Planning for Pregnancy, Birth & Beyond*, 2nd ed. Washington, DC, © ACOG (American College of Obstetricians and Gynecologists) 1995

delivering at less than 34 weeks of gestation is higher. Interestingly, African-American women may be an exception to this rule. In a large study, even when they had the more severe kind of bleeding episodes, they didn't have more preterm deliveries; only white women did. So if you're African-American, you can feel more reassured.

Often the reason for bleeding is a mystery; about half of the time, doctors never discover one. But your obstetrician will probably want to do an ultrasound to check for two common causes of bleeding: placental abruption and placenta previa. Both of these conditions can be harmful to the mother if she loses a lot of blood, and anything that interferes with good functioning of the placenta (which provides the fetus with oxygen and nutrients) can interfere with a baby's development. If the danger becomes too great, the doctor will recommend delivering the baby early.

The most common symptom of placental abruption that you would notice, besides vaginal bleeding is abdominal or back pain. Placental abruption means that part of the placenta has detached from the wall of the uterus. When that happens, the detached part can no longer get oxygen and nutrients from the mother's blood. If the area of abruption is small and the rest of the placenta is working well, everything should be fine: It won't make much difference for the growth and well-being of your baby, and your pregnancy can continue. But if the area of abruption is large, it can be dangerous, seriously disturbing the blood and oxygen supply to your baby and sometimes requiring an emergency preterm delivery. Ultrasound and other tests of fetal well-being can usually assess how extensive the problem is.

Placenta previa means that the placenta partly or completely covers the cervix, so that when your cervix dilates or your baby pushes against the placenta during labor, it can tear and bleed. Bleeding may also occur as pregnancy advances and the lower part of the uterus stretches. The usual reason for a premature delivery for a placenta previa is to prevent a serious maternal hemorrhage, which is dangerous for both mother and baby.

If you've been diagnosed with a placental abruption or placenta previa, depending on its seriousness, you may be placed under close medical observation or hospitalized. The aim is to give your baby a chance to stay in the womb as long as it is safe for him and for you. Your doctors will want to prolong your pregnancy as long as possible but also need to be ready to intervene with an elective delivery if the risks suddenly increase. (You can read more about elective delivery on page 32.) Thankfully, there are good ways to evaluate a fetus's well-being in the womb, giving your doctors the best chance to guide you and your baby safely through the dangers of a placental condition.

Hidden Infections and Preterm Birth

Do I really need to take medicine for an infection that doesn't bother me? If it isn't causing me any problems, how dangerous to my pregnancy could it be?

When you're feeling fine, it's natural to think that you *are* fine. But in this case, if your doctor is suggesting treatment it's really important to listen. There's a growing understanding that low-grade, often asymptomatic infections may play a significant role in preterm birth.

It has long been known that some infections during pregnancy can cause a premature delivery. The reason is that a mother's immune system responds by producing substances that can trigger changes in her uterus, cervix, and amniotic membranes that lead to preterm labor. An infection in the womb is doubly dangerous because it can reach the fetus, in some cases disrupting his development or causing him to be ill at birth. And there is some evidence, though it's not conclusive, that chorioamnionitis—an infection of the amniotic sac—may increase a preemie's risk for developing some serious complications after birth, such as chronic lung disease or certain kinds of brain injury.

But obvious infections don't occur very often, certainly not frequently enough to explain why the membranes of the amniotic sac are found to be infected at delivery in up to one-half of all preterm births and up to 80 percent of births before 30 weeks of gestation. Of course, simply finding an infection at the time of delivery doesn't tell you whether it came before, and maybe caused, preterm labor or whether it came afterward. (During labor, when the cervix opens and the membranes of the amniotic sac rupture, some natural barriers to infection are removed.) But an abundance of data indicates that hidden infections in expectant mothers' genital and urinary tracts are a major cause of premature birth. For example, bacteria in the urine are more common during pregnancy than usual, often without the symptoms of burning, itching, or fever that make an infection apparent. Many studies have now shown that the risk of delivering prematurely is much lower if pregnant women with asymptomatic urinary tract infections are treated with antibiotics.

Another well-known culprit for causing preterm delivery is group B strep. This strain of bacteria lives peacefully in many women's vaginas, but during pregnancy it can be dangerous. If it climbs up to the cervix and into the womb, it can cause preterm labor, premature rupture of membranes, infection in the mother's uterus before or after delivery, and severe illness in the baby. (If you go into preterm labor and your obstetrician hasn't screened you for group B strep, you'll probably be treated with intravenous antibiotics just in case you have it. Fortunately, even a single dose of a penicillin-type antibiotic while you're in labor can protect your baby.)

More recently, researchers fingered a hidden infection called bacterial vaginosis, or BV, caused by an overgrowth of some common bacteria that normally live in the vagina. It is silently present in about 10 percent of white women and about 25 percent of African-American women; only a few get symptoms, such as pain and whitish vaginal discharge. BV is not a sexually transmitted disease, although women who become sexually active at an early age are more prone to it, as are those who douche (douching can destroy the useful bacteria of the vagina, which help to keep other bacteria under control). Doctors believe that bacterial vaginosis can almost double some women's risk of delivering prematurely.

BV is easy to diagnose (your doctor painlessly swabs your vagina with something like a Q-tip), and it can be effectively treated with oral antibiotics or a vaginal antibiotic cream. The dilemma is deciding who should be treated. Several studies have shown that treating BV in women who had a previous unexplained preterm birth can lower their risk for another preterm delivery by up to 70 percent. But in women who haven't delivered prematurely before, it's not clear that having BV is harmful or that treating it will help. That may be because it doesn't often lead to a uterine infection, and there's even a small chance that treating it could hurt: Any time you take antibiotics, there's a slight risk of an allergic reaction or of developing an overgrowth of other bacteria that may be hard to treat. Some researchers even question whether in some cases antibiotics not only kill the bacteria causing BV but also enhance the inflammatory response, triggering preterm labor instead of preventing it. You can talk to your obstetrician about the pros and cons in your case.

Believe it or not, another hidden infection that

can cause prematurity is gum disease. So don't be surprised if your obstetrician tells you to floss—to prevent prematurity as well as cavities! If you've been diagnosed with gum disease, you should be treated by a dentist with deep cleaning as soon as possible.

There are several other infections that can cause serious illness in a fetus and occasionally lead to preterm birth but are sometimes so mild that a mother doesn't realize she has them. It will be your doctor's responsibility to decide if you need to be treated for any of these. Most obstetricians screen for sexually transmitted diseases, such as syphilis, gonorrhea, and HIV, and for such viruses as hepatitis B and rubella (German measles). Depending on your situation and exposures, your doctor may also add tests for herpes, cytomegalovirus, or other infections that can harm a baby without his mother always being aware of them.

For many of these infections, prevention is the key: You'll be advised by your doctor to practice safe sex, to avoid douching, not to eat raw or undercooked meat, fish, or shellfish, and not to touch dirty kitty litter (a great excuse to let your partner do that job!). You should try to stay away from anyone who's sick with something contagious. If you have Lyme disease in your area, try to follow the precautions you already know even more carefully. Before your next pregnancy, if you haven't had rubella, mumps, or chicken pox, you should get vaccinated against them. (These vaccines usually aren't given to women who are already pregnant, for fear they could harm the fetus.)

If you had a preterm birth in the past, it may be tempting, but painful and probably useless, to go back and torture yourself about an undiscovered, hidden infection that may have been to blame for what happened. Even if you or your baby had signs of infection after delivery, there's no way to tell, in retrospect, whether it was a cause or a consequence of your preterm labor.

It is also impossible to know what would have happened if you had been diagnosed with an infection and treated with antibiotics during your pregnancy—everything, or nothing, might have changed. Right now, if you can, try to focus on the present and future. Doctors are constantly learning more about the links between infection and inflammation and premature birth. Hopefully, this will soon lead to better tests and treatment. You and your baby might be among the first to benefit from them.

If Your Water Breaks

My water broke. Have we lost the battle?

Not necessarily. It's true that you may have to be in the hospital for a while, and it's likely that you'll deliver prematurely. But pregnancies often go on for some time after premature rupture of membranes (the medical term for water breaking), and it's quite possible that your baby will gain some additional, very valuable time in the womb.

It's understandable that you would feel scared. There's something about the rush of fluid out of the womb that creates a feeling of great helplessness: There's nothing you can do to stop it while it happens, and nothing you can do to put it back. All you can do is wait and hope. One thing you should not do is blame yourself or your partner for what happened. We've known mothers who believed they brought it on by getting up from bed rest and fathers who thought they were to blame for not carrying that last bag of groceries. In fact, nothing so simple has been found to be the cause of premature rupture of membranes.

Researchers don't have a full understanding of why some women's water breaks early, but most believe it's the culmination of a long-term process in which many medical factors combine. Women who smoke are at increased risk, as are women who have had bleeding during the pregnancy, and those whose water broke before they went into labor in a previous pregnancy (at term or before). Uterine contractions, too much amniotic fluid, pressure and stretch from the baby's growth, or the presence of more than one baby can all cause the membranes to weaken. Certain nutritional deficiencies and previous surgery on the cervix may play a role. Experts suspect that infections (some without any symptoms) are often important factors, with bacteria from a mother's genital tract climbing up through the cervix and irritating the membranes. New research suggests that genetic differences may be a key part of the story, such as in the way a woman's immune system responds to psychological or physical stress or to the presence of bacteria or viruses in her body. Although it has been suspected that sexual intercourse might contribute to early rupture of membranes, studies have produced no clear evidence of that.

The first thing your doctor will want to do is to test the fluid that leaked out to confirm that it was indeed amniotic fluid, rather than urine or vaginal secretions. Usually when membranes rupture, there's a large gush of fluid, followed by a continuing trickle. In a few cases, though, women have some less dramatic dripping that goes on for a while. Once the doctor establishes that your water did break, he'll decide whether to deliver your baby right away or wait.

Why shouldn't every pregnancy go on as long as possible? Because after membranes rupture, there are some real risks:

* **Infection.** The membranes that surround your baby act as a barrier to the bacteria that normally live in the vagina. When the membranes are broken, the bacteria can swim up into the uterus, infecting the mother and possibly the baby as well. A mother's infection can almost always be effectively treated, but for a fetus or newborn, an infection can be life-threatening or cause long-term health and developmental problems. A premature baby who is born a little younger but not infected is often better off than an older preemie who is.

Fortunately, fewer than 20 percent of fetuses become infected after premature rupture of membranes, and usually not until after their mothers have had symptoms themselves, like fever or abdominal pain. So your obstetrician may not feel that it's necessary to deliver your baby unless you or your baby show signs of infection.

* **Inadequate growth of a fetus's lungs.** Called pulmonary hypoplasia, its causes aren't fully known, but it is thought to occur because without much amniotic fluid, the uterus presses tightly against the fetus and prevents the lungs from expanding well. Lung expansion is one of the signals that prompts a fetus's lungs to grow and develop. (It's one reason fetuses in the womb practice breathing movements.) There may also be growth hormones in amniotic fluid that are no longer getting into the fetus's lungs. No matter how old a baby is at birth, if her lungs are too small, it will be difficult or impossible for her to breathe.

The risk that a baby's lungs won't grow large enough for her to survive outside the womb is greatest when a mother's water breaks early in the second trimester of pregnancy. Most babies whose mother's water breaks after 26 weeks of gestation are fine. The outlook is also better the more amniotic fluid remains in the womb.

* **A greater risk that the umbilical cord could slip into a dangerous position.** This could cut off some oxygen and blood flow to the fetus.

* **A baby's movements can be constrained.** With little amniotic fluid to expand it, the uterus may press tightly against a fetus, constraining her movements. Lack of movement

could cause her joints to become stiff and contracted, so that she can't bend fully or straighten some of them. Over time, these contractures may resolve, sometimes with the help of orthopedics or physical therapy.

You can see that these risks have to be balanced against the risks of your baby's prematurity, to come up with the right timing for delivery. In some situations, the decision is easy: As soon as there are obvious signs of infection or fetal distress, your baby will be delivered immediately. Before 32 to 34 weeks of gestation, in the absence of infection or fetal distress, most obstetricians believe that the risks of prematurity outweigh the risks of continuing the pregnancy. Most believe that the reverse is true after 34 weeks, when most preemies are nearly as mature, if not as hefty, as full-termers.

So how long can you expect your pregnancy to last? There's nothing more frustrating for parents to hear, but it is impossible to predict what nature will do in any individual case. Occasionally you're lucky and the best possible outcome occurs: Your membranes reseal within a few days and amniotic fluid builds up again around your baby. No one knows why this sometimes happens, but when it does, the pregnancy can go on with nearly the same risks and benefits as if the membranes had never ruptured in the first place. Sometimes the membranes partially reseal, leaving the door still open to infection but providing the important advantage of an adequate amount of amniotic fluid around the fetus.

A majority of women give birth within a week after their water breaks. But if labor doesn't occur within several days, your pregnancy has a good chance of lasting considerably longer. About 15 percent to 20 percent of women go four weeks or more before delivering.

Between now and delivery, you will most likely be kept in the hospital, where you and your baby can be monitored carefully, and taken care of if delivery occurs very quickly after labor starts. You will probably be kept on bed rest, partly to cut down on the amount of amniotic fluid that leaks out. Don't be alarmed, though, if no matter what position you're in there is some continued leakage. Unless your membranes reseal, it's normal and unavoidable. Bed rest can also improve blood flow to the baby, which may help produce more amniotic fluid, and can lower the chance of the umbilical cord's falling into a dangerous position through the cervix. A few doctors occasionally use a technique called amnioinfusion (infusing fluid into the womb with a catheter), particularly to help a fetus tolerate labor, but the fluid tends to leak out so quickly that it can't help with lung growth unless it is done repeatedly.

You will probably be given antibiotics to treat any infections you may have and to prevent them in your baby. Antibiotics given after preterm rupture of membranes have been found to lengthen pregnancies and to give preemies a health advantage after birth. You may be given a course of steroids (see page 34) to speed up your baby's maturation. You probably will not get anti-labor medications, which have not been proven to lengthen pregnancies after a woman's water breaks and may mask signs of infection. You will need to abstain from sexual intercourse, which could introduce infection or bring on preterm labor. A cerclage increases the risk of infection, so if you have one, your doctor will consider whether or not to remove it.

To monitor for infection and fetal distress, your temperature and your baby's heartbeat will be checked several times a day. Your doctor may suggest an amniocentesis (taking a tiny bit of amniotic fluid out with a needle) if there's enough fluid to do it safely. The fluid can be checked for infection and can show how mature your baby's lungs are. You will probably get an ultrasound every few days to observe your baby's breathing, heartbeat, and body movements as well as to measure the amount of amniotic fluid.

One thing of which you can be sure: This period, when you have so little ability to predict or control the future, is going to be difficult for you and your partner. Try to keep your mind calm and optimistic, perhaps with the help of stress-relief strategies, such as guided imagery, breathing techniques, meditation, or (if your doctor OK's it) massage. Live in the present, taking a day at a time, because every day you gain in your pregnancy is valuable.

When a Baby Needs to Be Delivered Early

My doctor says my baby isn't doing well in the womb and that he may decide to deliver him early. How does he know when the right time has come?

Few things are harder for an expectant mother than hearing that your baby would be better off being born prematurely than spending more time in your womb. Along with worrying about your baby's health and your own, you may feel inadequate, or betrayed by your own body. At a time when you should have been cheered by the tumbling presence of your baby inside you, instead you're undergoing checkups and tests, observing him with trepidation and alarm.

It may help you to know that you're far from alone in this difficult experience. Elective preterm deliveries—done early for medical reasons—bring nearly one-quarter of all preemies into the world. The most common reason for an elective preterm delivery is preeclampsia (see page 14), which is usually done primarily to protect the health of the mother. But preeclampsia and many other maternal medical conditions can also adversely affect the health of a fetus. Sometimes, even when

a mother is well, her uterus may not be the best environment for her baby.

These are the major reasons that an obstetrician might decide that the time has come—sooner than expected—when your baby would do better outside the womb:

* **His growth has become very poor**. If a baby isn't growing well in the womb, he may not be getting enough nutrients and oxygen, which can affect his long-term development. If your baby's growth is already slow, and slows down even further or stops altogether, most obstetricians would decide that it's time to deliver him.
* **He has signs of fetal distress.** Fetal distress is a signal that a baby's supply of blood or oxygen is inadequate. It can be caused by problems with the placenta or by anemia, infection, or a severe illness of the mother or baby. Doctors recognize fetal distress when a baby moves a lot less, is unresponsive to stimulation, or has an abnormal heart rate, or when there is an abnormally low level of amniotic fluid. Obstetricians usually decide to deliver a baby urgently if there is fetal distress, because it usually means that conditions in the womb are dangerous enough to jeopardize your baby's life or health right now.
* **Congenital conditions.** Babies with congenital conditions may sometimes do better if they get prompt medical or surgical treatment. If so, your doctor may opt for an elective preterm delivery.
* **A mother's health is seriously at risk.** Complications of pregnancy, like preeclampsia, placenta previa, and placental abruption, can be not only harmful to the baby but truly life-threatening to the mother. Other illnesses, such as heart disease, can worsen during pregnancy, compromising both fetal and maternal health and requiring an early delivery.

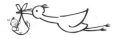

If Your Water Breaks Before Your Baby Has Reached Viability

Sometimes, a woman's water breaks very early, before the baby would be ready to survive if she were born. If this happens to you before around 22 weeks of gestation, your doctor may present you with an excruciating decision. He may ask whether you want to try to go on with the pregnancy or think it would be better to go through with delivery immediately. Choosing delivery now means that you know your baby will not survive. Choosing to go on means that you are willing to accept the risks that your baby may not thrive in the environment she's in, even if the pregnancy lasts much longer. Many babies who are born after extremely early rupture of membranes have poor outcomes, dying shortly after delivery, or suffering from short-term or long-term health problems or lasting disabilities.

Don't hesitate to ask your doctor for his recommendation and for all of the information you need, such as: What gestational age range your baby is likely to reach by the time she is born, what the outcomes are like for babies in her situation (how great her chances of survival and living a healthy and normal life will be), and how much intensive medical care she is likely to need. When you read about general outcome statistics for babies born at various gestational ages on pages 55–59, keep in mind that your baby is facing additional hurdles, such as lung hypoplasia (see page 30), which can make her situation worse.

After weighing the facts along with their deep feelings and beliefs, some parents conclude that the decision to deliver now, although incredibly painful, is the right one for them and their baby, given the risks ahead. Others want to try for more time. Either choice can be the right one for you and your family.

Your doctors will assess how your baby is doing in the womb using one or more of the tests described in *Checking on a Baby's Well-Being Before He Is Born* (page 42). To decide whether he would be better off if he were born now and cared for in a newborn intensive care unit, they'll take into account your baby's gestational age and size (crucial elements affecting how he will do after birth) and weigh the risks he'll face if he's born prematurely against the risks he faces by staying inside the womb. If your baby is still very immature and small, your doctor probably won't recommend delivering him unless he or you are facing life-threatening dangers. As he gets older, the risks of prematurity lessen.

You should know that there's always a good deal of guesswork in a decision like this. Unless you're past 34 weeks, when most of the major hurdles of prematurity are behind your baby, there's hardly ever a definitive "right" time for an elective premature delivery. Doctors usually discuss with parents the pros and cons of an elective preterm delivery and try hard, using the tools and experience they have, to make the right choice.

Baby's Fighting Spirit

My baby kicks a lot. Does that mean he is a fighter?

Some fetuses, with a constant stream of left hooks and right jabs, give their mothers the distinct impression that they have a future as heavyweight boxers. Others seem a lot more relaxed, moving more softly and fluidly, or, it sometimes seems, not that much at all.

There's no doubt that different fetuses have different movement patterns, but nobody knows whether they foretell who will be "fighters," those able to face down the challenges and hurdles of prematurity with particular vigor. First of all, strong children (physically and emotionally) come in many different packages: strong, silent types; feisty, impish types; or assertively physical types. In addition, at this point researchers don't even know whether movement patterns established in the womb persist into infancy and childhood. Plenty of parents are surprised to see their in utero prizefighter turn into an easy, calm baby—and vice versa. Many factors can affect fetal movements, including a mother's diet, mood, and activity level (when mothers are busier, they tend to concentrate less on their babies' movements and think they're moving less, even when they're not), the time of day (fetuses sleep sometimes, too), and the stage of pregnancy (as fetuses grow and have less room to move around, their movements tend to involve more wriggles and fewer kicks), along with the baby's own physical strength and temperament.

It's safe to say that whatever is going on in your belly now, you will be amazed by your tiny baby's spunk and spirit. Almost all parents of preemies are. In the nursery, you see one fighter after another after another. To adults, it is inspiring. To babies, it just comes naturally.

Steroids

My doctor is giving me a medication to make my baby's lungs mature more quickly, because she may be born any day now. How much difference will it make?

You've probably been told that every extra week, in fact every extra day, in the womb is valuable, allowing your baby's organs to mature just that much more so they'll have a better chance of functioning well when the moment comes that she enters the world. Luckily, we live in an era when modern medicine can sometimes fill in for nature, at least partially, when nature isn't cooperating. Studies show that when a mother takes steroids before delivery, her premature baby's lungs and other organs mature faster, giving them the equivalent of about a week's longer stay in the womb. The benefits of taking steroids are so great in reducing some major complications of prematurity and increasing the odds of survival that the National Institutes of Health recommends them for every expectant woman between 24 and 34 weeks of gestation who is at risk of giving birth within seven days.

Steroids are hormones that everyone's body produces, especially during periods of stress. These hormones surge naturally in pregnant women just before delivery, speeding up maturation of the fetus's organ systems—a kind of developmental boost just before they have to function independently.

Getting steroids can be incredibly valuable to a preemie. One of the most common illnesses in the intensive care nursery is respiratory distress syndrome, or RDS, which arises from lung immaturity. A baby with RDS is dependent on a ventilator or other breathing assistance and is at risk for other potentially serious complications until her lungs are able to breathe well on their own. The risk that a newborn will have RDS

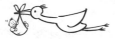

Are There Medications Other than Steroids You Can Take to Help Your Baby?

Researchers are always on the lookout for medications that a mother can take before a premature birth to help her baby mature faster or to prevent some of the complications of prematurity. Various drugs have been studied because they looked promising. Now there's one, in addition to steroids, that has been proven effective.

Doctors have found that giving magnesium sulfate (a medication prescribed for preeclampsia and preterm labor) to expectant mothers also helps to prevent cerebral palsy in their preemies. In one large study, it cut the risk of cerebral palsy in half. Since this disorder, in which a child has trouble controlling his muscle movements, is one of the most serious complications of prematurity, there's reason to rejoice at this news. Many doctors think magnesium sulfate will soon be given to most women who are likely to deliver before about 28 weeks of gestation. (Even if their mothers don't get magnesium, fewer than 3 percent to 4 percent of preemies will develop cerebral palsy, but these youngest babies are most at risk.)

It's not yet known how magnesium sulfate works to prevent cerebral palsy, although it is known to be important for the normal functioning of cells throughout the body. It may help by maintaining good blood circulation in the baby's brain and keeping harmful molecules at bay.

If you're going to be given magnesium sulfate, there are a couple of other things you may want to know. The medication may be unpleasant for you—it can cause nausea, sweating, and palpitations—but most mothers consider these side effects worth it in light of the possible benefit for their babies. Also, since it acts like a sedative and relaxes muscles, your preemie may be born floppy and possibly not breathing deeply, but this side effect wears off soon, usually within a day or two. (Don't worry—your baby's doctors can give her any help she needs in the meantime.)

As for other medications, there's been speculation that phenobarbital and vitamin K, given to a mother before delivery, might reduce the risk of bleeding and damage in her premature infant's brain. But the evidence isn't there. Other possibilities have been investigated and will continue to be, with the hope that one day, some will be successful.

drops lower and lower with increased gestational age at birth. While virtually all preemies born before 26 weeks of gestation have to deal with respiratory distress syndrome, only about a quarter of 30- to 34-weekers, with their more mature lungs, do. (If you want to know more about RDS, see page 109.)

When steroids are given before delivery, the rate of RDS in newborn preemies between the ages of 28 weeks and 34 weeks of gestation is cut in half. For infants born before 28 weeks, the incidence of RDS doesn't seem to be reduced but the severity certainly is. Now that some 22- and 23-week babies survive, doctors are debating whether steroids should be given to expectant mothers who may give birth even before 24 weeks of gestation; not all fetuses that young have bodies mature enough to respond to the boost from steroids, but those who do might have an improved chance of survival. Beyond 34 weeks, the risk of RDS is so low that a mother isn't given steroids unless her fetus's lungs are known to be especially immature.

Being exposed to steroids in the womb has beneficial effects that go beyond helping a preemie's breathing. Steroids also speed up maturation of the brain and intestines, substantially lowering a preemie's risk of brain injury and NEC (inflammation of the intestines), some of the most worrisome potential health consequences of prematurity.

If your doctor is giving you a course of steroids (betamethasone is the kind given to pregnant women), you'll get two shots, 24 hours apart. The maximum benefit comes when you get both shots at least 24 hours before giving birth, but there's some benefit even if you've had only one shot, or if you deliver less than 24 hours later. The effects last for seven days or more. If you get steroids when your baby is less than about 26 to 28 weeks of gestation and more than a week passes without your giving birth (which is good news!), you may be given another course, in case his body was too young to respond to them the first time. Most doctors would not give any more than that, however, because too many courses of prenatal steroids can adversely affect the long-term growth of a baby's brain and possibly other organs, offsetting their beneficial short-term effects.

What about other risks from prenatal steroids? Some mothers have medical conditions, such as diabetes, which steroids can worsen. Your obstetrician will judge whether taking steroids is safe for you. The fear that one course of steroids before delivery would increase a mother's risk of getting an infection or have some negative effects on her baby has been extensively researched in studies that followed the preemies until they were 12 years old. Thankfully, research hasn't shown any adverse effects from one course of these extraordinarily valuable drugs. Steroids are given around the world today to large numbers of expectant women, and the benefit to their babies is one of the biggest achievements in prenatal medicine in the last 30 years.

MULTIPLES

Likelihood of Prematurity After Assisted Reproduction

I'm pregnant after an IVF cycle, and I'm having twins. Am I likely to deliver prematurely?

You may know that if you're having more than one baby you have a higher chance of a preterm birth and the risk increases with the number of babies you're carrying. The risk of prematurity is about 12 percent for a singleton pregnancy, but it's nearly 50 percent for twins and nearly 90 percent for triplets. The average length of a twin pregnancy is 36 to 37 weeks, and each additional fetus shortens it by about three and a half weeks.

Most couples who are treated for infertility with assisted reproduction therapies (in vitro fertilization or other treatments) are aware of the high rate of multiples—roughly 30 percent—that result. But it's easy to be so focused on just getting pregnant that you push the possibility of having more than one baby into the back of your mind. Some couples even hope for twins or triplets to see their desire for a big family finally come true all at once while they have the chance.

Although having multiples is sometimes an unavoidable consequence of infertility treatments, from a medical standpoint it's not a desirable one. Multiple pregnancies have higher rates of miscarriage, stillbirth, and prematurity. A preterm delivery is much more likely for a simple reason: the amount of space in the womb. When the human uterus, which was not meant to carry more than one fetus, gets very distended, it starts contracting. That may be nature's way of trying to deliver a baby when it's well grown; but, not surprisingly, with multiple fetuses the womb gets overcrowded and tends to contract before term. Also, because of the space and nutritional resources they have to share, multiples tend to be smaller than singletons. (You can see how much smaller on the growth chart, page 583.) And women who are pregnant with multiples are more likely to have pregnancy complications, like bleeding or high blood pressure, which can lead to an early birth.

Considering that you face extra risks from a multiple pregnancy, it's nice to get some good news, too: The length of your pregnancy is likely to be no different than if you had conceived your twins naturally. Only a few years ago, doctors were convinced that assisted pregnancies were shorter by two or three weeks than natural pregnancies with the same number of fetuses. Although true when you're having a singleton, this turns out not to be true when you're having twins. In fact, studies show that twins conceived through infertility treatments are more likely to survive than twins conceived naturally. Doctors haven't yet been able to clarify why, but it may have to do with better care during pregnancy and a higher incidence of fraternal rather than identical twins.

So if you don't have other risk factors for prematurity, your twins are likely to enjoy a long enough stay in the womb to be born after 34 weeks of gestation—when a preemie's outcome is excellent, very similar to babies born at term.

Twin-Twin Transfusion Syndrome

My doctor said my twins aren't doing well in my womb because they share a blood vessel. What problems will they have, and can anything be done to help?

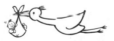

If You're Pregnant with Just One After Infertility Treatments

If you are expecting one baby after infertility treatments, your risk of delivering a preemie is twice as high as that of a mother who became pregnant naturally. Doctors can't point to the exact reasons why; it could be due to some still unknown side effects of assisted reproduction therapies or to whatever caused the infertility in the first place.

Fortunately, having a preemie is still not very likely for you. But after clearing all of the emotional, practical, and financial hurdles of infertility treatments, it can be very hard to hear something worrisome again. Your infertility specialist will refer you to an obstetrician with experience in managing high-risk pregnancies who can help you feel more in control, and can give you and the baby you desire so much the best possible care.

Your doctor probably suspects a condition called twin-twin transfusion syndrome, which can affect the health and growth of identical twins during pregnancy. A twin-twin "transfusion" occurs when shared blood vessels in the placenta cause too much blood to circulate out of one twin and into the other.

To understand how this can happen, it's necessary to look at events that occur at the very beginning of life. A fertilized egg, to develop into a fetus, needs a placenta to supply it with vital amounts of oxygen and nutrients from the mother's blood and to get rid of its waste. The placenta begins to form right out of the fertilized egg the moment it attaches to the uterus, quickly growing into a net of fetal blood vessels connected to the fetus by the umbilical cord. Around the fetus, a sac of membranes—the amniotic sac—forms and gradually fills with amniotic fluid, consisting mostly of fetal urine.

What about twins? Fraternal twins come from two different eggs and always have two separate placentas and amniotic sacs. Identical twins come from the same egg, which splits sometime after fertilization, forming two fetuses. When that split happens very early after fertilization, before the placenta has developed, each identical twin will make its own placenta and amniotic sac. When that split happens later, after the placenta has already formed, the twins will share the same placenta. Depending on whether the fertilized egg splits in two before or after the amniotic sac forms, each twin may make its own sac, or they may share one.

In a placenta shared by identical twins, there are almost always some blood vessels connected to both umbilical cords that allow the circulation of a little blood from one twin to the other. As long as the blood vessels are small and the amount of blood flowing from one to the other is minor, it's not a problem. But if the connection involves large blood vessels, a substantial amount of blood may flow from one twin (the donor) into the other (the recipient).

The recipient twin gets more blood, with its oxygen and nutrients, so it becomes bigger. But a lot of blood can be too much of a good thing, and bigger is not always stronger. The recipient twin can get overloaded with fluid, putting a strain on her heart to pump all that blood. When twin-twin transfusion syndrome is really severe, the recipient twin is at risk of dying in the womb or in early infancy of heart failure. The extra blood will also make her urinate a lot, filling her sac with excessive amounts of amniotic fluid (a condition called polyhydramnios; see page 44), which is one of the main causes of preterm labor.

The donor twin can also get into trouble. She gets less blood than she should, so lacks some oxygen and nutrients. This can restrict her growth, making her smaller than the other twin. She won't urinate as much, so there may be too little amniotic fluid in her sac (a condition called oligohydramnios). Not having enough amniotic fluid increases the risk that the umbilical cord can get compressed in the uterus, leading to a dangerous interruption of blood flow to the fetus. In severe twin-twin transfusion syndrome, the donor twin is also at risk for heart failure, from profound anemia.

It's hard to generalize about the effects of this condition. If it's mild, both babies will probably do well, perhaps differing in size or blood cell counts, but with few or no other consequences. If it's moderate, an early delivery and prematurity are the likely consequences. But if it's severe, the disturbances in blood flow can potentially damage the vital organs of both fetuses, leading to death or long-term disabilities.

Twin-twin transfusion syndrome is diagnosed by ultrasound, usually in the second trimester of pregnancy. The primary indicators are: twins of

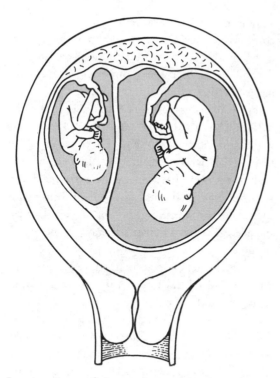

In twin-twin transfusion syndrome, one twin receives too much blood and is bigger, with more amniotic fluid. The other twin receives too little blood and is smaller, with less amniotic fluid.

the same sex, a shared placenta, and too much fluid in the bigger twin's sac with too little fluid in the smaller twin's sac. Sometimes ultrasound measurements of fetal blood flow can pick up abnormal circulation patterns in the twins and show the blood vessels that are causing the problem.

When twin-twin transfusion syndrome is diagnosed, the obstetrician usually rates its severity from Stage I (mildest) to Stage V (most severe). Every case is different, and research statistics vary, but some experts estimate that only about half of all cases at an early stage will progress to a higher one. About 30 percent of cases will stay the same, and a lucky 20 percent will even improve and move to a lower stage as the pregnancy goes on.

There are a few options for treatment. The right one for you will depend partly on how severely your twins are affected and how early it is in your pregnancy, and partly on your personal choices.

The traditional treatment for twin-twin transfusion syndrome, which some obstetricians consider useful, is to drain amniotic fluid from the sac of the recipient twin. It has been suggested that this may slow down the passage of blood from one twin to the other and may delay preterm delivery. This procedure, in which a needle is inserted in the mother's abdomen, has to be repeated often, though, and other doctors don't think it works, especially when the twin-twin transfusion syndrome is moderate or severe (Stage III, IV, or V) or when it appeared before 26 weeks of gestation. Occasionally drugs may be given to the mother to help the babies' hearts or to reduce their urine output (so the recipient twin won't make as much amniotic fluid), but they are not without risks. Once the obstetrician thinks that the babies' problems in the womb are worse than the possible complications of being born prematurely, an elective preterm delivery is commonly done, by 29 weeks or 30 weeks, on average.

A more recent and very promising innovation is laser surgery on the placenta. This involves closing the blood vessels connecting one twin to the other while both babies are still in the womb, then removing the excess fluid in the recipient twin's sac and going on with the pregnancy. This procedure carries a higher risk of complications, like preterm labor, preterm rupture of membranes (water breaking), or infection, and only a few hospitals have the expertise to do it. But for certain babies with rapidly advancing disease who are younger than about 28 weeks of gestation, it has become the therapy of choice. In recent studies of severe, early twin-twin transfusion syndrome, laser surgery led to survival of both twins in one-third of cases and survival of one twin in about

75 percent. Some 10 percent to 15 percent of the surviving babies had long-term disabilities—about half as many as after the traditional treatment of draining amniotic fluid.

In the most severe cases of twin-twin transfusion syndrome, when it looks like one or both babies will almost surely die, some doctors suggest that parents consider the difficult option of selective reduction—aborting one fetus to give the other a better chance. For parents, this is a terribly painful decision. There is a hopeful 80 percent chance that the twin who continues developing will survive, although there are no statistics yet on long-term health.

When Only One Twin Needs Early Delivery

One of my twins is having trouble in the womb, and the doctor says she'd benefit from an early delivery. But the other is doing fine and could go to full term. Whom should I put first?

The dilemma that arises when one of your babies is doing well during pregnancy and the other is not can be gut-wrenching. While your womb is the best possible place for one of your twins, for the other it's dangerous, leading your doctor to believe that she would be better off being born prematurely and cared for in an intensive care nursery. Doctors often want parents' input in deciding what's best: to deliver both twins now, before term, or both twins later—a decision that requires parents to help one of their babies at the expense of the other.

If you are faced with a painful decision like this, the first thing you need is information. It's important for you to understand as clearly as possible the risks and benefits of each course of action for each of your children. For your baby

who is doing fine now and may abruptly become a preemie, you can read about a premature baby's prospects for survival and long-term health depending on her gestational age at birth on pages 56–59.

For your baby who is not doing well now, the best thing is to discuss her risks and prospects with your obstetrician and a neonatologist (a pediatrician who specializes in the care of premature and sick newborns; your obstetrician can refer you) since she may have medical problems that make the statistics different for her than for the average baby, whether she stays in the womb or not.

Unfortunately, even when you've armed yourself with all of the information that's available, there is rarely an obvious "right" answer. If one choice is clearly better in balancing the welfare of both of your children, your obstetrician will direct you that way. Very rarely, the problem can be solved with a delayed interval birth (see page 75), in which one baby is delivered days or weeks before the other, but this requires that certain conditions be met and is never a sure bet.

The only way that most parents can make a decision like this is to follow their values and their hearts. Some parents instinctively want to protect their child who is most sick or vulnerable and feel compelled to do whatever will help her. Others feel that it is their job as parents not to hurt their children who are thriving. So, for example, if one of their children is fine while the other will face daunting survival or developmental risks no matter what, they would not make a choice that would hurt their healthiest baby's chances. Some parents lean toward accepting the most natural course of events, believing that as long as the pregnancy would keep going on its own, they and the doctors should not intervene to stop it.

You will probably second-guess your decision

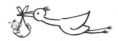

Pregnant with More than Two:
A Note about Multifetal Pregnancy Reduction

If you are pregnant with three or more fetuses, you have an extremely high chance of delivering prematurely, often at a very early gestational age when tiny and immature babies face great hurdles. Your obstetrician might have talked to you early in your pregnancy about the possibility of a multifetal pregnancy reduction. This procedure, in which one or more fetuses are aborted on purpose, is done to give the babies who will later develop a better chance to survive, so that they can reach an age when they can be born without such high risks of an early death and future disabilities.

Couples who are faced with this choice, no matter what decision they make, may feel certain and comfortable that they did the right thing or may be left with deep sorrow and excruciating doubt. It's important to remember that for this path, there is no absolutely right or wrong choice. Even the future cannot prove that your decision was good or bad, because not even time can tell you what would have happened if you had chosen differently. Try not to let your joy for the lives that are developing in your womb be shadowed by past choices or future statistics. Give yourself credit that whatever happens, you've done what was in your power, or what your conscience allowed, to best help your babies and your family.

many times over the coming months and years, no matter how things turn out. Just remember that the very nature and essence of a family is that several people are in it together. As parents, it's impossible for us to do what's best for every one of our children all of the time—much as we wish we could. We are forced to weigh everyone's needs and to make decisions that are best for one member of the family in one situation, for another in another situation, always thinking about what's good for the family as a whole.

Take all the time you can to think and talk through your decision. Later, give yourself credit for trying to make the best choice for your family that you could, in an exceedingly difficult situation.

IN DEPTH

Checking on a Baby's Well-Being Before He Is Born

There are various ways an obstetrician can "visit" a baby in his mother's womb to find out how he's doing. Some are high-tech and may require a hospital visit. Others are simple ones you can do at home or your doctor can do in his office. Depending on your particular medical situation, your obstetrician will decide when to monitor your baby's well-being and which tests will be most helpful.

Each of these tests has pros and cons, and, unfortunately, the cons often include a high number of false alarms. They cause a lot of anxiety until the test is repeated or a different kind of test is performed and everyone is assured that things are actually all right. But even though nobody likes unnecessary scares, when there really is a dangerous situation such focused medical attention can help to pick it up early while there's still time to intervene and lessen the harm to your baby.

* **Kick counts.** This is the most basic kind of monitoring—something you can do yourself at home—based on the assumption that an active baby is a healthy baby. There are several different methods. A simple one is to lie down comfortably on your side once a day and count how many times your baby kicks you. Some fetuses are generally more active and others quieter—some mothers swear they could tell their child's personality *that* early!—but if you feel at least ten movements in two hours, that's good. (A fetus may be sleeping for 20 to 40 minutes but then should wake up.) If you don't feel any movement or your baby is moving much less

than usual, you should immediately call your obstetrician. Although this is one of the tests with a high rate of false alarms, you shouldn't be afraid to cry wolf. Some studies have shown that when expectant mothers do kick counts, they lower their risk of miscarriage or stillbirth.

* **Ultrasound.** Ultrasound uses sound waves to see inside your womb. An ultrasound scan is painless and safe for both you and your baby. Doctors use it to estimate fetal weight and gestational age, monitor whether a baby is growing normally, check on how a baby's organs are developing, measure the amount of amniotic fluid (too much or too little fluid can indicate a problem), make sure the cervix is staying closed, assess whether the placenta is properly attached to the uterus, and evaluate a baby's position and movement patterns. The accuracy of ultrasound depends on the expertise of the person doing the test and on the precision of the equipment. So if your obstetrician suspects a problem, he may refer you to a special ultrasound clinic to confirm the diagnosis.

* **Fetal heart rate monitoring.** The most basic form of fetal heart rate monitoring is done at every prenatal visit. Your doctor spreads some gel on an ultrasound probe that is attached to earphones (like a stethoscope) and moves the probe over your belly until he can clearly hear your baby's heartbeat. A heart rate that is too slow or unchanging is worrisome, possibly signaling that the fetus is not getting enough oxygen. A heart rate that is too fast can be a sign of infection. And an irregular rhythm

could indicate a heart problem that might need treatment, before or after birth.

A more sophisticated version of fetal heart rate monitoring is done routinely during labor to detect any signs of fetal distress. You'll be asked to lie down, and a belt with a probe that detects when your uterus contracts will be wrapped around your belly. At the same time, an ultrasound probe, also on your belly, will monitor your baby's heart rate. The probes will be connected to a machine that continuously records your contractions and your baby's heart rate on a long strip of paper. Your doctors will assess whether your baby's heart rate is normal and how it responds to contractions.

✳ **Non-stress test.** A non-stress test—checking on a fetus in a natural situation without adding any extra stress or stimulation—is performed the same way that fetal heart rate monitoring is done during labor, but the doctors will be specifically watching to see that your baby's heart rate speeds up periodically. The human heart normally speeds up in response to various bodily functions, especially movement—as when you dash to catch a bus or a fetus kicks—thereby assuring that the body gets more oxygen and blood flow when it is needed. When doctors see that a fetus's heart rate speeds up periodically, they know that your baby is active, his neurologic connections are intact, and his heart is able to respond appropriately. If your baby's heart rate accelerates two or more times within a 20-minute period, the non-stress test is "reactive" and your baby is probably doing fine. If not, your doctor probably will want to do other, more specific tests. A non-stress test can last up to 40 minutes, because some babies may be peacefully sleeping and not move at all for some time. Some hospitals, to speed things up (and to spare you unnecessary worry), may try to wake up the little sleeper with a buzzing device to

finally get him to kick. But even then, some babies don't wake up, which leads to a high rate of false alarms with this test.

✳ **Contraction stress test.** This is also a kind of fetal heart rate monitoring, but unlike a non-stress test, which merely involves observing your baby, a stress test puts him in a stressful situation to see how he reacts. That stressful experience is a series of uterine contractions—a preview of labor—because contractions have the power to temporarily decrease blood flow through the placenta. If a baby is healthy and everything is going well, he has a reserve of oxygen that allows him to sail through a contraction unscathed—after all, that's what he'll have to go though during labor. But if that reserve doesn't exist because there's already a scarcity of oxygen, his heart rate will slow down. To stimulate uterine contractions, you may be given intravenously a medication called pitocin, a man-made form of oxytocin, which can make your uterus contract, or you may be asked to gently rub your nipple, because that stimulates your body to release oxytocin naturally. If you're having spontaneous contractions (which may or may not be a sign of preterm labor, depending on their regularity and intensity), you may not need any medication or stimulation. For a stress test to be accurate, you'll need to have at least three contractions within a ten-minute span, each one lasting at least 40 seconds. To achieve that, the test may last for up to two hours if you're waiting for natural contractions; using intravenous pitocin requires less time, usually about an hour. Since uterine contractions can be the enemy for some mothers—those with preterm labor or vaginal bleeding, for example—a stress test may not be advisable for them. An excellent alternative is a biophysical profile.

✳ **Biophysical profile.** This is a multifaceted exam in which your baby's behavior is observed with ultrasound for 30 minutes. The doctor will score your baby on five elements:

- **Breathing.** A healthy fetus will make breathing movements for at least 30 seconds.
- **Body movements.** A healthy fetus will move his body or limbs at least three times.
- **Tone.** A healthy fetus will have at least one episode of extending his limbs or trunk then returning to a flexed position (such as opening and closing his hand).
- **Heart rate acceleration.** A non-stress test should be reactive, or the examiner should see by ultrasound that your baby's heartbeat speeds up at least twice in 30 minutes, when he moves.
- **Amniotic fluid volume.** The amount of amniotic fluid around your baby should be normal.

If two or more of these elements are abnormal, it could mean that your baby isn't getting enough oxygen or blood flow. On the other hand, you can truly feel safe if the results indicate your baby is fine.

(A simpler, modified biophysical profile consists of only two elements: the non-stress test and the amniotic fluid volume. Some doctors consider it almost as precise as a full biophysical profile.)

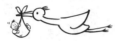

Amniotic Fluid: A Telling Sign of a Baby's Health

An intact sac of membranes filled with the right amount of amniotic fluid protects and nourishes a fetus until delivery. Too little or too much fluid immediately catches a doctor's attention because it sometimes—although not always—signals that something is interfering with the fetus's normal development in the womb.

In medical parlance, too much amniotic fluid is called polyhydramnios, and too little is called oligohydramnios. Using ultrasound, doctors can easily measure the amount of amniotic fluid. By calculating the depth of the fluid surrounding the fetus in four sections of the uterus, they derive a number called the "amniotic fluid index." A normal index is around 8 to 18 cm. If an expectant mother's index is less than 5 or 6, she has oligohydramnios; if it's more than 20 to 24 cm, she has polyhydramnios.

Polyhydramnios can lead to preterm delivery because the excess fluid can overly distend the uterus, stimulating it to begin contracting too early. Since the fetus normally swallows large amounts of amniotic fluid, anything that impairs the fetus's ability to swallow (such as problems with his mouth, neck, or stomach, or neurological conditions) can cause too much amniotic fluid to build up. But only 20 percent of fetuses with polyhydramnios are found to have a congenital abnormality. A variety of other maternal and fetal conditions have been associated with polyhydramnios, and your doctor will discuss with you any that apply. In many cases, no reason for the extra fluid is found. If your case is severe, your doctor may drain some of the fluid out with a needle and syringe, in a procedure similar to an amniocentesis, to lower the immediate risk of preterm labor and delivery.

Oligohydramnios, or too little amniotic fluid, can be caused by premature rupture of the membranes (when your water breaks, most of the amniotic fluid leaks out), abnormalities of your baby's urinary system (because the amniotic fluid is made mostly of fetal urine), or a poorly functioning placenta, as can happen with preeclampsia, for example (because babies who get less blood flow through the placenta will urinate less). Often oligohydramnios is accompanied by signs of fetal distress or poor growth be-cause your baby is no longer cushioned by a fluid-filled sac, and less blood flow from the placenta means less oxygen and fewer nutrients are delivered to the fetus. If your doctor determines that your fluid is too low, she'll keep a close eye on your baby's growth and well-being. Sometimes a sufficient amount of amniotic fluid can be reestablished with bed rest, drinking more water, time, and possibly medical treatment. Some doctors occasionally use a technique called amnioinfusion (directly infusing fluid into the womb with a catheter), particularly to help a fetus tolerate labor and diminish the need for a cesarean section, but whether it is beneficial is controversial. If your doctor thinks your baby will have a better chance of growing and developing well outside of the womb, she may recommend an elective preterm delivery.

* **Doppler studies.** These ultrasound tests—the newest in prenatal monitoring—measure blood flowing through the umbilical cord between the placenta and fetus. With doppler studies, doctors can detect whether blood flow is normal, mildly abnormal, or very abnormal and thereby pick out babies who may not be getting enough oxygen and nutrients in the womb. Doppler studies are especially helpful in distinguishing between babies whose growth is restricted because they aren't receiving enough maternal blood flow and those who are simply constitutionally small. Babies with marginal or inadequate placental blood flow need to be closely monitored, and most likely will benefit at some point from an elective delivery. Babies who are merely small can safely stay in the womb to grow at their own pace until the end of gestation.

Doppler studies of a different blood vessel, in the brain, can also help doctors diagnose severe anemia in a fetus, which may occur if there is a blood-group incompatibility between a mother and baby.

* **Percutaneous umbilical blood testing (PUBS).** This test involves taking a sample of your baby's blood from the umbilical cord. It is more risky than most other fetal diagnostic tests because the cord could be damaged, and obstetricians do it only when they need very precise information about your baby that can be obtained in no other way—for example, to evaluate your baby's blood counts if there's reason to believe they may be abnormal or to see if he has an infec-

tion or genetic problem. You will be given local anesthesia, and a long needle will be inserted in your belly. Your doctor will watch exactly where it's going with ultrasound as she guides it through your uterus and into a blood vessel in the umbilical cord. Normal results could confirm that your baby is doing well in your womb, perhaps allowing you to avoid an elective preterm delivery.

✳ **Amniocentesis.** You may already know that amniocentesis is offered to many women as a test for some birth defects (like Down syndrome). But amniocentesis—taking a sample of amniotic fluid by passing a needle through your belly and into your uterus—has other useful applications as well. In cases of preterm labor, amniocentesis can detect a uterine infection sooner than maternal blood tests and other cultures. If your amniotic fluid were infected, it would probably convince the doctors to do an elective delivery. Moreover, amniotic fluid can be used to assess your baby's lung maturity. When a fetus's lungs have developed enough to breathe well on their own, certain substances are released into the amniotic fluid. If your baby will be delivered soon and those substances aren't present, you'll probably be given steroids to speed up the maturation of your baby's lungs. If, instead, your baby's amniotic fluid says "lungs OK," your doctor may opt for an immediate delivery.

Part II

IN THE HOSPITAL

CHAPTER 2

WELCOME TO THE WORLD

Your Baby's Delivery

. . . .

Your baby's transition from the womb to the world.

Preparing for and understanding a premature birth.

. . . .

PARENTS' STORIES: DELIVERY*

A premature delivery may occur unexpectedly, to parents who haven't had a chance to prepare for that life crisis. In other cases, a pregnancy is known to be at risk, and parents deal with uncertainty and fear for long weeks. Some parents cope by actively seeking more information. For others, denial works best.

Today is Thanksgiving and I'm in a hospital bed. My baby and I are all right, she's moving a lot and kicking me more vigorously than ever. But my obstetrician decided to keep me in the hospital a little longer. "Just to be safe . . ." she said. Two days ago I began to bleed, so I came in and was rushed to a labor room. My contractions stopped, and since then, everything has been fine. Only I wish I could go home. It's so upsetting here. There are only curtains between beds, and little or no privacy. The woman to my left came in last night. She was in her first trimester, but they couldn't find her baby's heartbeat anymore. He was gone. I heard her story unwillingly when she talked to a doctor before surgery. I was shocked: She and her husband didn't sound very upset. Maybe they didn't really want this baby. Or maybe they have exceptional self-control. I can't even think what I would be like in their shoes. In the bed across the aisle, there's a woman who cries a lot. She just gave birth to premature twins, and they are upstairs, in intensive care. "You don't know what I see there," she told me in tears, when we exchanged a few words. I tried to be nice to her, but I didn't want to hear what she was saying. My due date is in three months. Tomorrow, my baby and I are going home.

(P.S. This mother went into premature labor ten days later at 29 weeks of gestation. Her child, now three years old, is doing great.)

---

* *Parents' Stories* describes events and feelings that really happened or that can happen. Every situation is unique, and you may relate to some parents' experiences and reactions more than others.

Obstetricians can prescribe bed rest and medications to expectant mothers, to try to prolong their pregnancies. But there are no simple instructions when it comes to taking care of older children, leaving jobs responsibly when you have to do so suddenly and earlier than you had planned, and surviving the siege of worry and ominous waiting with one's psyche and relationships intact. Sometimes, an early delivery (though not as early as originally feared), is almost a deliverance.

Yesterday, Mark and Louise came over for lunch to celebrate my birthday. She'd been on and off bed rest for several weeks and looked surprisingly round in her long maternity dress to have two more months to go. "I gained too much weight," she said, faking some shame. "Lawrence is going to be a big boy, like all the men in my family!" Mark, who's slight, joked about having to build up some muscles to be able to hold his son at birth. They seemed glad to join our family reunion but looked weary and tense. It hasn't been easy for them. Yesterday was their first social outing—with the doctor's permission—in a long time. That's not how you should spend your pregnancy, poor Louise. She grew more tired and pale as the party went on, and they left after the cake. Then that night the phone rang. It was Mark, telling us that Lawrence had been born, at a mere four and a half pounds. Louise's water had broken, and labor this time could not be stopped. Mark managed to tease me over the phone: "We told you he was going to be a big boy!" He sounded worried but in some way relieved. Lawrence was in an incubator and breathing oxygen through a little tube when we saw him today in the nursery. This little guy and I share a birthday, I realized. He'll do well, I know it.

"We have to deliver your baby." Depending on the medical circumstances and the stage of gestation your baby has reached, this news may merely increase parents' anxiety or plunge them into pure terror. Even if the doctors say encouraging words, some parents can't allow themselves to be hopeful. The fear of the unknown is just too overwhelming.

I don't want to see. I don't want to be awake. Put me to sleep and, please, don't wake me up. I will not hear my baby crying, I know it. He'll be too exhausted after this long run. His heart has been racing so fast in the last hours, like a little crazy horse who's desperate to be freed. They say it's better for him to be born, even so early. Inside, I'm poisoning him. Outside, they can take care of him. I'm choking in my tears when they make me sit up, gently pushing my back from behind. "You'll feel a needle stick and some burning," a doctor says. The anesthesia is quickly working, taking the pain out of my body but not out of my head. Behind the drape, under the glaring lights, they're pushing and pulling strongly on a body that happens to be mine. "I'm giving you the kind of C-section that will allow you to deliver your next baby naturally," the obstetrician says. "But I'll never have another baby. I don't want another baby," I cry out with no voice. How can he tell me that when my baby is fighting for his life? Seconds fly, voices overlap. "Oh . . . he's not so small after all . . ." "Did you hear him crying? Did you hear his voice?" This is my husband talking. No, I didn't. "This is your son, he's beautiful, you know?" somebody says, putting a little face all bundled up in a blanket really close to mine. But not close enough.

Premature babies are fragile, and the youngest of them need the kind of special care that only a few hospitals can provide. To get it, some of them have to travel right after delivery, leaving their shocked parents behind.

—Are you Mr. Wood? Hi, nice meeting you. I'm Alice Lewis, a transport nurse from St. Anne Metropolitan Hospital, where your twins are being transferred. My colleague, Donna, a neonatal nurse practitioner, is getting your babies ready for the ambulance trip. Do you know where our hospital is located?

—Yes, I've been there several times. My brother lives nearby.

—Oh, great, so you'll have some family to help you out. Will you be staying with him?

—I thought so. But now I'm concerned about leaving my wife. She's sick, with a very high fever.

—What does her doctor say?

—He says they're treating her with antibiotics and that she should be better soon. Let's hope so. . . .

—Does she know that the babies are being transferred?

—Not yet. She's only barely awake from the pain medicine and can't handle any more bad news, I think. . . .

—But moving them to St. Anne isn't bad news. . . . It's a hassle, we know, having them 40 miles away, but you should think of it as a safety measure. This hospital doesn't have the expertise to treat preemies like your twins. Has your wife seen them yet?

—No, only some instant photos, but you could barely see the babies with all the wires and tubes. She's too sick to get out of bed.

—If she can't come to the babies, the babies will come to her. Once we've put them in the transport isolette, we'll just make a stop upstairs to say good-bye to their mom before leaving. Would you like to go up and tell her?

—Are you sure it's a good idea?

—Absolutely. Trust me.

Do preemies run in families? There's some evidence for that. Knowing what you may be in for, because you've had a preemie before or because your sister had one, has both good and bad sides. You may live for months in apprehension, but you can take preventive steps as well. You know the risks but also know when it's safe, cautiously, to relax.

Stephanie and Tommy are fine. I'm a little shaken, but . . . so happy. . . . Don't cry, Laura, everything is all right. Your sister was so good, I'm so proud of her. . . . We were together, she had a natural delivery . . . and after all, the baby is only six weeks early . . . OK, OK, just kidding. You're right. We should have stayed in the city. But we needed some fresh air . . . and the doctor said we could go, so. . . . Have you ever been up here? You should see the view from Stephanie's room. We have the whole valley at our feet. . . . There was a helicopter ready to take Tommy to a city hospital. But he didn't need to go . . . exactly . . . he's already a mountaineer, like your father. . . . Of course he's breathing on his own! I could hold him already. He's small, but beautiful. I can't wait to take Stephanie to see him. . . . No, she hasn't yet, she can't move, the stitches they gave her are killing her. . . . Breastfeeding? Yes, I think. . . . Tomorrow we'll have a cell phone, so you'll be able to talk to her. She has to begin pumping her breast milk right away. Of course I'll tell her. Listen, don't say that. How could it be your fault? Preemies run in your family? . . . Maybe . . . but to me . . . it's just that you and your sister . . . do all your things in a rush. . . . Don't laugh, that's true! But this time you have to admit that Stephanie was much more patient than you were with your daughter. By the way, can I talk to my former microniece? Hi, Raphaelle! It's Uncle Ray. Did Mummy tell you that you have a little cousin?

THE DOCTOR'S PERSPECTIVE: DELIVERY *

It's the moment you've been waiting for—although not quite long enough! Like alxl delivery days, the birth day of your child will be full of pain and joy, a remarkable, momentous occasion. But it will be different, too, as your baby will be met with more trepidation and more technology than the average full-term baby. No amount of advance information can predict exactly how your preemie will do when he's born. We're always ready to be surprised in the delivery room—by tiny babies who remarkably come out kicking and screaming, and by bigger babies who unexpectedly need more help to get going. One expectant mother asked her obstetrician after an ultrasound, "How can you know so much about him when he's in there and you're out here?" Well, we do know a lot, from assessing you and your baby before delivery and from having dealt with many other preemies of his age and size before, but until he's out here too, there will always be an element of mystery. It all becomes real when your baby arrives.

Physical Exam and Laboratory Assessment

In the delivery room, doctors initially focus on the basics—a baby's essential signs of life—leaving the rest of the physical exam until later. From the moment a preemie is born and delivered into our hands—as we carry her to the warming bed, dry her off, and clean out her nose and mouth—we're constantly assessing her breathing, heartbeat, and circulation. We're hoping that she cries (which means that she's vigorous, alert, and taking a deep breath—good on all fronts). We're checking her color (if she's gradually getting pink it means she's getting enough oxygen) and watching to make sure that she continues to breathe regularly (many preemies don't, in which case we'll have to help her out). We're also making sure that her heartbeat is strong and regular and that she doesn't have any life-threatening conditions we need to treat immediately. Occasionally in a baby born extremely prematurely, we're also assessing whether she appears mature enough to survive for longer than a few hours outside the womb, even with

our best medical treatment. Based on your baby's vital signs and vigor and how well she responds to medical treatment, we'll assign her Apgar scores (see page 70).

After we're certain that a baby is breathing well (by herself or with our help), and has a normal heart rate, we do a quick physical exam to make sure all her body parts are there and normally formed. We'll neatly cut her umbilical cord, examining that, too, to make sure the blood vessels that nourished her in the womb are normal. Then, we'll weigh her—in grams (the measure we use) and pounds (to tell you).

Your obstetrician may take some blood, painlessly, from your baby's umbilical cord after she's born to check for such things as her blood type, whether she has certain infections (nearly all newborns in the United States are screened for syphilis, for example), and whether she was getting enough oxygen right before delivery. Other than that and maybe measuring her oxygen level, we usually wait until a preemie is safely ensconced in the more controlled and closely monitored atmosphere of the nursery before getting X-rays and lab tests.

---

* *The Doctor's Perspective* describes how your doctor may be thinking about your preemie's condition and what she may be considering as she makes medical decisions. All of the medical terms and conditions mentioned here are described in more detail elsewhere in this book. Check the index.

Don't worry if you're having more than one baby. Each of your preemies will get the same attentive care. As soon as each one is born, she'll be taken to her own warming bed in the delivery room or in a special stabilization room for newly born babies, where she'll be evaluated and treated by her own, dedicated medical team.

Common Issues and Decisions

Seeing and holding your baby: Given their early births, we don't expect that all preemies will come out rarin' to go. The reason a neonatologist (a doctor who specializes in the care of newborns) may be in the delivery room, along with the rest of the medical team, is to insure that your preemie's transition from the womb to the world is as quick, easy, and safe as possible. I know it can be agonizing to get only a quick glimpse of your baby as we whisk her away out of your sight, and sometimes out of your earshot, too. We know that you want to be with her and are wondering when she'll be back with you and how long she'll be able to stay.

The answer depends on how young your preemie is and how quickly we get her stabilized. (Some babies will be intubated and given surfactant, a medication that can help a premature baby breathe more easily, or resuscitated in other ways at delivery, as you can read more about on page 69.) The wait, usually twenty minutes or so, difficult as it may be for you, really is for your baby's welfare. Once your preemie is warm and dry, her heart rate is normal, and she's breathing regularly (by herself or with our help), we no longer have to watch her quite so intensely and can bring her back to you. If you have an older preemie who's doing well on her own, she can probably linger for a while in your arms—a joy for her and for you. But if she's younger than about 34 weeks of gestation or needs help with her breathing, her stability is still fragile, so it's safer to take her quickly to the intensive care nursery. There we'll

continue to monitor and assess her, and give her any therapies, such as antibiotics or oxygen, that she may need. Above all, we'll make certain that she stays stable. It shouldn't be too long—usually about an hour—until she'll be ready for you to visit her there.

Babies at the edge of viability: Viability means the ability to survive. Some preemies are born so immature that they absolutely cannot survive, no matter what kind of medical treatment they get. Nowadays, that's the case for babies who are born at less than 22 weeks of gestation. Other preemies are far enough along in their development to survive, although they may need intensive care for some time. That's the case for most babies who are born at 25 weeks of gestation or more. Between those ages are preemies who are born at the edge of viability, where we aren't very good at predicting whether a baby is mature enough to survive.

Rarely do neonatologists believe that we should aggressively treat every newborn. Most, after giving the matter careful thought and weighing the outcome statistics for premature babies, have adopted policies of initiating intensive care at delivery for all preemies who are beyond the age of viability and providing comfort care only—without invasive or aggressive treatment—to preemies who are below it. For a baby born in between, though, at the edge of viability, you and your doctor will have to make difficult decisions about how much treatment to offer your baby at delivery. (Whether to continue or stop intensive care later, after seeing how your baby is doing, is a separate question, which you and your baby's doctor will consider together when appropriate.)

Because there are some real, unpredictable differences in how rapidly children develop, we usually don't know for sure how an individual preemie who is born at the edge of viability will do. In general, we know that a 23-weeker has a poor chance of surviving without disabilities while a 24-weeker has a better outlook. But chronological age and physical maturity don't always go hand in hand. Other factors, too, play a role in how mature a preemie is. For example, girls tend to mature faster than boys, singletons may have an advantage over multiples, and heavier babies usually do better. Babies who were given prenatal steroids jump about a week forward in their development.

It's occasionally obvious in the delivery room that a baby born at the edge of viability isn't mature enough to survive outside the womb. We may find that we can't get air into her lungs or that her skin is so fragile that any touch injures her. More commonly, though, it takes hours or days—and sometimes longer—before it's clear that a preemie is getting worse instead of better. This uncertainty about whether your baby has developed enough to be able to survive can be excruciating, for you and for us, because it makes it so hard to know what the best thing is to do.

I usually tell parents that we have three options. Although I may recommend one, based on what I know about your preemie's medical condition, I believe that any of these can be the most appropriate choice for you and your baby.

The first option is to do everything in our power to support your baby's life, even if that will take a great toll on her and you. I've met many parents who feel that there is nothing they wouldn't do to try to keep their baby alive. They want their child to live, whether or not she is very sick and suffers for a long time, may die soon, or will have disabilities in the future. Her survival is all that counts for them now, and they'll love and cherish her no matter what.

The second option is not to provide intensive medical treatment, but instead to make your baby feel as warm, comfortable, and loved as possible in the brief time that she's alive. (Without intensive care, most babies this young will live for only a few hours, although some will live for several days.) Many parents feel that it is kinder and more loving not to extend their infant's life if it's only for a short time, will involve suffering and pain, and there's very little chance that their child could be healthy or happy.

The third option lies somewhere in the middle: to start by giving your baby all possible medical treatment, but to reevaluate, and maybe stop, if things are not going well. That painful point may be reached as early as in the delivery room or hours, days, or weeks later. Parents and doctors who choose to do things this way usually believe that their uncertainty about a baby's future will diminish over time. If you decide that this approach is the right one for you and your baby, let your baby's doctor know if you want to play an active role in making a decision about whether to stop treatment if necessary, or would rather trust her to make it for you.

Some hospitals and doctors won't feel comfortable with all of these options, and they won't all be appropriate in every situation. Each doctor will have her own, particular way of approaching you about this. But if you feel strongly about what you want done if your baby is born at the edge of viability, be sure to talk about it with your obstetrician and neonatologist before delivery so that your wishes are heard and you know what your doctors are willing or able to do. Most will want you to be an active partner in making such a momentous decision, because it is you and your family who will be living with its reverberations for the rest of your lives.

Family Issues

If we were lucky, we had a chance to introduce ourselves to you before your baby was born, to begin to prepare you (if that's really possible) for the experience of having a premature baby. Some parents, though, will be meeting their baby's doctors for the first time at delivery. You may not even recognize us later, when we shed our masks and gowns. Try to excuse us if we don't say much to you in the delivery room. Most likely we'll need to get down to work and will have time to update you only briefly about how your preemie is doing before taking him back to the nursery with us for further care. Most parents aren't in top shape for asking questions and taking in a lot of information in the delivery room, anyway. Mothers may be medicated or unable to see what is happening, and the attention of fathers is often torn between their wife and their new baby. But be assured that you haven't missed any opportunities. Soon we'll be talking a lot more, including about what happened in the delivery room. We'll simply do it in a calmer place and time.

Few things lift our spirits more than being at a birth where a newborn is lovingly welcomed by his mother and father, with grandparents, aunts, uncles, and cousins all waiting outside the door. That's a lucky baby! But much as we value your presence at delivery, right after your preemie is born we'll want you to hang back, to give us some time alone with him. That's so we can focus all of our concentration on observing his physical condition and quickly providing any medical treatment he needs. I know that's a hard thing to ask you to do. Naturally you'll be wondering what's going on, and you may be worried. But if we talk to you then, we'll have to be less attentive to your baby. You may have to bite your tongue for a while, or miss out on some great photographs or videos, but I promise you, it's a trade worth making.

We've seen parents of preemies react in all sorts of ways to their baby's birth. You may be thrilled and excited, with an unshakable faith in the future. Or you may be overwhelmed with doubt, afraid for your child. If your preemie's condition is really tenuous, you may be afraid for yourself, too, wondering how you're possibly going to handle what will happen next. Some parents are stunned and numb, going through all of the motions but not feeling much of anything. But no matter how you're feeling now, your preemie's birth is a time for hope and faith, for deep looks inside to find sources of strength, for accepting things that you can't possibly change, and for figuring out what really matters. The Chinese philosopher Lao-tzu said, "A journey of a thousand miles must begin with a single step." Your journey is just starting, and like all new parents, your destination isn't clear. It's our job to help you on your way. Remember that all you have to do now is take that single step.

YOUNGEST PREEMIES TO OLDEST PREEMIES: SURVIVAL AND LONG-TERM HEALTH

We have mixed feelings about disclosing statistics on the survival and long-term health outcomes of premature babies. It is not easy for anyone to hear this kind of information, let alone the already worried parents of a newborn preemie. And our own experience in the NICU has taught us that numbers are not only terrifying—they can be misleading, too. For example: You read that 50 percent of preemies get a certain long-term health problem, and you conclude that your preemie has a 50 percent chance of getting it. Not necessarily true! No baby is "average," so the numbers that apply to preemies in general don't always apply to yours. There are numerous different factors and symptoms that can transform a grim forecast for preemies as a whole into a much more positive prospect for your baby.

So as you read the section below that applies to your baby, please keep two important caveats in mind. First, this part of the book is meant to help you develop balanced, realistic expectations—but not to make predictions about your baby. Even within each of the four gestational age groups, the range of medical outcomes for individual babies is very wide. Your baby is not a statistic, and the only guide you have to how he is doing is your baby himself. Spend time with him, look at him and how he's behaving, and, of course, ask the doctors about the results of their evaluations so far.

Second, the following statistics are merely estimates. Although gestational age is the most important factor, other things affect your baby's chances, too. A recent large study found that a combination of five factors—gestational age, birth weight, sex, whether a baby is a singleton or multiple, and whether steroids were given before delivery—more accurately predicted survival and long-term development than gestational age alone. (Being older, bigger, female, a singleton, and having gotten steroids all help a preemie do better.) Also, accurate projections for today's preemies are elusive in part because neonatal intensive care is constantly improving. Ten years ago, babies born at 23 weeks of gestation did not survive at all, and all preemies receive better care today than ever before.

Less than 23 Weeks of Gestation

Survival

Most doctors still consider babies who are born this early to be too immature to survive, even with medicine's best efforts. There have been some recent reports of 22-weekers who have survived, but although these cases are encouraging—and have been reported with great excitement by the news media—at this point it's best to remember that they are rare exceptions. Current estimates put the survival rate at less than 5 percent for preemies born at 22 weeks and at zero for preemies born earlier than that.

Long-term health

Because it is only recently that babies this young have survived, no reliable data is available yet on their long-term health. The earlier a baby is born, the greater the risk of some kind of disability, since his bodily systems are less mature and less ready to function in the world outside the womb. If your baby is one of the rare 22-weekers who survive, it is estimated that he has about a 25 percent chance of developing normally in early childhood and about a 75 percent chance of having one or more disabilities. It's unclear whether those numbers will change as these very tiniest preemies grow up. You might want to read the section below on 23-weekers for an explanation of what is meant by a disability, keeping in mind that no one knows for sure how your little baby, in particular, will do.

23 through 25 Weeks of Gestation

Survival

Preemies this young, born at the edge of viability, are the ones who benefit most from the recent advances in neonatal medical care. Ten years ago, babies born at 23 weeks of gestation did not survive. Babies born at 24 weeks survive today in greater numbers than ever before. But for the parents of these very, very premature babies, the numbers are still hard to hear: Survival rates vary from about 25 percent for 23-weekers to about 75 percent for 25-weekers.

A baby's ability to live outside the womb depends on the maturity of his organs—whether his lungs can take in enough oxygen, his skin can hold in vital fluids, and his brain can withstand the perturbations of handling and medical treatment. The younger and smaller a preemie, the more defenseless he is. Every extra day in the womb can make a difference at this stage, and an extra week is a tremendous advantage. But gestational age is not everything. Other individual factors can also influence a baby's maturity and prospects, including how big he is (although by no means exact, there's some correlation between size and maturity), sex (females have about a one-week advantage over males), whether he's a singleton or multiple (singletons do better than twins or triplets), and whether his mother was given steroids before delivery (steroids speed up maturation of a preemie's organs).

When can an extremely premature baby be considered safe? Doctors typically warn parents that it may take weeks or even months to know. But if your baby responds well to treatment during his first week, indicating that he is somewhat self sufficient and resilient, his chances of eventually coming home with you improve dramatically.

Long-term health

Because their bodily systems are so immature, babies born at 23 through 25 weeks are at risk of developing long term health problems. The earlier a baby is born, the greater that risk. But to quantify it—or predict what it is for a given, individual little baby—is not an easy task.

According to the best available estimates, about one-third of surviving 23-week gestation babies and about one-half of 25-week babies will grow up normal. Another one-quarter to one-third in this age group will have mild or moderate disabilities, such as having weak muscles or awkward movements, vision or hearing impairments that are correctable with glasses or hearing aids, learning difficulties that may require special tutoring or education, or behavior problems like

hyperactivity or excessive anxiety. Finally, about one-quarter will suffer the heaviest consequences of their premature birth, such as having lasting, severe respiratory problems requiring chronic oxygen or ventilator support, having severe cerebral palsy that calls for a wheelchair, or being blind, deaf, or mentally retarded.

It's impossible on the first day—and sometimes even for the first few months or years—to tell which preemies will be fine and which will be affected by one kind of disability or another. But not all babies are equally at risk. The main risk factors are very poor growth in the womb (particularly head growth), evidence of brain damage on a head ultrasound or MRI scan before hospital discharge, severe chronic lung disease (called BPD, for bronchopulmonary dysplasia), and ROP (retinopathy of prematurity, an eye disorder) severe enough to require surgery. Preemies who have a severe infection or a severe case of NEC (necrotizing enterocolitis, an intestinal disorder) while they are in the hospital are also at higher risk of having developmental problems. But even with one of these conditions, many babies turn out just fine.

26 through 29 Weeks of Gestation
Survival

The increasingly high survival rates of babies born between 26 and 29 weeks of gestation leave room for great optimism. Your baby's odds of surviving vary with his gestational age, from about 80 percent for 26-weekers to 95 percent for 29-weekers.

Babies at greatest risk are those with severe infections (acquired in the womb or after birth) or whose lungs, brain, or intestines are particularly immature and have trouble withstanding the perturbations of intensive medical care. It can take weeks to know for sure that he is out of danger, but given the really good prospects, you should be prepared for that happy day when you'll take your baby home.

Long-term health

Many babies born at 26 through 29 weeks of gestation grow up perfectly healthy, but there is still a considerable risk that they will develop some sort of disability, usually a mild or moderate one that will not prevent them from leading a happy and productive life. For this age group, the worst consequences of a premature birth are less likely.

The best available estimates—which do not take into account the most recent improvements in neonatal intensive care—indicate that about 65 percent of surviving 26- to 29-weekers will be normal. Another 20 percent will have mild or moderate disabilities, such as abnormal muscle tone or poor control of some movements, vision or hearing impairments that necessitate glasses or hearing aids, learning difficulties that require special tutoring or education, or behavior problems, such as hyperactivity or excessive anxiety. About 15 percent will have a severe disability, perhaps requiring oxygen or ventilator support for chronic lung disease, having severe cerebral palsy and needing a wheelchair, or being blind, deaf, or mentally retarded.

Being realistic is probably a good thing, but assuming the worst is not. Not all babies this age group are at equal risk of developing a long-term disability. The closer to 29 weeks your baby was born, the smaller his risk. Even more important is whether your baby has certain risk factors: having been born very small for his gestational age, especially in terms of head size; having suffered from severe chronic lung disease (or BPD, short for bronchopulmonary dysplasia), severe ROP (a preemie eye disorder), a major infection, or severe NEC (an intestinal disorder); or having had a head ultrasound or MRI scan that shows evidence of brain damage. If not, his chances of being normal are very high. And even with one of these conditions, many babies turn out fine.

30 through 33 Weeks of Gestation

Survival

Today, with modern neonatal intensive care, the overwhelming majority of babies born between 30 and 33 weeks of gestation survive: around 95 percent to 98 percent. In this age group, as with term babies, those whose lives are most at risk are those born with major abnormalities in their vital organs, such as their heart, kidneys, liver, or intestines. Their prematurity alone is almost never life-threatening. So you should be ready to take your baby home with you, probably in six to eight weeks, just before his full-term due date.

Long-term health

Babies born at 30 through 33 weeks of gestation have very good odds of growing into perfectly healthy, thriving children, despite their early entry into the world.

According to the best available estimates, fully 75 percent of preemies of this age will develop normally. Another 15 percent will have mild or moderate disabilities, such as mild abnormalities of muscle tone or movement, or having a common learning disability or behavior problem, such as dyslexia or hyperactivity. Unfortunately, about 10 percent of these babies still end up suffering from severe disabilities, perhaps needing chronic oxygen support at home, having cerebral palsy so severe that they need a wheelchair, or being blind, deaf, or mentally retarded. These figures are scary, but be sure to keep them in context: Even among full-term babies, about 5 percent have severe disabilities.

As in all gestational age groups, the earlier

the birth, the higher the incidence of long-term problems. If your baby is 32 weeks or older and does not have respiratory distress syndrome (RDS) severe enough to be on a ventilator or a severe infection, he will almost certainly be normal. But even younger and sicker babies in this group are at minimal risk unless they have a major birth defect, severe growth delay, show signs of brain damage on a head ultrasound or MRI scan before hospital discharge, or develop severe chronic lung disease or severe NEC (an intestinal disorder that affects some preemies) during their stay in the hospital nursery. And even many preemies with these risk factors turn out just fine.

34 through 36 Weeks of Gestation

Survival

Although preemies born at 34 through 36 weeks of gestation are less mature than term babies, the immaturity of their organ systems is so mild that in this era of excellent neonatal care they are nearly as likely to survive as if they had been born at term. In other words, you can feel safe. The approximately 99 percent survival rate for these older preemies is nearly identical to the survival rate for term babies.

Long-term health

After a preemie reaches 34 weeks of gestation, even if he has some medical problems initially, such as respiratory difficulties, problems starting to feed, or jaundice, he is very unlikely to be left with any long-term health problems stemming from his prematurity. These near-term preemies have a very slightly increased risk of learning disabilities, social difficulties, behavioral problems, or neurodevelopmental problems (such as cerebral palsy)—a rate of about 5 percent, compared with about 3 percent for term babies. So you can take heart: Although no one can promise that his first few weeks will be problem free, your preemie's overall prospects are almost the same as those of any full-term baby newly facing the world.

QUESTIONS AND ANSWERS

Moving the Mother to Another Hospital

Why do they have to take me to a hospital far from home?

Your obstetrician is probably choosing to transfer you to a hospital where you and your baby, during and after birth, can be taken care of by doctors and nurses specially trained to handle very premature labor and delivery. Following professional guidelines, hospital nurseries are classified according to the level of care they can provide. Only in some hospitals—those with a Level III nursery—can the smallest, youngest, and sickest newborns receive the highly specialized, intensive medical care they need.

* Level I hospital nurseries (also called well-newborn nurseries) provide basic neonatal care and can assist mothers and babies through uncomplicated full-term or slightly preterm (35 weeks or more of gestation) labor and delivery. The vast majority of community hospitals' nurseries are in this category. They have the medical personnel and equipment to perform an emergency C-section, evaluate a healthy baby, or resuscitate a baby at birth if the need arises. They also can stabilize an ill infant until she is transferred to a hospital

nursery where neonatal intensive care is available.

* Level II hospital nurseries (also called special care nurseries) can handle most high-risk labors and deliveries and can take care of moderately premature babies (usually those born at 32 weeks or more of gestation) who are expected to recover quickly from mild complications. They also take care of older preemies who have spent time in a Level III nursery but don't need intensive care anymore and are recovering well. Many Level II hospitals have a neonatologist on staff.

* Level III hospitals have intensive care nurseries (usually abbreviated NICU, for Neonatal Intensive Care Unit), and are staffed with full-time obstetricians, neonatologists, neonatal nurses, and respiratory therapists. These hospitals are equipped to assist mothers and babies with the most severe complications of pregnancy and prematurity. Most Level III hospitals are located in cities or affiliated with universities or medical schools. Sometimes Level III hospitals are subdivided into further categories (Level IIIA, IIIB, IIIC) depending on the equipment, procedures, and expertise they can provide (special kinds of ventilators, diagnostic studies, pediatric surgery, for example). The highest level hospitals have the ability to evaluate and manage babies with the most complex conditions and complications. Normally, an expectant mother would be referred to a Level III hospital if she has a serious obstetric, medical, or surgical complication, if she is at risk of a premature delivery at less than 32 weeks of gestation, or if her fetus is diagnosed with a condition that is likely to require surgery or other complex medical care after birth. (Depending on where you live, you may hear of slightly different classifications. But there's general agreement on the concept of three different levels of newborn care and

on the helpfulness of this classification for directing mothers and their babies to the hospital where they can get the kind of treatment they need.)

Research has shown that very premature babies are more likely to survive and have fewer complications when they're born in a Level III hospital. So ideally, as soon as an obstetrician knows that a woman is at significant risk for a very premature labor and delivery, he would refer her to a Level III hospital in the region and arrange for her to be admitted there before she delivers.

If an expectant mother is already in a hospital with only a Level I nursery, her obstetrician must decide whether it's best to keep treating her where she is and deliver and stabilize her preemie there, or to transport her to a Level II or III hospital. Sometimes delivery is too imminent for a transfer, since it's more dangerous for a preemie to be born in an ambulance or helicopter than in a hospital.

Father's Role When the Mother Is Moved

My wife is being transferred to another hospital. What should I do?

The best thing you can do is to wait with your wife before she leaves, to comfort and reassure her on this sudden change of location, and to meet with the transport team when they arrive. Since your wife may not be able to move much (she may be in bed, attached to an IV line), you should help her pack the small bag she'll be allowed to carry on the ambulance or aircraft. Ask her what else she needs you to bring to her in the new hospital. Mothers in preterm labor or with complications of prematurity often rush to the closest hospital or emergency room without even a toothbrush or a change of underwear.

How a Maternal Transport Is Done

Most maternal transports to hospitals up to 100 miles away are by ambulance; a helicopter or airplane may be used for greater distances. The choice of transportation will also be influenced by:

* the urgency of medical treatment;
* the availability of a helicopter or plane;
* how close the helipad or airport is to each hospital;
* the weather (whether it's safe to fly);
* space constraints (whether a helicopter has ample room to carry an expectant mother and the equipment needed for her baby in case the birth occurs during transport).

The medical team accompanying you will include two or more medical professionals (usually emergency medical technicians, nurses, respiratory therapists, or doctors) who can treat you if your condition suddenly worsens, deliver your baby if necessary, and stabilize your newborn until you reach your destination. Usually your partner or spouse can't ride with you, but will meet you at the hospital. Your baby's and your vital signs will be constantly monitored, and your condition kept stable with fluids, medication, and portable medical equipment (including ventilators, oxygen tanks, and an incubator). Pain medication or sedation can be given if you should deliver. Before leaving and while on their way if need be, the transport team will be in touch by mobile phone with the doctors at the receiving hospital, updating them on your condition, getting instructions about treatments, and arranging for your speedy admission.

You or your wife will probably be asked to sign a written consent form for the transfer. Also, make sure you give the transport team and your obstetrician your cell phone number and any other numbers where they can reach you in case of an emergency. Be sure to write down the name and telephone numbers of the hospital and ward your wife will be admitted to and the name of the doctor who will be in charge of her care. On the new hospital's web site, you'll be able to find and print out telephone numbers, directions, hospital rules, and practical tips you'll want to know right away (such as visiting and cafeteria hours, whether your other children can visit, where to park or stay overnight nearby).

Family members will probably not be allowed to ride in the ambulance because the lack of room may make it impractical or unsafe. But you might want to plan to leave at the same time as your wife and drive behind the ambulance, so you can be with her soon after she gets to the other hospital. (These transports aren't the sirens-blaring, speed-through-red-lights kind!) Ask the transport team if your wife is allowed to carry and use her cell phone in the ambulance. If you do plan to drive, be careful. Remember that your wife is in good hands. And keep in mind that you are going through a time of stress, which can play havoc with your concentration and attention and may have taken a toll on your nerves or sleep over the last few weeks, days, or hours. It might be a good idea to ask a friend or relative to drive you, or to take public transportation.

Although you'll have to travel now, and probably for some time after your baby is born, take heart: Once your preemie has gotten over the most serious complications of prematurity, he can likely be transferred back to your community hospital and spend the last part of his hospitalization closer to home.

Meeting with Your Baby's Doctor

My obstetrician told me that the neonatologist is going to come meet with me to answer my questions. Why is she coming, and what am I supposed to ask her?

A meeting with the neonatologist is often arranged for parents who are expected to have a premature baby. Having a premature newborn can be quite different from having a full-term one, and the neonatologist mainly wants to help you prepare for it and get your questions answered. Since childbirth classes and parenting books seldom prepare parents for having a preemie, she hopes to help you become a little more comfortable with what is going to happen after delivery. If you are having an especially small, young preemie, there's a second important reason for the meeting: Decisions may need to be made about your baby's medical treatment soon after birth, and the neonatologist wants to start you thinking about them.

If you have a sense of dread about this meeting, you're not alone. Many parents don't feel emotionally ready to deal with all of these issues in advance. They are still focusing their energies and hopes on trying to make it to term, and their anxieties about having a preemie may be just too painful to discuss.

Nonetheless, this meeting is important. It's the beginning of your relationship with your baby's medical team. Right now, the neonatologist seems like part of the bad news you're getting, but she is going to be one of your baby's most important allies. There's even a good chance that the meeting will make you feel better, because you'll learn that your baby's prospects are better than you think, or because it uncovers and addresses some of your anxieties.

Neonatologists all have different styles, of course, and approach this meeting differently. Yours will probably cover some of the following topics. If she omits any that concern you, feel free to ask about them.

* **Delivery.** What will happen when your baby is born? What medical professionals will be there to take care of your baby? Will you be given your baby to hold, or will she be taken right away to the intensive care nursery? Will you hear your baby cry, and if not, what does that mean about her condition?
* **Your baby's outlook.** What are your baby's chances for survival? What are her chances for doing well in the long run, despite her early birth? What are the key medical hurdles that babies of her size and gestational age typically encounter?
* **Feeding.** How will your baby initially be fed? When will she be able to breastfeed or bottle feed? Is there a lactation consultant to help you with the essential steps in providing breast milk for your preemie?
* **Spending time with your baby.** How soon can you or your partner visit your baby in the nursery? How soon can you hold her? What

are the visiting policies: Are any times off limits; are children or other relatives allowed?

* **Keeping you informed and involved.** How will the staff of the nursery give you updates about your baby? Can you be present on rounds, when the doctors and nurses report to each other about her health and progress and make their daily plans? What kinds of medical decisions can parents participate in? (In intensive care nurseries, dozens of medical decisions are made around the clock, and parents, who may not be there, are usually not consulted about routine or minor changes in advance. No matter what, your permission will be obtained before any major procedure is performed on your baby, unless it's an emergency and the staff can't reach you. But you should feel free to let the doctor know, now or later, if there are some other things you particularly want to know about before they happen—a blood transfusion or a new medication, for example. And even if you don't help to make every decision, you should expect to be kept informed about your baby's care.)

* **Homecoming.** How long is your baby likely to be in the hospital? If you're far from home, when might your baby be transferred back to your community hospital?

* **In advance.** Can you or your partner get a tour of the neonatal intensive care nursery before your baby is born? Does your NICU have a handbook or other resources for parents?

* **Decisions for extremely premature babies.** Will the neonatologist be making decisions in the delivery room, or early on, about how much medical treatment your baby should be offered? (Doctors don't all agree, and neither do all well-meaning loving parents, on whether it is good or bad for extremely premature babies to be put through intensive medical treatment if they have only a small

chance of surviving and growing up healthy. For help in understanding these decisions, you can read *The Doctor's Perspective: Delivery* on page 53.) What are the options? How will your wishes be taken into account? Can you meet with a hospital social worker or chaplain, separately or with your partner, to get help in sorting through your feelings and working out any differences of opinion you may have? These are momentous, wrenching choices that you and your partner both have to live with, and you don't have to feel that you need to give answers on the spot. Unless your baby's arrival is imminent, you should feel free to say that you need time to reflect on them.

One thing you cannot expect from this meeting is any definite answer as to how your own precious baby is going to do. That is impossible to predict with certainty before she is born. But this is not your only chance for information. On the contrary, it's just the beginning of your relationship with your baby's doctor. Most likely you will be traveling down a long road together, and as questions or issues about your baby come up along the way, you will have plenty of opportunity to talk about them in more depth.

Why a C-Section?

I was dreaming of a natural childbirth, but now my obstetrician is telling me a C-section might be safer for my baby. Why?

Your disappointment is understandable. Not only has your pregnancy been cut short, now you may have to miss the natural childbirth for which you've been preparing. But at this point, there's something more important at stake: your baby's well-being. You should try to focus on that and keep in mind that a C-section, although unpleasant, can't beat the immense joy of bringing your child into the world, no matter how. For one thing, remember that as many as one in four babies in this country are delivered by C-section. Most of their mothers would probably tell you that they were utterly overwhelmed by their baby's presence and quickly made peace with the fact that their birthing experience was different from what they'd imagined.

You can be sure that your obstetrician has considered the pros and cons carefully. She is probably suggesting a C-section because it gives your child the best chance of survival and a good outcome. A C-section is usually faster, and may be less stressful and traumatic for a baby than a vaginal delivery. Your obstetrician will explain to you why a C-section is indicated in your case. Here are some of the most common reasons:

* **There are signs of fetal distress.** Fetal distress is usually diagnosed when a fetus's heart rate is too fast, too slow, or too flat (meaning that it doesn't respond to changes in his condition). Whatever is causing the fetal distress—an infection, imperfect supply of blood or oxygen from the placenta, or other illness or complication—a prompt cesarean birth allows a baby to escape any condition in the womb that may be causing problems and to receive medical treatment sooner, possibly preventing damage to his brain and vital organs.

* **Labor hasn't begun or isn't progressing normally.** Sometimes a pregnancy is purposely cut short because of the mother's or baby's health. Your obstetrician may elect to do a C-section if prompt delivery is the goal and labor-inducing medications won't work fast enough or if she anticipates that a vaginal delivery is going to be difficult. Forceps and vacuum extractors—devices that can help pull a baby out of the womb—increase the risk of bleeding in the brain (what doctors call an intraventricular hemorrhage) in babies born under 35 weeks of gestation. If your doctors try to induce labor but end up doing a cesarean, you may hear them use the term "failed induction." Please don't take it personally! In fact, when babies are preterm, starting off trying to induce labor but ending up with a C-section is extremely common. It makes perfect sense once you remember that neither the mother's body nor the baby is naturally ready to go through labor yet. Your doctor won't be surprised if this happens and certainly won't think it's *your* failure—and you shouldn't, either.

* **Your baby is in a breech or other abnormal position.** Normally, babies are delivered head first. Breech babies, who are head-up instead of head-down in the womb, would be born buttocks or feet first if delivered vaginally. But coming into the world head last is considerably more dangerous, especially for preemies. That's because an infant's head is its largest part, and if it gets stuck inside after the rest of the body has come out (because the cervix hasn't yet opened wide enough to let it through), the flow of oxygen and blood through the umbilical cord can be cut off. And if it becomes necessary to use forceps or a vacuum extractor to help get the head out, a preemie's delicate brain can be injured. According to several studies, a vaginal delivery for preemies in breech position carries a higher mortality risk, as well as a higher risk for brain damage, than a cesarean section. (An exception is twins when the first twin can be delivered headfirst, and only the second twin is breech. In that case, the cervix may be sufficiently dilated by delivery of the first twin's head that the second one isn't in danger of getting stuck.)

How a C-Section Is Done

After making an incision in your skin and separating your abdominal muscles, your obstetrician will examine your uterus, check your baby's position, and decide what kind of incision she will make in the uterus to deliver him. The first choice is usually a horizontal ("transverse") incision in the lower, thinner part of the uterus (just above the pubic bone), because that segment bleeds less and heals with a stronger scar. The second choice is usually a vertical incision, again in the lower part of the uterus. These low incisions are preferred because they don't prevent a mother from delivering another baby vaginally in the future.

Sometimes, because of the position of the placenta or your baby or if you're delivering earlier than about the 28th week of gestation before the lower part of the uterus is well developed, your obstetrician will opt for a higher, vertical ("classical") incision in the uterus. That incision heals well, but the resulting scar is not as strong, and your uterus might tear during the stress of labor, possibly leading to very dangerous complications for a mother and a baby. Therefore, women who have had classical C-sections are not able to deliver subsequent babies vaginally. Still, that shouldn't prevent you from getting pregnant or carrying a future pregnancy to term. Since the position and shape of the scar on your skin doesn't necessarily correspond to one made in your uterus, make sure to ask your obstetrician what kind of C-section she's performed. If it was a classical C-section, you can be sure that she chose it to make your baby's delivery as easy and gentle as possible.

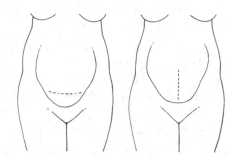

C-section: uterus with horizontal, or "transverse," incision.

C-section: uterus with vertical, or "classical," incision.

* **You are having twins or higher-order multiples.** If your twins share the same sac of amniotic fluid, then a C-section is recommended to avoid possible tangling or mixing up of the two umbilical cords during delivery, with a risk of diminishing the blood flow to one twin or cutting off the wrong cord. Triplets or more are delivered by C-section to give all of the babies the same chance for prompt delivery (there's a chance the cervix will start to close before all of the babies are delivered) and medical attention.
* **There are other indications, such as a maternal illness that make it unlikely that a**

(*Continued on page 67*)

The Crowd in the Delivery Room

Some births, when there are no complications and the pregnancy goes to term, are private affairs: an obstetrician or midwife coaching a woman and her partner in a secluded room as their baby gradually emerges. A premature birth, however, is usually a different story. If you give birth in a hospital, you can expect your preemie to be welcomed by at least a few strangers—sometimes a crowd of them—often in masks and gowns, all there to help your baby as she enters the world. Most parents look around the room and wonder: Who are these people? Why are they needed? Is this a bad sign for our baby? Don't worry. All their presence really means is that you and your newborn will get the best possible assistance.

Although every hospital and birth is somewhat different, here is a quick introduction to the typical members of that crowd in the delivery room:

* **If you are having a cesarean delivery,** more people will be present than for a vaginal one. In addition to your obstetrician and labor nurse, one or more anesthesiologists, several nurses to assist during the operation, and possibly an obstetrics resident may all be involved in the delivery itself.
* **At every hospital birth,** whether premature or full-term, there is a medical professional who's designated to take care of the newborn infant. When it's a term baby, that may be your labor nurse or midwife. When it's a premature baby, either a pediatrician or a neonatal nurse practitioner will be called in, often with an extra nurse to assist if it's a younger preemie who might need extra medical care.
* **When you give birth in a teaching hospital,** you may really draw a crowd. Every teaching hospital has a pediatric team that is called to the delivery room whenever there is a premature birth. The team generally includes—at a minimum—a pediatric resident or neonatal nurse practitioner and a pediatric nurse. It also may include a neonatologist and a respiratory therapist. In addition, the group may be joined by a pediatric intern, a medical student, and a nurse in training, all of whom can help out and learn. If you're having multiples, you can expect even more company; most hospitals try to have a team for each baby.

A warning: It can be pretty scary to see some half a dozen people wearing surgical scrubs come running into the room when you're on the verge of giving birth. But this rarely indicates an unexpected emergency. Usually it's just the routine pediatric team, in a hurry to get their equipment set up before your baby makes her appearance.

What are they setting up? Everything they need to welcome your baby into the world:

* A special warming bed, which needs to be switched on a minute or two in advance. (Preemies don't maintain their body temperature as well as full-term babies, and this will keep your baby from getting cold.)
* Equipment that can help your baby breathe, if necessary.
* Warm blankets: several to dry off the just-born baby, who comes out covered with amniotic fluid, and others to lay her on and wrap around her after she's been cleaned and dried off.

During or after the setup, don't be surprised or alarmed if you hear the doctors and nurses chatting or joking quietly among themselves.

Although you may be put off by their less than reverent attitude, you needn't worry: They're well trained to do what they have to do and know exactly when concentration is required.

After the obstetrician delivers your preemie and cuts her umbilical cord, he'll hand her to the pediatric team. While the obstetrician continues caring for you, the pediatric team will take care of your newborn, cleaning out her nose and mouth so she can breathe well and making sure she's warm and dry. They'll also be continually assessing her condition. If your baby looks a little blue or is breathing irregularly, as many younger preemies do at first, the doctor may decide to give her some extra deep breaths by pumping air or oxygen into her lungs through a soft mask placed over her nose and mouth. She may perk up and become pinker as she becomes accustomed to breathing on her own, or she may need more resuscitation. If that's the case, you can read about it on pages 67–70. Once your baby is stable, the doctor or nurse will weigh her, dress her in a hat and a clean, warm

blanket, and place her in an isolette (a closed, heated crib).

Most likely, you'll have a chance to see or hold your baby in the delivery room soon after she's born—and you'll be amazed by what a complete and tiny thing she is! But it may be only for a minute or so if the doctors feel that she'll get cold or need immediate care. If the pediatric team is caring for your baby right in the delivery room, your partner can watch what they're doing—though it may be hard to get a good view, and he certainly should be sure not to elbow any of the doctors or nurses aside! In some hospitals, just-born preemies are taken immediately to separate stabilization rooms, where your partner may or may not be allowed.

Before you know it, your baby will be taken to the nursery and the crowd in the delivery room will disappear, with just a nurse left to clean up and a doctor to jot down some notes about what went on. They all did their jobs to ease your baby's transition into the world.

mother can tolerate going through labor, or pregnancy complications, or fetal birth defects, that make a highly controlled delivery the safest option. A cesarean section can be safely performed under either general anesthesia (which will "put you to sleep" for the procedure) or regional anesthesia (spinal or epidural, in which you stay conscious but have little sensation of your body from your chest to your toes). Regional anesthesia offers you the great advantage of being awake during your baby's birth and seeing him shortly after he's born. But it's slower than general anesthesia, so it won't be used if you have to deliver quickly and unexpectedly. You can discuss the choice of anesthesia with your obstetrician and the anesthesiologist. Since a C-section is surgery, you should also feel free to discuss your own

health risks and what to expect for yourself immediately after this delivery and in the future.

If Your Baby Needs Resuscitation

I didn't hear my baby crying at birth, and they told me she had to be resuscitated. What does that mean?

Although the word "resuscitation" is terrifying to parents, it probably doesn't involve anything as dramatic as you may think. Parents often associate the word with bringing a person back to life, but when used in the delivery room, resuscitation usually means simply giving extra support to an already very much alive newborn baby so she can breathe more deeply and regularly than she's ready to do all by herself. In other words, it means something you already knew: that your baby is a preemie, and preemies are not always ready to breathe completely on their own when they are born.

The conventional wisdom—that all newborns come into the world with a loud wail—is based on experience with full-term babies, not preemies. A newborn needs to be strong, vigorous, and breathing deeply to be able to cry. The main reason that a preemie doesn't cry in the delivery room or gives a weak initial cry and then stops is that below a certain age, most premature infants just don't have the strength or drive to breathe deeply. It's part of their immaturity.

For those same reasons, many preemies need to be resuscitated—given some extra breaths of room air or oxygen or put on a ventilator that gives them deep, ongoing breaths to supplement their own. Most of the time, the breathing problems arising from prematurity are a combination of underdeveloped lungs (called respiratory distress syndrome, or RDS, a condition that is extremely common among preemies), weak muscles, and an immature breathing control center in the brain. In short, immature respiration.

Since that's usually the only problem, your newborn's prognosis is probably no different from what it was before you entered the delivery room, knowing you were about to give birth to a preemie.

Occasionally, though, the problem is not just immaturity: Something else is depressing a premature newborn's vital functions. If this is the case for your baby, it can, but doesn't necessarily, mean a worse prognosis. You'll need to discuss this with your obstetrician and neonatologist, because your baby's prospects will depend on what the problem is.

Some things are quickly reversible. Say you were given magnesium sulfate just before delivery to treat preeclampsia or preterm labor. It passes to the baby through the placenta and can cause respiratory depression. The more magnesium

sulfate you were given, the more relaxed and limp your newborn may be; she may be barely breathing at all. Don't worry: The doctors can place her on a ventilator, which will breathe for her until the magnesium sulfate wears off (usually in a day or less) with no long-term effects.

Some other drugs, like general anesthesia or certain pain medications given to a mother for delivery, can affect the baby in a similar way. They, too, should wear off without any lasting consequences.

On the other hand, there are some reasons a baby needs to be resuscitated that can be more serious. For example, infections can decrease a newborn's drive to breathe and cause her heart to beat too slowly. If she is sick from an infection, her prognosis will depend on what kind of infection it is and how soon the doctors are able to control it. Some infections are more likely than others to cause lasting damage to a baby's brain or other organs, and the longer an infection goes on, the more chance that it could be fatal. Children whose mothers had an infection of the membranes and amniotic fluid inside the uterus, called chorioamnionitis, have been found to have a somewhat higher incidence of cerebral palsy. When chorioamnionitis is detected during a pregnancy, an early delivery is often performed in the hope of catching it before the baby also becomes infected. Most babies whose mothers have chorioamnionitis, though, grow up with no long-term developmental problems.

There are situations in which resuscitation is necessary because the supply of blood and oxygen to the baby was disrupted before delivery. This could be due to various things, from very low maternal blood pressure, to a tear in the placenta (called a placental abruption), a knot or blood clot in the umbilical cord, or the umbilical cord's lying in a position where it gets squeezed hard with the baby's movements in the womb or with contractions during labor.

(Continued on page 70)

How Is a Baby Resuscitated?

Since premature newborns need to be resuscitated mainly because of breathing problems, doctors usually start by trying to stimulate the baby to breathe on her own, often just by rubbing her. They'll clear her nostrils and mouth of amniotic fluid, and if she doesn't breathe deeply or regularly enough herself, they'll give her some extra breaths. To give her breaths, they place a soft plastic mask over the baby's nose and mouth and pump room air or oxygen through it from an attached bag or a device called a T-piece (you'll hear the medical staff refer to it by its brand name: usually NeoPuff or NeoPip). Doctors and nurses call this "bagging" or "puffing" a baby.

These initial breaths may be all it takes to get her breathing well on her own. The doctors may keep the mask on or put some little plastic prongs in her nose to give her continuous positive airway pressure, or CPAP, which will help keep her lungs well expanded. If she's breathing really well then, they may see how she does without any assistance, or with just a little oxygen blowing by her nose. But if after a few minutes the baby is still not pink, with a strong heartbeat and breathing regularly, the next step is for the doctors to intubate her. This means inserting a tube through her mouth or nose into her windpipe to send air directly into her lungs. The tube can be connected to the oxygen bag or T-piece, or to a ventilator, a mechanical breathing machine that can continue to help breathe for her.

At some hospitals, all very young preemies are intubated immediately, since doctors know that most of these babies aren't yet ready to breathe on their own. One of the great advantages is that after a baby is intubated, she can be given a substance called surfactant, which coats the tiny air sacs in the lungs and helps them to stay open. Getting surfactant has been shown to dramatically increase the chances of a very young preemie's survival.

Most of the time, a preemie's heart will respond with healthy beats as soon as she is breathing well. Rarely, when this is not the case, the doctors will do chest compressions (CPR) or administer medications to make the baby's heart beat stronger and faster.

Occasionally other problems require treatment as part of the resuscitation. If there was a large placental abruption, for example, the baby may have lost some blood and need intravenous fluid or a blood transfusion in the delivery room. Another example: If a small tear in a baby's lung has occurred, allowing air to escape around it and interfere with her breathing and heartbeat, the doctors may try to remove the free air with a needle or tube. Your doctors will tell you about any of these unusual situations when they explain how your baby is doing and what happened in the delivery room. Otherwise, you can assume that your preemie's resuscitation was a straightforward process of helping her to breathe better than she was ready to do just yet by herself.

Most infants can withstand a short period of low blood flow and oxygen (which often occurs intermittently during delivery or for several minutes after birth) and will be fine. But when the problem goes on longer, either around the time of delivery or earlier during the pregnancy, there can be damage to a baby's brain.

How would you know if your baby had a period of low blood flow or oxygen before delivery? A fetal heartbeat that is too slow or unresponsive (as seen on a fetal heart rate monitor), the passage of meconium—a baby's first stools—while she's still inside the womb (this occurs only in older preemies with more mature bowel function), an excess of acid in the fetus's or newborn's blood (this can be measured painlessly from your baby's umbilical cord when the obstetrician cuts it at delivery), low Apgar scores, or pulmonary hypertension (high blood pressure in the lungs) that persists after birth are some of the signs. The doctors will let you know if your baby shows any of these and what it might mean for her. Just remember, a great many newborns show one or more of these signs and never go on to have lasting problems.

If you are worried about the possibility of damage to your baby's brain from lack of blood flow or oxygen, keep in mind that the signs of a recent severe injury will usually show up within the first week of life. A baby may have seizures, be hyperalert and jittery, or comatose. Or her other organs, such as her heart, kidneys, or liver may be damaged, leading the doctors to believe that her brain was injured, also. Babies who start recovering within a few days will most likely be fine. Occasionally, though, if the injury occurred earlier in gestation or was less severe, neurological problems may not show up until a baby is older.

Apgar Scores

Do preemies always get low Apgar scores? Our son's were only four and seven, and we're very worried.

The Apgar score, developed by Dr. Virginia Apgar in the 1950s, is a tool to assess whether a newborn infant needs resuscitation. It consists of five signs: the newborn's heart rate, respiration, reflex irritability, muscle tone, and skin color. Each sign receives from zero to two points, indicating a negative, mediocre, or optimal finding.

Preemies don't always get low Apgar scores, but they often do. The earlier a baby is born, the lower his Apgar scores are likely to be, simply because of his immaturity. Whereas in a full-term newborn, very low Apgar scores are likely to mean there's been some asphyxia (insufficient blood flow or oxygen before, during, or right after delivery), in a premature baby, low Apgars often have to be interpreted differently. That's because some findings that are typical for a preemie, such as irregular respiration or low activity, can take points off his Apgar score but don't tell much about how he's really doing. In one large study, the average five-minute Apgar score for preemies born at 26 to 27 weeks gestation was between six and seven, versus between eight and nine for those born at 34 to 36 weeks.

A baby's first Apgar score is assigned at exactly one minute after birth (but if his heartbeat is slow or he's not breathing well, the doctors will begin to resuscitate him before then). Scoring is repeated at five minutes and, in some cases, again at 10, 15, and 20 minutes after birth to check on a baby's improving or worsening condition. The highest score (rarely obtained by a preemie) is ten. A one-minute score of less than seven usually indicates that an infant needs to be resuscitated; resuscitation then continues until the score is seven or higher.

Sign:	0	1	2
Heart rate:	Absent	Slow	Normal
Respiration:	Absent	Irregular	Strong
Irritability:	No response	Grimace	Cry
Muscle tone:	Limp	Some flexion	Moving
Color:	Pale or blue	Body pink/extremities blue	All pink

The five-minute Apgar score is a much better predictor of survival than the one-minute score because it reflects how well a newborn is recovering in response to resuscitation. The fact that your baby's Apgar score rose rapidly is a good sign, showing that he responded well. Studies show that the survival rate through the newborn period is highest for infants whose five-minute score is seven or more.

Apgar scores were never intended to predict future development or disability, so not surprisingly, the one-minute and five-minute Apgar scores by themselves are rarely helpful in predicting how a baby will do in the long run. Only if a baby's score is very low—zero to three—for ten minutes or longer is there an increased risk of future disabilities. And even then, the vast majority of babies do not suffer long-term consequences as long as their score improves within 20 minutes. Most of the time, other information doctors gather about a preemie's condition in the first weeks of life is far more important than the scores he was given in the delivery room immediately after birth.

It is still too early to know what the future is going to bring for your baby, but soon you're going to find out much more detailed (and hopefully reassuring) information about him. In the meantime, you shouldn't focus on his Apgar scores, because for a preemie, things are much more complex than simply counting up to ten.

Birth Weight Predictions

They told me before delivery that my baby would weigh over two pounds, but he's a lot smaller than that. How could they have gotten that wrong?

No matter how skillful the doctor, the estimate of fetal weight is always at best a good approximation. Until a baby leaves his mother's womb and can be put on a scale, there's no way to measure exactly how much he weighs. Doctors can only make predictions, using different tools, knowing that a baby's actual birth weight can always be higher or lower than their estimate. Studies show that doctors' estimates of fetal weight are rarely off by more than 15 percent but only about two-thirds of the time are they within 10 percent of the baby's actual birth weight. The smaller and more premature a baby is, the greater the chance that his weight will be overestimated.

Even an imperfect weight estimate, however, can be helpful in a high-risk pregnancy for planning what kind of medical assistance a mother and her baby may need before, during, and right after delivery. For instance, when the dating of a pregnancy is unclear, estimated fetal weight can help determine a baby's gestational age. It can help assess how well a baby is growing in the womb and lead to efforts to find out what's wrong, if growth is poor. Identifying babies before birth who are small for their gestational age allows doctors to make important clinical decisions like whether to perform an elective delivery, and can influence the choice between a vaginal delivery and a C-section. These options can give a baby a better chance of thriving, even if his birth weight turns out to be a few ounces more or less than predicted.

The most common methods of estimating fetal weight are:

✳ **Carefully feeling the uterus.** With her own hands and a good dose of clinical experience, an obstetrician can assess the size of the fetus in the uterus and make an estimate of his weight.

✳ **Measuring the fetus by ultrasound.** The size of a fetus's head and abdomen and the length of his femur (the long bone in the thigh) correlate with how much he weighs. An ultrasound is done to obtain these and other measurements, which are then combined using mathematical formulas to calculate the fetus's weight.

If a pregnancy is close to term, doctors consider a clinical estimation as reliable as an ultrasound. For premature, smaller babies, an ultrasound is more accurate.

Even ultrasound, though more precise than it was only a few years ago, is not a perfect tool. That's because the fetus's size is used to estimate his weight, but babies of the same size may have different proportions of muscle and fat (fat weighs less than muscle) or heavier or lighter bones. Occasionally a weight estimation is off because the baby is in a position in the uterus where the size of his head, abdomen, or femur can't be accurately measured. Factors such as low levels of amniotic fluid or maternal overweight—which can lead to difficulty seeing subtle physical features well on a prenatal ultrasound—also can affect estimates of fetal weight.

It may seem unsatisfying in this age of medical miracles to learn that a series of educated guesses about a premature baby's condition is often all that doctors have in their hands before delivery. Still, that's usually all it takes to get ready to meet their little patient and to make the choices necessary to take care of him in the best possible way.

Bonding

My baby was rushed to the NICU as soon as he was born rather than being placed on my chest. I'm so upset about the loss of bonding.

Your sense of loss is natural and actually a healthy sign that your bonding with your baby is already well under way. You only got a peek at your newborn and then he was gone, leaving your arms painfully empty. Although right now the stress and confusion around his early birth probably feel like they will affect your whole relationship with your newborn, you really don't have to fear that. Just because you couldn't have the picture-perfect experience of feeling him skin-to-skin on your belly after delivery, you aren't likely to be less attached to him, nor he to you.

The theory that mothers go through a bonding period shortly after their infants' births and that if they miss that crucial window their relationship is forever flawed, has been widely criticized since it was first proposed in the 1970s. Goats or ducks may reject their offspring by instinct, as the theorists observed, if they're taken away right after birth and then given back. But the growth of love and attachment between a parent and a child can begin before birth, immediately after, or even months or years later (as adoptive parents and their children know well). It can amaze you with its immediate power or slowly grow over time.

This doesn't mean that contact between parents and their new babies during the first few days and weeks has no value. Many studies have demonstrated that early, ongoing contact can foster stronger parental involvement in their child's care later on. In fact, research on bonding has helped to humanize perinatal medical care: for instance allowing fathers to be present at delivery and new mothers to keep their babies with them in the hospital unless a separation is necessary for medical reasons. In the neonatal intensive care unit, parents are now welcome with few if any restrictions (many nurseries allow parents to be at their baby's bedside 24 hours a day if they want) and are involved as soon as possible in the hands-on care of their fragile premature infants. But clearly, parents can love their babies desperately—and their love will be returned—even if they don't touch or see each other immediately after birth.

The tempo and pattern of your relationship with your infant will depend on his temperament and maturity (preemies are not always as ready as full-term babies to be fully responsive to human contact and stimulation), your own needs, fears, and personality, the time you spend together, and many other factors. Biology probably comes into play, too; recent research has shown that women who have higher levels of a certain hormone, oxytocin, starting early in pregnancy are generally more attached to their newborns in the first weeks after birth. We'll have to wait for further studies to learn just what effect a premature delivery has on the level of a mother's oxytocin.

If your premature baby needs intensive medical care now and you won't be able to hold him or take care of him for days, or even weeks, be assured that it won't be difficult to make up for the lost time. Even the feel of his soft little hand or heel under your fingers—if that's all you can touch for now—can be a miraculous sensation that intensifies the love you feel. And as soon as your baby can tolerate it, you can begin "kanga-

roo care" (see page 249) to feel your baby's naked skin on yours—that special, intimate experience you are now missing so much. We can promise you that by simply being at your preemie's side often throughout his hospitalization, talking to him, touching him, and holding him when you can, the bonding you're longing for will take place.

Many parents of preemies think they are even closer to their child precisely because they went through the same painful forced separation as you, and the whole experience of prematurity together. They say their love for their child turned out to be more intense and fulfilling than they ever imagined—even if that didn't happen in the baby's first minutes of life.

Moving Baby to Another Hospital

My baby is being transferred to another hospital. I'm terribly upset.

Even though you have understandable reasons to be anguished about her separation from you, your daughter's untimely travel is in her best interest. She's going to be taken to a neonatal intensive care unit, or NICU, at a Level II or III hospital (see page 60), that has the special expertise and equipment to treat infants who are born prematurely or are at high risk for medical complications. If the hospital where your baby was born does not normally take care of preemies or her doctors are concerned about some additional complications, there's no doubt that the benefits of being cared for by neonatologists in a specially equipped NICU amply exceed the risks of being transported there. Portable medical equipment allows even the tiniest baby to travel while receiving the critical care needed to keep her stable. And thanks to the training and experience of the medical team that will accompany your baby, the therapies provided to preemies in the NICU may even begin as soon as the team arrives to pick her up.

The transport team for your baby will probably be sent by the hospital to which she is going, supervised by phone by the neonatologist who'll be directing her care when she arrives. Most neonatal transport teams are composed of two or more experienced medical professionals—usually nurses, or a nurse and a respiratory therapist—who have worked in neonatal or pediatric intensive care units. They have additional training in stabilizing and transporting critically ill babies and in performing emergency procedures.

The transport team will create a traveling mini-intensive care nursery for your baby. She will be kept warm and comfortable in a portable incubator, a battery-heated clear plastic box with fold-down sides that is tightly attached to the vehicle for safety during transport. This isolette will enclose and protect her, and at the same time allow the team to monitor her condition and provide any medical care she may need during the trip. The transport team will take copies of your daughter's medical records, X-rays, and a note from her doctor summarizing the care she's received so far.

It's important that both parents (or at least the father, if the mother is still too weak after delivery) talk to the transport team. One of you will be asked to sign a written consent form agreeing to the transfer and to leave telephone numbers and addresses where you can be reached in an emergency. The transport team may also want to ask you some questions about the pregnancy or your family's medical history. In turn, they will tell you about the medical assistance your baby will receive and the logistics of the transfer. They'll also try to make sure you get a chance to see your baby before she leaves—bringing her to your room if you can't get to the nursery—so

you can say "see you soon" and send her off with love.

You'll feel better and more connected if you have a tangible memento of your baby—a photo or maybe a lock of her soft, newborn hair—to keep close to you while you're apart. If you haven't been able to take pictures of your baby yet, try asking your baby's nurses to take a few pictures for you. Some nurseries have digital cameras for parents to use. The nurses may also be able to make a card with your baby's footprints on it for you to keep.

It's perfectly normal to feel distressed right now, and anxiety can make understanding and remembering information difficult for anyone, so don't be shy about asking for help. The transport team and your nurses will make sure that you receive written information on the hospital your baby is going to, its address, the location and phone number of the NICU within the hospital, the name of the doctor who will be in charge, ways to get there by car or public transportation, and parking and lodging options in the area. If you have access to a computer, you'll also find much of this information on the new hospital's web site.

Sometimes, if there's enough room and the transport team feels it is safe, one or two family members are allowed to accompany the baby in the ambulance or aircraft during the transfer. A suggestion from others who have been there: Although it's a parent's first impulse to want to stay with their baby, if you're given this opportunity, first take your own pulse! Remember, the transport team needs to focus all of their attention on keeping your baby stable and safe and on getting her to her new nursery as quickly as possible. If you're very emotional or talkative, or become faint or sick during the trip, they will be distracted from their primary task. Also, consider whether you might need a car once you get to the new hospital and how you will travel back home.

Often parents choose to follow behind the ambulance in their own car. (Don't worry, you won't need the skills of a race-car driver. It's very rare in this kind of transport to have to speed through red lights or weave through traffic.) That way they won't get lost and will be at the new nursery at the same time their baby arrives.

If the mother needs to stay in the hospital for more than a few days, it may be possible for her to transfer to the same hospital as her baby (although with a different transport team and in a separate ambulance) so the family isn't apart for long. If you're in that situation, you can ask your obstetrician whether this can be arranged. But most likely you will remain in the hospital where you delivered until it's time for you to be discharged, and your partner or family members will be the first to visit your baby in her new nursery. Frequent phone calls, news, anecdotes, descriptions, and pictures will help you feel connected until you can see her. A few NICUs even have a web camera connection so you can see your baby live through a computer if you can arrange access to a laptop or computer at the hospital. Your baby's new doctors in the NICU will keep you updated on her condition, and you'll be encouraged to call and speak to the nurses taking care of her as often as you want.

Yes, be prepared to miss your baby a lot. But keep in mind that the best thing you can do for your daughter now is to get your health and stamina back. While you rest, you can read on pages 101–107 about what a NICU is like and about the specialists who are taking care of your baby. And remember that this forced separation will probably last only a few days. Soon you'll be able to walk through the doors of your baby's new hospital to be with her again.

MULTIPLES

Twins Delivered at Different Times

My doctor said that although it looks like one of my twins will be delivering early, she's going to try to give the other more time in the womb. How is that possible?

It used to be only a twist of nature recorded by medical historians: quadruplets all born on different days over a ten-day span; a boy born an amazing 95 days before his twin sister. But today this surprising occurrence is becoming more common, as obstetricians become more aware from case reports and studies published in medical journals of the possibility of delivering some babies in a multiple gestation later than others, to give them extra days in the womb.

To be sure, what's called "delayed interval delivery" is still unusual. Normally when one baby in a multiple gestation is born, the obstetrician makes sure to deliver the other babies right away. That's because the risks of not doing so are substantial, primarily from placental tears or separation, bleeding, and infections that can quickly become life-threatening for both the mother and the babies who remain in the womb.

There are no official records (a good guess would place the number of cases so far in the hundreds), and delayed interval delivery has not been studied thoroughly by medical researchers yet, so its relative risks and benefits are not clearly known. It requires a lot of courage and motivation from expectant parents, and not all doctors are willing to chance it.

Of the multiple pregnancies at risk for a premature delivery, which few can take advantage of a delayed interval delivery? It's possible only when whatever threatens the continued gestation of one baby doesn't affect the others. If your doctor believes you are a good candidate, it probably means that although the premature birth of one of your twins appears likely—perhaps because his amniotic sac has ruptured or he's already pushing through a slightly open cervix—you are healthy and your other twin looks stable and secure in his own sac.

The decision to attempt a delayed interval delivery is best considered before the birth of the first baby so that a treatment plan can be made in advance, but your doctor won't know if it's really possible until you deliver. Most doctors consider these to be some of the necessary requirements:

* The twins each have their own placenta and amniotic sac (as all fraternal twins but only some identical twins do);
* Their gestational age is at least 16 weeks, so that the baby who stays in your womb has a good chance of holding on long enough to reach the point of viability (when he can survive outside the womb), but less than 29 weeks of gestation, in the range when even a few more days in the womb can greatly improve a premature baby's outcome;
* You do not have chorioamnionitis, an infection of the amniotic fluid;
* Your first baby is delivered vaginally, not by C-section, and you are not bleeding heavily after delivery;
* After your first baby's birth, your uterus stops contracting and your cervix begins to close (meaning that your body will cooperate and continue the pregnancy).

Your obstetrician will explain why it may be feasible in your case and what her treatment plan is, since there is no standard medical protocol for this procedure. You will probably be treated with antibiotics to try to prevent infection. Immedi-

ately after delivery, some doctors start intravenous medications to stop contractions and perform a minor surgical procedure called a cerclage (see page 25) to keep the cervix closed. Others don't prescribe anti-labor drugs or do surgery on the cervix, preferring not to mask any signs of labor, which could indicate an infection.

If you've reached at least 23 weeks of gestation, you will be given a two-day course of prenatal steroids to boost the maturity of your baby who is still in the womb, giving him the best possible chance once he is born. (Earlier in gestation, a fetus isn't developed enough to respond to steroids.) This alone can be a benefit of delayed interval delivery.

If after the first delivery your condition stabilizes and the baby still in your womb is doing well, you will probably be kept in the hospital on complete bed rest, under strict medical observation. Occasionally an expectant mother is put on an inclined bed with her feet higher than her head to reduce pressure on the cervix, but this maneuver has not been shown to be beneficial, so is rarely prescribed anymore. Eventually, if your pregnancy continues to proceed well, you may be allowed to go home—although probably still on bed rest—until the second delivery occurs. Despite the best medical care, though, nobody can predict whether and for how long your pregnancy can be sustained.

In the meantime, you'll have to cope with a very confusing and stressful situation: being new parents of a premature baby who may be in the hospital in an intensive care nursery while still continuing a demanding high-risk pregnancy. Parents who face a delayed interval birth should be prepared for a time of great anxiety and tension, and of strong, contrasting emotions. You will worry about the first twin you've delivered prematurely. If he is on a ventilator and can't be moved and you are confined to bed, you may not be able to see him for several days or even weeks. At the same time you'll be struggling to keep your stress to a minimum and to be optimistic. You probably won't have much emotional energy to spare. Couples who have gone through this experience say they got through it by keeping hopeful and by trying to take one day at a time.

Who's A, Who's B?

Throughout my pregnancy my sons were triplets A and B, and my daughter was triplet C. But now in the NICU, it's changed—she's B. What happened?

When you're having multiples, each fetus's growth and health is assessed and followed individually to make sure each one is developing well. To do that, doctors have to keep each baby straight, so they label them with letters. "A" is always the one at the bottom of the uterus closest to the cervix, "B" is the next one up, and so on. In a multiple gestation, as many letters as fetuses are used. For instance, septuplets born in 1997 to the McCaughey family were known to their doctors before delivery as Babies A through G. Baby A, a boy, was given the nickname Hercules, because he was at the bottom of an inverted pyramid of seven fetuses, with the weight of all of his siblings on top of him!

Sometimes, if there are more than two fetuses, doctors can't be sure exactly who's higher than who. In that case, they may simply (sometimes randomly) decide to call the baby on the bottom right "B," on the bottom left "C," and on the top "D," etc.

These letters are then reassigned at delivery according to the babies' birth order. If it's a vaginal delivery, Baby A will remain "A" because being closest to the cervix, he will be born first. But when babies are delivered by C-section, occasion-

ally the first baby to emerge from the womb isn't the one who was at the bottom. So the letters you knew your babies by before birth can become scrambled. That's what happened with your triplets. Your girl was born second, so she changed from Triplet C to Triplet B, while one of your boys now has a blue sign on his bed saying Triplet C after his last name.

During a C-section of twins or triplets, the obstetrician is usually certain about which baby is coming out. With higher-order multiples, though, it's possible that matching the original letters to the babies won't be crystal clear at delivery. That can be confusing and upsetting for parents. During pregnancy many parents attribute personality traits to their babies, using clues from their growth and behavior in the womb or from differences they detect after seeing their babies' sizes, favorite positions, and activity levels on ul-

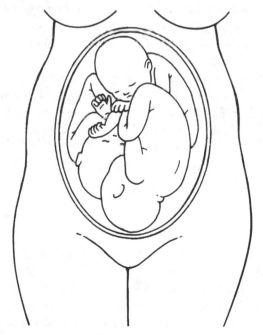

Triplets in the womb: doctors label the one at the bottom "A," the one in the middle "B," and the one at the top "C."

trasounds. For instance, they may talk about their smaller girl, who moves around more and kicks vigorously, as the feisty one with an active, outgoing personality, while thinking of their bigger boy, who is quieter, as a more contemplative, peaceful child. After delivery, if the letters get mixed up, it can feel like your babies are mixed up, too.

Luckily, you needn't worry about any confusion in medical treatment. Any serious condition that was being followed before delivery should be readily identified in a baby soon after birth, so the new letters shouldn't interfere with your babies' receiving good care.

Soon even the doctors and the nurses will begin calling your babies by the names you've chosen for them, and those fickle, anonymous letters will become a thing of the past.

Identical or Not?

My obstetrician could not tell from the sonograms during pregnancy if my twins are identical. Now that they are born, can we finally know for sure?

When parents learn that they are expecting twins, their first question is often: Are they identical? All couples are eager to know if the additions to their family are two genetically identical individuals whom they may some day have a hard time telling apart or two much more different siblings who by chance are spending their prenatal lives together.

Sometimes the answer is apparent even before the birth. If prenatal tests reveal two fetuses of the same sex sharing the same amniotic fluid sac, then the twins are almost definitely monozygotic, or identical. Identical twins come from one fertilized egg that divided in two, so they carry the same genes. (At birth, the obstetrician can confirm this finding by looking at the placenta. If it has only one chorionic membrane, it almost always means that only one sac formed around the fertilized egg; then, only after the sac had formed—surprise!—the egg split in two.)

On the other hand, if ultrasound and other prenatal tests reveal that the fetuses are a boy and a girl, then they obviously don't share all the same genes. They are dizygotic, or fraternal, twins. There's also a high likelihood that your twins are fraternal if they were conceived after treatments for infertility because fertility drugs stimulate the ovaries and often cause the release of more than one egg, and because more than one embryo is usually implanted during in vitro fertilization.

But sometimes the answer is more elusive. Say that you learn your twins are the same sex and are in two different sacs. Chances are they're fraternal, but you can't be sure; they could be identical twins who come from a fertilized egg that split into two so soon after conception that each embryo went on to make its own sac. In these ambiguous cases, examining the placenta after birth doesn't help. But you can ask your babies' doctor to check their blood types. If they don't have the same blood type, they're not identical.

What if your doctor still can't reach a definite conclusion? Looking at the babies themselves after birth may not tell you much, either. Even many parents of full-term twins find it a hard call, and preemies have slightly more immature facial features that can make many of them appear strikingly similar to inexperienced eyes (although it doesn't take long for parents to learn to identify their tiny offspring).

At that point, the only remaining option is genetic testing. A swab of the inside of each of your babies' cheeks can be sent to a laboratory for analysis, where they'll match and compare the biological markers that are different in each person—*except* identical twins. This is a complex and costly analysis that health plans don't cover unless the information is needed for medical reasons, like organ transplantation. But don't worry; except for your own curiosity, there's no rush. The test can be done anytime, even when the twins are adults. And you may find that the answer soon becomes obvious, as your preemies develop into two very similar or very different little tots.

Is it worth it to get your babies tested? That's up to you. But most people find that the intense curiosity of the first few hours or days soon fades as they are overtaken by the joy of watching their twins grow—and discovering, day by day, who they are going to be.

IN DEPTH

Your Baby Is Small-for-Gestational-Age: What Does It Mean?

There's enough to absorb and understand when you're having a premature baby. On top of that, some parents are told that their baby is small for her gestational age. How could a tiny preemie be even smaller? Does it matter?

First, a definition. Of course, many infants—full-term or premature—are slightly smaller than average. A full-term or premature infant is labeled small-for-gestational-age, or SGA, if her weight falls below the tenth percentile on the standard growth curve for her age, meaning that she weighs less than 90 percent of all infants her age. This means that your baby didn't grow as much as expected in the womb, and it's important to know why. She may just be normally small. But it's also possible that something slowed down her growth. (Obstetricians call this intrauterine growth restriction, or IUGR.) By contrast, an infant is considered appropriate-for-gestational-age, or AGA, if her weight falls anywhere between the tenth and ninetieth percentiles for her age. (Babies who weigh more than the ninetieth percentile are considered large-for-gestational-age, or LGA.)

For example, a preemie who is born at 28 weeks of gestation is AGA if her weight ranges between 750 grams and 1,500 grams. If her weight is less than 750 grams, she is SGA. You can check the chart on page 582 to see where your baby falls.

Why do doctors make this distinction? Because in general, newborns who are small-for-gestational-age are more likely to have certain health problems after delivery. Some, whose growth was severely restricted in the womb, are also at greater risk of having long-term development problems. Whether and how your baby is affected is going to depend largely on what caused her growth to be restricted and how long-lasting and severe the restriction was.

Why Some Babies are Small-for-Gestational-Age

There are a wide variety of reasons why a fetus may not grow properly in the womb. Your obstetrician may already know or be able to tell you soon, after doing some tests, if any of these most common causes seem likely:

* **Insufficiency of the placenta.** The fetus gets its supply of nutrients and oxygen through the placenta, so anything that disrupts an efficient flow of oxygen and nutrient-rich blood through it can slow the fetus's growth. Placental insufficiency, as it is called, may be caused by an illness that affects the pregnant mother's circulation, such as preeclampsia, diabetes, or heart disease. It can also be due to any of a number of possible problems with the placenta itself, including a placental abruption (separation of part of the placenta from the wall of the uterus), a placenta that's poorly functioning because it is small or malformed, one that has an inadequately attached umbilical cord,

or one that has been damaged from inflammation, infection, or a lack of blood flow and oxygen. Placental insufficiency is often the reason that an obstetrician recommends an early delivery if he thinks a baby will get better nourishment and face fewer health risks in the nursery than in the womb.

* **Chromosomal or other congenital abnormalities.** Many different genetic and congenital anomalies, which may be discovered during the pregnancy (through amniocentesis or ultrasound, for example) or after birth are associated with fetal growth restriction.

* **Infection of the mother and fetus.** Common colds and flus rarely harm a fetus. But some infections, which may be transmitted to the fetus if a mother gets them during pregnancy, can affect the baby's growth and development and cause other serious problems. Some of the more common ones are rubella (which causes German measles), herpes, cytomegalovirus (called CMV), toxoplasmosis, and syphilis. In some cases, infections are discovered through diagnostic tests done during pregnancy, and in other cases after birth. (Symptoms in adults may be so mild that they go unnoticed.)

* **Smoking, drugs, alcohol, and some medications.** Pregnant women who smoke, drink heavily, or use drugs such as cocaine, heroin, or amphetamines, have a tendency to deliver small-for-gestational-age babies. The same is true for mothers on certain medications, such as some anticancer and antiseizure drugs. These substances can be toxic to the developing fetus and have direct adverse effects on fetal growth, or they can cause growth restriction by interfering with the flow of blood and oxygen through the placenta.

* **Malnutrition.** Mothers who are poorly nourished and gain too little weight during pregnancy are also at risk for having malnourished and poorly grown infants. That's because the fetus relies on the mother for the nutrients it needs to grow and develop well.

Being African-American, a very young or older mother, having multiples, and living at high altitude all increase the chance of having smaller babies. Studies also indicate that women who were themselves small-for-gestational-age are at greater risk of having small-for-gestational-age infants than their peers.

Of course, some newborns end up in the smallest 10 percent for no other reason than normal variation in size. Remember that if you are small, your babies are more likely to be, too. In fact, some doctors prefer to use a stricter, alternative definition of SGA: that a baby is small-for-gestational-age only if she falls below the third percentile on the growth curve, thus weighing less than a full 97 percent of babies her age. The rationale is that some perfectly well-nourished and healthy newborns (premature or full-term) will fall in the smallest 10 percent due just to the genetic luck of the draw—say, their parents and grandparents are small—and the medical problems associated with being SGA won't apply to them. Supporting that stricter definition of SGA are many studies showing that it is only babies in the smallest 3 percent who are likely to have problems due to significantly restricted growth.

How Your Baby Will Look

Above all, your baby will look like a preemie, so the best description is in *Your Beautiful Newborn: a Portrait*, on page 93. Only a few things in her appearance may differ because she is small for her gestational age. Some babies have so-called symmetric growth retardation, meaning that all parts of their bodies were affected fairly equally. These babies are often described as looking "old" despite their little size, because they're short and skinny, and their heads are small. Usually, these babies' growth has been restricted since the early stages of pregnancy.

Alternatively, your baby may have asymmetric or "head-sparing" growth retardation. If that's the case, she'll still be scrawny and maybe short, but her head will be normal in size for her age—disproportionately big for her small body. Usually, head-sparing means that the baby's growth restriction was less severe and occurred only in the later stages of pregnancy: There was at least enough nourishment for the brain to grow. One of the truly amazing aspects of fetal development is that when there are not enough nutrients to go around, the body knows to give preference to the brain, protecting it by giving it more than its fair share.

Sometimes growth restriction is accompanied by very low levels of amniotic fluid. (That's because a fetus's urine is the main component of amniotic fluid and when a fetus doesn't get enough blood flow, usually because of placental insufficiency, she doesn't urinate as much.) Without amniotic fluid to expand it, the uterus can press tightly around a fetus, constraining her movements. When a baby doesn't move around enough in the womb, her joints can become stiff and contracted. If this has occurred in your baby, you'll notice that she can't bend or straighten some of her joints as freely and fully as she should. Over time, and possibly with the help of orthopedics or physical therapy, these contractures often can resolve.

What Being SGA Means for Your Baby in the Short Term

Unfortunately, being small-for-gestational-age does carry increased risks. The best way to think about it is that your preemie has two conditions to deal with rather than one: prematurity and the problem that caused her growth restriction. This means that for SGA babies on average, the chances of survival are not quite as good as for appropriately grown preemies of the same gestational age. It also means that your baby may have a more complicated and somewhat longer hospital course than bigger babies of her age.

If the underlying problem is that your baby has an ongoing medical condition, such as a chromosomal or anatomic abnormality, or an infection, that condition is likely to be the dominant factor determining her prognosis during her hospital stay. Of course, your baby's prematurity and size are going to count, too, but probably less than the other problem. Since there are a wide variety of congenital and genetic conditions that can affect a fetus's growth, ask your baby's doctor to go over your baby's specific problem and its prognosis with you.

If the underlying problem was solely pregnancy-related—placental insufficiency, with subsequent malnourishment of the fetus—her prognosis will be determined by two things: how the lack of nutrients affected her before she was born and what normal hurdles her prematurity brings.

There are certain health complications that affect many SGA babies in their early days and weeks of life. Your baby's doctors will look out for and manage them. Because many SGA newborns weren't getting quite as much oxygen as they needed from the placenta during pregnancy, more of these smaller babies have low Apgar scores and need oxygen and breathing assistance right after they're born. (Be reassured that in preemies, a need for resuscitation at delivery is much more common and less grave than most parents think.)

Many small-for-gestational-age infants develop low blood sugar (hypoglycemia) during the first day or two; they have particularly high energy needs but their own energy stores are low after they used up every bit they could in the womb. This is a temporary problem. Hypoglycemia is only serious if it isn't recognized and treated promptly. Your baby's doctors and nurses will know to watch for it, so you don't have to worry. If she needs it, they'll give her extra calories, usually in the form of intravenous sugar water or additional feedings of preemie formula, for several days until the problem resolves.

Small-for-gestational-age infants also tend to have more feeding intolerance than usual. It makes sense—Mother Nature knows to send scarce nutrients and oxygen to the organs that need them most, and intestines aren't of much use to a fetus, who doesn't need to eat in the womb. The result is that the intestines make do with less, leaving them a little weaker and less developed than normal. So it takes longer for SGA babies to move from intravenous feedings to full feedings of breast milk or formula, and they are at higher risk for NEC (an intestinal disorder). Once they do become adept at digestion, they often eat very large quantities for their tiny size, as if they are making up for lost time. (Their parents like nothing better than seeing them eat like little piglets, as they deserve to do!)

It won't be surprising if your baby is born with an excess of red blood cells, a condition called polycythemia. This happens when the body doesn't get quite enough oxygen over a long period of time. It responds by making more red blood cells in a valiant attempt to deliver as much oxygen as possible to the organs and tissues. (Red blood cells transport oxygen throughout the body.) But an excess of red blood cells can be too much of a good thing, causing the blood to be too thick, which can then make breathing harder, jaundice worse, and blood sugar lower, among other problems. If your baby has this condition, the treatment is to thin out her blood, usually by simply giving her extra fluid or occasionally (if the polycythemia is severe) by taking out some of her blood and replacing it with another fluid. (This is called a partial exchange transfusion or a reduction transfusion.)

Another thing the doctors watch for—in all premature babies but especially in those with intrauterine growth restriction—is hypothermia (or in everyday language, being cold). Babies who are SGA have a harder time holding in body heat because they have less body fat and so less insulation. This is nothing to worry about but may mean that your baby has to stay in an isolette a little longer than other babies of her gestational age.

Breathing is one of the main initial challenges for all premature babies. The younger they are, the more likely they are to have respiratory distress syndrome (RDS) and to develop chronic lung disease, which means they are dependent for longer on supplemental oxygen or other breathing assistance. Recent research seems to indicate that SGA preemies may have worse breathing problems—more severe respiratory distress syndrome and more chronic lung disease—than appropriately grown babies of their gestational age. It is not known why that may be the case, but it might have to do with a lack of protective nutrients or prenatal changes in lung structure from lower than normal oxygen levels, or both. Some studies, but not others, have found that SGA babies are more likely to develop an eye problem called retinopathy of prematurity, or ROP. In any case, if your baby is a very young preemie, she will be given an eye exam when she's four to six weeks old, time enough for early signs of ROP to appear. Some SGA babies may also have weaker immune systems, which may get better fast or may persist into adulthood.

All of this can sound pretty overwhelming, but remember that most SGA babies won't have all of these complications, and most of them are highly treatable. While your baby's hospital course may be more complicated because of her small size, be assured that the nursery's tiniest babies can be a lot stronger and more resilient than you might think, and with good care, most do well.

What Being SGA Means for Your Baby in the Long Run

The long-term prognosis for a baby whose growth was restricted in the womb also depends heavily on what caused the problem in the first place. If your baby has a lasting condition, such as a genetic or anatomical abnormality, or had a congenital infection, you should ask her doctor to explain her prognosis, which will depend on the specifics of her case.

As a general rule of thumb, when it comes to long-term development, SGA preemies as a group face risks comparable to preemies who were born a few weeks younger and share their birth weights. In other words, a 32-weeker who is small-for-gestational-age and thus was born with the weight of a typical 29-weeker has long-term prospects similar to those of a typical 29-weeker.

What that means is that SGA babies have somewhat lower IQ scores, on average, and a somewhat higher incidence of long-term neurological problems (such as problems with movement, hearing, and vision) than appropriately grown preemies of their same gestational age. An exception are SGA babies who are born extremely premature, at less than about 26 weeks; their outcomes are comparable to their bigger peers of the same gestational age. That's because their extremely early birth brings greater risks, with consequences that tend to outweigh the effect of their smaller size.

You shouldn't assume here that having a lower IQ means being mentally retarded. Although mental retardation is more common in SGA preemies than AGA preemies, mild cognitive deficits are more frequent than severe ones, with a loss of some of the intellectual ability a child might have had if her growth hadn't been restricted. Most preemies who were born small for their gestational age are not intellectually impaired by any objective measure, but they may have slid down a few points—which could perhaps mean going from "superior" to "normal," or from "average" to "low average"—on the IQ scale. It is a loss, but only a theoretical one, that nobody, including you, is apt to notice. There is also some evidence that more SGA babies have learning disabilities and behavioral problems (such as difficulties with concentration and more mood swings and irritability).

It's important to realize, however, that grouping all small-for-gestational-age babies together can be deceptive. These smallest babies fall broadly into two groups: those whose lack of nourishment or underlying reason for restricted growth was relatively mild and occurred late in gestation (usually causing asymmetrical or head-sparing growth retardation) and those whose lack of nourishment was severe and occurred early (causing symmetrical growth retardation).

The chances of being untouched by developmental problems are not as good for babies with symmetrical growth retardation. When the brain doesn't get enough oxygen and nourishment to grow normally before birth, or development is disordered because of a disease or genetic error, there is a high risk of lasting neurological impairments. When there is head-sparing, the brain may well have gotten the appropriate developmental signals and enough nourishment to grow normally, or suffered only a mild injury from which it is still able to recover. Thus if your baby has asymmetrical growth retardation with head-sparing, her chances of coming through with no long-term consequences are much better. The same goes after she's born: If her head circumference (a proxy measure for brain growth in infants) catches up to her AGA peers by the time she's eight months old, it's a good sign—her intellectual development is likely to be normal.

What about your child's size? She's tiny now, but will she always be? Some small-for-gestational-age babies remain shorter and lighter than their peers, although many—especially those whose birth weight was low but whose length and head circumference were normal—do catch up. Those who do often reach a normal weight and height for their adjusted age within the first 6 to 12 months of life, the most critical period for catch-up growth. Those who don't catch up on their own are now able to get some valuable help: Growth hormone treatment was recently approved for SGA babies who remain short at two years of age and has been shown to be successful in boosting their growth. And when adolescence comes (far ahead, but sooner than you think!), even if your child is small, she'll go through puberty at the usual time, with normal sexual maturation.

Incredible as it may sound now, there is some evidence that SGA babies who have very rapid catch-up growth are more likely to be obese later in life. It's not known whether trying to slow down their growth in the weeks and months after birth will prevent this, but it does suggest that pushing extra-big feedings on your baby just because he is small is not a good idea. Research also indicates that smaller-than-normal babies have a higher likelihood of developing high blood pressure, diabetes, and heart disease as adults, especially if they remain small. (This may be equally true for preemies who are not SGA but who were, of course, born smaller than term infants.) But try not to worry too much now about this connection given that strategies to prevent and treat cardiovascular diseases—through diet, exercise, and medications—are already very effective and are likely to become even more successful in the years to come.

As your baby grows, don't forget to put away her little newborn socks or hats. Keep them in a safe place: No matter how big your baby eventually grows, you can be sure that from time to time you'll want to pull out those mementos to remind yourself of how tiny she once was and how much you went through together.

CHAPTER 3

THE FIRST DAY

. . . .

Entering the foreign world of the neonatal intensive care unit.
Why it's the best place for your baby to be.

. . . .

PARENTS' STORIES: THE FIRST DAY *

When a preemie is born, his family's world freezes in expectation. At the beginning of the first day, little is clear and certain, most questions cannot be answered yet, and contradictory feelings come to the surface in turmoil. Deep inside the parents' souls, a painful sense of separation arises.

The first hours of the first day of my daughter's life feel unbearably slow. In this limbo—a nowhere—we wait for the doctors to assess our baby's condition, to stabilize her, to come up with some news. The little creature they showed us after delivery before rushing her to the NICU was the baby I was carrying in my womb. Why is it already so difficult to remember her face? I know that my nurturing and nesting instincts must be put on hold, because medical care is now the top priority. By my hospital bed there's no bassinet, while women all around are nursing plump, full-term newborns. Instead of my baby, the nurse brings in an electric pump for breast milk. She says it is comforting to express your milk and freeze it for later, when your baby will be fed. If you intend to breastfeed, she says, you have to start pumping now. But along with my first milk, I express tears. Are they bitter tears or tears of joy? Visitors and flowers seem so inappropriate. There's a birth to celebrate, but where is the baby? Are we allowed to be joyful?

Sometimes the trauma of having been unwillingly separated from your premature newborn lingers in the subconscious, and can unveil itself later, as a mother recalls:

* *Parents' Stories* describes events and feelings that really happened or that can happen. Every situation is unique, and you may relate to some parents' experiences and reactions more than others.

For some time after the premature birth of my son, I had a recurrent dream. I knew he was born, but I couldn't see him or even imagine him. I was standing at the edge of a crevice in front of a long, narrow, suspended bridge. All around, just a quiet, dark, empty space: I didn't fear any danger. The baby must be on the other side, I thought; I should go and find him. But I couldn't take a step onto the bridge because my foot wouldn't move. That didn't make me panic or even worry, though: No baby was crying, after all. Meanwhile a voice inside me, the dreamer, was screaming aloud, to shake that woman who looked like me out of her crazy, incomprehensible stillness.

A father's reaction to the stress of a premature birth may be different from a mother's, perhaps to compensate for his partner's excessive pessimism or optimism. If they don't become too extreme, these differences are healthy, helping the couple to hold up in a time of crisis. There are plenty of good reasons to rejoice today: Most preemies' stories have a happy ending despite the difficult start. A new life together has begun.

My son was born tonight, eight weeks too early. "My son!" I've never said those words before. They make me think of the baseball games I'll take him to, the talks we'll have about manhood, the car I'll teach him to drive when he turns sixteen. I just wish my wife could feel happier tonight. The doctors say Max is healthy, just immature. And they say a three-pounder is a big preemie. My wife is so worried. Okay, I admit it, I'm a little worried, too. The doctors say it's still too soon to tell how everything will go. But our family, we're fighters. Max is our son, and I bet he's a tough little guy. Setbacks happen to everyone sooner or later—so for Max it's a little sooner. I know he'll be fine. He's great! Hey, I wonder if I can find some tiny, preemie baseball caps and pass them out instead of cigars?

The nurses know how important it is to break the parents' solitude on the first day, helping them to bond with newborns who don't seem real yet because they cannot be held, cuddled, or breastfed. But possessing just a symbol of the baby can create a strong sense of belonging.

A new mother is lying in her hospital bed, her husband at her side, after an emergency C-section. She is still drowsy and slightly nauseated. He looks pale and tense. A nurse comes by and places something in their hands: the first photos of their twins, a boy and a girl, who are now in the NICU. She kindly points out that the two babies look beautiful and not even too small, despite having been born ten weeks before term. But what the parents see are two rag dolls lying among tubes and tape, with snorkels coming out of their mouths, lips redder than wounds. Why is the nurse doing this to us, they think? Why this torture? It will take them time to realize what a great gift she has brought. It's the first link, a paper-thin, narrow bridge that connects them with their babies. When the nurse leaves, the parents cry together and look again at the photographs. It is already less painful. And their children are just two floors above, in the NICU. All they need now from their parents is that they pull themselves together and go up and meet them for the very first time.

Is it helpful to put the emotional journey of giving birth to a premature baby into a rational perspective? Some psychologists have tried doing that, giving parents some additional tools for understanding their experience.

Worry, anguish, anger, terror, feeling cheated by life, guilt, loneliness, desire to escape. Just plain numbness. Joy, hope, excitement, trust, relief. And much more. There's a wide range of emotional reactions parents can experience after the premature birth of their children, from the first day of their lives through the many later stages. Whatever you feel today may be influenced by the circumstances of your baby's delivery, by whether it was expected or not, by how early the birth was, by the medical condition of your baby, by your temperament, values, religious faith, personal history, and family relationships. It's hard and maybe wrong to generalize about what feelings are normal or to predict how your feelings will evolve. Some experts talk about a first stage of denial, when you unintentionally refuse to realize what's going on. Something called projection is said to follow: blaming someone else or something else for what happened. Then there may be a stage of detachment, when you pull away from your situation because it is too painful—before finally coming back to accept reality. Is all of that true? For some parents of preemies, it is. For some, only partially. Others may think it's just nonsense, psychobabble. Until they have done it, nobody really knows what it means to give birth to a child and to let him go off alone, in a high-tech medical world.

Your first meeting with your preemie in the NICU is going to be much different from the ideal picture described in ordinary pregnancy books. At least for today, before your baby's condition has stabilized, you'll have to forget about privacy, hugs, her warm skin on yours, sucking at the breast. It's normal to be scared of what you may see and feel in the NICU; many parents are. But most of them feel relieved after having finally met their babies. Overcome by tenderness and desire to protect their tiny offspring, mothers and fathers pull themselves together, finding the energy to face this life challenge and to overcome it.

During my twin daughters' first day of life I couldn't find the strength to go and see them in the NICU. My husband and sister had already been there several times and had talked extensively to the doctors. I kept repeating to them and to myself: I'm going to be a good mother, I just need more time to adjust and muster my strength. But I knew they must be worried about me, and I was, too. How am I going to survive all this? I thought. What if we lose our babies? What if something bad happens to them, and they end up severely disabled? I wasn't ready for all that, I wasn't. But as the hours of that long day passed, I felt something switching inside me. My maternal feelings were struggling with and gradually overtaking my fears. Whatever happened, my husband and I had each other; we would make it. My babies were downstairs, they needed me. That evening, when I went to see my beautiful daughters in the NICU, I was a better person. All that mattered was giving love and strength to my babies. It's as if inside me the essence of mothering had been tested and revealed.

THE DOCTOR'S PERSPECTIVE: THE FIRST DAY *

We may have had a dramatic meeting at delivery, but now is the time when doctor and baby really get acquainted. I approach each new tiny patient in the nursery with curiosity, excitement, hope, and trepidation, guessing at what I'll find but not really knowing what's in store for either of us until I take a closer look and some time passes by. Even if you've had twins (or triplets, or more), each baby will be evaluated as a separate, distinct individual. Your babies may have been together in the womb, but just as their personalities may be different later, their medical and physical conditions may be very different now.

---

* *The Doctor's Perspective* describes how your doctor may be thinking about your preemie's condition and what she may be considering as she makes medical decisions. All of the medical terms and conditions mentioned here are described in more detail elsewhere in this book. Check the index.

Physical Exam and Laboratory Assessment

As soon as your baby reaches the nursery, she'll be placed on a cardiorespiratory monitor and we (the doctors and nurses) will check her vital signs—her temperature, how fast she's breathing, her heart rate and blood pressure—and determine how much oxygen is getting into her blood. We want this information immediately, because significant problems with any of these would need quick attention. At the same time we watch her intently for signs of health or distress. Is she moving (active and vigorous—a good sign) or limp (lethargic, exhausted, maybe sick)? Is she pink and resting comfortably or blue and struggling to breathe? Most of the time, we're relieved to find that she's acting just as we expect babies her age to act, and often we're delighted that all looks so well.

Next your baby gets a thorough physical examination, more extensive than the brief exam done in the delivery room. We'll scrutinize your baby from head to toes, asking and answering questions as we go, aiming to be complete in noting what's normal or abnormal. This is done for all newborns, of course, but our eyes are drawn to details that are especially important for premature infants.

We evaluate her physical features: feel her head, including the fontanelles, or soft spots. Are they normal size? Is her head swollen or molded, as commonly happens from moving through the birth canal? We need to know the size and shape of her head now to determine if it's growing normally later. We look at her eyes, ears, and chin and feel her palate—are they well formed? We press deeply into her belly. Is it soft and gently rounded, with normal-sized liver, kidneys, and spleen? What is her skin like—clear and intact or bruised or thin? Thick, unbroken skin helps protect against infection and prevents her from losing important fluids. We look at her color to assess whether she might have lost or gained too much blood, as sometimes happens during delivery or between identical twins in the womb: Is she too pale or too ruddy? We listen carefully to the sounds of her heart beating and feel her pulse to make sure her blood is flowing well. We check that her joints move smoothly and count her fingers and toes.

We also evaluate how well your baby is adjusting to being out in the world: Is her breathing quiet, deep, and comfortable, or is it shallow and labored, a possible sign that her lungs are not quite mature yet? Is she responding appropriately to all of the stimulation and handling she's getting? We're happy to see her resisting sometimes or crying; it's a sign of neurological health if she's aware of what's going on and can respond vigorously.

If your preemie's breathing is labored, we'll probably get a chest X-ray to make sure her lungs are open enough and to see whether something other than immaturity is affecting her breathing. We'll take blood to insure that all her organ systems are functioning well and that important substances like oxygen, carbon dioxide, salts, sugar, and blood cells are at normal levels. Over the course of this first day and intermittently for as long as your baby remains in intensive care, we'll do blood tests—as often as every few hours if your baby is very young or very sick—to make sure that her vital functions are in a safe range so we can treat them if they're not.

We don't expect everything to go perfectly right from the start as babies make the difficult transition from life in the womb to life in the outside world. In fact, in the first few hours after birth, when mild functional abnormalities are common and usually transient, an infant is said to be "transitioning." For example, a little bit of grunting and hard breathing may resolve as soon as some extra fluid moves out of her lungs. (After all, your preemie has been living in amniotic fluid for quite a while.) A pale, mottled skin color could indicate insufficient blood flow, but more likely your baby will turn a nice, even pink when her blood flow shifts from the routes it took when she was a fetus to the pathways needed for a newborn. As her circulation improves, any extra acid in her blood that may have built up during labor and delivery will likely soon be cleared. We'll decide what needs to be addressed immediately and what can be watched for now and followed up on later.

Features that may seem strange and unusual to you may be commonplace to doctors who care for so many premature newborns, so sometimes we may not think to comment on something you're worried about. If you have questions, ASK! The answer will usually be less than earth-shaking, like "That bump is just the tip of her rib cage" or "I don't know what that rash is, but it doesn't mean anything; it will disappear soon." Most of the time you'll be reassured that your baby is just like other babies her age.

In addition to checking her physical features and general functioning, we'll also examine your baby to determine her gestational age (how many weeks have passed since the menstrual cycle when she was conceived). To do so, we'll look at how thick—and hairy and wrinkly—her skin is, feel for the size of her breast buds and the stiffness of her ears, note how fully formed her genitals are and how mature her neurological functioning is. This method of calculating your baby's gestational age after she's born is called a Dubowitz or Ballard examination. It's less accurate than an ultrasound exam in the first trimester of pregnancy or the dating of your pregnancy if you were certain about when she was conceived. But if the dating of your pregnancy is less exact, we may tell you that your baby appears to be several weeks older or younger than you thought—

which can affect how she does in the hospital and later.

Although the first physical examination is the most extensive, it's just the first. Your baby will be examined several times today and at least once or twice a day by each of her doctors and nurses (she'll have several) for as long as she remains in a special care nursery. They will perform ongoing evaluations of her breathing and circulation, activity and muscle tone, and comfort or pain in order to make sure she's doing well and to respond quickly to any problems.

Common Issues and Decisions

Respiratory Distress Syndrome: It won't be surprising if your premature baby has some breathing difficulties, since that's a natural consequence of having immature lungs. The breathing difficulty that occurs when a baby's lungs are immature is called respiratory distress syndrome, or RDS for short. Probably the most important decisions her doctor will make on your baby's first day is whether or not she has RDS or some other problem (like pneumonia) that prevents her from breathing well, and what kind of treatments would best help.

If your baby has to suck her chest in deeply to pull in enough air, if she's grunting and her nostrils flare with effort, or even if she looks comfortable but her oxygen saturations and blood tests tell us that her lungs aren't taking in enough oxygen or getting rid of enough carbon dioxide, she may need the help of a breathing machine (either CPAP or a ventilator). Most of the time, we'll try nasal CPAP first, which just requires putting some soft plastic prongs in her nose because it's safer and less disruptive than a ventilator. But if after a few hours—or sooner, if a baby isn't breathing sufficiently—it looks like CPAP isn't helping enough, we'll intubate her. Intubation is a minor procedure that involves placing a plastic tube through her mouth and into her windpipe. Once she's intubated, we can give her a medication to help her lungs stay wide open (called surfactant) and connect her to a ventilator.

If your baby needs more than a little help with her breathing—if she's on a ventilator or high amounts of CPAP or oxygen—we'll probably draw blood fairly frequently (usually several times a day until she's stable). In that case, we'll probably put a catheter into one of her arteries so that we can take blood without hurting her each time. We'll also probably decide not to feed her right away, since that would be an added stress. So you can expect that she'll be nourished with intravenous fluids for now.

Baby's Comfort: One of the things your baby's doctors and nurses will be monitoring on the first day—and throughout her stay in the nursery—is her comfort or pain. If she can get by without a breathing machine, then once the nurses and doctors are finished drawing blood and putting in catheters, she'll probably be pretty comfortable in her warm bed in the nursery. The nurses can turn down the lights and make a little nest around her body, or swaddle her in blankets so she feels cozy and protected. We really don't know whether being on a ventilator is painful for a baby or if it's just a mild discomfort that resolves quickly as the ventilator provides welcome breaths. We also don't know how much anxiety a baby feels from relying on a ventilator to breathe for her. Probably this differs from baby to baby, depending on her maturity and temperament, the general atmosphere in the nursery around her bed, how sick she is, and what kind of breathing support she's getting. (For example, some babies wriggle around and try to pull out the CPAP prongs that blow air into their noses; others calmly tolerate nasal prongs but don't like having the tube in their throats that connects them to the ventilator.)

Depending on how comfortable your baby seems, we'll decide whether or not she needs medicine to control pain or to calm her down, or even to stop her from moving and "fighting" the ventilator. (If she fights too much, the ventilator's breaths can't get into her lungs.) It can be hard to tell when a premature baby is in pain, especially a very young one whose normal behavior is most different from a term baby's, but clues that we use are agitation, excessive crying, and a high heart rate and blood pressure. We don't want to medicate your baby unless she needs it. So, we'll keep monitoring all of those things and adjusting our care to make sure your baby is in as little pain as possible.

Infection: An infection in an expectant mother or her baby is probably the most common reason for a baby to be born prematurely; in addition, infections often cause breathing difficulties that are indistinguishable from simple RDS. For that reason, unless her early delivery was planned, we'll probably treat your preemie with intravenous antibiotics, especially if she needs help with her breathing. That decision is based on the philosophy "better safe than sorry"—infections are dangerous (life-threatening if they remain untreated), and we usually can't know for sure whether she's infected until several days after she's born, and sometimes not even then.

Some signs that your baby may have an infection are persistently low blood pressure, abnormally high or low numbers of blood cells, or an especially dense patch of lung on her chest X-ray. We'll be watching for those things and take some blood for a culture to see if any bacteria grow—a nearly certain sign of infection. Other cultures may be taken, too, such as a skin swab if she has suspicious blisters or a spinal tap if her activity or movements are abnormal. Based on whether her cultures turn positive (bacteria grow) over the next couple of days and whether or not she has other signs of infection, we'll decide how long to continue the antibiotics. If it looks like she didn't have an infection, the antibiotics will be stopped after two or three days. Otherwise, the antibiotics will be continued until the infection is cleared—usually for one to three weeks.

Family Issues

We may be meeting you and your family for the first time on the first day. We need to understand what you really care about so that we can take your concerns into account when we tell you what's happening and what we think is in store for you and your baby later. We'll be trying to figure out (and you may be, too) your deeply felt values and concerns as together we make treatment plans and decisions. You can help by talking about the desires and hopes that mean the most to you—what you most want for your baby and family.

One of the most difficult—and sometimes most important—things to talk about is whether you want your baby to survive at all costs, even at the risk of her having severe medical problems or disabilities later, or whether you would rather not take extreme measures to keep her alive if the chances for her to have a good quality of life are very small. Don't be afraid that your feelings

are unacceptable. Very loving parents have felt strongly either way. Other wishes or worries you have may just be practical, or may seem trivial to you, but are still important for us to know, and I hope you will express them all to us. You may want to move to a hospital closer to home as soon as possible; you may want your twins to be kept together in the nursery; you may not want to make any decisions until Grandpa arrives; you may want to pray with a chaplain, even if things are going very well. You can't communicate (or even know) all these things at once, but the first day is a start. And although we won't always be able to make your wishes a reality, at least we'll know what to aim for.

Overall, for most families, and for those of us helping to take care of your baby, the first day is a time of uncertainty, waiting, and hope. It's often not clear whether a premature baby's condition is going to improve or worsen. If your baby is an older preemie and doing well, things will probably settle down quickly and mild problems will disappear in a matter of hours or days. If your baby is younger or sicker, realize that the first day is a time to discover what treatments your baby needs and to get support systems (such as ventilator tubes, catheters for blood drawing, intravenous fluids, and medications) in place. Time is often needed before things become clearer.

QUESTIONS AND ANSWERS

Afraid to See Your Baby

I haven't even seen my baby yet. The nurses have offered to take me from my room to the NICU, but I'm too afraid of what I'll find there.

Most parents of premature babies feel unprepared for, and scared of, the first sight of their baby in the intensive care nursery. Those feelings are

nothing to be ashamed of; they're normal. After all, you've already been through a lot—preparing for a premature birth or being surprised by it, and possibly experiencing medical problems of your own or undergoing a C-section, a major operation. The next few weeks or months are going to be demanding, and if you feel you need an extra day to muster your emotional or physical strength, you should certainly take it.

(Continued on page 95)

Your Beautiful Newborn: A Portrait

Parents seeing their premature babies for the first time often have conflicting feelings. Pain and pleasure. Shock and a touch of relief. Most parents are shocked by how tiny their babies are—but impressed by their complete, perfectly formed little bodies. It's not unusual to see mothers and fathers staring in awe at a beautiful set of micro-sized eyelashes, fingers, or toes, complete with all of the knuckles. Everything is already in place, just waiting to grow.

Obviously, though, preemies are not full-term babies, and you can't expect them to exactly resemble 40-weekers any more than you can expect 40-weekers to exactly resemble older, two- or three-month-old babies.

What are some of the differences you may notice?

* Preemies younger than 30 to 32 weeks have thin skin, lacking the layers of body fat that they would have put on during the final weeks of pregnancy. When skin is thin, the arteries and veins below it are easily visible, so the skin has a reddish-purple tint, regardless of the infant's ethnic background. (So don't be concerned that your baby was switched accidentally with someone else's! Babies born to African-American parents often look very similar in color to white babies at this stage. Natural pigmentation may not be obvious until around the eighth month of gestation.) Until those layers of fat appear and fill out the skin's folds, babies also tend to look a bit wrinkled. But their slender fingers and toes look unusually long and graceful.

* In extremely premature babies (born at less than 26 weeks gestation), the coarse, top layer of skin hasn't formed yet. So their skin looks smooth and shiny and is too fragile to caress and rub for the time being. (You can touch it gently.) This usually changes by three days or so after delivery, as exposure to air quickly toughens up the skin.

* The very youngest preemies don't have any body hair at all, and the hair on their head is just a fine fuzz. An older preemie, though, is covered by lanugo—soft, fuzzy, fetal hair—over much of her body. It is particularly heavy on the back, upper arms, and shoulders, and dark hair is more noticeable than light. Don't worry if your baby has more lanugo than the baby in the bed next to her; some preemies have more, some have less, but it always goes away. Even some full-term babies are born with some lanugo. Most preemies gradually shed theirs by their due date or at the latest a few weeks after. It's not until approximately 36 weeks of gestation that the hair on a preemie's head becomes thick and silky.

* A premature baby's eyes may still be fused shut if she is born before the 26th week. But around that time, they will open on their own—already framed by beautiful little eyelashes.

* Fingernails and toenails may look like tiny buds at first. By roughly your baby's due date, her nails will reach the ends of her fingers or toes, and it will be time to pull out the scissors or emery board.

* A preemie's ears still have a little developing to do. Many parents get worried when they see one of their baby's ears doubled over, as if it's folded. Actually, that's a common sight in the NICU and nothing to worry about. Before the 35th week or so, ears are very soft, without

the thick, firm cartilage that develops later. So an ear that gets folded (perhaps when a baby is laid on her side) may stay that way rather than springing back on its own. A mere touch from your gentle fingers can fix that.

* Breast nipples usually don't appear until the 34th week, although both boys and girls may already have hints of their areola, the circles of dark skin around where the nipples will be.

* Most likely, your baby's buttocks will be quite flat (remember, he has very little body fat to cushion the muscles underneath and his muscles have yet to develop much bulk and tone). Because his buttocks are so flat, the crease between them may look wider and deeper than you're used to. Just keep in mind that putting on some weight will soon give your baby the sweet bottom roundness you expect to see.

* Sexual organs are clearly differentiated even on extremely premature babies, but they aren't mature yet, as most parents quickly notice. A premature boy's testes have not yet descended from deep in his abdomen into his scrotum. So his scrotum looks small and unusually smooth. A premature girl's outer labia (the mounds around her vagina) are still small and spread widely apart, leaving the inner labia and clitoris looking large and fully exposed. This will change when the outer labia fill in with fat and come together. Some girls also have a little tag, as the doctors call it, protruding from their vagina. Strange-looking? Yes. But don't worry; it will soon disappear. Both boys and girls will look just like full-term babies around their due date. In fact, neonatologists can often estimate a preemie's gestational age by looking at his or her genitalia.

* Whether a newborn is full-term or premature, it's hard to tell on the first day whether she has inherited your nose or Grandpa's chin. And if your preemie is on CPAP or a ventilator, it will be hard even to get a good look, because parts of her face may be covered and stretched by tape holding the equipment in place. When she finally comes off the ventilator, you'll see your baby's little face unobscured at last.

* A premature baby's posture and movements depend on how old she is at birth. Younger babies have less muscle tone. So while full-term newborns hold their arms and legs flexed and can curl themselves up into the fetal position, a very young preemie tends to lie flat on her back, with her arms and legs splayed out, frog-like.

* Before around 28 weeks, a premature baby doesn't move much. She'll sometimes curl her fingers into a fist, or stretch or flex an arm or leg—reminding you of those pokes your belly got while she was still inside you. A slightly older preemie, between 29 and 32 weeks of gestation, moves more often, but her movements are often jittery and jerky. She can turn her head from one side to the other to get comfortable, and she can grasp your finger (although not strongly enough to hold on if you try to pull her up to a sitting position).

* By around 35 weeks, a preemie has enough muscle tone to tuck herself into a fetal position, just like a full-term newborn. Although she startles more frequently than a full-term baby, her grasp is strong enough to keep hold of your fingers while you lift her, and her movements are more fluid and purposeful. Some babies are even coordinated enough to get their hands in their mouths and suck on them. Sounds easy? Many 40-weekers wish they could do it!

Soon you'll get so used to seeing your preemie that you may forget what it's like for a newcomer to the NICU. So if you send a photo of your beautiful little one to family or friends, expecting "oohs" and "aahs," don't be surprised—and try not to be hurt—if they seem shocked instead. They're just newbies!

The Appearance of Extremely Premature Babies

Extremely premature babies, born between, say, 22 and 26 weeks of gestation, look different from more mature preemies. As you might expect, they look more like fetuses: Their eyes might still be fused shut; their skin and head, not yet covered with lanugo, might look translucent and red and be too delicate to touch; and their ears may be soft and folded where the cartilage hasn't thickened yet. Some parents don't find these babies of theirs beautiful—*yet*. By a few weeks later, the babies' eyes open, their skin thickens, and their looks change—and so do their parents' sentiments.

Your baby is in good hands with the doctors; right now, that's the kind of care he needs most. There will be plenty of time and opportunity for bonding between mother and father and baby in the days to come.

Rather than getting overwhelmed by your fears, you can begin to prepare yourself for your first trip to the NICU.

* **Know what to expect.** If you already saw your baby in the delivery room, you know what he looks like. Parents of preemies are often shocked by how tiny their newborns are. Some are so small that they can fit in the palm of an adult hand. But usually parents are also surprised by how fully formed their babies are. And love is blind. It's uncanny the way a preemie's parents soon find their baby the most graceful and beautiful in the world and come to view full-term newborns as ungainly giants.

    Even if you saw your child in the delivery room, you probably got little more than a glance before he was whisked away by the doctors. So take a minute to read *Your Beautiful Newborn: A Portrait* on pages 93–94. It describes some of the typical traits of premature babies, such as lanugo (a soft layer of hair covering some of his body), thinner than normal skin, and not yet fully developed sexual organs, among others. It's good to know about these things in advance so they won't worry you.

    Once your baby is settled in the intensive care nursery, he'll be attached to various monitors and machines. The first sight of them is disturbing, but once you understand why they're there, they're a lot easier to take. So reading *Through the Doors of a Neonatal Intensive Care Unit* on pages 101–107 is another good thing to do before that first visit.

* **Ask for a photo and a description.** A close friend, family member, or a helpful social worker or nurse can take a photograph of your baby for you to look at and can tell you about things the photo doesn't capture. There may seem to be more tubes and wires than baby in the picture, but what matters most is that you'll have a link to your infant. After you've looked at his picture, you may find that going to see him in person feels like less of a big step.

* **Knowing is more comforting than not knowing.** Try to keep in mind that for most parents

the first trip to see their baby in the NICU ends up being a great relief. They find that their baby's actual appearance is more comforting than the fantasy and fears their minds had concocted. And being with their baby—seeing his tiny fingers and toes, caressing his soft skin, and in some cases looking into his little eyes or feeling his firm grasp around their adult finger—brings a rush of love that makes wires and tubes practically disappear.

Chances are that after a few seconds or minutes to adjust you'll find your baby very beautiful—parents usually do. And remember, your preemie just needs some time before all those wires are history and he looks like a roly-poly, full-term newborn.

Micropreemies

Someone referred to my daughter as a micropreemie. What does this say about her and whether she's going to be OK?

The term "micropreemie" has no precise definition and doctors rarely use it, but you'll often see the word used by the media to describe the very youngest and smallest of all premature babies. That generally includes babies who are born between 22 weeks and 25 weeks of gestation.

If your baby was called a micropreemie, she probably falls in that category, so in reading our book, when you come across certain facts or observations about the tiniest or youngest preemies, you'll know they apply to her.

It would be so helpful if only someone could tell you now how your precious, tiny newborn is going to do. You could prepare yourself emotionally for the road ahead; you could make the best decisions for her when her doctors tell you there are medical choices to be made. Unfortunately, on the first day of life of any preemie, but especially a preemie born this early, no one can.

The doctor can give you statistics that apply in general to preemies of her age, size, and sex and can describe how she is doing right now, based on her very first physical exams and her response to the medical care she's been given so far, but at the same time he'll probably tell you that you and he both will have to wait and see what the future holds. That's because for the smallest, most fragile premature babies, the range of possible outcomes is extremely wide. On the first day, it's often unpredictable; watching her body's reaction to the world outside of the womb each day or week, it will become gradually apparent how mature and resilient her lungs, brain, skin, and other organs seem to be, giving you more information. Merely letting time pass to see what ups and downs it brings—because all preemies go through unforeseeable ups and down—will complete the picture. (If at any point your baby's doctor becomes concerned for her immediate survival, you can be sure he will tell you. Doctors know when a baby's condition is that serious. Try to let go of this worry as long as he tells you your baby continues to be all right.)

If you've seen stories about "miracle" babies in the press, it's important to keep in mind that it's the nature of the media to play up the most extreme stories. Personally, we shake our heads when we read about preemies who were born at extraordinarily young gestational ages yet somehow flourish without serious medical hurdles or problems. That's absolutely wonderful and moving, but it can be misleading to other parents: The reason this baby is in the news is that she is an exception. Few preemies can expect to have a similar course. Parents shouldn't feel that they or their babies are inadequate in some way if their roads are tougher.

In truth, as the parent of one of the youngest, tiniest preemies, your road may be tough. But we will keep you company throughout, answering your questions, explaining what you and your baby are going through, and assuring you that you can get through it.

We have mixed feelings about giving you statistics on the survival and long-term health of premature babies, because they cannot, and do not, tell you what is going to happen with your baby. They are useful in helping you form balanced, realistic expectations, but not as a crystal ball. Understanding and absorbing them will help you know what to hope for, what to prepare yourself for, and how to help the doctors make the best possible decisions for your baby. But many unknowable and unpredictable factors make your baby unique, and unless the doctor has told you about something that lets him know she is unlikely to survive, it is impossible to tell in advance whether her outcome will fall within the majority—or far outside it.

Preemies born this young are surviving in greater numbers than ever before. A decade ago, it was unheard of for a 22-weeker to survive. Now, some 5 percent survive. For 23-weekers, the number rises to 25 percent. More than half of 24-weekers survive, and a full 75 percent of 25-weekers do. This news can be very heartening for you to hear, but your next question is going to be: survive at what cost? with what quality of life?

You can get a better sense of the short-term and long-term health statistics that apply to your baby with a tool that was recently put online by the National Institutes of Health at http://www.nichd.nih.gov/about/org/cdbpm/pp/prog_epbo/. By entering five factors—a newborn preemie's gestational age, birth weight, sex, whether the baby is a singleton or a multiple, and whether the mother was given steroids to boost the baby's maturity before the birth—you can generate an estimation of her chances of survival, and her chances of survival without severe disabilities. Because this tool is based on a large database of extremely premature babies born at many different hospitals in the United States and because these five variables together yield a more accurate prediction than any single variable (such as gestational age), it is the best estimator of statistical outcomes now available. Still, you should remember that it gives you general information about groups of preemies, and not about the future of your own particular baby, who is unique. If she has features her doctor can point to that make her outcome likely to be better or worse than those of average preemies in her group, he'll tell you.

(Keep in mind that the estimator's statistics do not apply to preemies who have major birth defects or genetic disorders, because babies with these conditions were excluded from the database, so if your baby has these, be sure to ask her doctor for information. Also keep in mind that no estimates are given for minor disabilities such as learning or behavior problems, which tend to show up at school age, and for which all preemies have a higher risk, especially the smallest and youngest.)

One of the purposes of knowing how likely various outcomes are is to help doctors and parents make difficult decisions about when and how aggressively to treat the youngest premature babies, like yours. You should be sure to be open with the doctors about your deeply held values so that they can use medicine's power wisely, in a way that you feel will help your baby best. Sometimes trade-offs must be made between trying to prolong the life of a very tiny baby and making sure she doesn't suffer. Let the doctors know whether you want them to do everything technologically possible to keep your baby alive for as long as possible or whether you feel more strongly that she should not suffer if her chances are very poor. You can read about the decisions that doctors are faced with, and that you will have a voice in, in *The Doctor's Perspective* on pages 88–92.

Now back to the nursery, where your baby is beginning to get settled. As parents of one of the youngest preemies, what can you expect of your experience there? Some of her neighbors may be as tiny as she is, while others were born older and bigger. You'll find that the bigger, more mature preemies will be the ones who move faster from one step to another in the NICU. Your baby and other "micropreemies" are the ones who are more likely to be breathing with the help of a ventilator, who must wait longer before their parents can hold them, who are slower to learn to eat, and who are more apt to develop complications of a premature birth—which slow them down further. But they are also the ones to whom the doctors and nurses get emotionally attached, as together they go through so much. The resilience and strength of the youngest preemies inspire awe in adults.

Because it is going to be a long hospitalization, you will need to figure out how to organize the next few months of your life. Some mothers of the youngest preemies take some time off from work for just a little while when their babies are first born, and then go back to work, saving the rest of their maternity leave for when their baby comes home. Others feel that they want to keep their baby company in the intensive care nursery every day and make whatever arrangements it takes to allow that. For example, if their baby is in a NICU far from home, some even move into a Ronald McDonald House (a charitable organization that offers low-cost housing near hospitals for families of hospitalized children) until their baby is discharged or sent to a nursery closer to home. One way or another, when you have an extremely young preemie, you will need to rearrange your life temporarily. It isn't easy—especially if you have older children or a job or other things you need to take care of—but at this time of crisis, you'll find strength within yourself and support from others that you didn't know you had, and find a way to do it.

The pace of the next few weeks may be dramatic, because the adjustment of an extremely premature baby to the outside world involves many medical events, frequent changes, and usually some ups and downs, each of them causing a shift in your baby's outlook. During this period you may be woken in the middle of the night to be told that your baby has had a setback or has become unstable or even that there is a chance she might not survive. You'll have moments of fear, calling on all of your inner reserves, and moments of hope, when you have faith that things will turn out for the best. You may find that what you're hoping for changes, depending on what the doctors tell you. To get through this period, it's important to take things hour by hour, day by day—and to remember that other preemies who were born so young and went through what your baby is going through ended up happy and thriving.

After the first month or two, things tend to slow down a bit, although what some people call the roller coaster of prematurity is still not over and your baby may yet go through some upturns and downturns. This can be painful—your wounds are still fresh, but you have started to let your guard down. Even if you tell yourself to expect it, it's hard to be prepared.

Then at some point, usually during a baby's last month in the hospital, things quiet down. Parents can barely believe the sense of calm. Not only the traumas but the big, euphoric events—such as coming off the ventilator, graduating to full feeds, or moving into an open crib—are also past. During this period, you might get frustrated: It can feel like no changes are occurring, yet your baby is still not coming home. Remember, she still has maturing to do. If your baby has been in a NICU far from home, at this point she may be able to move to a nursery in your community hospital, one that is able to take care of bigger, more stable preemies like she is now. You may be able to start to relax, take your family and friends to see her, introduce her to the pediatrician who will be taking care of her in the years to come, get her crib and car seat ready for use.

Your baby's hospitalization will be a long, tough, eventful, and momentous journey, for you and for her. When she finally comes home and you can share the fullness of ordinary, everyday life together, you'll rejoice and your wounds will begin to heal. Your attachment and love for your preemie will be unimaginably strong after what you've been through. This is a precious baby you will never take for granted.

Baby's Bed

I thought preemies were put in incubators, but my baby is lying out in the open. Is this a good sign or a bad sign?

Probably neither. While preemies in some hospitals are put straight into isolettes (a modern incu-

bator), when premature babies are first born they are usually placed on an open bed, referred to in the intensive care nursery as a radiant warmer. This allows the doctors and nurses to have easy, free access to the baby in the early period when they are getting him stabilized and conducting tests to determine what kind of medical care he needs. While he is on the open bed, an overhead heater keeps him nice and warm. (Most preemies have very little fat tissue as insulation and still can't regulate their internal body temperature on their own.)

Some nurseries keep preemies on open beds for their entire stay, but if that's not how your hospital does things, then the decision to put your baby in an isolette later on is a good sign. You can assume it means that his condition is stable and he doesn't require frequent medical interventions. In an isolette he can enjoy lying in a comfortable, warm little home, protected from drafts, dust, and strange odors.

The Plastic Spa

The tiniest preemies—those with the least amount of body fat who are born at less than 26 weeks gestation or weigh under, say, a pound and a half—are more susceptible to fluid and heat loss because they have the thinnest skin and greatest proportion of skin surface to body mass. Therefore, when they are on an open bed, the bed may be enclosed in plastic, a material that's very efficient at preventing too much fluid from evaporating and holding in the heat their bodies generate. This can take different forms: It might

be a soft plastic box that you'll hear referred to as a mist tent, because a tube running into it supplies a regular spray of mist. Or, in a much simpler but also effective approach, the bed might be wrapped in cellophane,

To parents who aren't used to seeing it, the plastic tent or cellophane wrap looks alarming. But they soon get used to it, and in the future might even look back on it with some humor—after all, it was their baby's first steam room. A baby spa!

You or the nurse can even place a cover over it to give him some peaceful dark time.

Unless your baby has to undergo surgery, goes back on the ventilator, or for some other reason needs frequent medical attention again, he'll probably stay in the isolette until he's almost ready to go home. You'll see that over time, as your baby matures, the amount of heat the isolette provides will gradually decrease until the temperature inside it is just a little higher than the air in the room outside. Then he'll move again to an open bed, but this one won't have a heater overhead.

This move is a good sign, too: It means the doctors think your baby is ready to try maintaining his body temperature on his own. Intensive care nurseries typically wait until preemies are about 34 weeks old and around four pounds before moving them out into the open air. (Don't be worried if your doctor decides to wait a little longer. It's a judgment call, and some babies flourish best when they're given a chance to devote their energy to growing or perfecting their feeding for a few more days rather than expending some of their precious energy on keeping warm.)

Some babies do fine on their first try in the open air; others need to return to an isolette briefly and try again a few days later. Every day that your baby gets older (and fatter), his ability to keep himself warm improves. Doctors and nurses can't tell for sure when a baby's ability to regulate his body temperature is mature without trying him out in the open, and sometimes they jump the gun a little. But at that point, chances are you'll be taking your baby home soon.

Touching Your Baby

I want to touch my baby so badly, but I'm scared to. She looks so fragile, like I might hurt her.

Your baby may look breakable to you, but that's one thing you *don't* have to worry about. Just look at how the nurses and doctors move her around and you'll understand. As long as she is 26 weeks of gestation or older, your little one is ready and eager for loving parental handling.

Premature babies born before 26 weeks of gestation still have fragile skin, and although a gentle finger in her palm or a touch on her leg can help cement that irresistible physical connection between parent and child, it's best to let her skin mature and toughen before touching it much more than that. The nurses can let you know when her skin can take more handling. If your baby is 26 weeks or older, your touch, far from being painful or harmful, is likely to help her. Some studies show that consistent gentle touching leads to better outcomes in premature babies, such as fewer episodes of apnea, faster weight gain, and earlier discharge from the hospital. And although no newborn appreciates vigorous rubbing, older preemies can benefit from—and usually love—a smooth massage (see page 329).

The only thing better than touching your premature baby is holding her. It may seem scary before you've tried it, but nothing could be more natural or enjoyable once you have. If your baby was just put on a ventilator today, has important tubes or lines that could easily be dislodged (like an umbilical catheter or a chest tube because of a pneumothorax), or is medically unstable for other reasons, you may have to wait. But as soon as the nurse says your baby is ready, you need not hesitate. The nurse will help pick your baby up, hand her to you, and arrange things so you don't knock any intravenous lines or other equipment out of place. All you have to do is support your baby's neck, be gentle—and relax. She'll be safe, and extremely happy, in her parents' arms. (And from then on, you'll be looking forward to holding her even closer to your body: Ask your baby's doctor when you can start kangaroo care, described on page 249.)

Through the Doors of a Neonatal Intensive Care Unit

When parents step through the doors of a neonatal intensive care unit for the first time, they often think: If my baby needs all that medical equipment attached to her, she must be very sick.

Thankfully, this impression is usually wrong. Most preemies are basically healthy. But they (and their organs and bodily functions) are immature and need a few more weeks or months to develop. In the meantime, your premature baby will get the extra help she needs from the medical staff and all of that high-tech machinery in the NICU. There are tubes that deliver nourishment to your baby until she is mature enough to eat on her own. There are machines called ventilators that provide breaths to preemies who haven't mastered the art of breathing by themselves yet. There are doctors, called neonatologists, who are intimately familiar with the normal behavior of preemies, though it may not always look normal to you. And so on.

Believe it or not, in just a few days you'll become familiar with the gadgetry and the staff, and they won't seem so threatening. In fact, despite all of those tubes and wires your baby is entangled in, you'll soon be able to hold her in your arms and even change her diaper. You'll come to know what the different beeping alarms emitted by your baby's monitors mean—and why you don't need to panic when you hear them.

To speed up your acquaintance with the NICU, here are some brief descriptions to browse through. First a quick tour of the equipment, then the staff.

What in the World Are All Those Machines?

Your baby will not have all of them. On the other hand, if she has some equipment we haven't mentioned, just ask your baby's nurse what it is and what it's there for.

Your baby's bed

Most preemies spend the first few hours or days on a special open bed under a device called a radiant warmer. The radiant warmer heats up the air around the baby and keeps her at a stable, healthy temperature. (Newborn preemies can't maintain their temperature well on their own.) A sensor taped to the baby's skin (usually on her belly) monitors her body temperature and adjusts the heat accordingly.

Once a preemie's vital signs have stabilized and she needs less constant medical attention, she may be moved to a new home: a transparent plexiglass box called an isolette. This is the modern form of what you probably know as an incubator.

The isolette is fully enclosed, protecting your baby from sudden shifts in air temperature. Most of the simple things that the doctors or nurses now need to do for the baby can be done by inserting their hands through the round portholes on the isolette's sides or on other models by partially sliding up the sides.

The isolette has a heating system, too. In some cases it is connected to a sensor on the baby's skin; the heating regulates itself according to the baby's temperature. In other cases, a fixed temperature is maintained inside the incubator. Some isolettes are also humidified so that the air inside doesn't get too dry. The isolette's front wall can be unlatched and opened easily so that you or the nurses can take your baby out. Soon you will learn how to do this yourself for feedings and diaper changes and to hold your baby.

Cardiorespiratory monitor

This machine is one of the most intrusive but also one of the most important. Your preemie probably will be attached to it as long as she remains in the NICU. The cardiorespiratory monitor keeps constant track of her heartbeat and breathing. It does this with three leads, or sensors, that stick on your baby's skin and attach with wires to the monitor. These leads—two on her chest and one on her leg or belly—count the number of breaths she takes each minute and measure her pulse, or number of heartbeats each minute. Both numbers are displayed prominently on the monitor's screen along with a graph of her breathing and heartbeat.

A preemie's pulse normally ranges from 120 to 160 beats a minute and breathing from 30 to 60 breaths a minute. The monitor sounds a loud, beeping alarm if either one strays too far outside of the normal range. (How far is "too far" will vary for preemies of different ages and with different medical conditions. Your baby's doctors and nurses will decide what's appropriate for him and program the alarms accordingly.) Very often a baby's own movements will displace the leads or cause false alarms—so try not to be terrified every time you hear the alarm go off. Nurses are trained to look at both your baby and the machine's readings to see if something is actually wrong. If the baby is pink and healthy-looking or wiggling around, they know it's a false alarm.

When there really is some irregularity, it may be an episode of bradycardia (a slow heartbeat) or apnea (a pause in breathing). You can read what these episodes mean and why they are common for preemies on pages 246–249.

Blood pressure monitor

If you see a small inflatable band wrapped around your baby's arm or leg, it is probably a blood pressure cuff (just a miniature version of the cuff used to measure blood pressure in adults). The nurses take a preemie's blood pressure several times a day, using a machine that can pick up heartbeats too soft to hear even through a stethoscope.

Another way to measure blood pressure is through a catheter in an artery. These blood pressure measurements are taken continuously and are displayed graphically on the monitor along with your baby's heart rate and breathing.

Pulse oximeter and carbon dioxide monitor

The amounts of oxygen and carbon dioxide in a baby's blood are important indicators of whether she needs help with her breathing. So your baby may have yet more monitors to keep track of these.

Most preemies will have a pulse oximeter, at least initially. This is another machine that requires a sensor on their skin, attached to a lead. (That's five leads so far—lots of wires!) This one, usually taped on the baby's hand or foot, measures the amount of oxygen circulating in her blood. The oximeter relies on a special red light inside the sensor; the light shines through the baby's skin and indicates how much oxygen is being carried by the blood underneath. One hundred percent means the blood is fully loaded with oxygen. The monitor's screen displays the preemie's oxygen saturation level (or "O_2 sat" in NICU parlance), and a beeping alarm is set off if it is too high or too low. (Believe it or not, doctors still don't know the optimal range for a premature baby's oxygen saturation, because too much oxygen can damage a preemie's delicate organs as much as too little can. Most NICUs aim for O_2 sats in the 88 percent to 97 percent range when preemies are getting supplemental oxygen. Once a preemie is off oxygen and just breathing room air, her O_2 sats will naturally rise as her lungs mature, and only then will the doctors allow her to consistently saturate at 100 percent.)

In order for the pulse oximeter to measure the oxygen in your baby's blood accurately, it has to pick up her heart rate. So anything that interferes with that—like something as simple as the baby moving around—can set off a false alarm.

The most common kind of carbon dioxide monitor is called a transcutaneous (meaning across-the-skin) monitor. A tiny plastic cup sits on your baby's skin and warms the area underneath it; the machine measures how much carbon dioxide diffuses from small blood vessels into the warm skin. Don't be surprised if the warmth from the cup leaves a small red mark on your baby's sensitive skin. The nurses or respiratory therapists will move the cup every few hours, before it causes a burn (or discomfort to the baby), and the red spots will fade within an hour or so.

These skin-based measurements aren't as accurate as measuring your baby's "blood gases" directly from a sample of her blood, but they can reduce the amount of blood the nurses have to take from your baby and can give up-to-the-minute information on her breathing status.

Intravenous lines and other catheters

Intravenous lines, or IVs as they're familiarly called, are common sights in all hospital patients, but it's still jarring to see them in the tiny hands, feet, arms, or legs of babies. Yet they're an essential part of your preemie's care. If you also notice a splint on your baby's arm or leg, don't worry: It's probably not because she broke something. Splints are sometimes used to keep these lines from being accidentally knocked out of place.

IVs—tiny tubes called catheters placed in veins to deliver liquids into the bloodstream—are used to sustain most premature babies during their first days in the NICU when they can't take all of the nourishment and medications they need by mouth. If your baby is very premature or has an infection, she may need an IV for longer. Many babies will have more than one IV line, because some medications can't be mixed together.

Because younger newborn preemies or those with breathing problems need to have blood taken frequently to make sure their blood gases, blood sugar, and other substances are at healthy levels, they may have an additional line—this one running into an artery. Arterial lines can do double duty: They are used to painlessly withdraw blood and to continuously monitor a baby's blood pressure.

For reaching an artery or vein, newborns have one great spot that the rest of us don't: the umbilical cord, still attached to their belly button. Not only are umbilical catheters painless to put in (there are no nerves in the umbilical cord), they go into major blood vessels. So an umbilical cath-

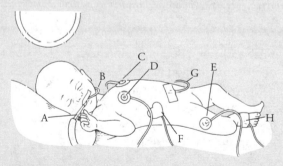

Tubes and leads attaching a premature baby to medical equipment. A: Breathing tube, connecting a baby to a ventilator; B: Feeding tube; C, D, E: Cardiorespiratory monitor leads, measuring heart rate and breathing; F: Temperature probe; G: Umbilical catheter, for fluid, medication, and drawing blood; H: Pulse oximeter probe, measuring oxygen saturation.

eter can deliver high concentrations of nutrients or medications that would irritate more delicate superficial veins.

Your baby will probably have one or two poles and pumps next to her bed holding bags of fluid or syringes of medication connected by clear plastic tubing to the catheters in her veins. The nurses will program the pumps to dole out medication in tiny increments so that it goes in slowly and gently and gives her exactly the right amount.

As your baby gets older and healthier, one by one these pumps will disappear and the lines will be taken out, until the happy day when she's free of them!

Feeding tubes

Preemies who are too young to breastfeed or drink from a bottle may get milk through a thin soft tube that is inserted in their nose or mouth and goes down into their stomach. This method is called gavage feeding. The gavage tube is very quick and easy to put in, and most preemies seem hardly to notice that it is there at all.

The ventilator, CPAP, and other breathing aids

The ventilator, also known as a respirator, is one of the most important machines in the NICU. Basically, it's a mechanical breathing machine. If your baby is not ready to breathe completely on her own yet, the ventilator will give her the extra breaths she needs until she's ready to take over.

When a baby is put on a ventilator, a small tube (called an endotracheal, or ET, tube) is inserted through her mouth or nose into her windpipe so that air can be sent directly to her lungs. It is secured by tape to her face. The ET tube is attached to bigger tubes, which are attached to the ventilator, a box on legs that stands next to your baby's bed. The doctors can set the ventilator to help a baby's breathing in various different ways: It can boost all or some of a baby's own breaths; it can give a certain number of extra breaths each minute; it can deliver a measured volume of air or provide a certain amount of force for each breath (enough pressure to keep the air sacs in the lungs open); and it can give varying amounts of oxygen (ranging from 21 percent—the amount of oxygen in normal room air—to as high as 100 percent, or pure oxygen). Some kinds of ventilators don't give a distinct number of breaths at all but oscillate the air in and out of a baby's lungs (a bit loudly, unfortunately). Babies on these "high frequency" vents look like they're jiggling rather than breathing deeply.

Don't assume that the ventilator is doing all of the breathing for your baby. It's far more common for the machine to be supplementing a baby's own natural breathing. For example, the ventilator might give your baby 30 breaths a minute while she takes another 30 of her own breaths in between. The ventilator may deepen or lengthen a baby's own shallower or shorter breaths. As she needs less and less help with her breathing, the doctors will gradually lower the settings on the ventilator. Finally, she will be extubated. (Some NICU language you're likely to hear: When a baby is put on a ventilator and the ET tube is put in, she is said to be "intubated"; when she is taken off the ventilator and the tube is taken out, she is said to be "extubated.")

This is a big moment in more ways than one. While a baby is intubated, the tube blocks her vocal cords and you can't hear her cry. So, many parents will now hear their baby cry for the first time since the delivery room. Let parents of full-term babies complain; for mothers and fathers of just extubated preemies, those cries are precious, sweet sounds!

CPAP

If a baby doesn't need all the help a ventilator can provide yet isn't quite ready to breathe completely on her own, she may be wearing prongs in her nose. The prongs are a way to give her something called CPAP. (Pronounced "SEE-pap," it's short for continuous positive airway pressure.) Translation: Your baby takes every breath by herself, but the air coming through the prongs—usually mixed with extra oxygen—flows into her airway under pressure and the pressure is maintained even when she exhales. That helps hold her airways and air sacs open, keeping them from collapsing after each breath. Various devices can deliver CPAP: Some look like small boxes, others like containers of bubbling fluid. A ventilator can also be programmed to give CPAP. Sometimes the prongs are replaced by a soft plastic mask over a baby's nose and mouth called a CPAP pillow.

Oxygen

Babies with mild respiratory problems—those who can breathe entirely on their own and just need some extra oxygen—may be given a set of smaller prongs, called a nasal cannula. Oxygen flows through the prongs into a baby's nose at a rate that can be turned up or down. When the rate is very high (referred to as "high flow"), there is enough pressure to hold the airways open and act like CPAP. The percentage of oxygen a baby actually gets through a nasal cannula isn't accurately measured because the oxygen flowing through the prongs mixes to varying degrees with the room air in her nose and mouth as she inhales. When doctors want to know precisely how much oxygen a baby is getting, they can use an oxygen hood. This big, clear plastic box may cover your baby's bed or fit snugly around his head. It may look bulky and not very pretty to you, but with warm, moist oxygen flowing into it, it can feel awfully cozy to a newborn.

The Professionals Caring for Your Baby

It's not just the machines that can seem overwhelming when you enter the NICU for the first time. It's also the staff: medical professionals everywhere, rushing around, all unfamiliar faces.

It's natural to feel anxiety about all of these people who are responsible for the health and comfort of your child. But be assured of one thing: The people on the staff of a neonatal intensive care unit are exactly who should be taking care of your premature baby right now. They all have specific areas of expertise and specialized jobs to do, and they work as a team to provide complete care for the youngest and tiniest, and oldest and plumpest, preemies. Within a few days, you'll know who the key players are and what they do for your baby. After a week or so, if your baby is still in the hospital, you'll probably feel more at home in the NICU—or if not quite at home, at least like part of the extended family.

Right now, though, you need some introductions. Keep in mind that not all NICUs are the same. Here are some staff descriptions that usually apply:

Neonatologist

The doctor who is primarily responsible for making medical decisions for your baby is called a neonatologist. Neonatologists have highly specialized training—at least five years beyond medical school—in pediatrics and in newborn intensive care. The neonatologist examines and makes a treatment plan for every infant in his care every day and supervises the rest of the medical staff in the nursery. You'll get to know your baby's neonatologist as he keeps you informed and answers your questions.

Neonatal fellows and residents

In teaching hospitals, there are often neonatal fellows: physicians who are already trained in pediatrics and are currently doing further training in newborn intensive care. (They will soon be neonatologists.) There are also residents: physicians who have completed medical school and are learning pediatrics. First-year residents are called interns. The neonatologist supervises the fellow, who supervises the residents. In most intensive care nurseries, at least one of these physicians or a nurse practitioner (see below) is in the unit 24 hours a day.

Neonatal nurse practitioner

A neonatal nurse practitioner is a neonatal nurse who has received advanced training so that he or she can perform many of the same tasks as a doctor. Neonatal nurse practitioners (or NNPs, as you might hear them called) prescribe medication, do medical procedures (such as putting in central intravenous lines), and help decide on your baby's treatment plan, among other things. If you have a medical question and a neonatologist isn't around, try the nurse practitioner.

Bedside nurse

The nurse is a very important person to your baby; one is by her bedside at all times, feeding her, weighing her, changing her diaper, giving her the medications prescribed by the doctors, responding to her cries, and keeping a constant eye on her and the machines. Neonatal nurses have specialized training in newborn intensive care,

too, and the doctors rely on their observations of how your baby is doing. You'll also learn to rely on them to teach you how to care for a premature baby and to take your calls asking for progress reports any time of the day or night.

Respiratory therapist

Many NICUs have respiratory therapists who are expert in handling the ventilators and other equipment that support your baby's breathing.

Social worker

Having a baby in an intensive care unit can be stressful, expensive, and a logistical challenge. Social workers are there when you need them to find resources and help you cope. Social workers can offer counseling or support groups and are the ones to consult for practical tips and financial matters, such as where to stay if you live far from the hospital, how to apply for financial aid, and how to get the community services you need after your baby's homecoming. An increasing number of NICUs also have a family support specialist from the March of Dimes to help you with these and other family-related issues and to connect you to other NICU parents who share some of your feelings and experiences.

Chaplain

For most of the members of the NICU team, your baby is the patient and her care is their primary concern. For the chaplain, your well-being is the primary concern. The chaplain's job is to help you with the powerful, confusing, and sometimes overwhelming emotional and spiritual aspects of your experience, through deep discussion and, if you want, prayer. They can also baptize your baby or lead a service at your baby's bedside. Don't dismiss the chaplain out of hand, even if you're not religious. Chaplains are trained to counsel and support patients and their families through critical illness, and they have much to offer that goes beyond religion.

There are many other physicians and professionals who may care for your baby at one point or another. We'll introduce you to them at later points in the book. But in the meantime, if you meet someone and want to know what he's doing, feel free to ask.

Baby's Twitches

My baby makes the strangest jittery movements. I'm afraid there's something wrong with his nervous system.

Remember those twitches you used to feel inside your pregnant belly? Now you're getting a glimpse of what your baby was doing to cause those tickling sensations! You didn't worry then, and you needn't worry now. Your baby's nervous system is probably functioning just as it should at this stage—which is to say, immaturely.

A baby's motor activity follows a predictable pattern of development as his nervous system and muscles mature. The earliest movements start just seven weeks after conception (though the mother doesn't feel them until later); complex movements, like putting his thumb in his mouth or reaching and grasping the umbilical cord, can be seen by 24 weeks. From 28 to 32 weeks, a preemie still has very little control, and his movements are expected to be uncoordinated and sudden, with lots of tremors and twitches. Sometimes you'll see jerky, flailing movements; other times you might see writhing or twisting.

Chances are that you'll get so used to seeing these movements you'll start thinking of them as normal, which they are! But if you have any questions, ask your baby's nurses, who are trained to distinguish a preemie's normal movements from abnormal ones that could indicate a medical problem. They can also tell you if your baby's movements are unusually frantic or diffuse, a sign of stress that often can be alleviated by holding the baby's arms and legs close to his body or swaddling him nice and tightly in a blanket.

Is Your Baby Sick or Just Immature?

There's something really basic I don't understand. The doctors keep talking about things like lung disease. Is my premature baby sick or just immature?

That's something that confuses many parents. The reason is that a premature baby can be either one, and doctors don't always make a clear distinction between the two. No wonder it isn't obvious to parents.

Some preemies are perfectly healthy, just immature. They're developing normally, but outside the womb rather than inside. But many newborn preemies (especially the younger ones) are sick or become sick at some point during their hospitalization, since being born early puts an infant at higher risk for certain illnesses.

How can you tell whether your baby is healthy or sick? Either way he'll have lots of wires and tubes attached to him, since even a healthy preemie has many bodily systems that are immature and not up to functioning on their own yet. Here's the way the experts look at it. Neonatologists consider a preemie sick if 1) he has medical problems caused by something other than simply being born too soon, or 2) his medical problems, although typical in premature babies, are unusually severe or have caused complications.

The most common problems stemming simply from immaturity—so even healthy preemies have to deal with them—are:

* **Fluid loss.** The youngest, tiniest preemies have skin that is thinner than a full-term baby's so it doesn't hold in water well and they can easily become dehydrated. But luckily, skin matures quickly after birth. For the first three or four days, a tiny preemie's bed may be wrapped in plastic to help keep moisture from escaping. After that, significant fluid loss is rarely a problem, and by two or three weeks, a premature infant's skin resembles a full-term baby's.

* **Inability to maintain body temperature.** With little fat for insulation, a large external surface area for their size (from which to lose heat), and brains that aren't fully ready to regulate body temperature, premature babies can't maintain their temperature on their own until about the 34th week of gestation. So they're kept in special heated environments: isolettes or radiant warming beds.

* **Apnea.** Because their respiratory and nervous systems are immature, preemies have different breathing patterns from full-term babies: They breathe irregularly and often stop for brief intervals. When a baby doesn't take a breath for 20 seconds or longer, it's called apnea. Various illnesses can cause apnea, but the version due to simple immaturity is called apnea of prematurity. Mild apnea of prematurity may be treated with just a tickle on the foot to stimulate breathing when necessary, or it may require more heavy-duty breathing aids, like a ventilator. As the nervous and respiratory systems mature, apnea of prematurity gradually disappears, usually by around 36 weeks of gestation.

* **Inability to feed.** Easy as they appear, eating and digesting are actually incredibly complicated processes. The stomach and intestines of very young preemies are not ready to digest all of the food they need, so most premature babies get some of their nutrition intravenously at first. Even when they can handle digestion, preemies younger than 32 to 34 weeks of gestation are still not ready to nurse from a breast or bottle because their sucking and swallowing reflexes are poorly coordinated. In the meantime, they are fed through a small feeding tube that runs from their mouth or nose into their stomach.

On the other hand, the ailments that most frequently make preemies sick on the first day are:

* **Lung disease, or respiratory distress syndrome.** It's very common for a preemie's immature lungs to make breathing difficult and cause an illness called respiratory distress syndrome, or RDS for short. The earlier a preemie is born, the more likely he is to have it. If the breathing problems are moderate to severe, he may need the help of a ventilator.

* **Infection.** The most common cause of premature labor and delivery is an infection in the pregnant mother's birth canal or amniotic fluid. If the germs spread to the fetus, he'll be born with an infection. Premature babies are especially susceptible to infection because they have immature immune systems. And since their infection-fighting capacity is easily overwhelmed, instead of getting mild, localized infections—say, in the ear or throat—they tend to get general or deep infections, like sepsis (an infection of the blood), meningitis (an infection of the fluid around the brain and spinal cord), or pneumonia. Chances are, your preemie will be tested at birth with blood cultures, a chest X-ray, and maybe other tests to see if he has an infection. Because the symptoms of infection can be hard to distinguish from problems due to simple immaturity, many premature babies are treated with antibiotics for a couple of days after delivery until the doctors are sure that they are not needed.

(Continued on page 113)

In Plain Language:
What Is Respiratory Distress Syndrome?

A premature baby's first—and often biggest—challenge couldn't be more basic: breathing. Mother Nature has programmed the lungs to be mature and fully functioning after around 35 to 36 weeks of gestation. What happens if a baby is born before that? Some preemies are lucky; for a variety of reasons, their lungs happen to mature earlier, so although they are young they are able to breathe successfully on their own. Other babies, whose lungs develop on or behind nature's usual schedule, develop respiratory distress syndrome, or RDS, the most common illness in the intensive care nursery. (You may also see it called hyaline membrane disease.)

RDS can range from mild to very severe. If a baby's case is mild, it will be no more than a bump on the road toward his hospital discharge. If it is severe, it can make that road a rough one. Fortunately, neonatologists have excellent success treating RDS nowadays. More than 99 percent of babies with RDS survive; those who don't tend to be the very youngest and smallest preemies.

Here's a simple description of RDS. In the tiny air sacs of the lungs, there's a foamy substance called surfactant. This substance—which is lacking in preemies with RDS—is crucial to the breathing process. When there's a lot of it lining the air sacs (or alveoli, as they are called), the sacs remain open and air slips easily in and out. When the air sacs don't have enough surfactant, they collapse between breaths. As a result, the lungs aren't as efficient at taking in oxygen or getting rid of carbon dioxide.

Picture the lungs as balloons. Blowing up a brand-new uninflated balloon is hard work, but once the balloon has expanded, adding air to it is easy. Similarly, a baby's first breath requires tremendous exertion as he opens the air sacs for the first time. If the air sacs remain expanded, it's easy to inhale after that. But the air sacs of a baby with RDS collapse between breaths, making subsequent breaths as difficult as the first one. So babies with RDS have to work very hard to breathe, and they can sometimes tire out if they don't get assistance.

The earlier a baby is born, the more likely he is to develop RDS and the more severe it is likely to be. Usually, surfactant starts appearing at around 24 weeks of gestation and gradually builds up to its full level by 34 to 36 weeks. (Before 28 weeks, the alveoli themselves have barely developed, so nearly every baby born before 28 weeks has RDS.)

What makes some preemies in each age group luckier than others? As with all medical conditions that affect some people but not others, we have only partial explanations; the rest we chalk up to the mysteries of individual differences. Here are some factors that play a role:

* In general, the bigger the baby the lower his risk. That's because size and maturity often go hand in hand.
* Boys are more likely to get RDS than girls because their lungs mature more slowly.
* Preemies with diabetic mothers and those with Rh blood-type incompatibilities are especially susceptible because the babies' lungs are slower to produce surfactant.
* If a preemie was under some stress in the womb—for example, from episodes of preterm labor—he is less likely to be susceptible to RDS. The body has a self-protective mechanism: When a fetus is under stress, it's as if his

body knows that he has to prepare for an early delivery and his lung development accelerates.

* On the other hand, if the stress was extreme—say the mother had severe preeclampsia or the baby became infected after his mother's membranes ruptured—the baby is more vulnerable to RDS because of disruption to his normal lung development and functioning.

* Babies whose mothers received steroid injections at least 24 hours before delivery are less vulnerable than those whose mothers didn't. Steroids (hormones that the body produces naturally in response to stress) speed up the maturation of the lungs, as if the baby had spent more time—according to estimates, an extra week—in the womb. For preemies born between 28 and 34 weeks of gestation, research shows that steroids reduce the incidence of RDS. For preemies born earlier, steroids may not reduce the incidence of RDS but may reduce its severity.

* Preemies delivered by C-section, particularly if delivered electively without labor, are at greater risk than those delivered vaginally. That's because substances produced during labor promote lung maturation and help remove some excess fluid that collects in a baby's lungs while he's in the womb.

* Interestingly, although you may hear people talk about older studies that found that black babies were less likely to get RDS than white babies, more recent studies have not found race to make a difference.

Does your baby have RDS?

There's no single easy test for RDS, like X-rays are for broken bones. To make a diagnosis, the doctor assesses your baby's breath sounds and behavior as he breathes, the levels of oxygen and carbon dioxide in his blood, and the look of his lungs on a chest X-ray. Then the doctor carefully moni-

tors how all of these things change with time and treatment. If your baby was given a lung maturity test before birth and his lungs were found to be mature, the doctor will take that into account, too; any signs he sees that seem to be due to RDS are more likely to have another explanation.

What are some of the signs of RDS? Because breathing is hard for him, a baby with RDS may suck in his ribs and chest deeply with each breath (these are called retractions) and grunt or moan as he exhales. His nostrils may flare, and he may breathe rapidly. Rather than a healthy pink he may be dusky or bluish in color. And he may get tired: His breathing may become shallow and less regular, and he may have episodes of apnea, during which he stops breathing altogether.

On X-rays, his lungs will look small rather than fully expanded, with less air in them than usual. And in his blood, he'll have too little oxygen and too much carbon dioxide.

The course that RDS takes

Most babies who are going to get RDS show signs of it right away, in the delivery room or within a few hours after birth. Occasionally, a preemie will seem fine at first, only to have the symptoms slink up on him gradually. If your preemie has no symptoms of RDS after a day has gone by, you can relax. He doesn't have it.

RDS often gets worse for two or three days before it gets better. That's expected, and though it's normal for parents to worry, you should try not to. After around 48 hours, your baby will start to produce more surfactant and his lungs should gradually recover. A good sign that he's recovering is that he'll urinate more as the fluid clears from his lungs and the rest of his body, and—of course—his breathing will get easier and easier.

A baby with mild RDS, who needs just a little assistance from CPAP (see below) or a ventilator, may be breathing entirely on his own within a few days. A baby with a very severe case (one who was born extremely early or who developed complications) will take much longer—several weeks, months, or in rare cases a year or two—to recover fully. If your baby is in this situation, try hard to take things day by day.

The wonders of modern treatment

The only cure for RDS is time. Treatment focuses on buying babies the time they need by providing breathing assistance and giving them replacement surfactant until they can produce their own.

There are different levels of breathing assistance. If your baby has RDS, at a minimum he'll need extra oxygen. If that's all he needs, his RDS is mild. Either he'll be given a little set of nasal prongs called a nasal cannula through which oxygen flows, or he'll be placed under a plastic oxygen hood. (You'll find descriptions of all the respiratory equipment and how it works in *Through the Doors of a Neonatal Intensive Care Unit*, page 101.)

If your baby's illness is a little worse and he needs more help keeping his air sacs open, he'll get a slightly bulkier set of prongs that delivers something called CPAP. On CPAP, your baby will take all his own breaths but a mixture of air and oxygen will flow into his lungs under pressure to keep them from collapsing when he exhales.

If your baby has a severe case of RDS or is extremely premature, it will be too tiring for him to take all his own breaths. He'll be put on a ventilator, which can do some breathing for him. The doctors will decide what kind of ventilator is best for him and how to set it: how many extra breaths your baby needs to supplement his own natural ones; how deep and long each breath should be; how much force, or pressure, the vent should deliver to get and keep the air sacs open; and how much oxygen should be mixed in. Once your baby's condition stabilizes, the doctors will try to gradually reduce the settings. The goal is to

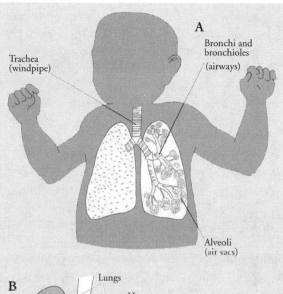

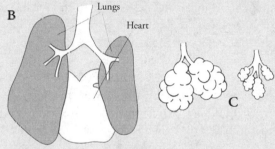

A: Airways, lungs, and detail of air sacs in the lung.
B: On the left, a lung without RDS is fully inflated. On the right, a lung with RDS does not fully inflate.
C: On the left, air sacs with surfactant remain expanded; on the right, air sacs that lack surfactant collapse.

have your baby do as much of his own breathing as possible, as soon as possible.

There are certain unfortunate things about ventilators. First of all, a baby has to be intubated—that is, an endotracheal (or ET) tube has to be inserted through his mouth or nose and down his windpipe (trachea) so that the ventilator can send air into his lungs. Some babies don't mind this tube; others who seem uncomfortable may be given sedatives or pain medication. Second, the ventilator itself can do some damage. Applying forceful pressure or inflating a preemie's delicate lungs too much can cause small tears and scarring and interfere with the lungs' development, and it takes a while for them to recover. There is a further risk of secondary complications, described below. As frightening as these things are, they are a necessary (and for most babies, a small) price to pay for the life-saving help a ventilator provides.

One positive thing about intubation: It allows a baby to receive replacement surfactant. A dose of it is sent down the ET tube, and within minutes to hours, it coats a baby's air sacs enough to significantly lessen the RDS, increasing his chances of survival and making secondary complications less likely. In fact, some neonatologists give surfactant in the delivery room to all babies who are likely to get RDS in hopes of preventing the disease, even though some of those babies won't need it and will never be connected to a ventilator. Once the surfactant is in, the ET tube can be removed if the baby is breathing adequately. Other neonatologists, who don't want to intubate any babies unnecessarily, wait until symptoms of RDS appear.

If your baby has RDS and is extremely premature, he probably will be given shots of vitamin A every few days; it helps lower the risk of longer-lasting breathing problems. For the same reason, some preemies may be given nitric oxide gas, a substance naturally produced by the human body, to inhale through the ventilator. Nitric oxide (different from nitrous oxide, or laughing gas, which is an anesthetic) relaxes the blood vessels carrying oxygen in a baby's lungs, and may decrease inflammation. Some studies, but not all, have found that inhaled nitric oxide may help certain preemies with RDS immediately, and may also lower their risk of developing persistent breathing problems. However, many experts feel there is not enough information yet to know how effective or safe nitric oxide really is for preemies and which babies with RDS can safely benefit from it. Feel free to ask the neonatologist whether your baby is getting this medication and for his views of the pros and cons.

Don't be surprised if your baby has ups and downs or if his progress is hard to predict; that's how RDS can go. Sometimes a baby on a ventilator can't handle a reduced setting on the first try and then does fine with it a day later. Basically, if your baby's ventilator settings are gradually coming down or if he is graduating from the ventilator to CPAP or from CPAP to oxygen alone, you know he is getting better.

Will your baby be OK?

It's natural for a parent whose baby has RDS to worry, but it's worth developing a realistic understanding of the risks—so you know what you're up against but don't suffer unnecessarily.

You already know that for all but the youngest and tiniest babies, the odds of surviving RDS are overwhelmingly good. Nonetheless, some babies—usually only those with severe RDS—may have to deal with some complications before they're discharged from the hospital, such as tears or bleeding in the lungs, or longer-term health problems, such as persistent breathing difficulties (known as bronchopulmonary dysplasia, or BPD), more frequent and severe respiratory infections in their first two years of life, and an increased likelihood of asthma. Fortunately, these complications affect only a small percentage of babies with RDS, and even the longer-term problems have usually successfully resolved before a child's second birthday. (Most are covered elsewhere in this book, but they're worth reading about only if they happen.)

What about long-term development? If your baby has a mild or moderate case of RDS, you shouldn't worry, because RDS by itself does not affect neurologic development. However, babies who are very sick with RDS are more likely to develop other medical conditions—such as an intraventricular hemorrhage or periventricular leukomalacia, retinopathy of prematurity, or BPD—that may be associated with developmental problems. Again, please don't worry about these unless your baby gets them—because most babies never will.

If you possibly can, keep in mind that most babies recover just fine—and in just a few days or weeks, they leave their RDS behind.

---

* **Intraventricular hemorrhage (IVH).** Some blood vessels in the brain are still fragile in a premature baby. The younger and smaller the baby, the more common it is for these blood vessels to rupture, usually within the first week of life. Doctors don't worry about very small intraventricular hemorrhages; they usually don't cause symptoms or serious long-term problems. But a baby with a larger bleed (diagnosed on a head ultrasound or MRI scan) would be considered sick and would be watched carefully to see if complications develop. Babies with large intraventricular hemorrhages tend to have breathing and blood pressure problems that are more severe than expected, and may need several medications and blood transfusions to keep them stable.

* **Major birth defects.** The vast majority of preemies have no such abnormalities. Your baby's doctors will tell you if your baby has any birth defects that are noticeable or affect his internal organs. Most will be picked up on prenatal ultrasound, the doctor's initial physical exam, or investigations of symptoms within the first week of a baby's life. Nearly all will be apparent by the time a baby is a few months old.

(All of these problems are described in more detail elsewhere in the book for you to read about if your baby has one of them. You'll find them listed in the index.)

Why does the distinction between immaturity and illness even matter? Because illness makes a baby's progress less predictable and a little slower than if there were no such hurdle to contend with. Either way, it's undoubtedly very hard on you. No parent can bear seeing their child uncomfortable—for any reason.

Why do some premature babies get sick while others don't? It's no easier to answer that question than to say why some toddlers get more colds than others or why some adults develop arthritis before their friends do. Risk factors such as lower birth weight, exposure to certain bacteria, or genetic predisposition are part of the equation, but they never tell the whole story. Even in twins one baby is often healthier than the other even though they both came out of the same womb at the same time. Just remember that all preemies have ups and downs on their way from birth day to going-home day—and that most of them, whether they started out healthy or sick, end up doing just fine.

Understanding the Doctors

I feel really stupid when I talk to doctors. A lot of times I just don't understand what they're talking about, or a half hour later I can't remember things they said.

You may be surprised to hear it, but the exact same thing happens to the vast majority of preemies' parents—even to those who are physicians themselves!

When a baby is born prematurely, his family is hurtled into a complex world of medical terms and devices that are familiar only to specialists.

Parents want to understand what is happening, but emotional turmoil makes it difficult for them to concentrate—especially on explanations that they dread may contain bad news. They sit quietly and listen to every word the doctor says, but with so much going on in their minds and hearts, they can scarcely remember the words a few minutes later.

It's important to realize that the doctors understand this well, so they expect you to ask the same questions as many times as you need to. Don't ever hesitate to request another—perhaps clearer—explanation. Sometimes doctors don't realize when they're using medical jargon, and if asked, they can rephrase things in a way that makes more sense to you. Some doctors will always be warm and reassuring, while others may seem impatient, but that has to do with differences in their temperament or mood, not with the appropriateness of your behavior.

If you think you're dealing with a doctor who is a poor communicator, don't hesitate to rely on the nurses in the NICU. They're very knowledgeable and can be great translators of medical information for parents. If you continue to have trouble understanding your doctor, you may want to consider kindly telling him so. Or ask to speak to a different physician or a nurse practitioner, whose communication skills might be more in tune with your needs.

Questions: Whom to Ask

I'm confused. I have questions about my baby, but I don't know which questions I'm supposed to ask the doctors and which I should ask the nurses.

On your baby's first day of life, the neonatologist taking care of her probably will talk with you at length, giving you a detailed picture of her health so far, and describing future developments you can reasonably expect at this point. Throughout your baby's hospitalization, her doctors will keep you informed of your baby's condition on a regular basis and will discuss significant new medical issues with you when they arise.

When you're with the doctors, ask any questions that come to mind. Some parents hold back, afraid that their questions are inappropriate or trivial. Every question is appropriate—and those you don't ask can make you feel frustrated or worried. Don't be inhibited by the fact that you don't know the medical terms. Few parents do.

What if you have questions at other times? Here are some rules of thumb.

The neonatologist is the one who determines what procedures and treatments your baby receives and when.

Ask the doctor if:
* You want to understand why a medical test is being done or what its results are.
* You want help understanding medical findings and putting them in perspective—whether the results are good or bad, serious or not serious.
* You are wondering why a particular treatment was chosen for your baby.
* You want to know whether something you've seen or heard about elsewhere might apply to your baby.
* You would like an overview of how your baby is doing and what the implications are for her long-term health.

While the doctors usually check on each baby only intermittently throughout the day, the eyes and ears of your baby's bedside nurses are constantly on her. It is from the nurses that the doctors get much of their information on your baby's breathing, feeding, sleeping, and crying patterns, as well as her daily weight gain, temperature, and signs of stress or well-being. All of this information is available to you, also; just ask.

(Continued on page 116)

Telephone Calls to the NICU: Do's and Don'ts

1 **DO** ask if there are any restrictions on when you can call. In many NICUs, phone calls from parents are welcomed by the nurses 24 hours a day. During the doctors' shifts (when they are not busy seeing patients), they are also available to talk to parents on the phone, with or without an appointment. This accommodating policy is intended to allow parents of preemies to stay constantly in touch with how their babies are doing.

2. **DON'T** be afraid of calling your baby's nurse for an update, even when you have nothing specific to ask. The nurses realize that parents want to feel connected even when they cannot visit, and the staff of the NICU encourages that. Talking to parents on the telephone as well as in person is an important part of the nurses' job. In fact, you'll find they are experienced at it. They understand the anxiety that parents feel as they dial the NICU's number, fearful of hearing bad news. They know how to start the conversation with reassuring words and to be forthcoming about your baby's condition.

3. **DON'T** be afraid of calling too often. There's almost no such thing. It's common for parents to check on their babies once or twice a day, by telephone or in person. Unless you're calling more than once per nurse's shift (about eight to twelve hours in most NICUs) about a baby who is stable and doing well or your phone calls last more than five or ten minutes, no reasonable nurse is going to find it inappropriate. If your baby is sick, everyone will understand if you want to call more often. It will help if you show that you're considerate of the NICU staff's time and realize that they have other obligations, also.

4. **DON'T** be offended or assume there's a personal reason if your baby's doctor or nurse can't come to the phone when you call. They may not be able to break away from what they're doing at the moment or may have stepped out of the nursery for a short time. **DO** feel free to call back or to leave your number and a message so they know to get back to you when they get a chance.

5. **DO** schedule a call with the doctor or nurse in advance if you think it will take a long time, or ask them to call you back when they're free to talk. (You should also consider whether a face-to-face conversation would be more helpful. You can always request a sit-down meeting with your baby's doctor to discuss complicated issues.) In general, staff members will appreciate your asking whether they're free to talk now or would prefer a call later.

6. **DON'T** encourage grandparents, aunts and uncles, or close friends to call. Information on babies is given only to parents, not to other callers, unless parents give their permission. If you really want Grandma to hear something directly from the nurse or doctor instead of from you, you can ask one of them to call her, but do this only if you feel it's very important, and don't do it more than once or twice. The reasoning: When doctors and nurses talk to too many people it can cause confusion and

misconceptions; parents should decide what they want to tell others and nurses and doctors should save their precious communication time for moms and dads, who need all of the attention and support possible during their baby's hospitalization. Repeating information

isn't a good use of the doctors' and nurses' time when they'd otherwise be with the babies. (An exception is when someone is designated as a regular stand-in for a parent—a grandmother who lives with the single mother of a baby in the NICU, for instance.)

Ask the nurse who is on shift if:
* You would like an up-to-the minute report on how your baby is doing and what has happened since your last visit to the NICU.
* You want to learn how to touch, handle, feed, or bathe your baby, either early in her hospital stay so that you can be as involved as possible in her care in the hospital, or later on, to ease the transition from hospital to home.
* You want help interpreting your baby's signals: how to know when she's content, or mildly stressed and in the process of soothing herself, or highly stressed (see page 234).
* You would like to hold your baby or do kangaroo care (holding your baby skin-to-skin; see page 249).
* You need assistance in your first breastfeeding attempts or in providing breast milk to give to your baby later. The nurse can answer questions about pumping, storing, and transporting breast milk.
* You have questions about the NICU's policies or facilities, such as visiting hours, parent sleep rooms, available computers, cameras, or books.
* You want help understanding the doctor's words, perhaps because they weren't completely clear to you or just because you would like to hear them again.

What if you have a question that doesn't fall into these categories and you're still confused about whom to ask? Don't worry. There's no wrong question to ask anybody—really. Everyone in the NICU is committed to helping you and your baby, and if they can't answer your question, they'll find someone who will.

Is a Baby on a Ventilator in Pain?

My baby is on a ventilator, and with that tube going down her throat she must be in pain. Are they giving her pain medication?

It may seem basic, but how to best recognize and control pain is still a controversial issue in neonatology (see page 117). While there are well-tested tools for assessing when a preemie is feeling acute pain—for example, from an injection or a procedure such as intubation—research on the signs of ongoing or chronic pain is still in its infancy. There are wide variations in practice among NICUs and neonatologists, so only the doctors and nurses taking care of your baby can give you a straight answer on their approach.

Worrying that your child is in pain is agonizing for a parent. But it's pretty safe to assume that if your baby is on a ventilator, she either is not bothered by it much or she's been given medication to help her relax so she doesn't fight the machine and resist letting its breaths into her lungs. Although an endotracheal tube (the tube that goes down your baby's windpipe, connecting her to the ventilator) is a distressing sight, parents sometimes suffer more than their babies, who may be less uncomfortable than it appears.

(Continued on page 120)

Pain in Preemies and Ways to Control It

Parents in the intensive-care nursery, watching their babies undergoing all kinds of medical procedures, are often in agony with worry over whether their baby is feeling pain. They wonder how they can tell, and since their baby can't speak up and ask for relief, whether the doctors and nurses are careful enough in preventing pain and treating it.

Pain is one subject on which it's especially useful for you to be knowledgeable because experts still disagree on when and how to control pain in preemies. Everyone gives preemies anesthesia for major surgical procedures in the operating room, but routine procedures in the NICU, from intubation to insertion of IV lines, may or may not be performed with pain medication. Medical views and practices are changing rapidly as new research results appear.

If you learn how a premature baby shows that he is uncomfortable and understand a few basics about what can and cannot be done to treat pain in preemies, you will be able to ask questions and raise any concerns you may have. Most satisfyingly, you will be able to take over some of the tasks of comforting your baby yourself.

A little background

Before the 1970s, the medical community assumed that premature infants, who still have immature nervous systems, were unable to feel pain. As recently as the mid-1980s, anesthesia was not routinely used when newborns underwent surgery because doctors feared that its risks outweighed its benefits and they believed infants would have no memory of the pain later, anyway.

Thankfully, these beliefs have been over-turned. Widely accepted research shows that by the time even the youngest preemies are born at 22 or 23 weeks, their sensory nerve fibers are already abundant and connected to a part of the brain called the thalamus. Some scientists believe that a baby still cannot have a conscious experience of pain until a pathway that is formed and starts functioning later—close to 29 weeks—links the thalamus to the brain's cortex, the seat of awareness and consciousness. This pathway from the thalamus to the cortex is the route for the awareness of pain in older children and adults. But other researchers think that preemies may be aware of pain through other mechanisms, even before the pathway from the thalamus to the cortex is formed. In any event, this connection may be up and running earlier than was previously thought. A recent small study looked at blood flow in the brains of preemies as young as 25 weeks. When their heels were pricked to draw blood, even the youngest of these babies had a surge of blood and oxygen to the cortex, raising the possibility that they might already be conscious of feeling pain.

Researchers still know very little about the emotional experience of pain in a prematurely born baby, that is, the intensity and memory of pain, the fear of it, and what lingering effects it may have. They don't know, but are trying to learn, what preemies remember of their time in the NICU (see page 423).

Relieving discomfort is doubly important because research has shown that pain and other stress can impede a premature baby's recovery, growth, and development. Of particular concern is the effect that stress might have on the development of the brain at a very vulnerable time. The brain grows at an especially fast pace in late pregnancy and early infancy, at the time when most preemies are hospitalized.

How preemies show they are in pain

It's true, preemies cannot speak up and ask for relief. They may not be strong enough to flinch, let alone kick the doctor away when he pricks their foot. So preemies depend on their caregivers to interpret their cues that signal when they are in pain.

What are some of the cues your baby may give? There are five signals that comprise the premature infant pain profile (or PIPP), one of the most reliable, widely used tools by medical professionals to assess whether a preemie is feeling pain:

* His heart rate increases;
* The oxygen level in his blood declines;
* He squeezes his eyes shut;
* His brow bulges outward;
* The furrow between his nose and his lip deepens.

Two other factors that the PIPP takes into account are a baby's gestational age and behavioral state (whether, for example, he was active, quiet, or sleeping beforehand), since preemies who are younger or asleep tend to have less obvious reactions to a painful event.

Other signals that a premature baby may give when he's in pain are: His blood pressure may rise and his breathing become shallow, he may become agitated, move jerkily, stiffen his body, arch his back, or cry. Sometimes, however, especially if the pain lasts a while, a preemie may do the opposite—become drowsy, lethargic, and passive; lose his muscle tone; and turn pale.

Please keep in mind that preemies can show the same behavioral changes when they're simply upset and irritable. Based on the medical context

and their experience, your baby's doctors and nurses will do their best to judge when pain is the problem and step in to relieve it. If you have any concerns, don't hesitate to ask for their opinions or give them yours. And you should always feel free to ask about the options for relieving your baby's discomfort.

Nonmedical ways to treat preemies' discomfort

When a preemie is feeling minor pain, the first choice is always one of the highly effective nonmedical approaches to relief. That's because all medications—pain relief drugs included—have side effects that can be dangerous. Many pain-relieving drugs diminish the drive to breathe. Other common side effects include decreased blood pressure, injury to the kidney or liver, delayed blood clotting, and drowsiness that can interfere with learning. Some of these medications could possibly alter brain development. So doctors will try to give as little medication as possible to alleviate your baby's pain and help him relax.

Wonderfully, there are a number of natural ways to soothe preemies. Many have been put to the test in research studies, and doctors and nurses believe that they are all effective. So when your baby looks uncomfortable or is about to undergo one of the minor procedures that are so common in the intensive care nursery—a heel stick, suctioning, removing tape, or others—it's worth trying these. (If your baby's nurse doesn't suggest them, don't be reluctant to speak up and ask.)

* **Sugar water.** Dipping a baby's pacifier in sugar water or placing drops of sugar water right on his tongue has effects that are similar to (and sometimes better than) pain-relief drugs for mild or moderate pain. The most extensively studied of the nonmedical pain treatments,

sugar water works best when it is given two or three minutes before a painful procedure, and can be repeated during the procedure itself. It is even now packaged under the brand name Sweet-Ease, which you may see your nurse get before a procedure. Of course, just as you wouldn't give an older child too much sugar, you shouldn't give sugar water to your preemie willy-nilly, either. Think of it as a lollipop, given to your own sweetie on special occasions!

* **Sucking.** Sucking on a pacifier or nipple even without the sugar water reduces pain, and it's effective immediately. Keep in mind that active sucking is required, so the pain-reducing effect stops as soon as the baby stops sucking. Luckily, babies become accomplished at sucking early, even when they're still in the womb.

* **Skin-to-skin contact.** Being held snugly against your bare chest, so your baby's skin touches yours, is not just pleasurable for him; it also provides pain relief, according to clinical research studies. Both kangaroo care (which you can read about on page 249) and breast-feeding have significant effects beyond regular holding alone. Did you know your body had such magic powers?

* **Other touch and distraction.** Seemingly simple comfort measures, like being rocked rhythmically, being patted, stroked, or massaged—or for the youngest preemies who can't be held or stroked yet, hearing the sound of your voice or music, smelling your scent, being given one of your fingers to grasp in his hand, or just feeling the touch of your open hand against his back in a gentle but firm way—can all lessen a preemie's response to pain. Why do they work? One reason, experts think, is that when an infant's attention is focused on a distraction, his brain's pain processing areas are blocked or less active.

* **Positioning.** Swaddling a preemie in a blanket or containing him in a little nest by placing blanket rolls around him with his arms and legs flexed close to his body can reduce pain and help him return to sleep more quickly.

* **Environment.** Premature babies tend to become more agitated when there is a lot of light and noise. If you can lower both, you will help your baby relax and soothe himself.

You can try any of these therapies on its own, or you can combine them for an even greater effect. Engaging more areas of your baby's brain and saturating his sensory channels reduces the effect of the painful event even more.

Medications to treat pain and stress in preemies

When pain is moderate or severe, it's time for medications that can alleviate it. Both analgesics (drugs that relieve pain) and sedatives (drugs that calm and relax) are given to preemies. The need for them often overlaps. For example, sometimes calming a baby with a sedative makes it easier and therefore less painful to perform a medical procedure; sometimes alleviating pain makes a baby's agitation go away.

Pain management varies a lot from one NICU to the next. Here's a quick run-through of the most commonly used medications and their effects:

* **Opiate narcotics,** such as morphine, fentanyl, and methadone, are among the most effective and commonly used drugs. They both relieve pain and are sedating.

* **Sedatives,** such as Valium and its relatives (like midazolam and lorazepam), barbiturates (like pentobarbitol and phenobarbital), and chloral hydrate are used to calm babies down but don't provide pain control.

* **Non-steroidal anti-inflammatory drugs (NSAIDs),** such as Tylenol, and sometimes

ibuprophen or indomethacin are used for mild or moderate pain. They have no sedative effects.

* **Local anesthetics,** such as lidocaine, can be injected into the skin to numb tissues for minor procedures like chest tube placement or circumcision. The injection itself hurts, however (think of a shot of novocaine at the dentist's), so neonatologists will want to make sure that the pain of the procedure is bad enough to warrant the pain of the injection.

* **Topical anesthetics,** such as lidocaine spray, or the creams EMLA and Ela-max, are painless to apply and cause loss of sensation in the skin or mucous membranes within an hour or so after their application. They can be used for drawing blood, inserting IVs, and other minor medical procedures like bronchoscopy. They are used sparingly, however, and mainly in older preemies, because the thinner skin of younger preemies can absorb too much of the anesthetic's chemical agent.

If you ever feel that your baby is uncomfortable and wonder whether her doctors are being callous by not giving more medication, just remember that neonatologists face a dilemma: They are aiming for a balance where the benefits of relief outweigh its risks.

By watching your preemie carefully, you'll begin to learn how he expresses pain and agitation. Remember that all babies get fussy sometimes! But don't hesitate to ask whether your baby can be given more relief if you think he needs it.

Many preemies tolerate it well, showing hardly any signs of agitation. Others need just a little medication in the beginning to help them become accustomed to it.

It's true that there are some preemies who don't like the ventilator at all; they gag, become agitated, or continue to fight it. Most NICUs give pain medication or sedatives to these babies to help them relax and ensure that every vent breath is as effective as possible. Calming the babies is also a precaution against a complication called a pneumothorax (a tear in the lung that is more likely to occur if a baby exhales against an incoming breath from the ventilator). Pain medication is usually administered as needed, typically every few hours as long as the baby shows signs of agitation or sometimes as a continuous infusion. Babies may also be sedated if they are on high-frequency ventilators, because their spontaneous breaths can interfere with the high-frequency oscillations, or if their ventilator is working at very high pressure settings. Because high pressure can be damaging to a baby's lungs, it's important for the vent to do its work of breathing as efficiently as possible.

Although it surprises many parents, some babies find CPAP (short for continuous positive airway pressure) more objectionable than being on a ventilator. (Ask a friend to blow forcefully up your nose, and you'll see why!) A preemie who persistently tries to pull the CPAP prongs out of her nostrils may be sedated, though usually more lightly because she has to initiate all her own breaths on CPAP and most sedatives slow down the natural drive to breathe.

You may be wondering: Why not give pain medication to every preemie on a ventilator, just in case there is discomfort? The reason is that pain-relief drugs have significant side effects. In a recent study, babies getting morphine infusions took longer to be weaned off the ventilator. Being on a ventilator longer means a greater risk of secondary complications, some of which can be serious.

Doctors and nurses are trained to keep a constant watch for signs of discomfort in each little patient, looking out for those who would benefit from relief. But if you think you notice that your baby is uncomfortable, *don't hesitate:* Speak up. Maybe something more can be done in your baby's case—and if not, at least you'll know the reason why.

Will Your Baby Become Addicted?

If my baby gets too much morphine, could she get addicted?

Not really. It's important to clarify what addiction means: It refers to a physical and psychological craving for a drug—because of its euphoric or calming effects—that produces an irresistible drug-seeking drive. Several studies have shown that adults who are given drugs in the hospital to control pain don't get addicted in the psychological sense and never develop that compulsive drive. In other words, once their pain goes away, they have no further desire for the drugs.

On the other hand, pain medications and sedatives can cause tolerance and withdrawal, indicating physical dependence on the drug. Tolerance means that higher doses of the drug are needed to get the same effects. Withdrawal refers to a wide range of negative symptoms that may occur when the drug is suddenly suspended. Tolerance and withdrawal are predictable side effects of many pain medications and sedatives, including those most commonly used in the NICU (such as morphine, fentanyl, methadone, midazolam, and pentobarbitol).

Neonatologists are well aware of these side effects and usually take some measures to minimize them, such as:

* Starting babies on low doses of pain medication or sedatives, and increasing the amounts gradually, only as needed;
* Using nonmedical methods to control pain and agitation as well (see page 118);
* When possible, choosing kinds and doses of pain medication that are less likely to cause tolerance and withdrawal;
* Reducing the dose slowly when it's time to wean the baby from medication.

Few preemies—usually only those who have been on high doses of an opiate or some sedatives for more than a week or two—ever need enough medication to cause withdrawal symptoms. Nonetheless, neonatologists are very used to handling this. They wean babies from the drug slowly, monitoring each baby's response to reduced doses of medication (sometimes using scoring systems with guidelines to help them know when it's time to reduce the dose again or when they've gone too fast). They watch carefully for signs of discomfort and use all possible measures to help calm the babies. Usually a preemie needs pain medication for only several days after the painful events have passed. But even when weaning takes a long time (parents may say, interminable!), once a baby is off the drug, she's off.

Many studies have shown that controlling pain can hasten and enhance a patient's recovery. Unfortunately, in today's society, where illegal drugs are a scourge, the use of the same substances to relieve pain is often surrounded by suspicion. Several studies over the last decade have found an unjustified underuse of morphine and other opiates in hospitals around the country. Only in recent years, after long campaigning by pain experts, are more adequate tools being employed to relieve the unnecessary suffering of patients of all ages.

So don't worry about drug addiction. When

pain medication makes your baby feel good, you can feel good, too.

If Your Baby Is Tied Down

They tied my baby down! Isn't that cruel?

Sometimes a preemie is restrained for a brief time, when the doctors or nurses are doing a procedure and movement could cause pain or potential danger to the baby. For example, restraint is often used when a baby needs a catheter placed in an artery or a deep vein, such as in his umbilical cord. It's considered a preferable alternative to heavy sedation or medication-induced paralysis and is generally used with some pain medicine to make the baby feel comfortable and ease his anxiety.

Restraining a preemie usually involves taping or tying down one or more of his arms or legs, or holding his head or torso in a particular position with a cloth that is pinned to his bedsheet. It might look uncomfortable to an adult, but doesn't seem to bother preemies much. Very young preemies—less than about 30 weeks or so—don't seem to mind restraint at all, while older preemies very quickly (in less than a minute, usually) stop fighting and relax. As soon as the procedure is over and it's safe, the restraints are removed and the baby can stretch and get comfortable again.

Father Feels Faint

As the father, I'm supposed to be the strong one, but I feel like I'm going to faint in the NICU. What's wrong with me?

Nothing at all. Because of the stereotypes in our culture, most fathers feel a sense of responsibility to be the strong one in the family and to be a support for their wives and children when times are tough. It's a common sight in the NICU: parents standing by their baby's bedside, the mother weeping and the father comforting her with his arm around her shoulders. How many of these fathers, even the most stalwart ones, feel like weeping, too?

Virtually all parents are unprepared for the way they feel when a preemie enters the family. Nothing in life can prepare them for walking into a neonatal intensive care unit, where infants not much bigger than the palms of their hands lie splayed under unnaturally bright lights and beeping machines, marred by needles and tubes. It's not uncommon for fathers *and* mothers to faint in the NICU. (Don't worry, the nurses are used to it by now!) Those who don't faint often have other physical symptoms. They feel woozy or nauseated, or their skin becomes clammy. Or they just feel emotionally overwhelmed. Not only are all of these responses normal, but they come from a wonderful source: the tremendous depth of emotion and protective instinct that parents feel for their children and all of the other babies there.

Studies of how couples have reacted to a premature baby's birth show that there were fewer divorces and marital problems in couples who openly discussed their feelings of anxiety, depression, and frustration. So don't feel that you are weak if you express your emotions or accept help from your spouse, other family members, and friends. One preemie's father, a psychologist, has spoken eloquently about his feelings. You can read two of his speeches at https://pantherfile .uwm.edu/hynan/www/LIFER.html and https:// pantherfile.uwm.edu/hynan/www/MINNAEP .html.

Difficult Start to Breastfeeding

My doctor said my preemie could begin breastfeeding, but we're on the third try and it doesn't seem to be going well.

Keep in mind that nobody should expect the first tries to be real feedings—just a tender, intimate way for mother and baby to get acquainted and stimulate the mother's breasts. Placing your little one by your breast, where she may just nuzzle or lick your nipple at first, is a successful way to start.

At birth, many premature babies aren't quite ready to breastfeed, because they can't yet coordinate the three necessary actions of sucking, swallowing, and breathing. Usually their reflexes become mature enough to perform such complex multitasking between 32 and 34 weeks of gestation (although every baby is different; a few may be able to breastfeed as early as 28 weeks, while some at 36 weeks still have trouble). Plus all newborns, and particularly premature infants, tend to be sleepy and not very interested in nursing during their first days of life.

Even full-term babies generally lose up to 10 percent of their weight in the first week or so, since breast milk doesn't come in right away, and some loss of extra body water is normal and expected after a baby is born. In preemies, who start out with an already meager body weight, doctors try to limit this initial weight loss because they don't want to interrupt growth and development at a time when preemies would have been growing at a rapid rate were they still in the womb. So while your baby is still practicing her breastfeeding skills, her doctors will make sure that her intake of fluids and nutrients is adequate by supplementing the breastfeedings with either gavage feedings of your breast milk, donor milk, or formula, or with intravenous nutrition.

You can be sure of one thing: The nurses and doctors want to help you and your baby in your breastfeeding efforts. Don't hesitate to ask whether your baby is doing what they'd anticipate at this stage or whether there seems to be a problem. Most likely you'll be reassured. If, however, breastfeeding really isn't going well, even for a newly born preemie, and doesn't seem to improve over the next day or two, the nurses may elicit the help of a lactation counselor if you haven't already seen one. (You should feel free to request that yourself, too. Many hospitals have such breastfeeding experts on their staff or can recommend someone locally.)

Chances are, though, that your preemie is acting just as she should—like a tired, not-all-that-hungry, not-too-coordinated newborn baby. In other words, perfectly normal!

Baby Is Not Being Fed Yet

They are not giving my baby any food yet. Won't that starve him and make him weaker at a time when he needs all the strength he can get?

What could be more natural than a parent concerned that his child isn't eating enough? But it's not something you need to worry about. Although you can't see it, your baby is already getting some nutrients today, just not in the usual way.

Many preemies remain NPO, as doctors put it—meaning nothing *per os* (Latin for "by mouth")—on the day they're born and for a few days after, until it's clear that they are medically stable enough to handle being fed. If a baby is breathing rapidly or hard, as many preemies with immature lungs do, it can be difficult for him to suck on a breast or bottle safely, without accidentally inhaling some milk into his lungs. And if blood flow to his intestines has recently been compromised (as can happen, for instance, from fetal distress during labor or low blood pressure as he makes the transition from the womb to the outside world), his doctor may think that having to digest food could put too much stress on his immature digestive system. Remember that a mother's breast milk doesn't really come in for a day or two, so all breastfed babies don't get much to eat on their first day.

Nonetheless, most doctors believe that the earlier you start feeding a preemie after birth, the better, so as not to stop the growth that would have continued in the womb. So on his first day of life, a preemie usually receives nutrients he can easily metabolize: a clear fluid made up of water and sugar, amino acids (the building blocks of proteins), and sometimes calcium, given to him intravenously through a small catheter. The goal is to give the baby enough sugar to fuel his immediate needs (the nurses will be checking his blood sugar periodically to be sure he has enough) and proteins of the same quality and in the same quantity as he would have received from his mother's blood for continued growth. By tomorrow, the doctor will probably add lipids (a separate white fluid), salts, other minerals, vitamins (which will turn the fluid yellow), and various trace elements to his intravenous "meal."

Intravenous nutrition, which doesn't pass through the mouth or digestive system but goes directly into the bloodstream, is called parenteral nutrition. (You'll probably hear the NICU staff refer to it by its initials, TPN, for total parenteral nutrition.) Most preemies continue to be fed this way—partially or totally—for the first few days, sometimes weeks, of life, because their gastrointestinal system is still immature and cannot yet digest all of the breast milk or formula they need. In the days to come, as your baby's metabolism matures, his doctors will adjust and increase the nutrients and calories in this intravenous nutrition to meet his changing needs.

Nevertheless, by the time he's one or two days old, your premature baby probably will start to be fed some drops of milk, also. This is an important experience that will be repeated every day, even if the milk just stays in his stomach and isn't absorbed. Smaller preemies will have their milk put through a soft tube that runs from the nose or mouth directly into their stomachs because they're too young to suck on a breast or bottle. (No matter how he gets it, his first feeding is a milestone! Ask the nurse to wait for you if you want to be sure to witness it.) Lucky, bigger preemies will get their first real taste of milk, in larger quantities, from your breast or a bottle.

The minimal feedings that very premature babies start with are called trophic feedings. They are not meant to provide much nutrition—your baby gets that intravenously—but to stimulate the development of his stomach and intestine. (You can think of trophic feeds as jump-starting a process—eating—that wasn't meant to happen until several weeks or months from now.) Gradually the quantities of milk will be increased. Once your baby can digest and tolerate breast milk or formula well, he will leave parenteral nutrition behind.

Today it's probably too early for doctors to say for sure how your baby will be fed a week from now, but most premature babies are off parenteral nutrition and enjoying complete feedings of formula or breast milk in a few days to a couple of weeks. Babies who are at least 32 to 34 weeks old may even graduate from tube feedings to feedings by mouth within that time. In the meantime, if you want to anticipate what will be served at your baby's table, you can read *How Your Baby Is Fed: A Journey from Parenteral Nutrition to Gavage Feedings to Breast or Bottle* on page 164.

Pumping Breast Milk

I'm trying to use the electric pump to express my milk, but I find it so awkward. Is there any other system I could try?

First of all, if no one has done it already, give yourself a pat on the back. Your breast milk (and particularly the first days' colostrum, which is especially rich in antibodies and nutrients), is top choice for your premature baby, as its health benefits are still unequaled by modern formulas. Unfortunately, giving your baby your breast milk right now is a hassle, since he's too immature to nurse from your breast yet. So you do have to learn how to use an electric pump—because the suction of this machine most closely resembles your baby's own sucking action, it's the most effective way to express your milk—and to start doing it within the first 24 hours after you gave birth so as not to miss the crucial time for building your milk supply. If you wait until your breasts become engorged, not only will you be uncomfortable, but the engorgement will send a signal to your brain to turn down your milk-producing hormones, making it more difficult for you to provide enough milk for your baby.

Until your baby is mature enough to latch on to your breast, the milk you pump can be frozen and stored, then given to your baby through a small feeding tube as soon as the doctors think he's ready for it. (He will probably get his first drops soon, not just for nutrition but also to help his stomach and intestines develop and mature.)

The first pumping sessions feel more or less comfortable to different mothers, depending on differences in their anatomics, aversion to machines, and other factors. You may also experience some psychological suffering, which is understandable. This is a time when you fully start to taste the frustration of not being able to take care of your baby yourself, as you expected during your pregnancy. But pumping your breast milk now is a gift you are giving your baby, the only way to make sure you'll be able to breastfeed him later, and possibly a way to lessen some of the risks of a premature birth. So it's certainly worthwhile.

Remember that it's hardly ever easy to start nursing, even with a full-term baby. The first breastfeeding attempts are often frustrating because of the mother's and baby's inexperience. It's normal to feel a slightly achy sensation in the areola (the dark circle around your nipple) during breastfeeding when your newborn is still learning how to latch on, and the same can happen with an electric pump. But if done properly, pumping your breast milk should not hurt, and you should become comfortable doing it after just a few sessions.

It is important to start with a hospital-quality efficient electric pump and to continue using it as often as you can, until your baby is ready to feed from your breast. Try to get used to double pumping soon (pumping both breasts at the same time) because it will cut the time you spend with the machine in half. Don't hesitate to ask a nurse to assist you in your first attempts or to get help from a lactation consultant.

There are some things you can do to make this easier. (Other tips are in *Practical Advice for Pumping and Storing Breast Milk,* page 173.)

* **Try to relax.** Try draping warm washcloths on your breast and massaging the nipple and areola before pumping. Listening to your favorite music while you pump may help soothe your nerves. If you have visitors, don't hesitate to kindly send them away. During your first pumping attempts, you need to be alone—or even better, helped and comforted by your partner or someone else you feel particularly close to.
* **Think about your baby.** To trigger hormones that help your breast milk flow, look at a picture of your baby or close your eyes, smile, and think of him, imagining that you're holding him in your arms.
* **Get comfortable.** Sit or lie comfortably, positioning the electric pump in front of you or at your side. Hospital pumps are often placed on a stand with wheels for this reason. (Remember that even if you had a C-section and are only comfortable lying down, you should still start pumping on the first day; otherwise it

becomes more difficult to establish your milk supply.)

✳ **Pump often.** Once you start, pump consistently at least once every two to three hours during the day, about 10 to 15 minutes at each breast. You don't need to wake up to pump at night until your milk comes in, but make sure you do pump before going to bed and first thing in the morning.

✳ **Start slowly—and stop if it hurts.** Start with the lowest level of suction and gradually increase it to a comfortable level. It should feel like a gentle tug. If you feel any pain, immediately stop the machine and reposition the funnel on your nipple until the pumping becomes more comfortable. If the entire nipple and surrounding area are well-centered and completely covered by the funnel, pumping should not hurt, and you should gradually get used to it. If you do have pain, ask for help from the nurse or lactation consultant. You may need larger pump flanges or to be assessed for a breast infection. After a few sessions, you'll become familiar with the machine and you'll get the level of suction right from the beginning.

✳ **Don't expect too much.** In the early days, most mothers can express only a few drops at each pumping session. This small volume is normal, because colostrum (the very first breast milk) is thick and extremely rich, and it doesn't flow as readily as the mature milk you'll make later. (If you have the help of a lactation consultant, she might be able to guide you in expressing some of the remaining colostrum by hand, which even a good breast pump can't extract.) Don't feel bad or give up because you're not making much milk. Even scant amounts of colostrum are great for your baby, and as your milk gets thinner, the volume you pump will increase.

✳ **Remember it isn't forever.** The first two weeks are a crucial time to become accustomed to the electric pump and to establish your milk supply. If your milk doesn't flow in sufficient quantities right away, your baby might be fed donor breast milk (see page 170) or special formula for preemies in the meantime, but this won't influence his preference for your breast milk (which babies always love best—and is best for them) or his ability to digest it later. In two to three weeks, when your milk supply is established, you can take more liberties: cutting back to pumping about five times a day (with occasional super-pumping days to increase your milk supply when your baby has growth spurts) and trying other methods to express your milk. For mothers who have to go back to work, there are lighter portable electric pumps that can be carried easily. Or occasionally you might decide to use a small hand-held pump or even simple, low-tech manual expression. But keep in mind that these methods, which may come in handy when you're traveling or at work, do not completely empty your breasts in as short a time or with as little effort as an electric pump. Using them routinely requires more time (and more manual labor) than most mothers usually want to commit. So whenever you can, try to continue using a hospital-quality electric pump—at least until your baby comes home and is breastfeeding well. At that point, while happily nursing your baby in your arms, you will feel very proud of what you've accomplished—and deservedly so!

Blood Transfusion

They told me my baby might need a blood transfusion and asked for my consent. Can I refuse? I'm terrified that he'll get AIDS.

It's completely understandable that you're scared; every loving parent worries about the safety of the blood their baby will get. But you really don't need to worry about AIDS. Nowadays, there's less than one chance in a million of getting HIV (the virus that causes AIDS) from a blood transfusion. It's true that no transfusion is 100 percent safe, but because of the many safeguards that are taken, the odds of your baby getting any other infection are very small, too.

First, by way of background, you should know that it's very common for a premature baby to need a blood transfusion. During their first days or weeks of life, many preemies, especially the youngest ones (those born at less than about 26 weeks of gestation) and those who are on a ventilator or receiving intravenous fluids, have blood drawn frequently. Monitoring the gases and chemistry of the blood helps the doctors keep a baby stable, but all of those draws deplete his circulating blood cells. Because a premature baby's bone marrow, which is responsible for making more blood cells, is still immature, it sometimes can't replace them fast enough. As a result, many preemies develop anemia (a low concentration of red blood cells). Red blood cells deliver oxygen throughout the body, so without enough of them, a baby's tissues won't get the oxygen they need to function well and grow. If anemia is severe, it can be dangerous, but fortunately one or more transfusions can easily solve the problem.

Thankfully, the U.S. blood supply is among the safest in the world because the Red Cross, which collects about half of all blood donations, as well as the other blood collection centers in the country, are regulated by the FDA, which has stringent safeguards that are constantly updated.

First, potential donors are screened with a detailed, lengthy questionnaire, which is rigorous and culls out people whose past experiences or behaviors might affect the safety of their blood, such as intravenous drug abuse, risky sexual be-

havior, exposure to various illnesses, or travel to parts of the world where certain infections are more common.

Next, every single unit of donated blood is tested and kept on hold until it is shown to be free of hepatitis B and C viruses (which cause liver disease), HIV 1 and 2, and other infectious agents on a list that is frequently reevaluated and revised.

Finally, in addition to these general rules, there are other special precautions taken when blood is to be given to a premature baby.

Blood for preemies is fresher, and is prepared and stored with fewer chemical additives, so it's less likely to disrupt a preemie's delicate metabolism. The white blood cells are removed from it, to reduce the already low risk of transmitting viruses that are carried by them (such as CMV, or cytomegalovirus, which is dangerous to anybody who doesn't have a fully functioning immune system, like a preemie). Most of the time the blood is also treated with radiation—a process that makes it safer, *not* radioactive—to inactivate the few remaining white blood cells and prevent them from reacting against the baby's cells (white blood cells are part of the immune system, programmed to detect and react against anything they perceive as foreign).

Another important safety measure most blood banks take for preemies is called single donor transfusion. Because most premature babies need only one, or a few, small transfusions and because red blood cells for premature babies can be safely stored for up to 42 days, it is often possible to get all the blood needed by a preemie from just one donor. This donor comes from a special pool of preselected donors; to be in this group, a person must have type O negative blood (meaning it is safe to give to people of all blood types) and been proved to be free of infection during all previous donations. Having just one super-screened blood donor, and therefore not being exposed to several donors if he needs more than one transfusion, gives a preemie the highest level of protection.

Occasionally, a preemie will need blood products other than red blood cells, for example, platelets or plasma to help his blood clot or IVIG (intravenous immunoglobulin), which contains antibodies to fight infection. These blood components are also given by transfusion. They're screened and tested for safety just as stringently as red blood cells but come from more than one donor.

The nurse might need to put in a new intravenous catheter to give the blood transfusion, because blood can't be mixed with any other fluid and it could clot and block off certain kinds of lines. While your baby is getting a transfusion, his nurse will be closely monitoring him to make sure he's tolerating it well. Luckily, the reactions that adults can have to transfusions, like fevers and chills, are extremely rare in preemies because a preemie's immune system is too immature to react strongly against the newly introduced blood—one of the times you'll be *glad* about your baby's prematurity!

Your baby's doctors will get your consent before giving him a blood transfusion, unless it's an emergency and you can't be reached. If you are convinced that a transfusion is not necessary, you can refuse. But remember that this is a very serious decision to make. If doctors believe that parents are refusing essential medical treatment for their child, putting him in a life-threatening situation, they can seek a court order from a judge to overcome the parents' opposition. Talk again to your baby's doctors if you need more information or assurance. Most likely the situation is not yet urgent, and you'll have time to work out a plan you're comfortable with, such as waiting another day or two to make sure additional blood is really needed or starting erythropoietin (a medicine that may help avoid transfusion; see page 308). There's no surefire test in preemies to know exactly when a blood transfusion is necessary, so many doctors are flexible. On the other hand, if the situation is urgent, you'll probably understand and accept that getting a transfusion is less risky than not getting one.

Can You Be the Blood Donor?

I would like to donate blood to my daughter since she's my blood type, but doctors say that a stranger's blood is better for her than mine. How could that be?

It is natural for you to be taken by surprise, or even offended, because you feel your blood is the best and healthiest she could get. But when it comes to blood transfusions for premature babies, it's better to rely on a special group of donors, identified by the Red Cross, who have a safety record built up over many donations in the past. This can be a great disappointment for mothers and fathers like you who are trying to protect their baby in any way they can. But once you know the reasons for this advice, you'll understand.

First, to reassure you about safety. The blood given to preemies (from a preselected pool of donors with O negative blood) is specially collected to keep each donor's gift separate from all the others, so a baby who receives it can continue to get blood from that particular donor and not be exposed to any more people's blood than is necessary. All of the donors in this pool have given blood in the past and have been screened many times during previous donations for infections, risky behavior, and exposures. With all that screening and testing, it's very unlikely that something dangerous has been missed or overlooked. Transfusions from this special pool of donors have actually proven safer for preemies than getting blood from people close to them who are well-meaning but not always aware of their own risks for infection—even parents.

Even if you are convinced that your blood is safe, there are other reasons a transfusion from a family member has disadvantages. Blood from the biological mother is more apt to react against a baby's own blood cells because sometimes the mother's blood forms antibodies against her infant's blood during pregnancy (if a little bit of the infant's blood gets into the mother's circulation and elements of it are viewed by the mother's blood as foreign). Those antibodies, in a transfusion from the mother, would attack the baby's blood cells. And research has shown that blood cells from fathers and paternal relatives don't circulate as long in a baby's body; so using the father's blood means your baby could need more frequent transfusions.

It's not a good idea to ask friends or more distant relatives for a directed donation (as a donation for a particular person—in this case, your baby—is called) unless they're already regular blood donors. Not every infection can be tested for, so honest and thorough answers on the detailed screening questionnaire for donors are an extremely important way to pick up possibly dangerous activities and exposures. Friends or relatives who feel pressured to donate—in their hurry or because they don't want to disappoint you—may forget or choose not to mention something that seems trivial to them (an old boyfriend, a summer job in a lab, a forgotten trip) that could affect the safety of their blood.

A directed donation may also raise timing problems. The Red Cross collects, processes, and distributes much of the donated blood in the United States, and needs several days at least for a regular blood donor—longer for a first-timer—to schedule drawing the blood and to screen, test, process, and get it to the hospital. Then the hospital's own blood bank has to do some testing and processing, too. You can ask your baby's doctor how long it will take in your case, but your baby might need her transfusion sooner than that.

Once she has one transfusion, you'll want to continue using blood from the same donor for any future transfusions because exposing her to blood from an additional donor (even a parent) increases her risk of infection.

Finally, there may be an additional cost for a directed donation. Because directed donations haven't been shown to be safer or more effective, most insurance companies won't cover the additional fees.

Still, there are some parents who want to give their own blood to their preemies, and most doctors won't turn them down. If you choose that for your baby, be assured that all possible precautions will be taken to make your blood a safe gift to your baby.

Experimenting on Preemies

Are they going to experiment on my baby?

While you were pregnant, you probably envisioned your newborn baby's first physical exam being given by a warm, smiling pediatrician in a colorful office with Dr. Seuss books in the waiting room. But now she is off by herself in a high-tech intensive care unit where the doctors and nurses are strangers. You have only the foggiest idea what they're doing to your baby—and little control over it.

Many parents get nervous under such circumstances. You're not the first to wonder if your baby might be treated with experimental therapies without your even knowing about it.

First, let us reassure you: Your baby cannot be used as a subject in a research study without your permission. The federal government imposes strict guidelines on medical research. Researchers must provide prospective subjects (or their parents, in the case of children) with information on all the significant risks and potential benefits of the study and must obtain their signed consent.

The government also mandates that hospitals have review boards to approve and monitor research protocols, ensuring that the interests of research subjects are protected and the government guidelines are strictly followed.

If your baby is in an academic medical center (a hospital affiliated with a university), there are sure to be some research projects going on there, and you may be asked whether you want your baby to participate in one or more of them. Don't reject the idea out of hand; there are some studies in which you might want your baby to take part. Say, for example, a promising new drug is being tested for an illness that has no good existing therapies, or some new services are being offered that she couldn't get outside of a research study. There's even potential benefit for research subjects who serve as controls: those who don't get new treatments but participate as comparisons with the research subjects who do. It turns out that controls often do better than similar patients who are not research subjects. It's not clear precisely why, but the effect is strong.

Still, research is nothing to rush into. Being studied can be intrusive, and many promising ideas in the past have not worked out, or have even caused more harm than good. So if your baby is asked to participate in a research protocol, you will need to think hard and use your best judgment. Do ask for lots of information. You can request written information and ask your family doctor or other people you trust for help in making a decision. And feel perfectly free to say no. Researchers are used to being turned down—it happens all the time—and your baby won't be treated any differently than if you hadn't been asked in the first place.

There's something else you might notice in the NICU that looks like experimentation: Doctors are now required to conduct regular quality-improvement projects to make sure they are keeping up with—and advancing—the best

practices in neonatology nationwide. The goal is to continually improve care for all of the babies there. For example, they might try setting the oxygen saturation alarms in a tighter range for a small group of babies because the tighter range is having excellent results in other nurseries. If the change works well with the small group of babies, it will be extended to all. These quality-improvement projects are based on proven or widely accepted medical principles and practices, so they are not really experimental, but they may be innovative practices for your nursery. You may or may not be asked to give your consent to a quality-improvement project that affects your baby's care, depending on what kind of data is being gathered from it.

Although you don't need to worry about your baby being enrolled in a research study without your knowing it, there is an aspect of neonatal intensive care that touches on your concern. Some of the therapies used as part of normal care in intensive care nurseries are less time-tested than would be ideal. Why? Because neonatology is one of the fastest changing fields of medicine, and most neonatologists feel that if they waited too long to use new treatments—it can take years to know how effective a new therapy is and decades before all of the long-term effects are discovered—they wouldn't be helping babies to the best of their abilities now. Your preemie's doctor might want to try an innovative therapy that she thinks could work, based on some positive case reports or because the underlying science makes sense, but without strong research to back it up. Even treatments that have been well-tested in older babies could be considered innovative when performed on 22- or 23-weekers, who have survived and been treated for only a few years now. Some people believe that there's only a fine line between using innovative therapy and experimentation.

There are some critics who say that neonatologists, in their desire to help babies, are too quick to rush new, unproven techniques into the intensive-care nursery. Others say that it wouldn't be right *not* to use a new therapy that could work. It's an important ethical question. What can you as a parent do if you're concerned about this? Talk openly with your baby's doctors, and tell them that you want to be kept informed. Listen carefully to them (remember, they have years of training and experience), and ask them to explain the rationale for their choices of treatment. But also trust your own instincts as a parent, and don't hesitate to speak up.

Most neonatologists are simply trying to do what's best for their little patients and look forward to establishing a partnership in decision-making with parents. An open relationship of mutual trust is the key to your preemie's best care.

Any Alternative to the NICU?

I don't like taking medications, and I don't trust doctors very much. Isn't there a less invasive, more natural way to take care of a preemie? Isn't it true that preemies did very well decades ago before NICUs existed?

While some parents of preemies find great comfort in the existence of NICUs and neonatologists—specialists in the latest medical techniques for taking care of premature babies—others, like you, react differently.

Maybe you longed to have a natural delivery at home with your partner and a trusted midwife. Maybe you wanted to welcome your child into the world while gently floating in water. Maybe you planned to breastfeed your baby within minutes after delivery, holding him on your belly, as your companion cut the umbilical cord. And then came a very different premature birth.

Those tubes and wires attached to your baby, the people in hospital uniforms, and the sights and sounds in the NICU may be horrifying to you. You ask yourself: Isn't this a perfect example of excessive medical intervention?

Here is a fact that may reassure you: Intensive-care spots are so precious that they are given only to babies who really need them as a potential life-saving measure. Once your preemie's medical condition stabilizes, he may go to a so-called stepdown unit—an intermediate care nursery—if your hospital has one, or be transferred to a hospital nursery closer to home. In this new, calmer environment, he can grow in a quiet isolette or crib with much less intrusive medical attention before he's sent home.

It's true that some preemies survived, decades or even centuries ago, before the era of isolettes and antibiotics, artificial surfactants and ventilators, but only a small fraction of the number who survive and thrive today. In fact, one of the spurs for the development and spread of neonatal intensive care units in the United States was the death of President Kennedy's 34-week-old premature son in 1963 from respiratory distress syndrome—a baby who almost surely would have survived in a modern NICU today.

As long as your baby is in a NICU, your options are limited. You could try to transfer him to a different hospital if you find one that's more compatible, but most insurance companies won't pay for an expensive ambulance transfer for this reason. You can't take your baby home if it is seen as threatening his life or health. (Parents have the legal right to withhold consent for medical treatment for their baby. But if a doctor feels that parents are preventing their child from being treated to a point that constitutes medical neglect, the doctor can appeal to a judge, who will decide whether the parents' choices are reasonable and if not, can appoint a temporary legal guardian to take over medical decision-making.)

You'll be interested to know that in the last decade neonatal intensive-care units in the United States have become more humanized, thanks to the concepts of family-centered care and developmental care. Experts in these fields have convinced doctors and nurses that babies can benefit if their families are present and involved in their care and if the technological environment is made more natural, soothing, and responsive to a baby's individual personality and needs. As a result, many NICUs now keep noise levels lower and lights dimmer; place babies more often in a flexed, fetal position; try to cluster caregiving activities and avoid unnecessary disruption of babies' sleep; and encourage parents to be at their babies' bedsides, with lots of loving physical contact. Some NICUs even have volunteer cuddlers to hold babies whose parents live far away or can't spend much time in the NICU.

If you want to learn about family-centered care and developmental care, you can read more about them on page 229. You can then observe, or ask your baby's nurses to point out, how these concepts have been integrated into your NICU. You may be surprised to see how much attention is devoted to protecting the babies as much as possible from the trauma and disruption of the intensive care they need, and you may feel better about the high-tech environment of the NICU, which although far from the intimate home nursery you wanted for your baby, for now is the best place for him to heal and grow safely.

Testing for Drugs

They are collecting my baby's urine to test it for drugs. I'm not a drug abuser and I'm deeply offended.

Nobody is trying to accuse you of anything unjustly. At most hospitals, it's the policy to screen for maternal drug use whenever the pregnancy or baby has certain characteristics. In other words, if specified criteria are met, your baby will be tested no matter who you are, what you look like, or what you do for a living. The idea is to identify the children and families who might need help without discriminating against anyone by guessing who would or wouldn't use drugs. So don't take this as a personal affront.

The specific criteria for drug testing vary from hospital to hospital. Many NICUs screen any baby born prematurely due to a placental abruption because cocaine can cause abruptions. (Many other things can, too.) Other reasons for testing may include a baby who is inexplicably small for his gestational age, a baby who has symptoms that could indicate drug withdrawal (such as marked irritability, seizures, jitteriness, or diarrhea), a baby who has an unexplained neurological complication (such as a stroke that occurred before birth), a baby with a major birth defect, a mother who has a history of drug use or sexually transmitted disease, a mother who received no prenatal care, or even a premature birth that cannot be otherwise explained.

The drugs tested for are those most commonly abused—usually amphetamines, Valium and its relatives (such as Xanax), cocaine, marijuana, opiates (such as heroin, oxycontin, and dilaudid), and PCP—but nearly any drug could be included. Some hospitals inform the mother before doing a drug test, even though obtaining the mother's consent may not be legally necessary. In other hospitals, parents sometimes discover that a test is being done by noticing a little plastic bag taped to their baby's groin collecting his urine. The newborn's feces, or meconium, can also be analyzed, as can his hair. Results from these tests usually take longer to come back, sometimes several weeks, compared to a day or so for urine analysis. Analysis of meconium or hair can reveal drugs used anytime in the last three to six months of pregnancy, whereas urine testing detects only drugs that a mother used within several days of delivery.

In most cases, the mother didn't use drugs and

the test results are negative. If they are positive, she is informed privately, usually by a social worker or physician. Not all drug use during pregnancy harms the fetus, but it can still have significant implications for a family. Nowadays, separating babies from their parents is usually a last resort. At the least, discussion or counseling can determine whether drug use is a serious problem—and a mother who is addicted to drugs may be able to get help before her baby is discharged from the NICU and she has to cope with the responsibilities of caring for a preemie at home.

When Your Baby May Go Home

Now that I've seen my baby, I feel so much more hopeful. She looks healthy to me. Maybe she'll be coming home soon after all.

If your parental instinct makes you feel optimistic, that's a great sign. As time goes by, you'll probably notice that even the doctors and nurses, who know so much about premature babies, give your judgment high regard. They've got the high-powered diagnostic tools, but nobody is more attuned to how a baby is feeling than Mom or Dad.

On the other hand, your preemie is only one day old now, and even if she's doing well, it may be a long time before you can take her home. She needs time to develop in the nursery just as she would have developed inside the womb. And since life outside the womb is not what Mother Nature originally planned for her at this point, she'll probably experience some ups and downs before reaching her due date.

This warning is not meant to scare you, only to give you realistic expectations. The earlier your baby was born, the longer she's likely to have to stay in the hospital. Most premature babies go home within two to four weeks of their due date, because that is when they've matured enough to

be safe and thrive outside a hospital. Requirements for discharge vary somewhat from doctor to doctor and hospital to hospital, but in general a baby is not considered ready to go home until she:

* weighs at least 1,600 to 1,800 grams (around 3½ to 4 pounds);
* is gaining weight at a rate of 15 to 30 grams a day;
* is able to maintain her body temperature in an open bassinet;
* has had no significant apneas or bradycardias for at least five to eight days; and
* is able to take all of her feedings from a bottle or breast.

Babies who undergo surgery or are on a ventilator for several months often need some extra time to convalesce and may have to stay in the hospital beyond their due date.

A piece of advice? Try to live this experience day by day. If you focus too much on taking your baby home, the hospital stay may feel even longer than the several weeks or months it generally lasts. You also may miss many moments of happiness with your developing baby along the way.

Born Almost at Term

Our newborn daughter was born 5 weeks early, but she seems perfectly fine. Why can't we take her home tomorrow?

You're right to say that she seems perfectly fine, since many preemies born at 34 through 36 weeks of gestation are the same size and just as vigorous at birth as full-term babies. But since your daughter was supposed to spend another month in the womb, she is still less mature and needs to be observed in the hospital for at least

48 hours before doctors can be assured that she'll continue to do well and be safe at home. In fact, in recent years doctors have stopped calling babies this age "near term" and switched to "late preterm," just to make sure that nobody takes their immaturity too lightly.

You shouldn't worry, but you also shouldn't underestimate the significance of your baby being a preemie, though a late one. Even if your daughter isn't having any problems now, it wouldn't be uncommon for subtle difficulties to arise soon. Hormones like adrenaline and other substances released during labor can initially make a preemie more active and alert than she'll be when they wear off, usually within 24 hours or so. For this reason, a late preterm baby's feeding and breathing might start off strong but become a little weaker or more irregular several hours later. As those hormones wear off, some preemies may also get cold sleeping in their bassinets—a combination of immature body temperature regulating mechanisms and less body fat than term babies—and need more clothing and blankets or even an isolette for a while. Since infection is the most common cause of preterm labor and its symptoms overlap with typical preemie problems, if your baby is having any difficulties with breathing, eating, or keeping a stable body temperature, her doctor may want to make sure that she doesn't have an infection. He can do that with blood tests, treating her with antibiotics until reassuring results come back (usually within 48 hours), or if he's not overly concerned, by simply observing her behavior over time. He'll be watching to see that she's acting normal for a baby of her age and that her condition isn't worsening.

While your preemie is in the hospital, she can take advantage of the experienced nurses and lactation consultants if her feeding becomes lackluster. Considering how much energy and coordination feeding requires, it's not surprising for a preterm baby—even a healthy one born almost at term—not to eat as avidly or as well as a full-term baby in the first few weeks. Parents report that feeding is one of their biggest worries and frustrations after they take their preemies home, so this is a great opportunity to get expert help and nip any problems in the bud. (If your baby has breastfeeding difficulties after she's discharged, it's still not too late; check in Appendix 6, *Resources,* or ask your pediatrician to help you find a lactation consultant in your community to help you out.) Sometimes a preemie's blood sugar falls too low if she's not eating enough—something the nurse can check for by drawing a drop of blood. This can be readily corrected: Your baby will be offered some extra milk or formula, and if she's too tired or sleepy to take it from your breast or a bottle, the nurse can give it to her through a little feeding tube. Some babies may even get sugar water through an IV.

Another potential problem is that poor feeding can make newborn jaundice worse. Jaundice is very common in both preemies and term babies; it occurs when the liver is unable to get rid of enough bilirubin, a substance formed by the body as it recycles red blood cells. Since newborn babies, especially preemies, have immature livers, they often become jaundiced. If they also have infrequent bowel movements or get mildly dehydrated because they're not eating much, jaundice is exacerbated. Luckily, it's easy to treat by simply laying a baby under a special phototherapy light or on a lighted "bili-blanket" for a few days—and it's nothing to worry about unless the jaundice becomes severe. But if jaundice develops after a baby goes home, it might not be recognized in time or she might need to return to the hospital.

Regular hospital nurseries are set up to handle phototherapy for jaundice but, depending on how your hospital's nurseries are organized, if your baby needs tube feedings, an IV line, an isolette, or a monitor to keep track of her breathing—even if she's not sick, but merely acting her age—she may be transferred to a neonatal intensive care unit or NICU. If that happens, her move and her new, intense environment will undoubtedly seem very scary to you. But try not to panic; chances are that her stay will be so brief that you'll hardly get to know the nurses and doctors there before she'll be ready to come home with you. Some late preterm babies in the NICU are so healthy that their parents even say they feel ignored by the doctors there! This is regrettable because research shows that parents of healthy preemies are just as anxious, sad, and distressed at first as parents of especially young or sick preemies. An unexpected premature delivery is a shock to *anyone*. Parents face dashed dreams and plans for their baby's delivery and the glorious days they thought would follow it, are confused about what's simple immaturity in a preemie and what's ominous, have pangs of fearing the worst whenever things are uncertain, and wish desperately that their child could be safe and sound with them at home. So don't let anyone minimize your emotions. You'll regain your equilibrium when you come to understand that your baby is not in real danger and as you readjust your expectations.

Now, please keep in mind that even though these potential problems are common when looking at large numbers of late preterm babies, your own baby's risk of having them is small if she's doing fine now. But being aware of them can help you understand why the hospital is the best place for your precious daughter to be for a few more days. Likely she'll be going home soon; most late-preterm babies are discharged a few weeks before their due dates. It's a good thing, since judging from her early birth, she is raring to go!

MULTIPLES

One Twin Doing Better

One of my twins was put on a ventilator, but the other wasn't. Why would one be doing better than the other when they both came out of the same womb at the same time?

So soon after delivery, it's natural to think of your twins as two little peas in a pod. And in a way they are. They shared the same uterus during pregnancy, they were born at exactly the same gestational age. That usually puts them in the same medical ballpark, but it doesn't mean they have identical medical conditions or prognoses.

To make sense of it, you have to consider all of the possible differences between them. To begin with, individual characteristics vary; if your twins are fraternal, they're as different genetically as any two siblings. And boys tend to mature less quickly than girls—anyone who thinks back to early adolescence won't be surprised by that—so if you have a boy and a girl, your son's lungs are likely to be less developed than your daughter's. Then remember that conditions in the womb weren't exactly the same for both babies. Stress tends to make the lungs of a fetus mature faster, so if one of your twins was subjected to more stress in the womb, he may be more likely to be able to breathe on his own. If one twin's membranes ruptured and he developed an infection, however, the illness makes him less likely to be able to breathe without a ventilator. Sometimes the twins' dissimilar medical conditions relate to their different sizes; if one twin got more blood flow and nutrients through the placenta, he will be bigger, and bigger babies tend to do better medically. On the other hand, his smaller sibling may be the one doing better if the stress made him mature faster.

You can see that it's impossible for anyone to predict how all of these factors will balance out. The two things that are entirely clear are: (1) different people develop differently, and that process starts as early as when they're fetuses in the womb; and (2) this is not the last time you'll marvel at how your twins have turned into two very different individuals.

One Bigger Twin

One of my twin daughters is much bigger than her sister. Does that mean my smaller baby is going to have a lot more health problems?

Although it's natural for parents to be anxious about their smaller baby, some difference in weight is almost universal among twins. Many times the smaller one is equally healthy, or even spunkier (and may surprise her bigger twin by catching up in size over time). Unless your twins are truly discordant (meaning differing in weight by 20 percent or more) or born before 26 weeks of gestation, when a baby's size may more closely reflect his degree of development and maturation, their different sizes don't usually indicate that your smaller baby is more apt to have health problems. A baby's weight is just one factor to be considered, together with other, often more important ones. (See page 135 for why one twin may do better than another.)

To make general predictions about a preemie's health and development, doctors determine whether her weight is in a range that's normal for her gestational age. A preemie whose weight falls between the 10th and 90th percentiles for her age is considered "appropriate for gestational age," or AGA. For example, twins born at 30 weeks of gestation are AGA if their weight ranges any-

where from 1,000 grams to about 1,750 grams. If your smaller twin's weight is within this AGA range (see chart, page 582), you shouldn't be particularly worried; any unpredictable turns she takes probably will be due more to her prematurity and factors other than her smaller size.

If your baby's birth weight falls under the 10th percentile (meaning that she weighs less than 90 percent of the babies her age), she's "small for gestational age," or SGA. SGA babies do tend to have more health problems after delivery, including low blood sugar and feeding difficulties. If the growth restriction is severe, there is also a higher risk for some developmental problems in the future. Your baby's doctor can help you determine your twin's particular health risks, depending on why and how severely her growth was restricted in the womb.

When fraternal twins have very discordant birth weights, one twin is usually normally grown and the other is SGA. This usually occurs because of insufficient blood flow to one fetus, perhaps due to a twisted, small, or unfavorably attached umbilical cord or an imperfectly developed placenta. Other possible causes of restricted growth in one twin are an infection in one sac or a birth defect that affects the normal development of that fetus. In all of these cases, the smaller twin would be at higher risk of health problems.

If identical twins are discordantly grown, it could also mean that during pregnancy there was a passage of blood from one fetus to the other because of shared placental blood vessels. This is called twin-twin transfusion syndrome. It is usually diagnosed during pregnancy but may not be picked up until after the twins are born.

In twin-twin transfusion syndrome, too little blood flows from the placenta into one fetus and too much into the other, causing one twin to be small for her gestational age, the other large.

When twin-twin transfusion syndrome is mild, there may be no serious effects. If it's severe or long-standing, though, it's hard to predict whether the smaller or bigger baby will do better, because both can be at risk for complications. If your twin daughters' different weights have been attributed to twin-twin transfusion syndrome, you can read more about it on page 37.

Your babies' doctors may not have all the answers ready for you immediately after delivery, but they should have more information shortly. Soon they'll be able to tell you if your twins' different sizes are a relevant issue, or just a natural occurrence of no concern.

Multiple Doctors for Multiples

I just delivered triplets. Today my husband talked to three different doctors, but he liked one of them more than the others. Why can't we just have that doctor for all of our babies?

While you thought you'd have to get three of everything for your triplets, you never imagined that included doctors. There's a reason, though, that many attending neonatologists assign twins, triplets, and other multiples to different doctors. The thinking is that each doctor will treat the baby he's taking care of as a separate individual rather than as "one of the triplets"—and give his patient the full amount of attention that any single baby would get.

Of course, the flip side is that this policy is somewhat harder on the parents, whether because the doctors give them conflicting advice, they have a preference for one of the doctors, or because they simply feel that having three doctors to get to know and three phone calls to make when they want updates isn't easy. If you feel strongly that three doctors is two more than you can handle, you should explain this to the attending physician in the NICU and ask if there's any flexibility in the assignments. Sometimes there is.

IN DEPTH

Breastfeeding or Formula Feeding Your Premature Baby: What Will Work Best for You?

The trauma and wonder are still so fresh a few hours after your baby's premature delivery that you should be spared any additional decision or worry. But there's an issue you have to face right away: making up your mind whether you want to breastfeed your preemie. In only a few days it may be too late, so if you're going to try you must take action now.

Chances are, you need more information. Maybe you already have an opinion on breastfeeding, or maybe you don't: After all, your pregnancy ended sooner than you planned, so you may not have had enough time to think about it. But even experienced mothers who breastfed an older child and intended to do it again don't know much about nursing a preemie. Some new moms who want to nurse their preemies but don't get the right advice on how to go about it may miss that opportunity and deeply regret it.

Women who earlier in their pregnancy had already decided not to breastfeed may now hear from their nurses and doctors that a mother's milk is particularly important for premature babies—many think of it as a medicine, not just a food—and they might want to reconsider their choice, carefully weighing the pros and cons. Even if you can't imagine breastfeeding your baby, there are other ways to give him your breast milk that may suit you better. Some mothers, for instance, decide that it is worth the effort to pump and establish their milk supply so their milk can be fed to their premature baby, even if they don't ever intend to nurse him at their breast. This is a perfectly fine choice, which leaves open all the other possibilities.

Now, before making up your mind, you should first know the facts.

Can a Preemie Be Breastfed?

Yes, it is possible to breastfeed a premature baby. However, if he was born before 34 weeks of gestation, because of his immaturity or other medical conditions he probably won't be ready to nurse at your breast immediately. But you can start on the day of delivery to express your milk with a breast pump and bring it to the nursery, where it will be frozen and stored for your baby. When the doctors say he's ready to begin to eat, usually within a day or two, he may still not be able to breastfeed, and may be allowed only a few drops of milk at first. But even when your baby can't nurse, he can be given your breast milk through a thin tube going from his nose or mouth to his stomach (a method called gavage feeding). As he grows, he'll be put to your breast to get acquainted with your touch, smell, and taste. Then when he's finally mature enough to coordinate sucking with breathing and swallowing (usually at around 33 to 34 weeks gestational age), he will really begin to practice his nursing skills, eventually stepping up to fully breastfeed or to enjoy a combination of milk from your breast and from a bottle. Breast or bottle feeding—usually a piece of cake for a full-term newborn—is a truly big accomplishment for a preemie. (See *How Your Baby Is Fed: A Journey from Parenteral Nutrition to Gavage Feedings to Breast or Bottle,* page 164.)

Advantages of Breast Milk for a Premature Baby

Mother's milk is universally accepted as the best food for normal full-term newborns, and this is even more true for premature babies. Early good nutrition for preemies is of vital importance because of the huge task they face: replicating the fast growth and development they would have experienced in their last weeks in the womb. During pregnancy, the mother would have provided all of the necessary nutrition through the umbilical cord; now the baby has to strive to do it himself, through his still immature digestive system.

Milk from a preemie's mother is particularly well-suited to his special nutritional needs. Nature seems to know what a preemie needs most and is smart enough to program his mother's breast to produce it.

* **Human milk is easier to digest than formula because of its protein, fat, and carbohydrate composition.** To a preemie, this means a lot. Digestion stimulates the development of his immature gastrointestinal system, and the sooner his gastrointestinal system matures, the sooner he'll be free of intravenous lines to give him fluids and nutrition.
* **The proteins in breast milk differ slightly in composition from those in formula.** Breast milk proteins are more quickly and completely metabolized than the proteins in formula, leaving fewer of certain amino acids that are

potentially damaging to a preemie's developing organs.

* **Human milk is different from formula in its fatty acid composition.** The so-called long-chain polyunsaturated fatty acids (or LCOUFAs) are considered the basic building blocks of the brain. They are especially important for preemies because the human brain goes through a period of accelerated growth during the last trimester of pregnancy. Interestingly, the preterm milk expressed by the mother of a premature baby has a higher content of LCOUFAs than term milk. Fatty acids contained in human milk have been proved to accelerate the maturation of the brain stem, a deep part of the brain that among other functions controls breathing and may help to reduce the frequency of apnea of prematurity (pauses in a preemie's breathing due to immature brain function). Fatty acids also stimulate the maturation of the retina (the back part of the eye that is crucial for vision) and the cerebral cortex (the part of the brain responsible for thinking and conscious awareness). These connections between nutrition and brain development may explain why in several controlled studies premature children who were fed their mothers' milk during their first weeks of life had better eyesight and higher IQs and developmental scores than entirely formula-fed preterm infants.
* **The milk of a mother who gives birth prematurely is different from breast milk expressed after a full-term birth.** It contains higher concentrations of nitrogen, proteins, fatty acids, sodium, chloride, magnesium, and iron—substances that preemies need more of.
* **Human milk, and particularly preterm milk, is rich in infection-fighting components.** These are especially precious to premature babies, who are less able than term babies to fight infections. Preemies who are fed breast milk—

totally or partially—have a lower risk of sepsis, diarrhea, urinary tract infection, upper respiratory tract infection, and necrotizing enterocolitis (or NEC), a disease of the intestine that is one of the possible serious complications of prematurity. Breast milk owes its infection-fighting power to such components as white blood cells, antibodies, and growth factors, and also to "good" bacteria passed from the mother's body to her baby's. These beneficial bacteria, which set up residence in the baby's intestine, assist with digestion and help keep some bad bacteria in check.

* **Breast milk can be particularly beneficial to a preemie if a mother has skin-to-skin contact with him (this is called kangaroo care; see page 249).** Spending time in the nursery and holding her baby close allows the mother to develop antibodies against the specific germs present in her baby's environment and to pass those infection-fighting antibodies along to him in her breast milk.

* **Colostrum, the first milk a mother expresses, contains substances that keep inflammation in check.** Inflammation contributes to some of the long-term developmental problems that preemies can develop.

* **Breastfeeding helps to create strong bonding and attachment.** Parents may feel frustrated or useless because their preemie is hospitalized and cared for by the medical staff. Expressing and feeding breast milk is a special, exclusive gift from the mother to her baby and a promise of a future, happier time together.

If a preemie's mother's milk is unavailable, donor breast milk can be a good—although not completely comparable—alternative. Human milk banks in the United States gather breast milk from healthy donors, pasteurize it, screen it for infection, and then ship it frozen, overnight, to hospitals all around the country (see page 170). Most mothers who generously donate their milk have delivered full-term babies, but some have had preemies, and their special preterm milk is processed separately and reserved for the smallest, most immature babies. Though some of the nutritional and infection-fighting components of human milk are altered by pasteurization, most of the enzymes, growth factors, vitamins, and minerals are unchanged or just slightly decreased in concentration. If a mother cannot breastfeed, many doctors believe that donor breast milk is the next best option for feeding a premature baby.

Why Formula Can Be a Good Choice, Too

When breastfeeding is not possible or advisable, a preemie can also thrive on today's new special formulas for preemies. (In fact, the majority of premature babies who are initially fed their mother's milk will get some preterm formula after a few days or weeks because often their mothers do not have enough breast milk to meet all their nutritional needs.)

* **Breastfeeding is not advised if you are taking a medication that may be harmful to your baby when passed on to him in your milk.** Most prescribed and over-the-counter medications are safe for a breastfeeding baby, but there are a few exceptions. Your doctor can tell you whether the medication you are taking is safe. (Some mothers express and discard their milk while they're taking medication, then resume breastfeeding when the risk of harm is past.) It is not wise to breastfeed if you use certain illegal drugs (such as methamphetamine) or if you drink large amounts of alcohol.

* **You should not breastfeed if you have untreated active tuberculosis or are HIV positive.**

Most other infections will not be transmitted to your baby through your milk, but be sure to check with your doctor if you're sick.

* **Today's new nutrient-enriched preterm formulas made expressly for preemies have been shown to promote much better growth and neurological development than standard infant formulas.** So you can rest assured that preterm formula is a good alternative to breast milk. Its mineral, protein, and caloric content is tailored to a premature baby's needs.

* **Supplementing formula with probiotics (commercial formulations of good bacteria) can help to prevent some infections and necrotizing enterocolitis (see page 267).** Probiotics, once the realm of alternative medicine, are becoming a focus of interest in neonatology. These good bacteria can be used to supplement preterm formula, endowing it with some of the protective infection-fighting properties of human milk. Researchers are still studying what kinds and quantities of probiotics are best.

* **Even if breast milk promotes cognitive development, research shows that the later intelligence of a child is highly influenced by his family's educational level and social environment.** To quantify the effect of breast milk on a former preemie's IQ is difficult because today's mothers who nurse tend to be better educated and belong to a higher socioeconomic class than mothers who don't. If you give your preemie lots of love and stimulation, you are also "feeding" him nutrition that is crucial for his development.

* **Premature babies who are fed formula tend to grow faster than those fed breast milk.** Preterm formula is often higher in calories with more calcium and phosphorus (minerals needed to develop healthy, strong bones), iron, zinc, copper, and magnesium than breast milk. (Some of the shortages of breast milk are exacerbated by the fact that, at least initially, a premature baby is not taking it from the breast. Expressing breast milk, storing it, freezing it, thawing it, and giving it to the baby through feeding devices can diminish important components. Fats can remain attached to tubes and syringes, and exposure to bright light can affect its vitamin content. Most breastfed preemies are given iron and multivitamin supplements, and special products called human milk fortifiers, to make up for the shortages in breast milk.) This point may have pros and cons, though. While fast catch-up growth has long been considered desirable for a small premature baby, some doctors now warn that entirely formula-fed babies may tend to become too fat whereas breast milk fosters the growth of a lean body mass.

Why Breastfeeding a Preemie May Be a Hassle

Even for mothers who are prepared to breastfeed, a number of factors can make breastfeeding a premature baby who is in the hospital a demanding enterprise.

* **The process of expressing milk through a bulky and noisy electric pump is not pleasant initially, though you'll get used to it.** To give your breasts the right stimulation, you have to start soon after delivery—if possible within 24 hours—when the hormones that stimulate lactation are at their peak. Your pumping should be frequent and consistent, every two to three hours during the day, to build up an adequate milk supply.

* **It's important not to miss a pumping session in the early days, even when you are exhausted, and maybe even sick after delivery.** If you are taking certain medications, your

milk may not be stored, but your lactation will be started.

* **The more premature your baby is, the longer you'll have to go on expressing your milk, for several weeks and maybe months.** You'll have to rent or buy a pump to use at home, store your milk, and get organized to carry it to the NICU. Figure on pumping even after your baby starts to latch on to your breast because initially his sucking may not be strong enough to keep your milk supply going.
* **If you have premature twins, breastfeeding them is obviously more demanding, although definitely possible.** (You can read more about breastfeeding twins on page 333.)

Remember: Even if you do everything you can, you may not produce enough milk for your baby and may need to supplement his nutrition with an increasing number of bottles of donor breast milk or formula. Studies show that more than two-thirds of preemies who are breastfed by their mothers eventually need some supplemental nutrition. In that case, you shouldn't feel inadequate, but instead congratulate yourself on what you've accomplished, because most of the benefits of breast milk are preserved with partial breastfeeding. You can justifiably see your glass of milk for your baby as more than half full!

So What Do I Do? Some Hints to Help You Decide

Considering all the patience and time it takes, most mothers who succeed in giving their preemies at least some of their milk are very proud of it. But should all mothers feel compelled to breastfeed their preemies even if they don't want to, or cannot do so for practical reasons? Should they risk their own well-being or health by discontinuing useful medications so as to be able to nurse? Of course not.

The best solution is one that benefits both mother and child and doesn't create a conflict in this intimate and precious relationship. So, for example, a mother might resolve to provide breast milk during the first several weeks to give her baby some infection-fighting antibodies and the gentlest nutrition. But as time goes on, she might supplement her milk with formula to assure that while her baby gets sufficient nutrition she doesn't overtax herself.

A practical approach to keep in mind if you're not sure of what you want to do on the first day: The first two weeks is a critical period, when breast milk is especially helpful to a delicate developing preemie. So you could start to pump, to at least give your baby the colostrum (the thick yellow milk first expressed after delivery, which is particularly rich in nutrients, infection-fighting antibodies, and substances that help dampen inflammation and promote good development). This will help protect your baby and give him the best start. Then in a couple of weeks, you can make a decision about whether to continue expressing your milk. If you decide not to continue, slowing down gradually will allow your lactation to taper off and then stop without causing pain or engorgement of your breasts.

Buying yourself some time by starting to pump on the first day will allow you to ask more questions of the doctors and nurses who are taking care of you and your baby. If you are on medication, you should ask your baby's doctor whether it's safe to breastfeed. It almost always is. If you want to breastfeed your premature twins or triplets, you should try to talk to another mother who has done it to find out whether it could work for you, too.

It's also important that you discuss the issue with your partner and perhaps with other people you love and trust so that whatever you decide you'll be surrounded by understanding and support.

CHAPTER 4

THE FIRST WEEK

. . . .

A time of crucial test results and waiting.

Understanding that things sometimes get worse before they get better.

. . . .

PARENTS' STORIES: THE FIRST WEEK*

The first week of a young preemie's life is a time of stress and upheaval for his family. Joyful excitement and anxiety often go hand in hand, one prevailing over the other depending on the baby's condition. Even if their baby is doing well, some mothers and fathers find it difficult to release their tension, and aren't yet ready to deal with relatives and friends who want to meet the new baby or know more about him. The happy events that all new parents take pleasure from may feel a little strange and out of place in a NICU. But they occur anyway, bringing relief and warming everybody's heart.

"Go ahead, your baby is stable now," the doctor told us. Steven was born a week ago, 11 weeks before term, at the bouncy—somebody said—birth weight of 3 pounds 2 ounces. We have been very worried for him, and still are, but today we're getting ready for something a bit vain: Steven's first photo session in the NICU. We owe my parents some pictures of him, since we asked them not to visit until he leaves the hospital. For the occasion, I'm making Steven wear some fine newborn clothes: an embroidered shirt, a matching blue knit cap. Under the supervision of Steven's nurse, I open one side of the isolette and carefully put a little hand and arm through one sleeve, then the other. Trying not to knock off any of the wires connecting Steven to the monitors, I turn him on one side and button the back. The shirt covers all of him, past his toes. The cap is so large it comes down to his mouth. "Wait, don't take pictures yet," I tell my husband, who looks amused. At this moment, I find Steven funny too, my little elf

---

hiding under a cap. Let's take it off, my baby, you're tiny, but perfect. With no giant clothes, and no adult hands in the picture, nobody will be able to figure out your size.

Adjusting to a premature birth means having to face a lot of emotional and practical problems at the same time. Daily engagements may seem impossible to reconcile with the need to stay at your baby's side. Most painful to deal with are the demands of older children who feel left out, creating in their parents a sense of inadequacy.

A father in the corridor outside a NICU, talking on a phone.
—Hi Sidney, honey, it's Dad . . .
—. . . Mom can't talk to you right now. She's with Nicholas. They took him out of his crib, the special one with see-through walls all around, and now she's holding him in a rocking chair. Yes, like the one in your bedroom, where we read books. She gave him all your hugs and kisses. Yes, she did.
—Oh, he loved it. I think I saw him smiling.
—No, we can't take Nicholas home tonight. I told you why. He's very small because he came out of Mummy's tummy too early. That's why he has to stay in the hospital, where tiny babies grow bigger and stronger before they go home . . .
—. . . No, sweetie, don't cry. . . . You'll meet your baby brother in a few days! The doctor said we can push Nicholas's crib into a little room, where you and Mom and I can visit with him for a while. Isn't that great?
—Yes, you can bring him the picture you drew . . .
—When is Nicholas's birthday? Next year, in March. He will be one then, and you will be four and a half. A big sister!
—Of course you can help him blow out his candle. We'll have a birthday party with cookies, cupcakes, and all of our friends. OK?
—. . . That's a wonderful plan, baby. We're missing you so much, Mom and I.
—. . . Sweet dreams, Sidney. I'll tell Nicholas you love him. Be nice to Grandma.

During the first week, most likely you will finally be allowed to spend some quiet time with your premature baby: holding her, looking at her, silently talking to her. This longed-for intimacy can release powerful, sometimes overwhelming emotions. But it can also make you feel an incredibly lucid sense of purpose. The bond between you and your baby, stronger than you ever imagined, is created.

Forgive me, daughter, for delivering you so soon. I'm holding you in my lap, a bundle of clothes, tubes, and wires, a snorting machine pushing air into your lungs. Are you really sleeping? Do you feel my love? Do you feel pain? Can I take over some of it? They tell me you're so strong, so determined to live, that I'm starting to believe it. One day, I know, we'll laugh and play together. Then guilt comes back to stop the good fantasies. To remind me that my body betrayed you when you were still needy. Still not able to open your eyes, feed at my breast, breathe air. It wasn't my fault, but who cares, it's now you who has to pay. My baby, forgive my weakness, my sickness, my haste. Give me a second chance. From now on, I promise, I'll be strong and patient. I'll hold you against my skin. I'll enclose you in my arms. I'll make you a new womb in the world outside. Take all the time you need to learn to breathe and grow. Then, when you're ready, I'll take you home.

Anxiety and hope, worry and relief, melancholy and happiness. The combination of contrasting feelings can be so draining that some parents of premature babies unplug their emotional connection to their problems in an unconscious attempt to maintain their stability. As a result, they may act unnaturally cool or detached. If these signals are misread, they can create frustration and misunderstandings in family relationships.

How could Paula ask me to take her shopping today? She only came back from the hospital three days ago after an emergency C-section. Her placenta tore, and our twins, Laura and Ben, were born. At 33 weeks gestation. Now they're doing well, the doctors say, but still. . . . They have tubes, wires, needles everywhere, they forget to breathe several times a day. And all my wife can think about is furnishing their nursery. "Don't you realize they won't be home for several weeks?" I tell Paula, upset. But it may take time to get the cribs she wants, and a certain brand of double stroller. I finally agree to take her to the biggest baby store in New Jersey. When we're finished with the furniture, it's almost four o'clock. "Time to call the NICU," I say. Paula looks up at me and says: "Come on, they were doing fine this morning, why should we bother the nurses?" I choke back angry words and head out of the store. Paula reaches me in the parking lot a few minutes later. "No apneas this afternoon. They started feeding them my milk," she informs me. And then she says in a softer tone: "You know why I never call the NICU? Because I'm way too scared." I'm driving back home now, and I can't see Paula's face. She's turned to the other side, leaning against the seat. Maybe she's asleep. Or maybe she wants to hide some tears in her eyes.

Calling the nursery, going to the nursery, spending time in the nursery. Meeting doctors and nurses, talking to them, trying to understand what they say. Delivery was only a week ago, but parents of premature babies don't have any time to relax and recover. No wonder they all, mothers and fathers, look and are exhausted. But they must keep going, and they do. Where does their energy come from?

Holding my baby for the first time, I am happy, truly happy, for the first time since his premature birth. He looks up at me to study my face. I look down at him to study his. He was crying in his bed, but as soon as the nurse handed him to me, he became calm and content. He seems at home in my arms. My arms ARE his home. I shield his eyes from the bright, overhead lights, protecting my baby for the first time.

THE DOCTOR'S PERSPECTIVE: THE FIRST WEEK *

During our first week together, your baby and I will become very familiar. We're learning some important things about her that help guide her treatment, such as whether she's basically sick or well, how gingerly we need to handle her (making small, gradual changes in her treatment or moving forward in leaps and bounds), and, if we've been able to spend time with her parents or grandparents, what special place she holds within her family. Just as with any new acquaintance, there can be lots of surprises, too. Pree-

---

* *The Doctor's Perspective* describes how your doctor may be thinking about your preemie's condition and what she may be considering as she makes medical decisions. All of the medical terms and conditions mentioned here are described in more detail elsewhere in this book. Check the index.

mies, in particular, have a reputation in medical circles for unpredictability! With that in mind, though, by the end of the first week we have a good idea about how quickly she's improving and often whether it's going to be a long haul or not.

Physical Exam and Laboratory Assessment

As long as your baby remains in intensive care, she'll be examined several times a day by doctors and nurses so we can respond quickly to changes in her condition. We'll be gauging how effectively your baby is breathing, listening with our stethoscopes to how much air moves in and out as she inhales and exhales, and watching how much effort she expends with each breath. If she's on a ventilator or CPAP, we'll try to evaluate how much extra "oomph" they're giving her, using measurements the vent provides or comparing her breaths with and without the CPAP prongs in her nose.

We'll also be assessing her circulation. Good circulation is vital because blood carries oxygen and nutrients to all her tissues and helps remove waste products. We'll be concerned if her skin looks mottled or saggy, her urine output or blood pressure is too low, her heart rate is too high, or she's losing too much weight. She may need more fluid, or medication to help her heart pump more effectively.

We'll watch your baby closely to make sure that she's as comfortable as possible. Depending on how well she's adjusting to her strange new environment, and how quickly she's recovering and shedding herself of encumbering equipment, her needs for pain control will change. It's a good sign if she's responsive without being too irritable.

A baby on a ventilator and IV fluids will get at least one chest X-ray and periodic blood tests. A chest X-ray shows that the ventilator is expanding her lungs well, the endotracheal tube is correctly positioned—not so high that it could slip out of her windpipe, not so low that it could scrape against her airway or block off part of her lung—and that fluid or air isn't accumulating where it shouldn't. We'll be checking the amounts of oxygen and carbon dioxide in her blood to assess whether she needs more or less help from the ventilator. Her blood will also be checked for calcium, electrolytes (or "lytes" for short, as you'll hear us say), and other substances that are crucial for the normal functioning of all her organs. Their concentrations must be kept within a narrow range, which we usually do by adjusting the composition of the fluid we give her. If we don't have to do a lot of tinkering with the fluids, it usually means that her kidneys, liver, and other organs are functioning well. She'll have other blood tests to count her blood cells, which helps us know whether she has an infection. If her blood counts are too low, she may need a transfusion.

As your baby's feedings progress and she comes off IV fluids, she won't need as many blood tests. Her digestive system can maintain tighter control over the composition of her body fluid than we can when we put IV fluid directly into her bloodstream (the intestines know to hold on to some substances and get rid of others). And when she comes off the ventilator, we won't need to check blood gases as often. As time goes on, we'll trust her body more to keep her stable and healthy on its own, with progressively less help from us and our high-tech equipment.

Some older preemies, those without respiratory problems who aren't getting intravenous fluids, won't need intensive monitoring and treatment for long. These "feeders and growers," as we affectionately call them, may graduate in a few hours or days to a step-down unit, where exams and lab tests are done less frequently. Other preemies will remain in the NICU for their first week of life or longer, receiving intensive medical attention until they've matured enough to do without it.

Common Issues and Decisions

Respiratory Distress Syndrome: If your baby has RDS, we'll carefully follow its course, watching for signs of recovery. Maybe she'll be one of the lucky ones who breezes through the first week, rapidly weaning from the ventilator or CPAP without blood pressure problems or significant lab abnormalities. Then, unless she's one of the tiniest preemies (say, 25 weeks or under) whose outlook is so hard to predict, we won't worry too much about her. In our minds, she becomes a "well preemie" who will still of course need close attention and careful handling—particularly as her feeding progresses. But her risk of incurring serious medical complications will fall precipitously, and we'll breathe a sigh of relief.

For babies who have a more difficult time with RDS—requiring high levels of respiratory support, stalling on their weaning from the ventilator, or having a lot of blood pressure problems and other laboratory abnormalities—something else may be complicating the picture. We'll investigate with blood counts and cultures whether she has an infection, and make sure it's treated with the right antibiotics at the right doses. We'll wonder about a PDA (a fetal blood vessel that can cause some instability until it closes) or an intraventricular hemorrhage (bleeding in the brain) and may ask for ultrasounds of her heart and head. We're always hoping that the amount of assistance she needs from the ventilator isn't damaging her lungs and watching for evidence of lung injury—primarily air leaks (caused by small tears in the lung; you can see them on an X-ray) and inflammation (which leads to worsening rather than improving respiratory function,

usually around the end of a preemie's first week of life). If she has an air leak, or if the vent settings are very high, we may decide to switch her to a different kind of ventilator—a high-frequency one—which may be gentler on her lungs or work better for her.

Except in the very youngest and smallest preemies (those born at the edge of viability) it's rare that a baby's RDS can't be adequately treated. Overall, our goal is to support her breathing now, and to prevent her from developing chronic lung or brain damage later. We want things to get better quickly, partly because we know that the more rapidly the RDS resolves, the less likely it is that she'll have complications from it, but also because doctors, like parents, can't wait for their tiny charges to get well. Luckily, patience is something that we learn with time and experience, and I remind myself that a few more days or weeks on a ventilator may mean nothing about a baby's final outcome. Even babies with far more than their share of complications and setbacks often turn out just fine.

Apnea: Apnea of prematurity—pauses in a preemie's breathing due to the immaturity of the respiratory control centers in the brain—makes its appearance in the first week of life. We'll be deciding whether to put your baby on apnea medication (usually caffeine—yes, it revs everyone up, even preemies!) or on a machine to help her breathe more regularly. We may just monitor her closely and stimulate her to breathe when she needs it. As with every medical decision, we'll weigh the benefits of treatment against the risks. The main benefit of caffeine is that it can reduce the number of breathing pauses she has and make them milder, so she's easier to rouse to start breathing again and less likely to need the help of a ventilator. Very young preemies whose apnea is treated with caffeine are less likely to develop chronic lung disease or have long-term disabilities. The risks of being on caffeine are slower growth (usually for just a few weeks), probably because it speeds up her metabolism, and possibly a longer hospitalization, because we'll need to know that all of the medicine is out of her system and she's breathing well on her own before we'll be comfortable sending her home. It takes five to seven days for the last dose of caffeine to be cleared from her body.

Machines that could help her breathe more regularly include those that provide "high flow" air or oxygen (the lowest level of respiratory support), CPAP (more support), or a ventilator (the highest level of support). Low levels of respiratory support bring only minimal risks and are easily removed when they're not needed, but higher levels can injure the lungs and airways, so we won't want to increase her respiratory support unnecessarily.

Since apnea is so common in very young preemies and in them it won't go away anytime soon, if your baby is younger than 30 weeks of gestation we'll probably start her on apnea medicine right away if she's not on a ventilator, or just before she comes off the vent if she's been on one. If she's older, we'll wait to see if she really needs it before starting medication. Some older preemies don't. Especially if your preemie is close to being discharged (say she was born at 33 weeks of gestation and just needs a week or two in the nursery to become good at nipple feeding), we might tolerate a few mild episodes of apnea a day without starting medication, as long as they resolve easily with a little stimulation. Or we may put her on "high flow" room air or oxygen, or CPAP, expecting that she'll soon outgrow the need for support. (Don't worry—we won't discharge her until about a week after her last apneic episode, giving her a chance to show us that her breathing pattern has matured.)

Patent Ductus Arteriosus: All babies are born with a patent ductus arteriosus (or PDA),

a blood vessel close to the heart and lungs that is open in the womb but closes in most term babies in the first few days of life. In preemies, however, it's not uncommon for a PDA to take a lot longer to close (several weeks or months). A PDA can be asymptomatic—and not need treatment—or it might make problems a premature baby has with breathing and blood pressure worse.

We can often tell from physical exams or chest X-rays when a baby has a PDA; she may have a heart murmur, overly strong pulses, low blood pressure and urine output, and extra fluid in her heart and lungs. An echocardiogram is a more certain test, and we'll ask for one to be done if, for example, we suspect that a PDA may be hampering her recovery.

When a preemie has a PDA and we think it might be causing problems, we'll usually first try to close it by treating her with medication (indomethacin or ibuprofen, which you probably know as Motrin or Advil). If the medication doesn't work the first time, it can be tried again. But if a baby still has a wide-open ductus after two courses of medication, we'll consider whether to recommend surgery to close it. This isn't an easy decision, because we're not always sure that the PDA is responsible for the baby's difficulties. There are almost always other possible causes. Although a large PDA can cause fluid to build up in the lungs, reduce blood flow to the intestines and other organs, and over time impede the strong pumping of the heart—all of which could cause problems, now or later—just how bad it is for a preemie to have a small or moderate-sized PDA for a fairly short time is a controversial issue in neonatology. Medical research hasn't yet provided a clear answer to whether surgery in that situation does more harm than good. I try to convey this uncertainty to parents, and try to avoid surgery unless the situation is untenable. Different doctors and parents will have different thresholds, however, and although no parents want their baby to go through an operation, there may be times when it ends up being a benefit.

Intraventricular Hemorrhage: Although an IVH (short for intraventricular hemorrhage, meaning bleeding in the brain) is a possibility in any baby born at less than about 32 to 34 weeks of gestation—and preemies who are at risk will get a routine head ultrasound at a week or two of age to check for one—we don't really expect to find an IVH in many of them. We worry that there may be an IVH when a baby is less than 30 weeks of gestation and is having trouble with severe RDS (air leaks, blood pressure problems, or too much acid in her blood, for example) or suddenly develops anemia, or bleeding in her lungs or elsewhere. In the smallest and most unstable babies, we may ask to see a head ultrasound sooner, perhaps within the first three days after birth. Most of the time our fears are allayed—there's no bleeding, or just a small amount that isn't expected to hurt the baby. If there's a large intraventricular hemorrhage, there is no specific medical treatment for it in the first week of life. We'll make sure that the baby's blood can clot appropriately, maybe give her a transfusion to replace the blood he lost through the bleeding, and try to keep him as stable as possible so he can heal. Then we'll watch the progress of the hemorrhage over the next days and weeks, hoping that it resolves without causing further problems.

However, in a very few babies—usually those who are younger than 26 weeks of gestation and whose respiratory and other problems are exceedingly severe and life-threatening—the added problem of a large intraventricular hemorrhage may cause us to believe that a baby's chance of surviving, or surviving without debilitating handicaps, is now very slim. In those rare cases, we would meet with the parents and discuss frankly the option of discontinuing aggressive medical treatment and focusing instead on doing everything we can to make their baby comfortable. Since some babies with very severe RDS and large intraventricular hemorrhages will not survive no matter what we do, this option is a way of not prolonging suffering. In babies who might survive, but with extraordinary difficulties and after much pain, it's a way of acknowledging that there are some things that are so hard and burdensome they are not worth going through when a baby's ultimate fate is so uncertain or dire. For most babies, these issues never come close to arising. But if such an agonizing decision becomes necessary, we will be at your side, trying to help you make the right choice for your baby.

Feeding: We have to decide when your baby is ready to start eating, and how quickly to advance her from small partial feedings to "full feeds," as we call them. Most preemies begin eating (by mouth or by means of a small feeding tube) early in the first week. Because intestinal function isn't fully mature in babies younger than about 34 weeks and because food is a stress (it requires energy to digest, and diverts some blood flow to the intestines), we'll first want to make sure that your baby's breathing and circulation are sufficient for her to get enough oxygen and blood flow throughout her body. This usually means that she's not on medications to keep her blood pressure up nor on extremely high ventilator settings with poor blood gases. Even if your baby is relatively stable, there are other reasons we may decide not to feed her temporarily. For example, some doctors won't feed babies if they're on medication to close a PDA, because both the medicine and the PDA may interfere with intestinal blood flow.

How quickly your baby's feedings are advanced will depend partly on how well she's tolerating them (does she digest all of the milk she's given, or does it sit in her stomach without moving on? is she comfortable after a feeding, or is she vomiting or bloated?) and partly on her doctor's judgment. Preemies need time and exposure to food before their digestion matures, but just how long that takes differs from baby to baby. Some neonatologists are more cautious, waiting up to ten days before beginning to increase feedings beyond just a few drops of milk. Others increase feeding volumes as soon as a preemie shows she might tolerate more. We'll always be balancing the short- and long-term benefits of good nutrition with the knowledge that feeding a preemie before she's ready could make her sick. You can read more about feeding throughout this book and, of course, ask your baby's own doctor what factors she's weighing in making these decisions for your baby.

Anemia: If your baby is very young (less than 30 weeks, say), on a ventilator for more than a couple of days, or has a severe infection, chances are that she'll become anemic during the first week of life. That's because the blood tests needed to monitor her condition also deplete her body of red blood cells. Anemia can cause problems because red blood cells deliver oxygen to her tissues; if she's anemic, she may not get all the oxygen she needs. We'll decide whether or not to give your baby a transfusion, trying to judge what level of anemia she can tolerate. (We don't want to transfuse her unnecessarily, even though nowadays the risk of infection from a blood transfusion is very low.) Unfortunately, there's no good test or constellation of symptoms to tell us precisely when a preemie needs more blood. If she's on a ventilator or showing signs of circulatory problems, we'll transfuse her sooner, thinking that she might need the additional oxygen-carrying capacity. If she's more stable and we know that we'll be taking less blood from her in the future, we may wait to see if her body can catch up and make enough red blood cells on its own.

Family Issues

We hope that you're delighting in your new baby, despite her early arrival and (for now) maybe less than perfect health. Even if you are, it's natural to feel frightened, angry, and tensely vigilant as well. It's easy to feel displaced by all of us (the doctors, nurses, respiratory therapists, etc.) who seem to know so much more about your baby and how to help and care for her than you do. Sometimes it may feel like this isn't your baby but ours, and you'll think that we believe that, too. We don't— we know that we're the professionals, not her parents, and that there's so much we can't possibly do for her that you can.

Although our first priority is meeting your preemie's medical needs, we also want to meet your needs, in part so that you'll be strong and knowledgeable enough to care for her now, and later, in the ways that only parents can. She needs love, affection, support, and attention—things that call for parents, not doctors. You can help us by getting to know us and letting us know you. It's OK to ask questions over and over. If we forget to explain something or don't explain it in a way you understand, ask again. I promise that we won't be offended. No doctor means to be obscure; it's just that sometimes it's hard to know what information you want to hear and how you need to hear it. And you may be surprised that all the information you may dread getting can also help you overcome your fear. The more you learn, the more comfortable you'll become. The initial shock of "this is my baby?!" will evolve into familiarity and togetherness as you learn what she's like and what to expect of her.

Try to trust that we're not purposely hiding things from you. If you ask us whether your baby is going to be OK and we tell you that we can't answer, it's not because we're keeping a secret from you. There are many things we honestly don't know, and although we can tell you about some good or bad signs, we're often far from certain what the future holds.

Finally, try not to judge the staff too harshly. You'd be amazed at how varied different parents' needs are. So please forgive us our lapses, let us know how to do better, and realize that we're in this together—trying to do what's best for your baby.

YOUNGEST PREEMIES TO OLDEST PREEMIES: WHAT YOUR BABY IS DOING AND SENSING

To help you understand what your baby is doing and sensing, we've separated preemies into four gestational age groups below. As you read the section that applies to your baby, please keep one important caveat in mind. The range of normal development is very wide; few babies are on an exactly average schedule. If you're worried that some aspect of your baby's behavior seems out of sync with his gestational age, ask the doctor. Chances are he'll reassure you that everything is fine.

During gestation, the sensory organs mature and gradually switch on: first touch, then smell, then the vestibular sense (the sense of balance and of position of one's body in space), taste, hearing, and, last of all, vision. A baby's behavior at birth depends partly on how developed his senses are, because the senses are connected to most activities: moving, eating, paying attention, and so on. Full-term babies are already good at eating, communicating their needs, getting love and attention, and understanding what's going on around them—in other words, at taking the star role in the family. But even they have a lot of growing to do, in more ways than simply adding inches and pounds. Their brains, nerves, muscles, and other organs continue to mature during infancy and childhood to allow them to blossom into self-sufficient young adults. Your preemie's developmental expedition is the same—you are simply watching it a few steps earlier than usual.

As your baby grows and jumps from one gestational age group to another, you can come back to this section and read about his new developmental stage. In the meantime, enjoy him!

22- through 25-Week-old Preemies

* **Behavior.** Preemies at this age, the youngest of all, sleep almost all the time. They never wake up fully, with eyes open and alert to everything around them, but they may reach a drowsy state from time to time when they are more responsive to external stimulation like sound and touch.

* **Touch.** Your preemie's sense of touch is already well developed. He knows when he's being handled—in ways he likes or dislikes—and he'll give you clues as to which is which (see page 234). At this age, his skin is very thin, fragile, and sensitive to touch, so you should wait until he is a little older before you stroke it. But as soon as the nurses give the OK, you can start touching him in other gentle ways that let him know you are there. Talk to him first, to prepare him for your touch, then gently lay a hand or a finger on his body. He will feel you even through the blanket and clothes.

* **Hearing.** Your baby can hear your familiar voice, which he knows well from before birth. The auditory organs are fully formed by about 20 weeks of gestation, and studies on fetuses show that they're constantly listening to the sounds inside the womb, most of which come

from the activity of the mother's body (such as her heartbeat and blood flow, which are pretty loud) and from voices filtering through from the outside. Since he can't yet perceive sounds under 40 decibels, the level of normal speech tone, he may not hear you if you speak too softly. On the other hand, be careful not to startle or stress him with sounds that are too loud, since sounds are amplified inside an isolette and preemies like only small amounts of stimulation.

* **Taste and smell.** Taste, also called the gustatory sense, begins to function early, too. Fetuses begin swallowing amniotic fluid at 12 weeks and can taste it at around 15 weeks. It is a very rich taste experience because amniotic fluid has sweet, sour, and salty components; if preemies could talk, they might sound like wine connoisseurs! The sense of smell is not completely formed until 29 weeks, but researchers think fetuses have some olfactory (as smell is also called) sensations even before that. The amniotic fluid filling a fetus's nostrils begins to move in and out when fetal breathing movements begin at 22 weeks, so most likely your baby has already smelled some of the ingredients of amniotic fluid as it passed by the receptors inside his nose. At this very early age, your baby might not respond in any noticeable way, but he can be bothered by strong perfumes or the smells of cleansing products and disinfectants. Don't use them on your hands or any other parts of your body you'll be placing close to your baby's nose.

* **Vision.** Vision is the last of the senses to mature. At this age, many preemies' eyelids are still fused, tightly or loosely, like a newborn kitten's; they will open any time now. In just two or three weeks, your baby will begin to see light and darkness, his first exposure to the visual world.

* **Movement and coordination.** Babies of this age don't have any muscle tone and can't flex their limbs yet, which explains their completely flat posture. But their arms and legs aren't totally still; they flutter slightly, as if they were still floating in amniotic fluid. Because nerves and muscles are still immature, your baby's movements are uncoordinated with a trembling or jerky quality. They increase or decrease depending on whether he is in lighter or deeper sleep.

26- through 29-Week-old Preemies

* **Behavior.** Babies of this age still sleep most of the time, but their sleep is becoming more rhythmical, with quieter periods in which body movements almost stop, alternating with more active sleep. Beginning at around 28 weeks, REM sleep (or rapid eye movement, when the eyes flutter incessantly beneath closed lids) gradually appears and is crucially important for learning, memory, and vision. During REM sleep, a preemie's developing brain is creating connections with his eyes, sending waves of stimulation to the cells of the retina to prepare them for sight and building the nerve pathways that will process visual experiences. Since REM sleep is when dreams occur, you may wonder if your baby is dreaming. According to sleep researchers he may be, though the landscape of his dream world is probably very simple, activated by the physical sensations he's experiencing, without feelings or thoughts. No nightmares, in other words, which children start to have only when they turn two or three. But dreaming, as a way of stimulating and exercising the mind, is part of the reason why REM sleep is so important for the development of a baby's brain and why

preemies of this age shouldn't be awakened unnecessarily. For brief moments, they do arouse to a drowsy, partially awake state, though not for long enough to focus much attention on their surroundings.

* **Touch.** As your baby's skin becomes less fragile and sensitive, you can touch him more, but still carefully. Before handling him, speak softly to him so your touch is not too surprising and arousing. The most fulfilling activity you and your baby can enjoy together now is kangaroo care (holding him skin-to-skin; see how on page 249). At this age, most preemies are ready for it. For your baby during kangaroo care, the feeling of loving touch will interact with smell (the familiar odor of your skin, and your breast milk if you are breastfeeding), hearing (your voice and heartbeat), and kinesthetic stimulation (being in a contained, flexed position). It is a perfect balance of rich but gentle sensory stimulation, just what your baby needs for his development right now.

* **Hearing.** When you're doing kangaroo care, you can talk softly or sing to your baby, or you can sit quietly while your baby listens to the most familiar sound he knows from the womb, your heartbeat. Studies on full-term newborns have concluded that babies who listen to recordings of adult heartbeats can gain more weight, more quickly, than other babies who are fed the same amount of food. Babies who listened to the heartbeat recording also spent less time crying. Try to avoid sudden, loud noises as much as possible. Remember that your baby's movements and senses are still not well coordinated, so he might not start when he hears them, but show his distress in some other way, or just not react at all.

* **Taste and smell.** If your baby is being fed solely by gavage or intravenously, he can't make the connection between the satisfaction of being fed and the smell and taste of the milk. So some experts advocate placing a few drops of milk on a premature baby's tongue, or on a pacifier he can suck while his gavage feedings drip in, to introduce him to its taste as his digestive system and oral coordination gradually mature. Taste and smell work together to stimulate nutrition. New studies show that gavage-fed preemies suck more vigorously on a pacifier (which is good practice for the nutritive sucking that will come later) when they are exposed to the smell of human milk. This means that preemies, like full-term babies, are born with an innate knowledge of the aroma of human milk—and a passion for it! Ask your baby's nurse if you can place a pad with a couple of drops of your milk near your baby's nose when he's being fed through gavage. The unique scent of your breast milk could help him make the transition sooner to breast or bottle feeding.

* **Vision.** Your baby's eyes might open occasionally now if you keep them well protected from direct light. The eyes are loaded with meaning—as "mirrors to our souls" or "windows to the world"—so it's very exciting and moving for parents to see their premature baby's eyes open for the first time. You should rejoice, but also be aware that this is just the beginning of a long developmental process. If he just flickers his eyes a little before shutting them again, you have to give him more time. Remember, he should still be in the womb. At this point, your preemie probably perceives blotches of light and dark but can't focus on any object or distinguish patterns yet. His eyes won't always stay centered or work together well, but don't be alarmed; most full-term newborns have the same problem until they're a few months old. Be aware that a young preemie's eyes are extremely vulnerable to direct light because his retinas don't have a fully developed system of cells called cones

(designed for daylight) and rods (for low light or night vision). His pupillary reflex—to shut out excessive light—is still limited, and his thin eyelids give little protection. So for now, his eyes should be shielded from direct light, even when they are closed (for this purpose, most NICUs use isolette covers), and any light he is exposed to during the day should be low and indirect. When you hold your baby in your arms, if the light in the room is very bright, you can make a tiny homemade visor for him, by folding a disposable washcloth and tucking it into the front of his hat. It works!

* **Movement and coordination.** Most of your baby's movements are still flimsy and uncoordinated. Don't worry; that's perfectly normal for a baby who was supposed to be giving you little kicks from inside your womb now. When not flapping or twisting, his arms and legs tend to lie flat at his sides. By about 29 weeks, his legs will begin to show more muscle tone, and he should be able to flex his thighs at the hip. Soon, you'll see more tone in his arms and trunk, too. And along with muscle tone comes nerve cell development, so more coordinated movements are just a few weeks away. One thing your baby is coordinated enough to do even by around 28 weeks is to curl his fingers toward his palm and gently grasp your finger. (His grasp will get stronger over time.) Though he isn't ready to breastfeed or bottle feed yet (coordinating breathing, sucking, and swallowing is still too complex for him), in the womb he was already practicing the art of sucking on his fingers or toes (as some sonogram pictures show). Now that he isn't floating in amniotic fluid and has to deal with gravity, those acrobatics are beyond his reach for a while. But you can help him by bringing his hand to his mouth or giving him the tip of your pinky to suck on. At 28 weeks, most preemies enjoy sucking on a finger or a paci-

fier to relax, comfort themselves when they are agitated, or even soothe mild pain. A few extremely precocious 28- to 29-weekers may even be ready for breastfeeding, weeks before most babies are mature enough to bottle feed.

30- through 33-Week-old Preemies

* **Behavior.** Although they are still seven to ten weeks from term, these premature babies can already sense a lot of the world around them and interact with it. Their sleep is now cycling regularly between active stages and quieter ones. While they can't reach a deep sleep yet, quieter sleep stages, which facilitate growth and restorative processes in the body, are getting longer. A 30- to 33-weeker also has a more mature type of wakefulness, remaining awake and alert for several minutes at a time, focusing his attention on the world around him. All of his sensory and motor functions become involved, and every new experience provides stimulation that helps him develop further.

* **Touch.** Now that your baby is opening up to his environment, he's also able to show you whether he's feeling pleasure or is stressed and overstimulated (see page 234 for how to read his cues). Special kinds of supportive touch, like the "hand womb" or cradling techniques (see page 233) that contain your baby in a fetal position, are a great way for you to comfort your baby and help him calm down inside his isolette.

* **Hearing.** Your baby's hearing is improving too, though whispers are still out of reach; until 34 weeks, a preemie's hearing threshold remains about 40 decibels, a normal speech tone. In just a few weeks he'll be able to hear the same soft sounds that full-term newborns can. Your baby needs to hear your voice talk-

ing and singing to him when he's awake, but don't disturb his newly achieved sleep cycles! If he were still in the womb, he would have many hours of silence and stillness every day when his mother was quiet or sleeping. At this age, your baby's vestibular system (which allows us to be aware of our position in space, maintain our balance, and move in controlled ways) is becoming developed enough for him to perceive and enjoy vestibular stimulation, such as being held while you are rocking in a rocking chair. The organs of hearing are involved in vestibular function (you might know that blocked tubes in one's inner ear can cause balance problems) along with vision, touch, and other nerves. Studies have found that rocking motions can reduce apnea, improve weight gain, promote sleep, and increase alertness in preemies.

✱ **Taste and smell.** Your baby's feeding journey is approaching a major destination: his first breastfeeding or bottle feeding attempts. His senses of smell and taste will work together with his new movement and coordination abilities to help him become a good feeder: Smell and taste cues will alert him when a meal is coming, stimulate his digestion, and contribute to the pleasure and satisfaction he will learn to expect at every meal.

✱ **Vision.** Vision takes a big leap forward at this age, and preemies start taking the time to scan the world around them. At 30 weeks your baby can fix on a simple pattern, such as black lines on a white background, if it is placed at a distance of eight to ten inches from his eyes. Research indicates that as early as 31 or 32 weeks, babies already show visual preferences, focusing on one pattern longer than another. Most likely, your face will soon become your baby's favorite visual object.

✱ **Movement and coordination.** Your baby's motor system is getting more efficient. By 31 weeks, a preemie has a fair amount of muscle tone and can flex his legs; as a result, his movements are more coordinated, with less twisting and writhing, and his posture starts looking more like the flexed position of a term newborn. He can even turn his head to the side (although he doesn't have the strength to lift it up yet). What independence! This new ability allows him to locate an image he wants to focus on or to find the source of a sound or smell. Preemies of this age begin to show some of the built-in behaviors, called automatic reflexes, which allow a newborn to fulfill his basic needs. At 32 weeks, a baby's sucking becomes stronger and better coordinated with swallowing. At the same time, the rooting reflex appears: If touched near the mouth a baby turns his head in that direction in search of a nipple to latch on to. Your baby is now developmentally ready to feed.

34 Weeks and Older Preemies

✱ **Behavior.** These older premature babies still sleep about 18 to 20 hours a day, a few hours more than full-term newborns, who sleep 16 or 17 hours a day. It's a good sign that your baby is a deep sleeper. At 36 weeks comes the first appearance of really deep, quiet sleep, which is crucial for growth and development of the body and brain. Remember that your baby needs lots of time when he is left alone to sleep peacefully. Even if you want badly to interact with him, wait until he wakes up by himself, or before a meal when he's more active and alert.

✱ **Touch, hearing, taste, smell, and vision.** Your baby at this gestational age may still need intensive care and may have the skinnier appearance of a preemie, but his neurological development is quite advanced. His sense of touch, hearing, taste, smell, and vision are almost as fully developed as those of a full-term newborn. (Remember that even full-term babies are very nearsighted until about three months of age, and believe it or not, only at three years of age does the visual system become completely mature.) Once your baby's breathing and vital signs are stable, he's pretty adept at organizing his behavior in the new world outside the womb and interacting with it. All in all, you've got a baby with abilities that will allow you to have a lot of pleasant experiences together, even if it's in a NICU or step-down unit. He can express his needs and his likes and dislikes. You can console him with the familiar sound of your voice, by caressing him, or by holding him and gently patting his back. But even though he thrives on your presence and enjoys play and stimulation, don't forget that he was supposed to spend these last few weeks quietly growing in the womb. Learn to read any signs of stress he may express (see page 235) and if possible, avoid taking him to that point.

* **Movement and coordination.** All the automatic reflexes are now at least partly in place. Most babies can coordinate sucking with swallowing and breathing. Their grasp is so strong that they can be pulled upward as they hold on to adult fingers. And their Moro (or "startle") reflex—they throw out their arms and legs and arch their backs when startled by a sudden noise or fear of falling—is strong enough to startle their parents! But don't try to test this or other reflexes on your own; if you don't know the correct method to use, you may scare or even hurt your baby. If you want to see how developed your baby's reflexes are, you can ask a doctor to demonstrate when he has some time. Your baby's movements are still less coordinated than those of a term newborn, since muscle cells are still developing, along with nerves and the motor cortex of the brain. But they are becoming smoother day by day. At 34 weeks a preemie's posture may still be a little frog-like, with unflexed arms, but by 36 weeks all four limbs are flexed. When you sit your 36-weeker on your lap, with his head hanging down on his chest, he can briefly straighten his neck and hold up his head (but it's still important to support his head with your hand!). This achievement, which allows him to see so much more of the world, may last for less than a second; in the next few weeks, you'll see his neck muscles slowly become much stronger. But it is a big step for a preemie, and you should be proud of him.

QUESTIONS AND ANSWERS

A Desire for Privacy

What's wrong with my husband and me? All of our friends want to know what's happening with our baby, but we just want to be alone right now.

When parents are dealing with the shock and stress that accompany the birth of a premature newborn, it's not uncommon for them to isolate themselves in a self-protective cocoon. They may not want phone calls or visits, even from close friends. If you've reacted this way, try not to feel guilty or to worry about your friends. Don't hesitate to tell anybody that you would rather be left alone. It's better to let them know that you need some time to yourself now than to be evasive or short with them when they call, visit, or e-mail.

Birth Announcements

Some parents of preemies who were planning to mail out birth announcements as a tangible way of marking their baby's birth now wonder: How can I? A joyous announcement saying my baby was born at 3 pounds?

But just a minute: Who decreed that a birth announcement must specify the baby's weight? No one! In fact, it's a tradition that many people ignore, even for full-term babies. They include their baby's name and date of arrival, the important things for their friends to know. That's what you should feel free to do, too.

Please don't misunderstand us: Your baby's birth weight is nothing to be ashamed of. In time, you'll probably end up openly discussing it and your hospital experiences, even bragging about your baby's extraordinary start in life and his mettle and fortitude. But at the moment, it may still feel private to you—like an intimate detail of your child's medical history. You may feel that it might cast your precious newborn in a nega-

tive light to people who've never had experience with a premature baby. (To those of us who know preemies firsthand, your baby's birth weight is more apt to be seen as a badge of honor, evoking admiration for the beautiful, little thing. What energetic, gutsy fighters those one-, two-, three-, and four-pounders are!)

We do urge you to send out those announcements. You don't have to do it this week or next; you're awfully busy right now, and your first priority is caring for your baby. Birth announcements are typically mailed out anywhere from a few days to a few months after the arrival, so you can certainly wait until your baby's health stabilizes. But if you let this birth go tangibly unacknowledged, you may regret it. Your baby's entrance into the world didn't go as you had hoped, but as things get back to normal, you will want to feel that you gave your child the celebration and honor that she deserved.

When you finally emerge and are ready to deal with the rest of your life again, you'll be able to explain to them why you reacted this way—and close friends will understand.

Why do you need this distance right now? Partly because it is easiest to cope with the tremendous fears and obligations of a premature birth by focusing on only one thing: what is happening in the nursery. Anything else seems like a distraction that saps the emotional and physical

energy you are trying desperately to conserve. Partly because you may feel that no one else could possibly understand what you are going through. Maybe because you want your friends to see your tiny baby as perfect—as you do—and don't think they'd be able to see beyond the tubes and wires and medical crises right now. Also because this wasn't how it was supposed to be—and all the social rituals that go on after a birth make that fact too painfully obvious.

You can decide, of course, just how much privacy you want. Some parents find they're willing to share news about their baby's progress but just don't have the energy to be in touch with their friends directly. If that's true for you, there are some useful options. You can set up a free personal web site (as many parents of full-term babies do, too) through many online services that make it as easy as logging on and following a few directions. Two specialized health services, CarePages.com and CaringBridge.com, allow parents of preemies to set up secure sites, accessible only to those on a list that they provide. Either way—or by just sending occasional e-mails to friends—you'll feel in control, able to communicate when you feel up to it. If it's helpful to sit down and process what you're going through, you can do the writing yourself; if not, you can be sure a close friend or relative would feel honored to do it for you.

Most important, though: Don't feel pressure to communicate any more than you want to right now. The most sensitive of your friends are probably letting you know that they're thinking of you, eager to help in whatever way they can, and that when you're ready, they'll still be here.

Holding Your Baby on a Ventilator

The nurses say I can hold my baby, and I really want to. But he's still on a ventilator, and I'm afraid of knocking the tube out. Shouldn't I wait until he's off the vent?

Of course you're nervous about holding your baby for the first time—any honest parent of a preemie would tell you that they felt anxiety, too. Some parents, like you, are particularly concerned about the ventilator tube. Others, whose babies are not on the vent, worry about dislodging intravenous catheters, getting wires tangled, knocking leads out of place, and, of course, hurting their tiny, fragile-looking babies themselves. What pregnancy book or class prepares you for an experience like *this*?

But we can assure you of two things. First, if the nurses tell you that it's OK to hold your baby, they aren't saying it lightly. Remember that their first concern is always your baby's welfare. They have the experience to judge which babies are stable enough to safely spend some time out of bed with their parents and which babies need to lie quietly without disturbances, even from loved ones, to conserve all of their energy for recovery. (On the other hand, you should feel free to ask the nurse or doctor whether your baby is ready if they haven't mentioned it themselves. Sometimes they just get busy and don't think of it, even when it would be quite OK to do.)

Second, despite all of the medical accessories, as soon as you've done it once, having your baby in your arms will feel like the most natural thing in the world.

So let's consider the risks. You're right that accidental extubation (the ventilator tube's getting dislodged) can and occasionally does happen. But according to one study, the most common cause of accidental extubation is regular care and handling by the nurses. The second most common is movement by the babies themselves. Third is loosening or wetting of the tape that holds the tube in place. The fourth, least frequent cause of accidental extubation is holding of babies by parents.

Parents tend to be extremely careful—and it's clear from your concern that you will be, too. Also the nurse will make things easy for you. Once you're sitting down, she'll place your baby in your arms. She'll show you how to hold him; try to keep him in the position that she recommends. She'll stay near you at first, and check frequently to see if your baby shows any signs of unusual stress, such as breathing difficulties or back arching. When he is first moved from his bed to your arms, he will undoubtedly show some signs of stress—a normal period of adjustment. But these should calm down after a few minutes as he gets comfortable. If they continue, your preemie is probably just overstimulated. The nurse will suggest that he go back into his bed for some quiet sleep, and you can try again later. Please do, since when the moment comes that he's able to settle calmly in your waiting arms, he will love being that close to you! For more on how to handle your baby and understand his signals, see pages 232–235.

The nurse will also be there in case your baby's tube does come out while you're holding him. If that happens, several alarms will probably go off, scaring you mightily, but the NICU staff will be ready to reintubate him almost immediately (if he needs it—it's not uncommon to discover that a baby does surprisingly well off the vent). The few minutes he must breathe on his own are unlikely to harm him. Remember that he isn't relying on the ventilator to do all of the work of breathing; he's doing a lot of it himself. If he needed very high levels of vent support, the nurse would most likely consider it too risky for you to hold him. And if he does run into breathing trouble, the nurse can help him breathe temporarily as well as a ventilator can simply by giving him oxygen and breaths manually through a little face mask.

What about intravenous lines? They're really pretty stable, secured with adhesive, and sometimes with supporting cotton, gauze, bandages, or even small covers. Just try not to move the IV catheter or pull the connecting tubing too tightly. If you think that's happened, let the nurse know, and she can check on the IV. And don't worry too much—a little knock or tension is unlikely to dislodge an IV line.

As for wires and leads, there's hardly a parent who doesn't tangle them up or knock them off at some point. (If it makes you feel any better, the doctors do, too, as they turn the baby this way

and that during physical exams.) But it doesn't matter. An alarm will sound, the nurse will see that your baby is fine but his wires or leads need fixing, and she'll do it. End of problem!

Although there are risks to holding your baby, there are benefits that override them. You will introduce your baby to something he greatly deserves: the feeling of being loved. You will teach him that not all touch is clinical and hurtful; it can be tender and sweet. And then there's something that you greatly deserve: resting your baby's little body against yours will confirm your feelings of parenthood. Our advice to you: Don't put these precious things off any longer than you have to.

Sores from Tape

My baby has sores on his cheeks where the nurses put tape on him. Will he have scars from them? Couldn't they be more careful?

Your baby's sores will probably heal completely without scarring—one of the benefits of having newborn skin, which regenerates beautifully. Even preemies with deep skin injuries usually end up with scars that are pale and barely visible. Luckily, the most serious skin injuries are rare today because of careful nursing techniques and gentle adhesives made especially for preemies.

Unfortunately, there is no way to avoid using adhesives in a NICU. Nearly all intensive-care equipment must be held fast to a preemie's skin so he doesn't accidentally dislodge it. Many adhesives can cause skin irritation and breakdown, and while tape or probes and leads (which come with their own adhesive pads) can be periodically changed and moved, even that's not as simple as it sounds, because removing them can itself damage the skin of a premature baby.

But here's the good news: We've come a long way in preventing skin injuries in the NICU. In recent years, some safe adhesive gels have been developed that help protect preemies' skin from injury. You'll see that most of your baby's probes and leads are attached to his skin with what looks like clear gelatin: This gummy, sticky cushion keeps the skin under it moist and is much more preemie-friendly than traditional adhesives.

Traditional adhesives still have to be used in a few situations. They're stronger, and necessary when the tape must not move even a few millimeters, such as when it is holding a baby's endotracheal tube that's connected to the ventilator in place. You can be sure that nurses know how to be extra careful when removing tape of this kind from a preemie's skin, gently lifting an edge, then rubbing the remaining adhesive away with cotton soaked in warm water or alcohol. Mineral oil or an emollient can help, but only if there's no need to reapply adhesive on the same area of skin. (Special solvents that dissolve adhesives aren't used because of their toxicity to preemies.) Sometimes barriers made of pectin (a natural gel extracted from plants) or other substances can be used beneath regular adhesive tape, easing its removal.

The problem arises because preemies have immature and delicate skin. For the youngest babies, under 26 weeks of gestation, an occasional superficial skin injury is almost inevitable, even when the nurses are extremely careful. Simple handling can cause abrasions or bruises. These babies can also develop pressure sores easily, so they are turned and repositioned regularly, and may be placed on water beds, gelled or furry mattresses, or thick foam pads.

Even preemies who are older are more susceptible to skin injuries than bigger children or grown-ups, because the layers of their skin are not as strongly anchored to each other. Studies have shown that changes in the normal functioning of the skin can be detected after ten consecutive removals of traditional adhesive tape in adults, but after only one removal of adhesive tape in a premature infant.

So even with special care and these new products, some preemies will still get skin sores. But these superficial injuries usually heal quickly. If this happens to your baby, try not to feel outraged. Nobody can be blamed for giving your baby the intensive care he needs to heal and grow. Once he comes home with you, his tender skin will get the soft, loving touch that it deserves, and before you know it you'll be putting colorful bandages on scraped knees without a second thought.

Why So Many IVs?

Why does my baby need so many IVs? It breaks my heart to see the poor thing with all of those needles sticking into her.

Of course it's painful seeing your tiny baby stuck with so many needles, not only in his little hands and feet but maybe in his umbilical cord or scalp, too. Your immediate reaction is probably: Take the extra ones out! One IV is enough! But as you might expect, the various lines haven't been put in arbitrarily. There's a good reason for each of them. Here are the main ones:

* More than one IV line is necessary if your baby is getting intravenous substances that are incompatible, meaning they must not go through the same catheter. A blood transfusion, for instance, shouldn't be contaminated by nutritional fluids or medications.
* Say that your baby is getting fed through a central line (like an umbilical catheter), but he also needs medications every few hours. The nurses may prefer not to open the central line for the medications, since every time you "break" a line, its sterility is compromised and the risk of an infection rises. So the medications may be given through a separate peripheral IV.

(Continued on page 162)

What Kinds of IVs Are Those?

Some of the catheters that you see in your baby may be IVs, or intravenous lines, and others may be arterial lines, ones going into arteries instead of veins. You wouldn't believe how different each kind of line is, with its own special advantages and uses:

✳ Some IVs go into small peripheral veins: superficial blood vessels, usually in the arms and legs. These are used to give your baby medicines, fluids, and some nutrients. To precisely control the amount of fluid getting into your baby's bloodstream, these catheters may be attached to machines called infusion pumps, which provide a continuous stream of fluid. Alternatively, an IV may be used intermittently—for a medicine given twice a day, say—and capped off between doses. **Peripheral IVs** don't tend to last long; tiny veins with catheters in them can become damaged or inflamed after a few days. So you might find your baby with an intravenous needle in her hand one day, her foot the next. (If a baby needs IVs for a long time, you might even see one in his scalp at some point. Doctors try not to use scalp IVs too often, simply because parents find them disturbing. See pages 270–272.)

✳ Other IVs, called **central lines**, are placed in larger veins in the arms, legs, or neck and passed into bigger, deeper blood vessels near the heart. The two most commonly used central lines are PICCs (short for percutaneously inserted central catheters), which neonatologists or nurse practitioners usually insert right in the NICU, and Broviacs, which are usually inserted by surgeons in the operating room. A Broviac differs from a PICC in that it's cuffed—meaning there's a small rim or cuff around it that gets stitched in place to secure it under the skin. (A PICC is uncuffed and simply taped to the skin to secure it.) Because

inserting a cuffed central line is a slightly more demanding procedure, it requires anesthesia or deep sedation. For that reason, a PICC is usually the first choice for a preemie, and only if the doctors can't get one in—it rarely happens—will they ask a surgeon to insert a Broviac. (An exception is when a baby needs surgery and anesthesia for some other reason so can be given a Broviac at the same time.) A Broviac can last for many months; a PICC can last for a few. But it's very rare for a baby to need a central line longer than that. There are two great things about central lines. One is that they can deliver highly concentrated nutrition or medications that could be irritating to more superficial, smaller veins. The other is that they can be left in place for so long, and can be used if a baby will need intravenous nutrition or medicines for a lengthy period of time.

✳ An **arterial line** goes into an artery instead of a vein. Arterial lines are used for measuring blood pressure and drawing blood for frequent blood tests. Doctors use them to keep an eye on levels of crucial substances like oxygen, carbon dioxide (you'll hear these referred to as blood gases), and calcium. Arterial lines may be placed in wrists or feet, but the most common kind in preemies goes into the baby's umbilical cord, or belly button. It's called a UAC, or **umbilical arterial catheter**. A UAC is painless to put in since there are no nerves in the umbilical cord, and can do triple duty. Not only can it be used for drawing blood and monitoring blood pressure, like other arterial lines; it can be used to deliver fluids and nutrition, too. And since it's a central line (going into a large blood vessel), it can deliver very high concentrations of nutrients, so it's often used for feeding babies on total parenteral nutrition. But nothing is perfect. A UAC can't be used for more than a week or two; after that it has to be taken out to prevent blood clots or infection. If a baby needs longer-term parenteral nutrition, this line will probably be replaced with a PICC or a Broviac.

* Your baby's umbilical cord has a large vein, too. A UVC, or **umbilical venous catheter,** is a central line that in addition to delivering nutrition and medication can also provide doctors with some key information: whether the baby has enough, or too much, fluid circulating in his body. The usual ways of telling, such as measuring urine output, don't always work well for very little babies, who can lose a lot of fluids from their skin. Estimating "central venous pressure" through the UVC is helpful. A UVC can't be used for long, though. Like a UAC, it needs to be removed within a week or two to avoid clotting and infection.

* One of those catheters may not be an IV, or intravenous, line—it may go into an artery. While intravenous lines are used for delivering substances like fluids and medications to the baby, arterial lines are used for drawing blood and measuring blood pressure.

Doctors can cut back on the number of IVs that a premature baby needs by using a catheter with two or three separate lines going through it. These double (or triple) lumen catheters can be used to simultaneously deliver nutrition through one line, for instance, and medication through the other. This is a big advantage, reducing the risk of infection raised by a second or third line, and eliminating the needle sticks to insert them. Multilumen catheters are slightly thicker, so they are used only in bigger blood vessels, like those in the umbilical cord. When a double lumen catheter is removed, it may be because your baby no longer needs it—hooray! But if it's taken out because it's no longer working well or the time has come to replace it (umbilical catheters shouldn't be left in for more than seven to ten days), two IVs may need to take its place.

What do the lines feel like to your baby?

Think about when you've had an IV in your hand. After an initial puncture, it wasn't painful anymore. You just had to remember to keep your hand still. When the IV was taken out, there was a bruise and some adhesive left behind, but a few days later, every trace of the IV had disappeared.

Your preemie's IVs are no different—except for the fact that managing them is more of a hassle for nurses, since they cannot talk a baby into keeping his arm or leg still. This is why IVs in little hands or feet are sometimes taped to a fat roll of gauze or a big clumsy board. All parents hate to see their preemie loaded with such a bulky swaddle, but it is necessary to keep him from flexing his joints and dislodging or causing kinks in the catheter.

One by one, your baby's lines will be taken out as he grows older and more stable. And then, one great day, you'll arrive to find that your baby is completely catheter-free.

Discolored Toes from Umbilical Catheter

My daughter's toes turned bluish-black, and the doctor said it was because of a blood clot in her umbilical catheter. How could they have let this happen? Is it serious?

It's an alarming sight, but not one you should have to worry about for long. Your daughter's nurse will watch to make sure that the blood flow in her foot is good and that her toes gradually return to normal over the next hour or so. If she has any doubts, or if your daughter's toes stay bluish-black, the doctor will remove the umbilical catheter or place it in a different position, which should solve the problem.

This complication of an umbilical artery catheter is so common that doctors and nurses even have a nickname for it: "cath toes." Cath toes occur when tiny blood clots form around the tip of the catheter, then break off and travel down to the toes. Most NICUs put heparin, an anticoagulant, into fluids infused through an umbilical catheter to help prevent the development of large blood clots in the catheter. But despite the heparin, some tiny blood clots are almost inevitable. Your baby's natural anticoagulants will work over the next few hours to get rid of the clot. To help them along, the nurse may apply some warmth to one of your baby's legs, encouraging the blood vessels to dilate and get the blood flowing.

Small clots, like your daughter's, hardly ever cause any lasting trouble. Very rarely a clot does not resolve on its own but grows bigger and obstructs a large blood vessel, seriously impeding blood flow to an organ or extremity. In that case, doctors would treat the clot with medication to help break it down. If medication didn't work, they might try surgery to remove the clot. Above all, they would give the body's own clot-dissolving mechanisms time to do their work.

Even when there's a rare more serious clot, treatment to dissolve or remove it is usually effective. Very, very occasionally, and only if blood flow is completely disrupted for many hours or days, a baby's toes or leg is irreparably damaged; but this is not something you should worry about now that your baby's doctors are watching her toes closely.

If only your daughter could put on a pair of socks to help you forget about this passing flaw, but the nurses need to monitor how her toes are doing. Before you know it, her little toes should be pink and perfect again.

High Blood Sugar

The doctors keep saying my baby's blood sugar is too high. Does this mean he has diabetes?

Don't worry: Your baby doesn't have diabetes. High blood sugar is just another, often inevitable, consequence of being born too soon. In a few days your baby's body will adjust, and his blood sugar level will probably come down to normal.

Very premature babies often develop high blood sugar levels (also called hyperglycemia, or too much glucose in the blood) as a result of stress and illness. This happens to adult patients in intensive care, too, as hormones cause fuel that is stored in the body to be released into the bloodstream as sugar—the body's way of making sure there's enough energy available in an emergency. Not surprisingly, the younger and smaller a preemie is when he's born, the more likely he is to have a still immature blood sugar regulatory system (controlled mainly by the liver, pancreas, and adrenal glands). As a result, his blood sugar levels are less stable and tend to fluctuate too much in both directions, too high and too low. To compound it all, hyperglycemia can be a direct consequence of the intravenous nutrition a tiny preemie needs in his first days of life before he's ready to be fed by mouth. Doctors want to give a baby enough glucose (together with other nutrients) to keep him growing and able to fight an illness or just the stress of his early birth.

(Continued on page 169)

How Your Baby Is Fed: A Journey from Parenteral Nutrition to Gavage Feedings to Breast or Bottle

It feels so natural to put a newborn to his mother's breast right after birth, or to bring the first bottle of milk to his eager mouth. Yet feedings, which most parents of full-term babies take for granted, can be a real hurdle for a preemie. Older premature babies who are born after 32 to 33 weeks of gestation and are healthy may be ready to breastfeed or drink from a nipple within a matter of days. But if your baby is younger or sicker, it will take longer for him to get to that point.

Why can't a young preemie just go ahead and eat? Because even though a fetus's intestinal tract is fully formed by 20 weeks, some important functions don't mature until later. For example, peristalsis—contractions of the intestines that propel food through them—doesn't start working well until about 28 to 30 weeks, and preemies don't yet produce sufficient amounts of some important digestive enzymes. And it's not on nature's agenda for preemies to feed by mouth before 32 to 34 weeks, when they develop the ability to coordinate sucking, swallowing, and breathing. Before a preemie masters this coordination, he could choke on his milk, or it might just dribble out of his mouth as he breathes.

A young preemie's feeding journey usually proceeds through three steps:

* **Parenteral nutrition,** meaning that it bypasses the baby's digestive system and goes directly into his bloodstream through an IV or other catheter;
* **Gavage feeding,** in which a baby is fed breast milk or formula through a tube that goes from his mouth or nose into his stomach;
* **Drinking from a nipple**—breastfeeding, bottle feeding, or both.

This progression allows a baby to be fed according to his developmental stage and medical condition. Keep in mind, though, that the passage from one leg of a preemie's feeding journey to the next is never clear-cut. Parenteral nutrition usually overlaps with gavage, and gavage usually overlaps with breast or bottle feeding, to allow the baby some time to get used to each new, more demanding step. Probably there will be ups and downs, too, and you may get frustrated at times. But you'll also get joy from watching your baby's progress and from many intimate moments along the way. Feeding your baby and watching him grow is one of the most basic pleasures of parenting—for parents of full-term and premature newborns alike.

The first step: parenteral nutrition

It is normal for preemies, as for all newborns, not to eat much and to lose some weight right after birth. (Some of this is water weight, which needs to be cleared.) But since premature babies have fewer body stores of fats and other nutrients, they need nourishment soon. The goal is for growth to resume, with the least possible disruption, to what it would have been in the womb, since appropriate growth is crucial for a baby's health and subsequent development.

The first nourishment for many preemies comes from IV fluids, usually a solution of sugar and amino acids (the building blocks of proteins) in water within 24 hours of birth. In the following few days, minerals, vitamins, salts, trace elements, and lipids are added and their concentrations increased until the solution contains all of the fluids, calories, and nourishment your baby needs to live and grow. It is called total parenteral nutrition, or TPN. Preemies usually are given TPN for several days to several weeks after birth.

While your baby is on TPN, his doctors will be on the lookout for possible complications, such as infection from the IV catheter, skin injury if some solution leaks out of the vein (when the calories in TPN are high, it is so rich that it easily damages small peripheral veins, so it is usually given through a PICC—a percutaneously inserted central catheter; see page 268—into a much larger blood vessel, taking care of that problem), excessive levels of glucose or fat in the blood (this is a problem only if the levels are too high for a long time), poor bone mineralization (the doctor will give your baby extra calcium and vitamin D if this happens), and liver damage (in the vast majority of babies, the liver heals after TPN is stopped). Chances are that your baby will not have any of these problems, but they explain why, despite TPN's many benefits, the NICU's little patients are kept on it only as long as they absolutely need it.

As your baby's feedings of milk or formula are increased gradually, to give her digestive system all the time it needs to accept and assimilate nutrition and prevent feeding intolerance, the amount of TPN she gets will be reduced, overlapping with them as a caloric supplement.

The second step: Gavage feedings of breast milk or formula

Although a young preemie may not be ready to drink from a nipple yet, putting nutrients in his intestinal tract will stimulate it to grow and mature faster. So on his first day or two of life, even though he's being nourished by TPN, a preemie will probably also be given his first drops of breast milk or formula by tube, or gavage. (Some neonatologists are investigating a new synthetic substance that is similar to amniotic fluid for the first few feedings, instead of milk or formula.)

The purpose of this small tasting, which will be repeated every day in gradually increasing amounts, isn't nutrition, but rather to stimulate a baby's intestinal tract to develop. Maturation of the intestine is a complex process that includes the release of some hormones and the development of digestive capability and coordinated movement so food travels down the intestines in the right amount of time and in the right direction. You may hear doctors call these little meals "trophic feeds" and this process "priming the gut": a descriptive though not too gentle expression. If you consider that gavage is a French word meaning cram or stuff, you might get even more of a sense of what's in store for your preemie!

The most advantageous milk for a preemie in his first days is breast milk from his mother. If his mother's milk is not available, he'll be fed donor breast milk (preferably preterm milk from a mother of a preemie) or preterm infant formula. A mother's breast milk doesn't fully come in for at least 48 hours, even if she starts using an electric pump right after delivery, and may take up to four or five days. But small amounts of colostrum, the thick yellow first milk a mother expresses after birth, are precious and sufficient for her preemie's first tryout feedings by mouth.

Gavage feeding involves a very small, soft tube going through your baby's mouth or nose down to his stomach. An OG tube (which goes through the mouth and stands for oro-gastric) is generally preferred because babies breathe through their noses. An NG tube (which goes through the nose and stands for naso-gastric) is good for some older preemies who have a strong gag reflex, and for those who are already nippling or breastfeeding, so they need their mouths free but need extra calories through gavage.

Inserting a gavage tube through a baby's mouth or nose is a painless procedure that usually doesn't bother preemies at all. The nurse slides the gavage tube down the back of the baby's throat, down his esophagus, and into his stomach. She secures the tube in place by taping it under his nostril or beside his mouth. The whole thing takes a matter of seconds, so if the tube seems to bother the baby—which it rarely does—it can be taken out and put in again for each feeding. (It is usually left in, since removing the tape can irritate a preemie's delicate skin, and a few babies gag or have bradycardia while the tube is being placed.)

When it's mealtime, the nurse connects a plastic syringe to the baby's gavage tube, pours in the right amount of breast milk or formula, gives the plunger a gentle push, and lets the liquid flow down into the tube by gravity. Alternatively, she may connect the syringe to a pump so the milk can be dripped into your preemie's stomach very slowly. (Sucking on a tiny pacifier while he's being fed by gavage can help a preemie rehearse for the next step on his feeding journey, nipple feeding.) If your baby tolerates the breast milk or formula he gets through gavage (meaning he doesn't vomit and the milk moves well through his intestines), he will be given gradually increasing amounts until he no longer needs intravenous nutrition.

The nurse may offer—if she doesn't, feel free to ask—to let you feed your baby by holding him and the syringe full of milk. If the milk is on a pump, you can hold the pacifier he's sucking on as the milk goes in. It can feel impersonal at first, but once you see how satisfied and peaceful your baby gets as he's fed in your loving arms, you'll probably change your mind. Many parents remember gavage feedings as some of the most moving moments of their NICU experience.

Feeding intolerance and ways to overcome it

Feeding may not always go smoothly. Some feeding intolerance is expected in preemies until their digestion matures, and although it may warrant a pause, it's rarely a cause for alarm. During this delicate stage of the feeding journey, your baby will be carefully watched for any of the following signs:

* **An incomplete emptying of the stomach.** Before starting a feeding, the nurse may use the syringe to gently pull out the contents of your baby's stomach, then evaluate them and return them to avoid the loss of any precious nutrients. Most of the time, more fluid than normal in a preemie's stomach just means that her immature intestines are moving slowly and need more time to digest their food completely or move it forward. But if the stomach contents (the NICU staff calls them aspirates) are very large and contain bile, the doctor may consider the possibility of an infection, obstruction of the intestine, or necrotizing enterocolitis (NEC). NEC is the biggest concern when a preemie starts feedings.

* **A tense or tender abdomen, or blood in the stools.** These can also be a sign of infection or NEC. They may be investigated with an X-ray of the baby's intestine. They may also be a reaction or an allergy to the cow's milk proteins in infant formula or milk fortifiers.

* **Vomiting.** Don't be alarmed if your preemie occasionally vomits—every baby does. But if the vomit contains bile (which is dark green), it could indicate an infection or intestinal obstruction. Usually, though, vomiting reflects less serious problems, such as overstimulation, constipation, or reflux. The doctors will see if the problem goes away when, for example, your baby is fed more slowly or placed on his stomach. They may also try thickening his feedings with cereal or try medication to treat reflux.

* **A bloated but soft abdomen.** This can be a sign of gas, constipation, or poor movement by the immature intestines. Full-term new-

borns usually have their first stool within the first 24 or 48 hours, and then stool several times a day, but preemies may take a week or longer and often go several days or more between bowel movements. A sliver of a glycerin suppository (a gentle laxative) might help him. There are also medications that can improve intestinal movement, but these have some side effects and are rarely necessary.

* **Diarrhea.** This can indicate incomplete digestion, usually because the feedings contain too many calories or nutrients that are too complex for the baby's immature intestines to digest. The remedy is to temporarily change the composition of the feedings. Infection is another possible cause, but less likely. Rarely, diarrhea occurs because of an inherited deficiency of lactase, an enzyme needed to digest milk, although this usually shows up later. (Don't worry; there are nutritious substitutes for milk that your baby can get.)

* **More episodes of apnea (a pause in breathing) and bradycardia (slow heart rate).** These may be brought on by the gavage tube itself if it slips out of the stomach back into the esophagus. Removing the tube between feedings might solve the problem. Sometimes if a baby's stomach gets very full and distended, that too could impede breathing. Doctors will also consider infection, NEC, and reflux as possibly contributing problems.

* **Excess gas.** Some babies who are on nasal CPAP have feeding intolerance because their stomachs fill up with gas. Some of this pressure can be relieved by placing a second gavage tube in the baby's stomach just to let the gas come out.

Changing any of the elements of a preemie's feeding schedule may improve his digestion, but it's a matter of trial and error. Your baby's doctor may adjust any of the following:

* **the quantity of milk:** going back to the amount previously tolerated by the baby;

* **the interval between feedings:** raising it from three to four hours, for example, or changing to continuous pump feedings;

* **the duration of feeding:** lengthening each feeding to 45 minutes or an hour, say, instead of 20 to 30 minutes, to give the stomach more time to empty;

* **the strength of breast milk or formula:** discontinuing or reducing the concentration of fortifiers or supplements to improve digestion, thickening milk or formula with cereal to help prevent reflux;

* **the type of formula:** changing to a predigested formula for babies with especially immature digestion or milk protein allergy, or to a special formula for babies with lactose intolerance (soy formulas are avoided in preemies because they contain hormone-like substances and don't support a preemie's rapid bone growth);

* **the location of the gavage tube:** bypassing the stomach if reflux or distention from CPAP is severe by placing the tube and the feedings going through it directly into the intestine.

Often a change that seems tiny to you will be all your baby needs.

Graduating to the breast or bottle

It's a great moment for all parents of very premature babies. Your preemie has reached the age of 32 to 34 weeks, when he might be capable of sucking, swallowing, and breathing all at the same time. He has already proved that he can suck vigorously on a tiny pacifier or the tip of your finger. His vital signs are stable, he's off the ventilator, and on less than about 40 percent oxygen. He has been tolerating and gaining weight on his gavage feedings. All of these encouraging signs lead the doctors and nurses to one conclusion: This preemie is ready to try nippling—nursing at your breast or drinking from a bottle. If you are breastfeeding, your preemie's first nippling attempts may begin even earlier, at 28 to 30 weeks, as studies have shown that a preemie may be able to nurse at the breast before he can drink from a bottle.

Since even preemies who are ready to try nipple feeding aren't usually able to take all of their feedings themselves yet, there are several subtle signals your baby's nurse will watch for during his early attempts, to determine whether to offer a feeding or continue it once it has started. She will make sure he's awake and alert, has good muscle tone and body flexion (showing that he's energetic enough for a feeding, a very tiring activity for a preemie), and promptly opens his mouth when his lips are stroked with a finger or a pacifier, his tongue descending to receive a nipple. After he latches on to your breast or starts sucking from a bottle, the nurse will watch to make sure that he is able to stay actively engaged in feeding and to coordinate breathing, sucking, and swallowing. If he falls asleep, loses interest in eating, or shows signs of breathing difficulties or distress, it's time to stop feeding him.

At this point, the nurse might give your little novice feeder some time to calm down and recover, perhaps swaddling him again to give him better support, and then after this pause resume the feeding. But if your baby seems too tired, his nippling session will stop for good, and he will receive the remaining milk he needs through gavage.

Remember that calories and nutrients are crucially important to support his growth and his ability to learn how to eat. This new task, nippling, can be so tiring for a preemie that in this short session, he may already have used up more calories than he took in! In a few hours, the nurse will reassess your baby, and if he shows signs that he's ready, he'll be offered a chance to try nipple feeding again.

You should know that most preemies who have just graduated to breast or bottle feeding are not very good at it! They may do it only once or twice a day at first, learning how to nipple while getting the rest of their feedings from gavage. At first, your baby may barely latch on to your breast or swallow only a teaspoon or two of formula and milk, and he may not be strong enough to do this at every feeding. Don't worry—and don't try to rush him. Your baby's feeding skills will improve gradually over time, with some inevitable (and often inscrutable) ups and down along the way. But eventually you'll discover that he's eating perfectly well on his own.

Studies have shown that a gentle, flexible approach to feeding preemies, called "infant cue-based feeding"—meaning the preemie is allowed to lead the way and choose when he's ready to breastfeed or nipple feed—is more developmentally appropriate, and more successful, than imposing a predetermined time schedule. Babies learn how to feed better when they are actively engaged in what they are doing and when the first feeding experiences are safe and pleasurable, focusing on the quality of the experience rather than the quantity of milk consumed. (Remember, all the calories he needs to grow can be given to him by gavage.)

Of course, if you are breastfeeding, you will be present at your baby's first feeding efforts, assisted by his nurse or a lactation counselor. Once your preemie has shown that he can breastfeed well, your expressed and stored breast milk can be bottle fed to your baby when you are not there, so he can become an expert at both kinds of nippling. (Even if he doesn't "cue" at every feeding and is still getting some milk by gavage, he may still be good at breastfeeding when he does it.) And if your baby is exclusively bottle fed, the nurses will be happy to help you participate in your baby's efforts by waiting for you to get to the NICU so you can hold and feed him. Just let them know in advance when you plan to be there.

Sometimes a baby may need a little extra help, such as switching to a slow-flow nipple (one that releases less milk and therefore makes swallowing easier for a preemie to coordinate), or having his supplemental oxygen, if he's on it, increased during feedings, or "pacing" his sucking by periodically taking the nipple out of his mouth to remind him to take a few breaths. (Preemies tend to take many more sucks between breaths than term babies do, a reflection of their immature respiratory control. Helping them to pace themselves while they're nippling can avoid some of the typical apnea, bradycardia, and desats that preemies have when they're learning to eat.) Even if your baby was born after 33 weeks of gestation, his immaturity might make breast or bottle feeding hard for him temporarily, so be prepared for the process to take a little longer.

Premature babies who were born at about 26 weeks or less, who were on a ventilator for a couple of months or more and have chronic lung disease, or who have some neurological issues (such as hydrocephalus or PVL) can have a harder time learning how to breast and bottle feed. Endotracheal tubes, suction catheters, and tapes on their faces can result in an unpleasant sensation in or around babies' mouths, which can disturb the natural association of mouth, sucking, hunger relief, and pleasure. Due to the hard experience of their first months of life in the NICU, these infants may refuse to nipple feed, or may be "disorganized feeders" who just can't seem to get the hang of it. These difficulties can often be effectively managed by having a baby evaluated early by a speech pathologist so he can receive feeding therapy sessions before and while he starts nippling. This kind of therapy, together with time and extreme patience by parents or caregivers, is the answer, and it nearly always works. In the rare cases when it doesn't, introducing the baby directly to feeding with a cup and spoon is sometimes successful, as is arranging for longer-term tube feedings while continuing to work on the oral-motor skills and psychological readiness necessary for feeding by mouth.

Your baby will reach the end of his journey when he has replaced all gavage feedings with breast or bottle feeding, can complete each meal in fewer than 20 or 30 minutes, and is gaining weight steadily. While you hold him snugly in your arms, just think of the long way your preemie has come, getting stronger and very well fed.

But they don't know in advance precisely how much sugar a preemie's immature body needs or will be able to handle. And exacerbating the situation for some babies, hyperglycemia is a frequent side effect of medications used to treat low blood pressure, a common issue in newborn preemies.

Your baby's high blood sugar poses no real problem if the level isn't extremely high and if it doesn't stay up for long. But it will be monitored closely, because when blood sugar remains too high, it can mean that not enough is reaching the cells to be used as a source of energy, and this could slow a baby's growth. Also, severe hyperglycemia can cause a baby to urinate too much, increasing the chance that he'll become dehydrated. When dehydration is severe, it can cause problems with a baby's blood chemistry and put him at risk for developing an intraventricular hemorrhage. Finally, probably because extremely high blood sugar levels over the course of many days impede healing in general, there is an association with higher mortality.

So the first thing your baby's doctors will need to decide is whether to try to lower his blood sugar immediately, by changing his IV fluids or with medication, or to wait for it to drop by itself. Simply adjusting the amount of glucose (and sometimes the concentration of protein and lipids) in his intravenous nutrition usually solves the problem. Occasionally, though, even when a baby is getting as little glucose as doctors consider safe, his blood sugar remains high.

Fortunately, soon after most babies start to be fed milk or formula, their blood sugar level stabilizes—often in a matter of a day or two—because digestion stimulates regulatory hormones. Therefore, if your baby is starting to be fed, his doctor may opt not to treat his hyperglycemia but just to keep a close eye on it.

If the doctor thinks treatment is needed, though, a preemie's high blood sugar can be treated with small doses of insulin (yes, just like a diabetic's). As always with medication, there are benefits and risks, and neonatologists haven't yet reached an agreement on how they balance out. The main risk with insulin treatment is that it can be so effective in lowering blood sugar that it works *too* well, sometimes causing sudden severe hypoglycemia (the reverse problem—too low a level of blood sugar), which is actually more dangerous than severe hyperglycemia, the problem you're trying to solve. To prevent this from happening, a preemie on insulin will be monitored with frequent blood tests, and the amount of insulin will be adjusted up or down, depending on his blood sugar level. If your baby's doctor is considering treating him with insulin, you should feel free to ask what he thinks are its pros and cons.

In short, if your preemie has high blood sugar, you can be optimistic. Most likely it's a fleeting concern and won't be a significant issue for you or his doctors again.

Human Milk Banks

I can't breastfeed my baby, and the doctor is recommending that we feed him donor breast milk. I've never heard of such a thing. Is it safe?

Yes, it is true that some mothers who have plenty of breast milk, more than their own babies need, generously donate it to human milk banks. If your doctor prescribes donor breast milk for your baby, it would be sent to your NICU by one of the nonprofit organizations that collect human breast milk, process and test it to guarantee its safety, and ship it to babies who need it. Premature babies whose mothers cannot breastfeed are candidates for donor milk because they can benefit from it, along with full-term babies who suffer from severe food allergies, feeding intolerance, or other illnesses.

Among the donors who give their milk to banks are some lactating mothers of preemies. Their preterm milk, which has a higher protein content and slightly different composition than full-term milk (see page 139), is reserved for the smallest, most immature preemies. (Only about 20 percent of preemies who are fed donor milk receive preterm donor milk, because it is so rare.)

After your own milk, donor milk is considered by many neonatologists to be the second-best choice for your premature baby because:

* Breast milk is easier to digest than formula, so it is less of a strain on a preemie's immature intestines. It also stimulates the motility and maturation of a preemie's gut, reducing feeding intolerance, and allowing him to move faster toward full feedings by mouth, thereby leaving intravenous nutrition behind.
* Babies fed donor milk have a lower risk of suffering from NEC (an intestinal disorder; see pages 266–270). Although babies fed their own mother's milk have lower rates of sepsis and other infections, studies so far have not shown that donor milk confers the same benefits, probably because some antibodies and other infection-fighting substances are lost or diminished when donor milk is processed.

If You Want to Be a Breast Milk Donor

If you are interested in donating your breast milk, you can be sure it will be a precious gift, particularly if your baby was born early: Your preterm milk is valuable nutrition for another premature baby whose mother cannot breastfeed. (Human milk banks consider milk to be preterm for four weeks after delivery from a mother who delivered at less than 36 weeks of gestation.)

You or your doctor should contact the nearest human milk bank. The bank will first establish whether you are an eligible donor. A staff person will interview you, have you fill out a questionnaire, ask your physician and your baby's doctor to certify that you are both in good health, and have you take a blood test to confirm that you don't have infections, such as HIV, hepatitis B or C, or syphilis, that can be transmitted through your milk. Once you get a clean bill of health, the bank will send you everything you need to store your milk and ship it back: containers, a cooler, packing materials, and labels. You will need to have your own breast pump, though.

You will receive clear instructions on how to store, pack, and ship your breast milk. You'll send it by FedEx to the human milk bank, where it will be pooled with other donors' milk (if it's preterm milk, it will be mixed only with other preterm milk). It will be pasteurized, frozen, and released only after all tests for infection or contamination come back negative.

You won't be paid for all of the time and energy you'll have to invest, but every time you pump your milk to help another unknown premature baby heal and grow, you will feel that special pride that comes from giving an anonymous gift—and the unspoken gratitude of the family who receives it.

Many hope that donor milk, like mother's milk, might improve a preemie's neurological development. At this point, however, research hasn't shown a difference in long-term development between preemies fed donor breast milk and those fed preterm formula.

* The Human Milk Banking Association of North America (which comprises six U.S. banks, one in Canada, and one in Mexico) follows guidelines accepted by the Food and Drug Administration that are identical to the strict regulations governing blood and tissue banking. Donor mothers are not paid, and they are screened in the same way blood donors are, to rule out infections, illness, ingestion of dangerous substances, and risky behaviors. The pediatrician of the potential donor's baby is questioned, also, to make sure the baby is healthy and growing well. After the milk is collected, it is pasteurized, then again screened for bacterial infection, so you can feel confident that it is safe. Despite pasteurization (keeping the milk at a temperature of 62.5 degrees Celsius—144.5 degrees Fahrenheit—for 30 minutes) and freezing, many of the precious components in human milk, such as

fatty acids, are preserved and many others, such as infection-fighting enzymes, growth factors, vitamins, and minerals are unchanged or just slightly diminished.

Pasteurized human milk does have somewhat less nutritional power than untreated mother's milk, both because of its processing and because preterm donor milk (which is richer in proteins) isn't always available. Before being fed to your preemie, donor breast milk will be mixed with the same things your own breast milk would be, products called human milk fortifiers, to increase its calories, vitamins, and minerals; in addition, donor breast milk may need to be supplemented with extra protein and other calories, often by mixing in a little preterm formula, if a baby's growth is slow. (Studies on preemies getting unfortified donor milk showed that they had slower growth in the NICU than preemies who were fed formula, although even then, their long-term growth was no different.)

If your doctor is suggesting donor milk for your baby, it probably means that your hospital has a standing arrangement with a milk bank, and you won't have to do anything special to get it. Some NICUs recommend donor milk for all preemies who are not breastfed, while others prescribe it only for some, such as preemies born at less than 27 or 28 weeks of gestation or those who are recovering from NEC surgery. If you would like your preemie to get donor milk and it hasn't been offered, you should feel free to talk about it with your baby's doctor. On the other hand, if you *don't* want your baby to get it—some parents have an aversion to the idea of their baby's being fed another mother's milk, no matter how safe or healthy it may be—be sure to tell the doctor that, too. Most NICUs, though not all, get parents' permission before giving donor breast milk to a baby.

What obstacles might stand in the way of your baby's getting donor milk?

* Occasionally the supply of donor milk runs low. When only a limited amount is available, it is rationed to babies who need it most, those with severe feeding complications or the very youngest preemies.
* Most banks will provide donor milk to any baby while he's in the hospital, as long as the doctor orders it. But after your baby is discharged, you may not be able to get it except in special circumstances. You'll have to show a doctor's prescription for it, and your insurance policy or Medicaid may or may not cover it, depending on the medical needs of your baby.
* Donor breast milk is expensive. It costs about $3 an ounce plus shipping and handling. The price arises from the high costs of running a safe, efficient bank. Some health insurance plans cover donor milk, but they may require a certificate of medical need.

Some mothers ask whether they can feed their baby breast milk donated by friends or relatives. Although human milk banks don't process milk for directed donation (from a particular donor, to a particular baby), a few are willing to screen and test a potential directed donor in the same way they do their other donors. If you're interested, you'll need to contact the nearest milk bank yourself (see Appendix 6, page 590) to make arrangements. But make sure to check first whether your baby's NICU will allow a directed donation. Most hospitals either don't allow or strongly discourage them because without pasteurization, safety can't be assured.

An important word of warning: You may see breast milk for sale over the Internet. Never feed this to your baby, because its safety and quality are completely unknown.

(*Continued on page 176*)

Practical Advice for Pumping and Storing Breast Milk

So you've started expressing your milk, and you want to breastfeed your preemie. There are many things you will learn by yourself during this highly rewarding experience, no matter whether you breastfeed for a short time or for many months to come. Here is some practical guidance to lead you through the challenging early stages of your preemie's nursing. After that, his feeding behavior will become no different from that of a baby born at full-term.

Expressing your milk

These days, most mothers who breastfeed eventually learn to express their milk for one reason or another, often because they're working, traveling without their baby, or fathers are helping with feedings. But as a mother of a premature baby, you'll become a true expert on breast pumps and expressing your milk from the very start.

In the first days: Prompted by hormones, the milk production system in your breasts develops during the very first months of pregnancy. Even if your baby was born extremely prematurely, just at the limit of viability, you'll be ready to provide breast milk for him. A remarkable sign that Mother Nature is looking out for you and your preemie is that your milk will be different from that of a mother who delivers at term: It is perfectly tailored to the nutritional needs of a premature baby.

For lactation to get started, your breasts must get a signal from the hormone prolactin, which is stimulated initially by the delivery of the placenta. It is also stimulated by the baby's sucking or the use of a breast pump. After the first week, your milk production is a finely tuned supply-and-demand system that responds to frequent emptying of the breasts: The more you empty your breasts, the more milk your body thinks is needed, so the more it makes. To start your lactation and keep it going if your preemie is not ready to nurse, you'll have to rely on the artificial stimulation of an electric breast pump, which provides the closest approximation to a baby's sucking.

Mothers of preemies who begin using a hospital-quality electric breast pump within hours after delivery, perhaps combined with expressing some milk by hand, have the best chance of producing enough milk to satisfy their babies' growing needs. With a pump, you can express your milk and store it so it can be fed to your preemie later, through a gavage tube, until he becomes mature enough to suck at your breast. The first attempts to express milk with an electric pump can be frustrating, due to the small volume of milk collected in the early days. This will get better if you keep at it! If you have pain or concerns, ask your nurse or a lactation consultant to help you identify and solve the problem. You can find suggestions to make the initial experience easier on pages 124–126.

In the hospital: In your room on the maternity floor or in your baby's nursery, you'll have access to a hospital-quality electric pump. Most nurseries have a quiet, secluded pumping room that gives mothers the privacy they need. Each mother is given her own personal pumping kit and containers to store her milk. Don't be shy about asking the nurses for help or advice. On the maternity floor or in the NICU, helping you express breast milk for your premature baby is an important part of a nurse's job. Many hospitals also have lactation specialists dedicated to teaching mothers and babies to breastfeed.

At home: Soon after delivery, find out where you can rent a high-quality electric pump to use at home (common brands are Ameda and Medela). Pharmacies near the hospital or medical supply companies often rent them; ask your nurse about that or contact a breastfeeding consultant. (You can get a referral through La Leche League, a nonprofit organization that advocates breastfeeding, at 800-LA-LECHE.) Since your baby was born prematurely, the cost of the rental may be covered by your health insurance.

You'll need a personal kit of collecting equipment (tubing, funnel, etc.) to use with a rented pump, which you should wash according to your hospital's instructions.

How soon and how often you should pump: You should start pumping as soon as possible after delivery, ideally within 6 to 12 hours. Pumping should be frequent, at least every two to three hours while you're awake, for at least six to eight daily milk expressions. You shouldn't go for more than six hours without pumping, even at night. (If you prepare all of the equipment before going to bed, you can set your alarm for an early-morning pumping session, then go back to sleep for a few more hours.) Some experts recommend that, a few days before your baby comes home, you get ready by waking up during the night and pumping every two to four hours, as often as you would breastfeed him.

You'll need to keep your breast pump throughout your baby's hospitalization and probably for another two or three weeks after he comes home. It can take a while for a preemie to become an efficient breastfeeder and completely empty your breast at each feeding. You should continue, for some time, to pump for a few min-

utes after breastfeeding to supplement his efforts and keep your milk supply going. You'll be able to stop pumping when you find that there's no milk left in your breast after your baby has finished nursing.

If you plan to travel or go back to work soon, you may want to rent or buy a lighter portable electric pump. It won't empty your breasts as completely as a hospital-quality pump will, but it has one big advantage: When it's packed up it looks like a briefcase, and many working mothers bring them to their offices with no one the wiser! When your milk supply is well-established, you'll occasionally be able to use other, less powerful pumps—battery-operated or manual ones that every pharmacy carries—or simply breast massage (see below).

How to get started: When you handle breast milk, good hygiene is a must. Wash your hands before touching your breast or the collecting equipment. At home, make sure that everything is washed and clean. Connect the tubing to the pump, to the collecting cup for your milk, and to the funnel you'll be applying to your breast. The first time you may want to ask a nurse to show you how.

The best way to express your milk is to use a double kit that allows you to pump from both breasts at the same time. Although it may feel awkward in the beginning, you'll find that it's convenient and saves time (something parents of preemies never have enough of). Most important, double pumping can stimulate your breasts to produce more milk; that's why mothers of twins who breastfeed both babies simultaneously are often able to produce enough milk for both of them. (If you're a mother of multiples, you'll find more breastfeeding advice on pages 333–337.)

Position the funnel on your breast: The nipple should be centered in the funnel of the flange. Before turning on the pump, adjust its suction to the lowest level. Then as you pump, gradually increase the suction to a comfortable level. Pumping should not pinch or hurt you. (Any discomfort that you feel during your first few pumping attempts should subside. If it doesn't, or if you feel sharp pain, even during your first sessions, ask your nurse or a breastfeeding consultant to help you figure out what is causing it.) Through the transparent funnel, check to make sure that your milk is trickling into the container. If the spray stops, switch off the pump and reposition the funnel on your nipple. With some adjustment, your milk will often start to flow again.

In the first few days, you should pump each breast for about 10 to 15 minutes. Later, you can gradually increase the time you pump each breast up to 15 to 20 minutes to completely empty your breasts every time. Some lactation experts recommend massaging your breasts during and after you pump to get even more milk out.

Why you might not get much at the beginning: It can take a few days for your milk to come in, so don't worry if you get very little in the beginning. You may express only a few drops, but they are precious. Your first milk, called colostrum, is yellow and very thick. Colostrum is important to feed to a preemie because it is particularly rich in proteins and antibodies. Transitional milk, which comes in about three to five days after delivery, is also rich in proteins but contains more water than colostrum. Mature breast milk, which resembles skim milk in its thin bluish appearance, has more calories and fats than the earlier milk, and generally takes one to two weeks to develop.

Why you should completely empty your breasts and not go too long between pumping sessions: Both of these are crucial for ensuring that your baby gets the best nutrition and achieves optimal growth. The first breast milk that comes out when you express, called fore milk, usu-ally has fewer calories, with less fat and more sugar, than the last milk you express, called hind milk. Since your baby needs all of these nutrients, it's important for you to completely empty your breasts every time you pump. Also, if you don't pump often enough, your body gets a wrong signal: It thinks your baby doesn't need as much nutrition as he really does and changes both the quantity and quality of the milk you produce. Not only do you risk making less milk, but the milk you do make will become less nutritious, with a lower calorie content than your preemie needs to grow and develop well.

Getting the milk from you to your baby

Bacteria can easily flourish in breast milk, so you should be very careful how you collect and store it.

Collecting your milk: Your baby's nursery will provide breast milk containers for you to use in the hospital and at home. Pump directly into one of these storage containers so you can detach the container holding your milk, close it with a lid, and bring it directly to the nursery. You should store milk from each pumping session in a separate container, because your baby will drink only small quantities at each feeding, and you don't want to thaw or discard any of your milk unnecessarily. Just be careful to choose a container that's big enough to store all of the breast milk from one pumping session to make sure your baby receives the nutrients contained in both the hind milk and the fore milk.

Every breast milk container must be labeled with your baby's name, hospital identification number, and the date and time you collected it; it is your responsibility to do so. Some nurseries will provide you with prestamped labels (to which you will add the date and time of collection) and won't accept handwritten ones. Ask your nurse about your hospital's policy.

Storing and preserving your milk: Ideally, breast milk is fed to a preemie fresh, right after pumping. If you're in your hospital room waiting for somebody to pick up your container of milk and take it to the nursery, place it in a pan with water and ice to prevent the growth of bacteria.

Breast milk for a premature baby can be safely stored in the refrigerator for 24 to 48 hours or for much longer in the freezer. Before feeding it to a baby, frozen milk should be thawed by putting the container in a room-temperature water bath. (High temperatures or microwaving can deprive breast milk of important components.) Freezing and thawing will lower the nutritional and infection-fighting qualities of breast milk slightly, but it's still the best choice for your baby when fresh is not available.

Once your milk is thawed, it will be used for your baby's feedings over the next 24 hours. You should learn how much milk your baby is taking at each feeding so you can fill each container accordingly (with just a little more than what is needed) and not waste any.

Transporting breast milk from home to the hospital: If you'll be taking your milk to the hospital within 24 hours of pumping, keep it in the refrigerator, then carry it to the hospital packed in ice. If you're storing breast milk for longer, freeze it immediately after it's pumped and bring it to the nursery packed in ice or an ice pack. Make sure it stays frozen until you give it to the nurse to put in the nursery freezer. Since there is limited space for each baby, you may be asked to store your extra milk in your home freezer, bringing it only when your baby's supply is running low.

When your baby begins feeding, your colostrum will be given to him first. After that, your frozen milk is generally used as a backup for your fresh milk. The oldest frozen milk is used first; that's why it's important to properly label each container. Because fresh milk is somewhat higher in nutrients and antibodies, many mothers try to bring some from home every time they visit, then pump more in the nursery before they leave. You should also check before each visit that there's enough breast milk left for times you're not around, and bring more if it's needed. If you are not pumping enough milk to meet your baby's needs, talk to your doctors and nurses about ways to increase your milk supply (you can read about this on pages 254–257) and about supplementing your milk with donor breast milk from a milk bank or with infant formula. And don't berate yourself when, despite trying your best, your baby occasionally gets formula if there's not enough breast milk or you didn't make it to the hospital on time; the advantages of breastfeeding will still be preserved.

While the idea of human milk banks may seem unfamiliar and strange to you as yet, you can feel comfortable about the safety, and potential value to your baby, of their special product.

Attention Paid to Diapers

Why are the nurses always examining our son's bowel movements and weighing his wet diapers?

Every NICU's golden rule is to closely monitor all preemies' vital signs and bodily functions, even those you may take for granted. For instance, most full-term babies pass their first stools, the peculiarly black meconium, within 24 hours of birth. But a premature baby may not have his first bowel movement for several days; the earlier a baby is born, the longer the wait, because of the immaturity of his intestines. Preemies who are sicker or who aren't being fed will also pass their first stool later. No wonder the nurses will proudly announce to you when that natural event has finally taken place for your baby!

Your baby's diapers will get a lot of attention because they contain such useful clues and information. In addition to a visual exam, the nurses may perform tests on your baby's stools to evaluate how well he's absorbing the nutrients in his feedings or to check for hidden blood. They will register the time, amount, and appearance of each stool in your baby's medical chart. If your baby has diarrhea (watery, frequent bowel movements), it may be due to incomplete absorption of his feedings—possibly because the caloric density is too high for his immature intestines, or because he has an intolerance to lactose or cow's milk protein. These problems can be treated by changing what he eats. Diarrhea could also be a sign of an infection.

On the other hand, constipation, in a tiny preemie, may cause enough abdominal distention to compromise his breathing! Don't worry—it's usually just due to immaturity, and he'll soon outgrow it. Infrequent, irregular bowel movements are expected in preemies because the mature, coordinated movements of the intestines that propel stool down and outward are sparse and uncoordinated until about 34 weeks of gestation. Even a week between bowel movements isn't uncommon in the NICU.

If your baby is constipated, the nurse may give him a glycerin suppository or a little rectal stimulation with a cotton swab or the tip of a gloved finger to encourage a bowel movement. Older preemies whose stools are both infrequent and hard may be given a teaspoon or two of prune juice every day to soften them—just like Grandpa! If constipation interferes with a baby's ability to tolerate his feedings and goes on too long, the doctor may decide to get a contrast enema—an X-ray study of his large intestine—

and to wash out any plugs of meconium that may be blocking normal bowel movements.

A little invisible blood in a preemie's stool is usually nothing to worry about; it's common and often results from minor irritation of the stomach from a baby's feeding tube. (The nurse knows the blood is there because it shows up as a blue color on a guaiac test. Pronounced "GWY-ak," this painless test is done at your baby's bedside. The nurse puts a tiny bit of stool on a special card then drips a chemical on it and watches for color change.) Small streaks of visible blood might come from a tiny cut in or around his rectum or a particularly bad diaper rash. If there's a lot of bleeding, though, or it lasts, it might be a signal of more severe inflammation, maybe due to a milk protein allergy or necrotizing enterocolitis. Doctors would want to treat these conditions early to prevent progression of the illness.

Most of the time, the color of a bowel movement isn't significant (even the green stools that surprise many parents), but in the rare cases that stools are pale gray or white, they may indicate that a baby is not passing bile appropriately.

Wet diapers get plenty of attention, too. Your baby's urine is monitored by weighing his diapers, as you noticed, and sometimes by performing dipstick tests. (A plastic stick painted with chemicals is dipped into the urine. It changes color if the urine contains certain substances, including blood, sugar, protein, and acid.) Dipstick tests may be done to check for mild metabolic disturbances (such as whether a baby is fully utilizing the glucose he's given) or infection, and to verify the overall functioning of the urinary system. The quantity and concentration of a baby's urine helps indicate the baby's level of hydration (whether he has the right amount of fluid in his system) and the effectiveness of certain medications he may be taking.

When you start changing your preemie's diaper, make sure that you leave it aside for the nurses, and don't drop it by mistake in the waste-basket. Remember: What may look like a common dirty diaper is actually a valuable piece of information about your preemie's health.

Meconium Obstruction

Our baby has constipation and feeding problems, and the doctor says she has meconium blocking her intestines. If she doesn't improve, she might need surgery. We are so scared.

Your baby is probably suffering from meconium obstruction of prematurity, also known as inspissated meconium, which is simply a kind of severe constipation with a perplexing name. Inspissated means thickened, and meconium is the first kind of stool a newborn baby passes after birth. When a fetus is in the womb, his intestines have already begun making stool, even though he isn't having bowel movements yet. This fetal stool, called meconium, consists of sloughed-off cells, amniotic fluid, bile, and mucus. It is black and thick, like tar—not at all like the stools babies pass later after they've begun eating—and fills much of a fetus's large intestine.

If meconium dries out too much, it can harden into a plug that literally plugs the intestine either partially or completely, not allowing gas or stool to get by it. Preemies with this sort of intestinal obstruction might have one big plug of meconium or smaller fragments that tenaciously stick to the inner walls of the bowel even after they've passed one or more small stools. Doctors don't know for sure why inspissated meconium happens, but they think it may come from a combination of diminished blood flow to the intestines (which can occur during pregnancy if, for example, a mother has preeclampsia or after delivery if a newborn is dehydrated or has a severe infection) and the weak, slow movements of the intestines typical of extremely premature babies, which allow meconium to sit there and the fluid in it to be reabsorbed.

The symptoms of meconium obstruction overlap with those of feeding intolerance: vomiting, big milk residuals in the stomach, a distended abdomen, and constipation. On regular X-rays, a baby's bowel will look dilated and blocked, but doctors can't know for sure what the problem is until they do a contrast enema—a special X-ray study in which dye is given to the baby in the form of an enema. The dye (contrast) makes the inner contours of the bowel visible, outlining the inspissated meconium. Most of the time, the contrast enema does double duty: It's good not only for diagnosing meconium plugs but also for treating them, because the extra water and pressure in the bowel from the enema helps the baby pass the plugs.

After a contrast enema, your baby's doctor may prescribe several more noncontrast enemas (usually with salt water) that the nurses will give in the NICU to flush out any lingering plugs. These enemas probably won't bother your baby much, and as they work, she'll feel more and more comfortable. In the vast majority of cases, this takes care of the problem, and the meconium obstruction resolves with no long-term effects.

In a few babies with inspissated meconium, the enemas don't relieve all of the obstruction, and since some plugs persist, the symptoms get worse. Unfortunately, these babies will need intestinal surgery, because unless the remaining meconium is cleared out, they are in danger of the bowel becoming so distended that it perforates (a perforation is a tear in the bowel wall, similar to what happens when a balloon is filled up with too much air).

Surgery to prevent or repair a perforation must be done urgently. The surgeon's goal will be to find the obstruction, determine its cause, and relieve it as much as possible.

(Continued on page 181)

Getting Acquainted with: Jaundice and Bilirubin

Many people know what jaundice is: a yellowish tinge of the skin. But it's less well known what jaundice comes from.

We all have a yellow substance called bilirubin in our bodies. It's made naturally all the time as used red blood cells are broken down and then it gets excreted in our stools. The reason so many newborns have jaundice is that they aren't good at getting rid of bilirubin yet, so it builds up. It's the liver's job to convert bilirubin into a form that can be passed out of the body, but it can take a few days after birth for the liver to switch this process on, and a preemie's immature liver can take even longer—a week or two. Plus, newborns produce a lot more bilirubin than older babies, since their red blood cells have shorter lives.

When doctors see jaundice in a newborn, full-term or premature, they rarely get worried. The jaundice is usually a result of immaturity, not illness, so it's just temporary, and small increases in bilirubin aren't harmful, anyway. Furthermore, there is a very effective treatment, phototherapy, to keep the bilirubin level from getting too high. If it does, it can cause brain damage—but your baby's doctor will treat her jaundice well before it gets to that point.

Which babies get jaundiced

All preemies, but especially the youngest and smallest ones, are apt to become jaundiced, because their livers and intestines are more immature than term babies. Their livers aren't as quick to start converting bilirubin into a disposable form, and they have fewer bowel movements to eliminate it (especially if they aren't being fed at first). Babies who have a lot of skin bruising from a difficult delivery, who are born with unusually high numbers of red blood cells, or who have intraventricular hemorrhages will be watched especially carefully, because they'll produce lots of bilirubin as those used red blood cells are broken down. Infants whose mothers are diabetic or have a different blood type, who have respiratory distress syndrome or an infection, or who suffered some birth asphyxia are also more likely to become jaundiced.

Diagnosis: Observation and blood tests

Compared to many other medical conditions, jaundice is easy to diagnose. As bilirubin levels rise, a baby's skin turns progressively more yellowish-orange, starting at her head and continuing on down toward her toes. Depending on your baby's color and how much of her body is jaundiced, the doctor can guess at her bilirubin level, or he may use a handheld tool that takes a reading of her skin color. If he wants a more precise measurement, he can measure the exact level in her blood.

If a baby's bilirubin level is high for her age and size or if it is rising quickly, her doctor will check out a number of possibilities, including whether something has caused more breakdown of red blood cells than usual (for example, an incompatibility with her mother's blood), whether bilirubin is not being passed out as feces quickly enough (depending on the reason, something as simple as a little suppository or starting feedings may solve the problem), whether breast milk could be interfering with bilirubin disposal (called breast milk jaundice, this develops slowly over several weeks, is rarely severe, and quickly resolves if the baby isn't fed breast milk for a couple of days), or whether the problem is actually a different sort of jaundice from liver damage (called direct hyperbilirubinemia; see page 317). Most of the time, though, there's no cause other than your baby's natural, to-be-expected immaturity.

The course that jaundice takes

Regular jaundice in preemies usually follows a typical pattern, becoming visible 36 to 48 hours after birth. Bilirubin levels increase gradually, peak at about five to seven days, then decrease gradually to normal levels over the following week or two.

How jaundice is treated

Enter any NICU and you'll see bright blue, green, or white lights called bililights shining on naked babies wearing eye shields, as if they were in a tanning salon. Other babies may be basking on green lighted pads called biliblankets. Phototherapy originated after some nurses in England noticed that babies near windows were less jaundiced than other newborns in the nursery. Like the sunlight streaming through those windows, the light waves from bililights change bilirubin into substances that can be eliminated easily from a baby's body—as the liver does when it is mature.

Phototherapy is very safe. Only a few babies may have some temporary side effects—diarrhea and skin rashes, in particular—but they go away when the lights do. During phototherapy, eye covers protect your baby's retinas from damage, and her reproductive organs are kept covered, too, by her diaper—although these precautions may not even be necessary. (When you're around, the lights can be turned off for a while and your baby's eye covers removed, to give you and your baby the joy of looking into each other's eyes.)

Most preemies remain under bililights for a few days or a week. If your baby is already being fed breast milk and her bilirubin level is very high, she may be taken off it and given formula for a day or two, because sometimes breast milk can raise bilirubin levels. (Don't forget to keep pumping in the meantime, since you'll be able to go right back to breastfeeding once your baby's bilirubin levels go back down. Breast milk jaundice isn't permanent—a baby's body would eventually adjust on its own—but a breastfeeding break can reduce high bilirubin levels quickly and easily.)

When your baby's bilirubin drops to a low level, the doctors will turn off the phototherapy. Often the bilirubin level will rebound higher again for a day or two after phototherapy has stopped, and the lights may be restarted. This isn't a setback; it merely means your baby wasn't quite ready to come off the phototherapy. Chances are that the lights will be turned off again a few days later and her bilirubin level will continue to fall.

Rarely, a baby's bilirubin will continue to climb, and her doctor may feel that the next therapeutic step is necessary: either an infusion of a medication called IVIG (short for intravenous immune globulin, this works when jaundice results from an incompatibility between the mother's and baby's blood types) or an exchange transfusion. In an exchange transfusion, the baby's blood, with its circulating bilirubin, is drawn out through a catheter and replaced with fresh blood from a donor. Exchange transfusions are hardly ever necessary in preemies because phototherapy and IVIG work so well.

Should you be worried?

Not unless your doctor tells you to be—and he probably won't. Up to 60 percent of full-term babies and 80 percent of preemies develop jaundice within the first few days of their lives. At low levels, there are no lasting effects of jaundice. In fact, a little jaundice may even be good, protecting the body against tissue damage caused by natural toxins called free radicals.

In the very rare cases when it reaches high levels, bilirubin can pass to the brain and cause brain damage, or even death. For full-term babies, doctors know how much bilirubin is safe. In preemies, though, they still aren't sure. (In a recent study, extremely premature babies whose jaundice was treated at lower levels than usual had better long-term development and less chronic lung disease than those who were treated at standard levels. But there were also more deaths among the tiniest preemies in the study, perhaps due to chance, but perhaps due to the earlier treatment of their jaundice.) The level at which brain or other injury will occur varies, depending on many interrelated factors having to do with a baby's age, size, and medical condition, among other things. You can ask your baby's doctor what level he would consider harmful for your child, but you should realize that until more research results are in, the number he gives you will be less than certain.

Although uncertainty like that sounds scary to a parent, it's important to put it in perspective. Fortunately, thanks to the widespread use of phototherapy, many NICUs haven't seen a case of serious brain damage from very high bilirubin levels in years.

So if your baby has jaundice, please don't worry needlessly. Be glad that she's bathing comfortably under those lights, which for the vast majority of preemies is no more than a little detour on the path toward home.

He'll have the valuable opportunity to closely examine your baby's intestines, noting whether they're connected correctly and in the right position, whether anything is pressing on them that might be hindering the passage of meconium, and whether they look generally healthy. If there was no perforation and the only problem the surgeon finds is meconium plugs, he'll open the bowel and wash out as much of the inspissated meconium as he can. If there was a perforation, he'll also cut out the damaged portion of intestine. Then, with the bowel safely cleared of plugs, the surgeon will decide whether he can sew it back together right then and there—he usually can—or whether it would be safer to make an enterostomy. With an enterostomy, the surgeon temporarily brings the two cut ends of the bowel through an opening in the baby's belly, where they can drain and heal (see page 357). After several weeks, when the intestine has had enough time to rest and recover, the surgeon can reconnect the bowel and close the ostomy. Most of the time, though, an enterostomy isn't needed, and in a few days, when the baby has recovered from the surgery, this whole difficult episode is, thankfully, history.

Try to remember, if you have to go through this, that while it's worrisome to see a preemie undergoing intestinal surgery for any reason, when the problem is inspissated meconium, parents should be very optimistic. The surgical risks are minimal, healing tends to be fast, and there are usually no long-term consequences. In fact, preemies with this condition are often so young that it doesn't even prolong their hospitalization—they're well recovered from it by the time they're old enough to go home.

You should be aware, though, that occasionally what doctors hope is only inspissated meconium turns out to be a different problem, NEC. The diagnosis of this other intestinal disease of prematurity (see page 266) can be confirmed during surgery. Meconium obstruction can lead to NEC if the distention from it is so severe that it affects the health of the bowel wall. Doctors may also want to test a baby with inspissated meconium for cystic fibrosis or Hirschsprung's disease because these conditions can cause overly thick meconium that leads to a bowel obstruction. But if you are being told about these tests, don't worry. It's extremely unlikely that your baby will have either one (there's no known link between them and prematurity), and many neonatologists don't even feel the need to rule out these disorders if a baby recovers uneventfully and has no unusual problems with feeding, bowel movements, and growth during the rest of his hospital stay.

For now, try to damp down your understandable fears, because most likely your baby is going to have clean, comfortable intestines—and a clean bill of health, too—within just a few days.

Nurses' Response to Alarms

I jump when one of the alarms goes off in the NICU, but I swear that the nurses act downright blasé. When I'm not there, they might not respond in time to save my daughter!

What can be more terrifying than the sudden beep-beep-beep of your baby's alarms? If you're like most parents, you feel a rush of panic and your eyes fly to the machine next to your baby's bed to see which of her vital signs is in a danger zone. A flashing light tells you that she has stopped breathing, that her heart has slowed, or that she is losing oxygen. You're on the verge of screaming for an army of medical reinforcements. And what does your baby's nurse do? She saunters over and, with a mere glance at your baby and the monitor, turns off the alarm and walks away again. Perhaps noticing your look of panic, she also reminds you: "Look at your baby, not the machine."

To you, the nurse may seem overly casual, but chances are she's not—she's just experienced.

Parents tend to think of the monitors attached to their baby as precise instruments, but they're actually subject to false alarms and unnecessary scares for any number of reasons:

✳ Your baby squirms around or the nurse moves her, causing one of the wires to the cardiorespiratory monitor to come loose, or one of the leads on your baby's chest to slide out of place or fall off. Since the leads are held on with very mild adhesive, this happens frequently. The result is that the monitor can't detect your baby's chest movements, and thinks she's having apnea (a pause in breathing) or can't detect her pulse, and thinks she's having a "brady" (short for bradycardia, a slow heart rate).

✳ Squirming often causes the oxygen monitor to alarm, also—either the sensor comes loose, or it's just unable to pick up your baby's pulse until she settles down. This machine needs an accurate reading of a baby's pulse to figure out whether there's enough oxygen in her blood; if it gets a low reading of her pulse, it thinks her oxygen saturation level is falling (she is "desatting"). It's easy to tell if the sensor isn't picking up your baby's pulse. If the cardiorespiratory monitor shows a heart rate of, say, 160, but the oxygen monitor shows a heart rate of 80, or if the red line that represents your baby's pulse is wildly gyrating (heart rates don't gyrate like that), you've got a false alarm for sure.

✳ Almost all preemies do something called periodic breathing. They may take a few deep breaths and then pause for five or ten seconds before taking another one. It's not apnea unless the pause lasts at least twenty seconds or is accompanied by a reduction in heart rate or change in skin color. But the cardiorespiratory monitor, because of the way it's programmed to calculate numbers of breaths, can sometimes misinterpret periodic breathing as longer apnea spells.

* Sometimes preemies do what's called shallow breathing: They pull their chests in slightly rather than deeply. If the lead can't feel these subtle chest movements, the monitor will think your baby isn't breathing.

Your baby's looks are far more reliable than the machines. So as the nurses urge, when an alarm goes off, don't stare at the scary numbers on the monitor's screen (which is everybody's instinct). Instead, look at your baby. If your baby is in distress, she'll show it. If her chest is moving in and out and her nostrils are gently flaring, she's breathing—even if the monitor says she isn't. If she's nice and pink, she has plenty of oxygen.

Even when they do have real apnea, a real brady, or real desatting, preemies often recover quickly on their own without getting into trouble. It's good to let them do that unless they're already showing signs of poor oxygenation or blood flow (we'll explain the signs in a minute). Why is it better for the nurse to wait to see what happens rather than rushing to intervene?

* It's important for the doctors and nurses to know whether your baby can recover on her own. This is an important piece of clinical evidence that will influence whether she needs further treatment (such as medication, supplemental oxygen, or other breathing assistance) and when she can be discharged.
* Whenever possible, your baby should be left alone and allowed to sleep undisturbed. It's far better not to bother her than to wake her if the episode is going to resolve on its own anyway.
* Sometimes it's the monitor that needs intervention, not the baby. As preemies get older, their normal heart rate slows down, especially during deep sleep. So if your maturing baby starts setting off lots of alarms with no signs of distress, it simply may mean that it's time to reset her cardiorespiratory monitor to sound

an alarm at a lower heart rate than before. Also, some babies just breathe faster or have faster heart rates than others. If the doctors are convinced these babies are healthy, they'll simply reset the monitor accordingly.
* Some preemies are particularly sensitive to stimulation. They become so easily stressed out that even loud noises, being handled, or their own movements can trigger apnea or desatting. When these babies are feeling overwhelmed, the last thing they need is more touching and handling. They really want to be left alone, and once the stimulation subsides, they recover. (You can read about how to interact with your baby and understand her signals on page 234.)

OK. What are the signs that your baby may really be in trouble and need help *now*? Her lips will soon turn bluish-gray if she isn't breathing or if her heart is pumping too slowly to send enough oxygen to the skin. After a little while longer, she may become limp, and her skin will become bluish-gray, too. This color change is called cyanosis. If the nurse sees it, you can be sure she will intervene to help your baby. (A bluish color of the hands and feet alone, in the first few days of life, is different; it is normal for newborns and goes away on its own.)

If your baby does need a reminder to breathe, the nurse's first step may be to touch her gently: A tickle or a tap on a preemie's foot is often enough. If she needs a little more rousing than that, the nurse can rub her arm, leg, or back slightly more vigorously. If that's still not enough, the nurse will provide the baby with oxygen. In an intensive care nursery, every baby has the necessary equipment right beside her bed. The nurse can blow oxygen from a tube near her face or place a mask over her nose and mouth and gently pump some oxygen into her lungs. (Since in some nurseries the oxygen comes out of a bag, you may hear this called "bagging" the baby, a terrible term, if you ask us! Other nurseries use a device called a Neopuff and say they are "puffing" the baby.) As soon as the baby is pink again and her pulse is back up, she's fine.

What does it mean that your baby is having apnea and bradys? Probably nothing more than that she's an official card-carrying preemie. The episodes are probably just a normal consequence of her immaturity (her doctor will let you know if he thinks otherwise) and will go away by about the 36th to 38th week of gestation. It's parents who suffer most from these alarms. For more information, see *Getting Acquainted with Apnea and Bradycardia* on page 246.

Afraid to Leave Your Baby

I'm afraid to leave my baby's side. What if there's an emergency and I'm not there?

That's a fear you share with many parents whose babies are in an intensive-care nursery. But there are a few things that should reassure you.

If your baby's doctor and nurse say she's stable, it's very unlikely that an emergency will occur suddenly. Just like other babies, if something is wrong, preemies usually provide their doctors and parents with a warning first, by getting sick and less stable.

In the rare event that an unexpected emergency does occur—say a baby needs to have an urgent medical procedure or CPR—an intensive-care nursery is set up to handle it. Although the incident may signal that there's an underlying problem, it would be very unusual for a baby to get sicker so rapidly that you wouldn't have time to receive a phone call and come in to be with her after the emergency intervention, when she'll need you.

If you have been told that your baby *is* unstable, you can ask her doctor whether there's any immediate danger; he can almost always tell you.

Many illnesses that preemies get have an acute period, then gradually resolve. (For example, babies can be very sick for one or two days after they have a major surgical procedure. The initial days after a baby gets an infection are usually the worst. Or when a baby has NEC—necrotizing enterocolitis—there is often a span of a few days when the need for emergency surgery could suddenly arise.) After the few days of uncertainty pass, the likelihood of a sudden emergency will largely pass, too—and you should try not to worry. This even applies to extremely premature babies whose parents fear they won't survive: After the first three or four days of life, they are out of the most dangerous period, and their chances of surviving go way up.

If the doctor thinks your baby is in a highly unstable or dangerous period, you would probably want to stay in or near the hospital to reach your baby quickly if anything were to happen. You can stay at your baby's bedside in the nursery or, if your hospital has one, in a special parent sleep-room (some NICUs offer this to families who need to be as close to their babies as possible for medical reasons) or in a nearby hotel. Be sure to ask the NICU social worker or your baby's nurse what the possibilities are.

Some parents whose babies are sick find they just can't shake the fear that their baby will die suddenly while they are away from the nursery. If this is what's worrying you, we can assure you: It almost never happens. Doctors can almost always tell when a baby's condition is becoming very serious, early enough to reach the parents so they can return to the nursery.

The most crucial thing is to tell the doctor and nurse that it's important to you to be with your baby if something happens and to give them any phone numbers they will need to reach you. That way the doctor will know to call you sooner rather than later, so you'll have plenty of time to get to your baby's side. You may have some false alarms—thankfully! But when your phone isn't ringing, you can relax a bit, knowing that everything remains all right.

Air Leak

We just got a terrible phone call from our baby's doctor. He said that our son, who's on a ventilator, had a setback: an air leak. I don't even understand what that means, let alone how worried we should be.

The first reaction a parent has after hearing about an unexpected complication is fear. That's understandable; like you, most parents have never heard of an air leak before. It will help you to understand what one is, why it happens, and why the doctor can't tell you yet whether your baby's air leak is merely a temporary setback from which he'll recover in a few days or one that will affect his health for a longer time.

When we breathe, air goes into our nose or mouth, down our windpipe, and into the many small airways and air sacs of our lungs. An air leak occurs when one of these tiny airways or sacs tears, leaking air into places where it's not supposed to be. There are different kinds of air leaks, depending on where the air goes.

The most common in newborn babies is a pneumothorax, when air leaks into the space between the baby's lungs and chest wall. Sometimes a pneumothorax is so small that it doesn't cause any significant problems and doesn't even need treatment. Roughly one out of a hundred newborns has an insignificant pneumothorax. If a pneumothorax is large, though, or if a baby's respiratory function is marginal, as it is in many preemies, a pneumothorax can cause the baby's condition to suddenly deteriorate. The level of oxygen in his blood drops, and his blood pressure and heart rate fall.

The doctor can quickly check for a pneumo-thorax by shining a bright transilluminating light on the baby's chest. The light shines through the chest wall, and pockets of air outside of the baby's lungs show up as luminous patches. A chest X-ray will confirm the diagnosis.

A serious pneumothorax must be treated. The tear itself is not the problem; like any minor cut, it will heal on its own. But air that gets trapped between the lung and chest wall must be removed because a large pocket of air will press on the lung, causing it to collapse. The doctor may simply try sucking the air out with a needle and syringe, but if more air continues to collect, a minor surgical procedure is required. Right at the baby's bedside, the doctor makes a little incision in his chest. He inserts a plastic tube into the space where the air has collected and with continuous suction draws the air out and prevents more from reaccumulating.

Once the chest tube is working, your baby's condition will stabilize and the emergency is over. The tube usually has to stay in for several days—until the tear in the lung heals. Then the doctor will turn off the suction and watch to make sure that no more air leaks out. If none does, the tube

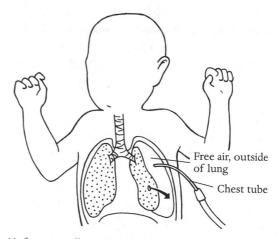

Air from a small tear in the lung (see arrow) leaks into the space between the lung and the chest wall. A chest tube can draw the air out, until the lung heals.

can be removed, leaving just a tiny bandage on your baby's chest.

A preemie who has just one isolated pneumothorax has a very good chance of healing quickly and being just fine. One complication that doctors always watch for is an intraventricular hemorrhage; the rapid changes in pressure accompanying the pneumothorax can cause some of the delicate blood vessels in a preemie's brain to rupture. Your baby's doctor may ask for a head ultrasound or may wait to see whether any symptoms of an intraventricular hemorrhage appear over the next few days. (If your baby does have an IVH, the doctor will tell you whether it was mild or severe. Mild hemorrhages aren't thought to cause lasting problems.) Most of the time, a baby's lung heals with no IVH. Once he is weaned from the ventilator, a recurrence of an air leak is extremely unlikely, and you can celebrate that this incident is completely behind you.

For some babies, recovery goes less smoothly. A pneumothorax is one indication that a baby's lungs are being damaged by the ventilator, so a baby on a ventilator who has had one pneumothorax has a higher chance of getting a second one, especially if he has pulmonary interstitial emphysema (described below). Doctors can't predict which path your baby will take, but they can tell you that once he has been weaned to low ventilator settings, the risk of any further air leaks is low, and you can feel more confident that he's on his way to recovery.

Pulmonary interstitial emphysema is also a sign that a baby's lungs are being damaged by the ventilator, but here the damage is not just in an isolated area of the lung; it's more diffuse. Many airways and sacs develop teensy tears, leaking air into the small spaces in the tissues of the lung. Pulmonary interstitial emphysema (or PIE, as you may hear this condition called) is more difficult to treat than a pneumothorax. The leaked air cannot be drawn out with a tube, so the baby is simply supported on a ventilator, waiting for his lungs to gradually heal and the leaked air to get reabsorbed. Doctors reduce the ventilator pressures as much as they possibly can for babies with PIE and don't aim for quite as high oxygen saturations as usual so as to minimize the lung damage caused by the ventilator. They may also switch a baby to a different kind of ventilator or mode of ventilation, one that may be gentler on his lungs (see page 187). Your baby's doctor may talk to you about possibly trying a course of steroids, medication that significantly improves lung function in some babies but carries some short-term and long-term risks. (You can read about the pros and cons of steroids on page 289, if your doctor recommends them.)

Because babies with PIE tend to have severe respiratory problems, they often require higher than average ventilator settings for longer periods, despite the fact that this is exactly what doctors want to avoid when they can. As a result, many babies with PIE develop bronchopulmonary dysplasia, or chronic lung disease. Try not to get too discouraged after reading this: Not all babies do, and some get mild cases that resolve before they're a couple of years old. Your baby's doctor can help you understand how your baby is faring now, and what he expects to happen in the future.

Why some babies get air leaks and others don't is one of the toughest questions to answer. The best we can do is explain why some babies are more susceptible than others. Preemies who are on ventilators at high settings are at higher risk because the levels of oxygen that are so beneficial to them, and the repeated stress of mechanically opening and closing the small airways and air sacs with high pressure, gradually does damage to their lungs. Weaker and more fragile areas of the lung are more apt to tear, as are those that get overstretched. Babies with more immature lungs sustain more damage, as do those who "fight" against the ventilator (exhaling against the vent's incoming breaths).

(*Continued on page 189*)

How Different Kinds of Ventilation Might Help

Today's premature babies who require high levels of respiratory support have resources that preemies of past generations did not have: new kinds of ventilators and new modes on conventional ventilators, which may be gentler on the lungs.

So if your baby is having problems such as air leaks, or just not responding as well or as fast as the doctors would like, it's possible that you'll hear them say something like: "Let's try her on assist control" (a different mode) or "Maybe she'd do better on the jet" (a different ventilator).

To help you understand what's happening, below are descriptions of the kinds of ventilation you are most likely to encounter in the nursery. Keep in mind that finding the right solution for each preemie can be a matter of trial and error. Every baby's medical challenges, maturity, size, and even breathing patterns are different. Moreover, research is still limited on the optimal use of each method, since the more advanced ones are relatively new and not all nurseries have the same equipment and capabilities. Your baby's doctor will make clinical judgments based on his knowledge of how each kind of ventilation works and the research evidence so far, and will make adjustments as your baby's needs become evident or change.

* **High-Frequency Ventilators.** Unlike conventional ventilators, which simulate normal breathing by using high then low pressures to deliver deep in-and-out breaths, high-frequency ventilators breathe for the baby in a completely different way: They provide tiny quantities of air and oxygen at rapid rates, using much lower peak pressures, and keep the lungs continuously inflated so they don't get strained by having to stretch open and close.

One type is a high-frequency oscillating ventilator, often called an oscillator; it works by gently shaking air in and out of the baby's lungs. You'll find it strange to see your baby being ventilated in this way, jiggled as if she were getting a vibrating massage. But it's nice to know that adults who have been on oscillating ventilators describe them as soothing. The other type, a high-frequency jet ventilator, uses an action like a tiny air gun, squirting minuscule jets of air into the lungs with slightly more force than the oscillator. If a baby's lungs are filled with fluid or trapped gas (as happens with pneumonia or air leaks), the jet action may help to clear them out.

Why shouldn't every premature baby who needs a ventilator be given the benefit of these gentler-on-the-lungs devices? Because research on the benefits of high-frequency ventilation has yielded contradictory results: Some studies have shown lower rates of air leaks and later complications, like development of chronic lung disease, and others have not. There may be risks associated with high-frequency ventilators, too. For instance, babies on these vents often have lower blood pressure, and a few studies, though not most, have found higher rates of certain signs of brain injury, IVH, and PVL. Also, a high-frequency ventilator may not work as well as a conventional one if a baby has a lot of mucus plugs, has obstructed airways for other reasons, or needs very frequent suctioning (because suctioning, which you can read about on page 200, interferes with these ventilators' special action).

Given the benefits and unknowns, different doctors make different judgments after carefully weighing the pros and cons. Some will put a baby on a high-frequency ventilator from the very beginning. Some will switch a baby from a conventional ventilator to a high-frequency one if he has an air leak (a pneumothorax or PIE). Very often high-frequency ventilators are tried for babies who are not improving on conventional ones or who require such high settings that doctors are concerned about the damage they could cause the baby's lungs. This arises most commonly when there are complications like persistent pulmonary hypertension, pneumonia, or a pulmonary hemorrhage.

* **Different modes on a conventional ventilator.** Modern conventional ventilators are more sophisticated and sensitive than their forebears and offer a variety of operating modes.

Some of these are synchronized modes: They can sense when a baby begins to take a breath and synchronize the timing of the ventilator breaths with the baby's spontaneous breaths. The benefits? The ventilator supports a baby's own breathing rather than replacing it, which is more comfortable and makes lower settings possible. And a baby is less likely to "fight" the ventilator (exhaling when the vent is pushing air in), so the vent is less apt to damage the baby's lungs and airways.

The options are many. In one mode, a baby takes all of her own breaths, but the ventilator deepens each breath with extra pressure. Another mode lengthens each of her breaths as well as deepening them. The vent can be set to insert extra breaths in between the baby's own breaths, and to do so until a certain volume of air, which is usually mixed with extra oxygen, is delivered. Several ventilator modes can even be combined. There are many permutations and they sound complicated, but the goal is always the same: to provide as little support as possible as gently as possible while giving the baby the assistance she needs.

* **Continuous Positive Airway Pressure, or CPAP ("SEE-pap").** One of the main benefits of CPAP is that it doesn't require an endotracheal tube. Instead, a steady flow of air and oxygen can be blown through nasal prongs, small tubes placed in a baby's nose. A baby on CPAP doesn't get any extra breaths, but the pressure of the incoming air is just forceful enough to keep the air sacs of the baby's lungs open even when he exhales so that each breath he takes is easier. CPAP is usually delivered from specialized CPAP devices (though a ventilator can also be specially programmed to deliver CPAP rather than doing any breathing for him). While clinical studies over the years have not pointed to one kind of ventilator or mode of ventilation as being consistently better than another, they have clearly shown that keeping a preemie off a ventilator altogether—thus avoiding the forceful way it pushes big breaths directly into the trachea and lungs—is the best way to avoid extra injury to his delicate lungs. Many neonatologists therefore put preemies on CPAP from the start (or intubate them only briefly right after delivery to give them a dose of that valuable medication, surfactant, after which the baby is put on CPAP), hoping that it will be enough and a ventilator won't be necessary.

But a preemie who still isn't breathing regularly or deeply enough will need more support. In that case, some doctors may try delivering pressured breaths from a ventilator through the CPAP nasal prongs rather than intubating the baby. This practice has not been well studied yet, so not all NICUs do it. But in theory it could be a gentler form of mechanical ventilation for preemies.

Babies whose lungs are smaller than normal—for example, some who are born weeks after their mother's water breaks—or those with pneumonia are also more prone to air leaks.

On the other hand, preemies who are given surfactant soon after birth are less likely to have air leaks. (Since surfactant works so well at improving a newborn preemie's lungs in the first days after delivery, some parents wonder why it isn't given again later if their babies have air leaks. Studies have not shown a clear benefit when surfactant was given after the first few days of life, probably because by then a preemie's lung problems are no longer caused primarily by inadequate amounts of surfactant.)

It is heartbreaking for many parents, seeing their babies with a chest tube, to wonder whether they are uncomfortable or in pain. We have some advice for you: Don't wonder silently. It's too hard on you, and doesn't help your baby. Instead, talk to your baby's doctor, and ask what is being done to keep your baby comfortable. The practice of pain control still varies widely from NICU to NICU. Most neonatologists give pain medication before putting a chest tube in, while it's in place if the baby seems at all agitated, and when they take it out, so most likely your baby is resting comfortably. Nevertheless, if you suspect that your baby is in pain, don't hesitate to say so. You may influence the doctor to give your baby more relief or alternatively will hear why he doesn't think it's needed—which may set your anxious mind at rest.

Seizures

The doctors say they can't tell for sure if my son is having seizures. I don't understand this. I've seen someone have a seizure, and there's nothing subtle about it.

Seizures in a premature infant can be so subtle that they're easy to miss, by parents or trained observers.

A seizure occurs when there are abnormal electrical discharges in the brain. Picture it as a kind of short circuit of the brain's normal nerve signals due to a brain injury or irritant. You probably saw an adult having convulsions in which the body shakes uncontrollably, but seizures can sometimes have milder, nearly unnoticeable symptoms. In a preemie, whose nerve connections are still immature, the same disturbances may show up in even less obvious ways, as just slight variations of normal preemie behavior.

There might be one or more of the following:

* Twitching of the arms or legs;
* Fluttering of the eyelids;
* Sustained opening of the eyes, with a fixed gaze;
* Trembling of the mouth, sucking motions, or drooling;
* Rhythmic movements of the arms or legs (called swimming, rowing, or pedaling);
* Stiffening or arching of the back, arms, or legs;
* A spell of apnea or sudden brief high blood pressure.

A preemie's normal jittery movements can be stopped by restraining the baby's arms and legs, or placing a calming hand on the baby, while seizure activity cannot.

If the doctor suspects that your baby is having seizures, he will probably ask for an EEG. This is a painless test for your baby (although his hair will get a bit messy) in which electrodes attached to little pads are placed on his head to record the electrical activity in his brain, usually for an hour.

Sometimes an EEG is definitive: Either it's absolutely normal, or there are some abnormal brain wave patterns that are clearly recognizable as seizures. But even EEGs can leave the doctors unsure.

(Continued on page 196)

In Plain Language:
What Is an Intraventricular Hemorrhage?

Since a premature baby's brain is still at an early stage of development, it is not quite ready to withstand all the stress of living outside of the womb. Some tiny blood vessels in an inner part of preemies' brains are especially fragile and vulnerable to changes in blood flow. If they rupture, bleeding occurs in or near the ventricles, which are fluid-filled chambers located within the brain. This is why doctors call this event an intraventricular (intra means inside) or sometimes periventricular (peri means near) hemorrhage. (You'll also hear the abbreviation IVH or PVH.)

An intraventricular hemorrhage is an often inescapable consequence of a premature birth. Fortunately, in most cases the bleeding is mild, and resolves without causing problems. Concern for a baby's health arises, however, when the bleeding is large and widespread, because in the worst scenario it can lead to permanent brain injury, or even to death.

When doctors find out that a baby had a moderate or severe intraventricular hemorrhage, they will inform his family about the possible consequences. From personal experience, we know that this is heartbreaking news. But after the initial, unavoidable shock, you should try to remember that a preemie's brain, which is still developing, has tremendous resilience, and how he is doing now counts for a lot. If he is stable, without significant respiratory complications or other abnormal symptoms, he has a good chance of overcoming a serious intraventricular hemorrhage—and being barely touched by it developmentally.

Why some babies have an IVH and others don't

As with many complications of prematurity, the younger, smaller, and sicker a baby is at birth the more likely he is to develop an intraventricular hemorrhage. Today, a baby with a birth weight of less than 1,000 grams has about a 35 percent chance of having an IVH and about a 20 percent chance of suffering from a serious one. The risk is a lot lower for older and bigger babies. Those born weighing from 1,000 to 1,500 grams have only about a 7 percent chance of a serious IVH. After 30 weeks of gestation, the risk of a serious IVH dramatically drops to less than 1 percent. For this reason, neonatologists don't even recommend screening preemies born after 30 weeks with head ultrasounds.

Abrupt changes or disturbances in blood flow or blood pressure to the brain can cause an IVH. The trauma of birth itself—labor and delivery—is a risk factor in a premature baby. Mechanical ventilation is another cause of IVH, particularly when the baby is breathing out of synchrony with the ventilator. Even common procedures, such as suctioning or weighing a preemie, can overstimulate him and increase the risk of a bleed.

Premature babies who were treated before delivery with steroids are less likely to have an IVH because steroids can prevent respiratory distress syndrome, one of the main risk factors for IVH, and speed up the maturation of a fetus's brain blood vessels. Although some studies have found that delivering the youngest premature babies (those born at less than 25 weeks of gestation) by cesarean section lowers their chances of IVH, other studies have not, and a cesarean section performed that early in pregnancy brings more health risks for a mother.

After a baby is born, all medical interventions in the intensive-care nursery that are aimed at stabilizing his breathing, oxygenation, blood circulation, and blood pressure are also effective in lowering his risk for an IVH. Because of greatly improved medical treatment, IVHs have been steadily decreasing in preemies.

Many different medications have been tested in recent years in the effort to prevent IVHs, such as substances that improve blood clotting, sedatives and muscle relaxants, and vitamin E (because of its antioxidant properties). But each of these drugs either didn't work or had serious side effects. Studies have shown that a low dose of indomethacin, a drug that alters blood flow, can reduce the risk and severity of an IVH when given to preemies within their first six hours after birth. Disappointingly, though, this drug has still failed to lower the risk of long-term neurodevelopmental delays. Since medical practices vary from hospital to hospital, you can ask your baby's doctors whether he has been given any medication to try to prevent an IVH.

Diagnosis: The head ultrasound

About three-quarters of all IVHs take place during the first five days of a preemie's life, and nearly all take place within the first 10 to 14 days. So if your baby doesn't have an IVH at two weeks of age, you can relax; he is unlikely ever to have one.

Premature babies who are at higher risk for bleeding in the brain—those born at or before 30 weeks of gestation or at less than 1,500 grams— usually get a routine head ultrasound in the first week or two of life. A head ultrasound is also performed on preemies born at any gestational age if doctors suspect that an IVH might have occurred, but serious IVHs are rare in older pree-

mies. The ultrasound scan, or sonogram, is a safe and completely painless test that allows doctors to look into a tiny baby's head without disturbing him. It doesn't involve radiation as an X-ray does; it uses sound waves to record images on videotape. A technician brings the ultrasound machine to the baby's isolette or bed, squirts some gel on the soft spot at the top of the baby's head (where his skull is still open), and with a transducer carefully scans the area. The whole thing takes only about fifteen minutes, and the resulting pictures of the brain are detailed and precise. Later, the videotape is analyzed, usually by a pediatric radiologist or neonatologist.

How intraventricular hemorrhages are classified

The brain, with its complex organization of different structures, may be the least familiar of all organs of the human body to those who are not physicians. The illustrations show, in cross-section, where IVHs occur.

IVHs usually begin with the rupture of delicate blood vessels in the germinal matrix, a primitive fragile nest of cells that is very active during the development of the brain. The germinal matrix becomes smaller as the fetus matures, disappearing by approximately 32 to 34 weeks of gestation. That's why IVHs rarely occur in older preemies.

The germinal matrix is located along the lining at the base of the lateral ventricles. The ventricles are a series of connected chambers that are filled with cerebrospinal fluid. This fluid, which functions as a cushion for the brain and spinal cord, circulates around the brain, is collected by the ventricles and flows down into the spinal canal. Cerebrospinal fluid is constantly being produced and reabsorbed; if not enough fluid is reabsorbed, it can build up to dangerous levels.

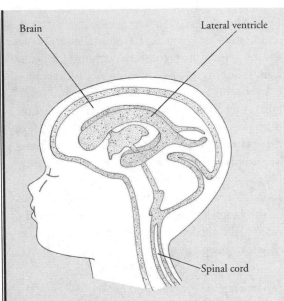

The cerebrospinal fluid (shaded), circulating around the brain, is collected in chambers called ventricles and flows down, into and around the spinal cord. The germinal matrix lies along the base of the lateral ventricles.

Intraventricular hemorrhages are given a grade depending on their location and size, and the right and left sides of the brain are graded separately:

* **Grade 1.** The mildest type of brain bleed, it begins and remains in the germinal matrix without getting into the ventricle.
* **Grade 2.** From a bleed in the germinal matrix, some blood leaks into the ventricle but doesn't cause the ventricle to swell significantly. (There may be minor swelling from a clot and some accumulation of cerebrospinal fluid, but only initially.)
* **Grade 3.** A large hemorrhage that fills more than half of the lateral ventricle, enough to distend it with blood. The bigger a Grade 3 hemorrhage is, the more likely it will cause chronic, progressive swelling of the ventricles (called hydrocephalus).

* **Grade 4.** A hemorrhage outside the ventricles, usually in the white matter of the brain, caused by bleeding from other blood vessels in addition to germinal matrix bleeding. Sometimes called a periventricular hemorrhage.

After a mild IVH

If your baby had only a Grade 1 intraventricular hemorrhage, you really don't have to worry. There's almost no risk of short-term complications, and the odds of your baby's growing up normal are just as high as those of preemies without bleeds. If your baby had a Grade 2 intraventricular hemorrhage, his outlook is nearly as good. Most studies show no long-term problems after a Grade 2 IVH, although one recent study did find slightly more disabilities in preemies who had a Grade 2 bleed. In a week or two, doctors will want to check whether the hemorrhage has gotten bigger, because a few do enlarge. But even if this happens, there's only a small risk that your baby's good prognosis will change. So take heart and don't focus on the next head ultrasound. Most likely, he'll have just one or two more, and you'll soon forget all about intraventricular hemorrhages.

After a Grade 3 or 4 IVH: Short-term outcome

Many babies with a Grade 3 IVH, and some with a Grade 4, will be fine in the short run. They will not have abnormal neurological symptoms, and their general health won't change significantly. This is great news, because it gives hope for a positive outcome.

But an IVH of Grade 3 can carry some immediate risk for babies, and the danger increases with an IVH of Grade 4. Babies with moderate to severe bleeds may have a sudden worsen-

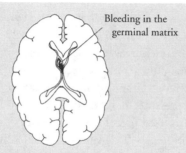

Bleeding in the germinal matrix

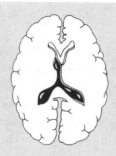

Bleeding in the brain

MILD—Grade 1. The mildest bleeding, it stays within the germinal matrix and doesn't reach the ventricles.

MILD—Grade 2. Some blood enters the ventricles without enlarging them.

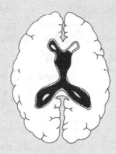

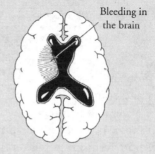

MODERATE—Grade 3. A lot of blood in the ventricles makes them swell.

SEVERE—Grade 4. Hemorrhage occurs beyond the ventricles, in the substance of the brain.

Adapted with permission from Rozmus C: Periventricular-intraventricular hemorrhage in the newborn, MCN 17(2):79, Lippincott-Raven Publishers, Philadelphia, PA 1992

ing of breathing, a drop in heart rate or blood pressure, and seizures or abnormal movements. These symptoms of brain swelling and inflammation are most commonly transient, but they can sometimes lead, within minutes to days, to death. The risk that this will happen is about 15 percent after a Grade 3 IVH and about 35 percent after a Grade 4.

Many preemies need one or more blood transfusions after a moderate or large intraventricular hemorrhage. If the doctor suspects that an infection in or around the baby's brain may have been responsible for any of his symptoms, she may start antibiotics or do a lumbar punc-

ture (also called a spinal tap). In this procedure a needle is carefully inserted between two vertebrae (back bones) in the lower, or lumbar, segment of the baby's spine. The needle withdraws a sample of the cerebrospinal fluid, which is sent for biochemical analysis and culture. Sometimes the bleeding causes problems with jaundice and abnormalities of electrolytes in a baby's blood, which the doctors will watch for and treat.

After a Grade 3 or 4 IVH, your baby's head circumference will be measured every day, a simple but crucial test to watch for progressive hydrocephalus (since an excess of cerebrospinal fluid in the ventricles can enlarge the skull). Doctors will also look out for other telling signs, such as a bulging or firm fontanelle and increasing episodes of apnea and bradycardia. Your baby will probably get a head ultrasound every week or two until the size of his ventricles is stable or decreasing, indicating that the inflammation from the bleed is resolving and that the drainage and reabsorption of cerebrospinal fluid is adequate.

Hydrocephalus: The most common complication of a Grade 3 or 4 IVH

For at least two weeks after a Grade 3 or 4 IVH, most babies' ventricles are enlarged. This is a hydraulic problem created by a serious bleed. Blood clots and scar tissue can plug the normal drainage of cerebrospinal fluid from the ventricles, disrupting its flow, and inflammation can interfere with its reabsorption. If too much fluid accumulates inside the ventricles, they can swell. Usually this condition eases and ends by itself within several weeks, with no need for intervention. But in about a third of cases the ventricles continue to swell, pressing on and stretching the brain around them. This progressive enlargement of the ventricles is called hydrocephalus, a Latin word meaning water in the head.

When an adult or older child gets hydrocephalus, perhaps from a head injury, the resulting high pressure on the brain can give him an instant headache, make him vomit, or possibly even send him into a coma. If the pressure is not rapidly relieved by removal of fluid from the ventricles in an emergency procedure, irreversible brain injury or death can result. Fortunately, babies have a natural defense system against hydrocephalus. Their tender skull bones are not yet fused together. So the swelling of the ventricles makes the whole head expand, enlarging its circumference. Much of the pressure on the brain is relieved.

What to do if your baby has hydrocephalus: Doctors will monitor your baby closely, watching for signs of excessive pressure on his brain: sleepiness, inability to nipple feed, vomiting, increasing episodes of apnea and bradycardia, and high blood pressure. If they occur, it is important to act quickly to prevent brain damage. The choice of treatment will depend on your baby's overall health and size. Today the only way to treat hydrocephalus permanently and effectively is with placement of a ventricular shunt, a procedure performed by a neurosurgeon (see page 360).

The ideal timing for a shunt placement is when your preemie is clinically stable, breathing on his own, infection-free, and feeding and growing well. The neurosurgeon will want to wait at least several weeks after the bleed to be certain that the hydrocephalus isn't going to resolve on its own, and long enough for the blood clot and inflammation in the ventricle to quiet down so the shunt doesn't get blocked with debris. Most neurosurgeons also wait until a preemie weighs at least 1,800 to 2,000 grams (less than that, and the shunt isn't likely to fit well or work properly).

Some babies, despite their expanding head, continue to do fine, sleeping, eating, and growing. They may eventually need surgery but not necessarily right away; they can grow a little older and stronger before going to the operating room.

But if doctors become worried about the increasing pressure on the brain—because of a baby's symptoms or because of a very rapid increase in ventricular size—there are temporary medical interventions they may try. Some NICUs do a series of spinal taps (lumbar punctures) in which the doctor inserts a needle in the baby's lower back and removes some cerebrospinal fluid. This may help relieve acute symptoms, such as apnea and bradycardia, but studies have not shown any long-term benefit from serial lumbar punctures. More effective is draining fluid directly from the ventricles by means of a ventricular tap, a minor procedure in which a neurosurgeon inserts a needle through the soft spot on top of a baby's head directly into the ventricle and removes some cerebrospinal fluid. It probably isn't safe to do ventricular taps again and again, however, so if a baby needs more frequent relief from his hydrocephalus, the neurosurgeon may recommend making a ventriculostomy (an artificial opening of the ventricles) from which excess cerebrospinal fluid can be drained. There are three main kinds of ventriculostomies the doctors will consider: an external catheter, a reservoir, and a subgaleal shunt. If your baby needs one, you can read more about it on page 361.

You should discuss with your neonatologist and neurosurgeon what chance your baby has of avoiding an operation and what the risks are of postponing surgery. If they tell you that your baby can wait, trust them and try to relax. It is normal for you to be very scared, but don't stop giving your baby all of the cuddling he needs from you. Remember that if his head is growing, it means he is defending himself well. If your baby has a ventriculostomy, you shouldn't be afraid to hold him. Don't give up on kangaroo care, if you are doing it, or on your breastfeeding attempts. Some parents become so obsessed by the daily rite of the head circumference measurement that they end up losing sight of everything else. Keep in mind that your baby can grow up and do well despite the hydrocephalus.

What you can expect in the long run

The long-term outcome of premature babies who had an intraventricular hemorrhage depends on the extent of the injury caused by the lack of blood flow and oxygen to the brain around the time of the bleed, and from its complications, such as hydrocephalus.

Although bleeding can be detected on the first head ultrasound, the kind of damage most closely associated with long-term problems takes several weeks to show up on a head ultrasound. Sometimes brain damage is invisible on a head ultrasound but can be detected on an MRI, or magnetic resonance imaging, scan. But even MRI findings are far from perfect predictors of a baby's outcome, because not all brain injury shows up on an MRI, either, and because it's not uncommon for a visibly damaged area on a brain scan to have no effect on a child's future functioning. Still, using head ultrasound or MRI scans, knowledge of a preemie's medical history, and observations of his behavior and development, doctors can generally make some reasonable predictions of what his family can expect before he is discharged from the hospital. You will learn more as time passes: By six months, most babies who are severely affected by their IVH will be identified, and by two years nearly all will. In very rare cases, hydrocephalus that appeared to have stabilized will over the course of the first year begin to worsen again, so the head circumference of any preemie with hydrocephalus will be followed closely by his pediatrician until his fontanelle closes.

It's important to remember that the statistics on babies' long-term developmental outcome after an IVH don't tell you how your baby in particular is going to do. Overall, approximately 65 percent of preemies who had a Grade 3 IVH and 25 percent of preemies who had a Grade 4 IVH were found normal in follow-up studies. But these percentages don't tell you all you can know about your baby; they don't separate babies who had bigger Grade 4 bleeds from those who had smaller ones, or babies who had bleeding on only one side of their brain from those who had bleeding on both sides. Nor do they consider other factors that can make a preemie's prognosis better or worse. Also, the consequences of a moderate or severe IVH can range in severity—they may be mild developmental problems, such as low-grade cerebral palsy, learning disabilities, or partial sight, hearing, or speech impairment, or serious handicaps, such as severe cerebral palsy, mental retardation, blindness, or deafness—and affect a child's life in lesser or greater ways.

Why do some preemies who survive a Grade 3 or 4 intraventricular hemorrhage grow up completely normal while others don't? It probably has to do with a variety of factors—some of them still undefined—that influence the brain's resilience and ability to heal itself. Among them are the size and location of the bleeding (smaller bleeds are easier to recover from, and sometimes there is bleeding in other parts of the brain in addition to the area around the ventricles); whether the problem that caused the bleeding also injured other parts of the brain (this associated damage often shows up later on a head ultrasound or MRI as periventricular leukomalacia); whether the IVH affected just one side of the brain or both (one side of the brain, as long as it remains uninjured, can often take over functions meant for the other side); and the stimulation a baby gets as he grows (statistically, a preemie's living and learning environment is an even more powerful influence than IVH on his future cognitive performance, which means some babies will surprise their parents by doing much better than expected).

Preemies who don't develop hydrocephalus, or whose hydrocephalus resolves on its own, do better than those who need a shunt. If a baby has a ventricular shunt, his development will be influenced by how many shunt revisions he needs during his childhood (the fewer the better) and whether he suffered from meningitis (an infection in the membranes around the brain) or has seizures.

Studies have shown that many preemies who are diagnosed with mild or moderate neurological abnormalities in their first two years substantially improve over time and often end up absolutely normal by the time they're six or eight years old, encouraging news testifying to the brain's self-repairing ability. On the other hand, some learning disabilities may become apparent only at school age.

You should always keep in mind that numbers and percentages from research studies or textbooks represent just the average outcome of large groups of babies. They don't take into consideration what really counts for you: Your baby's unique medical course, how he is doing now, and the attention and stimulation he'll be getting in his early months and years to give him the best possible start in life. These are the factors that make your baby's future different—and hopefully better—than average.

Certain brain wave irregularities may be seizures or may simply result from medications a baby is taking, stress, illness, or the very fact that he is a preemie with a brain that behaves in immature ways. Ideally, your baby's EEG will be read by a pediatric neurologist who has experience with premature babies.

If there is uncertainty that the doctor feels is important to clarify, he may suggest a 24-hour EEG or a video EEG. During these tests, whenever your baby makes unusual movements or has

an episode that may be of concern, the nurse will press a button to mark the event on the EEG printout. With the suspicious event captured, the neurologist will be able to examine what was happening in your baby's brain—whether its electrical activity was abnormal—at that time.

A normal EEG is a very good sign, but it can't tell you that an episode that occurred before it was performed was definitely not a seizure. The doctors may also want an MRI or CT scan of your baby's brain: detailed pictures that should reveal any swelling, bleeding, or malformation that might be causing seizures.

There are a few common causes of seizures in premature babies. One is a severe intraventricular hemorrhage, which most often leads to just one or two transient seizures at the time of the bleed—although occasionally, scarring in the brain causes the seizures to continue. Babies with severe birth asphyxia can have seizures beginning several hours after birth. Another common cause is infection, especially meningitis, an infection around the brain. With meningitis, seizures may continue if there is lasting damage to the brain, but otherwise don't recur. Metabolic problems— levels of glucose, sodium, calcium, and other substances that are too high or low—are another major cause of seizures. When the metabolic imbalances are fixed, the seizures stop. But some premature babies' seizures remain a mystery, and no cause is ever found.

You may be wondering: Why don't the doctors treat my baby for seizures just in case, whether they're sure or not? Because as usual, there are pros and cons to treatment. On the one hand, it makes sense to treat seizures since some of them may be harmful. During a seizure, the brain uses up a lot of oxygen and glucose, so it may not get enough of those crucial substances. While brief occasional episodes probably cause no trouble, a long, sustained seizure or very frequent ones could cause damage to some of the brain's cells. And if the seizures are accompanied by apnea, a baby may need to be put on a ventilator.

On the other hand, the usual treatment for seizures—medications called anticonvulsants— work by sedating the brain. The one most commonly used for preemies is phenobarbital. Phenobarb, as you'll hear the NICU staff call it, is usually effective in controlling seizures. The concern is that it may turn the brain down in bad ways as well as good, interfering with a baby's learning. In long-term studies, children who remained on phenobarbital for six months or longer tended to do no better, and sometimes worse, developmentally than their peers, with little difference in the rate at which their seizures recurred. Thus many doctors don't treat babies who have had a single seizure since it might be an isolated incident that won't recur. When babies have had several seizures, though, most doctors agree on treating them for a short time (usually three months or less).

Here's an important fact that's often misunderstood: One or two seizures in a preemie is not the same as epilepsy, which is an ongoing seizure disorder. Most premature babies with seizures have only a temporary problem and will never develop epilepsy, so treatment doesn't have to last long.

Most of the time, coming off medication involves some trial and error: The doctors try taking the baby off as soon as they think the seizures won't recur and watch to see how he does. If the problem is metabolic, as soon as it's fixed the baby can come off the medication. If the seizure occurred with an intraventricular hemorrhage or meningitis, many neurologists would keep the baby on medication for a month or two. If there's an underlying brain abnormality, or a scar from a severe IVH, treatment would probably continue longer.

How a preemie who had seizures will do in the future depends on the underlying problem that caused them. Lasting brain injuries may be associated with developmental problems that range from mild to severe. Your baby's development will be closely monitored after his discharge from the NICU to detect any problems early and help ensure that he reaches his maximum potential. But many seizures have temporary causes, and babies leave them behind with no signs of long-term neurological damage.

Since the doctors aren't even sure that your baby is having seizures, you should definitely try not to imagine the worst. He may have no problem at all, or he may have one that needs attention but will soon pass, never to return.

Pulmonary Hypertension

The doctor says my baby needs higher vent settings than he expected because of high blood pressure in her lungs. Why would she have that?

Normally when a baby starts breathing on her own at birth, the blood pressure in her lungs falls. If instead it stays very high, the condition is called persistent pulmonary hypertension and can be clearly diagnosed with an echocardiogram. Neonatologists usually suspect it when a baby's oxygen levels are lower or more erratic than they expected.

Actually, pulmonary hypertension is much more common in term babies and older preemies, because lungs usually have to be more mature to generate very high blood pressures. But persistent pulmonary hypertension can be caused by severe respiratory distress syndrome, or pneumonia, or even by a baby's having had recurrent episodes of fetal distress. A baby whose lungs didn't grow as big as they should have in the womb (as could happen, for example, if a mother's water breaks early in the pregnancy) is also likely to have it.

Why are your baby's vent settings high? Because the high blood pressure in her lungs creates an obstacle to the incoming blood pumped by the heart, blocking it from flowing into her lungs. So in essence, your baby's blood continues to circulate in its fetal route, partly bypassing her lungs, just as before birth. When blood doesn't get into the lungs, it can't pick up oxygen, so her oxygen saturations fall.

As long as your baby's blood keeps flowing in its fetal route, a fetal blood vessel that normally closes at birth (called the ductus arteriosus) thinks it is supposed to stay open and does. Much of her blood bypasses her lungs by going through the patent—meaning open—ductus arteriosus (or PDA).

Pulmonary hypertension is serious, but the good news is that it usually resolves in four or five days. The first treatment for your baby is more oxygen, to make sure she is getting enough and because oxygen helps to relax the tightened arteries in her lungs that are causing the high pressure. Some babies will need to be put on a ventilator to improve their oxygenation, or if a baby is already on a ventilator, the settings may be raised, as happened to your baby. She will probably be given a medication to inhale through the ventilator, nitric oxide, which will open up the blood vessels in her lungs, and possibly another medication to help her heart beat more strongly.

Most of the time, oxygen, nitric oxide, and the ventilator work well, and within hours you'll start seeing some improvement. After that, it's only a matter of time until your baby recovers. But if her problem persists, her doctors may decide to try one other medication: sildenafil, which you know by its brand name, Viagra. Yes . . . really! Sildenafil, which like nitric oxide relaxes the lungs' blood vessels so more blood can flow in, is already a proven treatment for pulmonary hypertension in adults. In preemies there are few studies, so it's too soon to tell how effective or safe it will prove to be, but early results have been promising. Occasionally a preemie's pulmonary hypertension can't be corrected. That usually happens only when the lungs haven't grown or developed appropriately or there's a very serious infection.

Once your baby's pulmonary hypertension decreases, her breathing should improve. Babies who had pulmonary hypertension are at a somewhat higher risk of developing chronic lung disease because of the extra time they spent on high ventilator settings that can be damaging to the lungs—but it's very possible that this will never become an issue for your daughter.

You might think that closing the PDA would solve the respiratory problem, but it won't. Some blood would still bypass the lungs through a small hole in the heart called the foramen ovale. Furthermore, the baby's heart could become so overworked from pumping blood into the lungs against high pressure, with no release, that it could give out. This is far worse than just waiting until the pulmonary hypertension resolves. Once it does, most of the time the PDA closes on its own.

X-rays

They are always X-raying my baby. I'm afraid she's going to be sterile or get cancer.

In our society, we all hear so much about health risks. That's helpful when it causes us to avoid serious unnecessary risks, such as when we stop smoking or strap our kids into car seats. But when it causes us to worry about insignificant or unavoidable risks, it's doing a lot more harm than good.

No one needs groundless worry less than an already stressed parent of a preemie, so let us alleviate your anxiety: The chances that the X-rays will cause health problems for your baby are minuscule.

While no amount of radiation is truly safe—the less the better—there is a natural background level of radiation that we're all exposed to in daily life from such sources as the sun, cosmic rays, the soil, and natural elements. Consider the amount of radiation (measured in units called rads) that your newborn gets from a chest X-ray compared with the amount of radiation people get from other sources:

* Natural, background level of radiation at sea level: 0.08 rad per year;
* Exposure of professional jet pilot and flight crews (from natural sources at high altitudes): 1 rad per year;
* The U.S. government's permitted exposure for workers: 5 rads per year;
* Radiotherapy done for curative medical reasons: 7,000 rads per week;
* Chest X-ray of a newborn: 0.004 rad.

In other words, only after your newborn gets 20 chest X-rays does he even reach the natural level of radiation to which we're all exposed—and the amount of radiation many cancer patients are treated with per week is equivalent to more than a million chest X-rays! Some tests, such as fluoroscopic studies like barium swallows, which involve X-raying continuously for the duration of the test, or CT scans, which are performed on preemies much less frequently than chest X-rays, have a higher radiation level (CT scans are equivalent to about two and a half years of natural background exposure), so most doctors don't order them lightly, only when they're very important to a preemie's health. Ultrasound and MRI scans, on the other hand, use no radiation at all. Experts have estimated that even in those preemies who receive the most X-rays in the NICU, because they are very tiny or sick, the risk of cancer increases by less than 0.01 percent. The dangers of withholding diagnostic X-rays from ill preemies would be far greater than that.

To guard against unnecessary exposure to X-rays of a preemie's reproductive organs and other areas of his body, X-ray technicians are instructed to pay particular attention to focusing the X-ray beam on the precise area the doctors want to look at, and your baby's nurse will help by positioning him carefully and correctly. Today's X-ray technology is very good at reducing "scatter," meaning that if they're focusing the beam on your baby's chest, hardly any radiation will reach her head or her toes. Essentially none will reach other babies in neighboring beds.

Why then do nurses often scurry from the room before the X-ray machine goes on? Partly from habit, left over from past years when X-ray machines did scatter more, and partly because, unlike your baby, who will be leaving the nursery to go home with you, the nurses may be around for thousands of X-rays a year over a period of twenty years or more. Interestingly, one study indicates that they still don't have to worry: The nurses in one intensive care nursery wore radiation badges to calculate the amount of radiation they received. After one year, the badges showed that the nurses' radiation exposure was not measurably greater than the natural background level of radiation that everyone is exposed to.

So don't worry about your baby's X-rays. The chance that a premature baby will be worse off because of X-rays is vanishingly small—and many have been far better off because of them.

Suctioning

Do the nurses have to suction my baby so often? He seems to hate it, and he always does worse while he's being suctioned and for a while afterward.

It is true that most preemies don't like to be suctioned. They may fight it, cough or gag, or respond with one of their special stress signals, such as apnea or bradycardia or a temporary loss of muscle tone. Their reaction is painful for parents to witness, but understandable. Who wouldn't hate having a catheter put down their nose or throat? It's irritating for sure, and the catheter, for the few seconds it's in, can impede the free flow of air and make breathing harder.

Of one thing you can be certain, though: The nurses don't like to see your baby react this way either, and they wouldn't suction him if he didn't need it. This unpleasant procedure is done to clear your baby's airways of secretions, something he cannot do yet without help. Babies who have prongs in their nose (to deliver oxygen or CPAP) need occasional nasal suctioning, and babies on ventilators need tracheal suctioning through their endotracheal tube. They do seem to appreciate it afterward; once it's over and they settle down, many babies breathe more easily and quietly, have better oxygen saturations, and seem calmer than they were before.

Just consider this. A preemie has a tiny airway, more than four times smaller than that of an adult, so it can easily get clogged by mucus and other debris that we adults are barely aware of, such as cells the body naturally sheds, bacteria, or particles in the air we breathe. Older babies and adults can effortlessly clear their throats and airways with a cough, but a preemie's cough is still too weak—and he obviously can't blow his nose!

The need is even greater because of a preemie's circumstances. When you're always lying down and not moving much, as preemies are, secretions tend to accumulate in the lungs, interfering with air flow and creating a risk of dangerous infections, such as pneumonia. Tubes in their nose or windpipe increase mucus production, and preemies with respiratory distress syndrome, bronchopulmonary dysplasia, or respiratory infections produce copious secretions. Because the vent's artificial airway prevents most self-cleansing activities, such as coughing or sweeping mucus into the back of the throat, it is vitally important to suction the ET tube, both to keep it from getting obstructed and to help mobilize and clear secretions farther down.

How is suctioning done? Preemies on ventilators have their endotracheal tube suctioned with a catheter connected to a suction machine, typically every three to six hours or when a change in their condition signals a need for it. Usually they're temporarily disconnected from the ventilator during suctioning. The nurse or respiratory therapist puts a few drops of saline down the ET tube to loosen and thin out the secretions, then carefully inserts the catheter just to the end of the ET tube and no farther, so it doesn't rub against the airway beyond the tube and irritate it.

Babies who are not on ventilators will have their nostrils or the back of their throats suctioned, with either a bulb or a catheter connected to a suction machine (called deep suctioning), when it appears that too much mucus has built up. Deep suctioning usually works better to clear the airways but can cause swelling and occasionally a little bleeding, so it's done only when needed. The baby's nasal prongs will also be periodically cleaned or replaced to keep them as wide open as possible.

Even with regular suctioning, a plug of mucus might at some point block a baby's airway or endotracheal tube, stopping air flow and setting off all of his alarms. Nurses and doctors call this a plug episode and are always ready to react with quick emergency suctioning (or by replacing the ET tube if it is thoroughly clogged). If the preemie's parents are present, they will surely feel panic and terror. But as soon as the mucus plug is removed and air starts flowing into the baby's lungs again, the crisis is over. So if this happens to your baby, try to remember that the NICU staff knows exactly how to handle such an unpleasant event.

Sometimes mucus plugs block off branches of small airways deeper in a baby's lungs. When this happens, his breathing may not be affected as dramatically, but his blood gases and oxygenation will worsen, and a chest X-ray may show patches of collapsed lung where air can't get past the plug.

Sometimes a medication that widens the airways, or chest physiotherapy ("chest PT") may help clear out these kinds of plugs.

Because the effectiveness and safety of chest PT in preemies is controversial, some nurseries use it and others don't. Chest physiotherapy involves percussion or vibration: The nurse gently taps or vibrates a small area of the preemie's chest or back to loosen the mucus in the underlying part of the lungs. Good pulmonary hygiene also involves changing a preemie's position every two or three hours, sometimes laying him on his back, sometimes on his stomach or either side. Varying positions, combined with gravity, allow the secretions to move from different parts of the outer lungs into the central airways, where they can be expelled more easily. Then comes suctioning to complete the job.

During suctioning, the nurses are always careful to watch for your baby's stress signals. If he's very uncomfortable, they'll stop to give him a rest if they can. Babies on ventilators might be given pain medication, and you can certainly ask about this since practices in different NICUs vary. As soon as the few minutes of discomfort are over, your baby can breathe more freely, and you can take a sigh of relief, too.

Bleeding in Lungs

I saw blood coming out of my baby's ET tube, and it scared me to death. The nurse tried to explain what was happening, but I was too shocked to understand. How serious is this, and why is it happening?

When a premature baby is on a ventilator and is being suctioned, it's not uncommon to notice some streaks of blood in the secretions coming from his ET tube. The intubation procedure, having an endotracheal tube in, and being suctioned can all bruise the inner lining of the airways, causing them to bleed a bit. This may be an upsetting sight, but it's nothing to worry about if the bleeding is slight and it only happens occasionally. Your baby's doctors will adjust the position of the ET tube if they think it's in too far. If the nurse thinks the bleeding was caused by suctioning too deeply, she'll advance the suction tube less far down next time.

Doctors and nurses will do all they can to avoid bruising a baby's airway, to prevent scar tissue from forming. (When a lot of scar tissue builds up in the airway, it can block some of the free flow of air and cause breathing problems later. Luckily, this happens only rarely nowadays because neonatologists and nurses are so diligent about avoiding continued bruising.)

Sometimes, though, a copious amount of blood mixed with secretions can come up a baby's ET tube. This is a visible sign of what doctors call a pulmonary hemorrhage. It comes from deeper in the lungs than the other, lesser bleeding that results from injury to the upper airways, and is thought to be caused by overly high pressure in the small blood vessels of the lungs (the capillaries), which then leads to an increase of fluids (water and blood) in the surrounding tissues. Eventually this excessive buildup of fluids can damage the delicate lung tissues of a preemie, bursting through them into the air sacs and the airways.

If this happens to your baby while you're visiting him, it's understandable that you'll be very scared. But you should try not to panic or despair. Although it usually requires medical intervention, this complication is most often treatable and is less serious than it looks to a shocked parent. (Some babies who have a pulmonary hemorrhage, due to their compromised respiration and the loss of blood and fluid, appear very pale, limp, and sick. Other babies will keep on doing surprisingly well during and after the pulmonary hemorrhage.)

Pulmonary hemorrhages are more likely to occur in extremely premature babies with severe respiratory distress syndrome. Most at risk are preemies who also have a patent ductus arteriosus (or PDA). The reason is that a PDA allows too much blood to flow into the lungs, leading to increased fluid buildup. Other complications that increase a baby's chance of developing a pulmonary hemorrhage include having suffered from a severe lack of oxygen or blood flow at birth, having an infection, or having a blood-clotting disorder. Being on a ventilator, an otherwise beneficial medical treatment, increases the likelihood of bleeding because it can damage a baby's lung tissues. Also, surfactant therapy, although effective in treating RDS, can predispose a baby to a pulmonary hemorrhage.

A pulmonary hemorrhage usually needs immediate treatment:

✳ The first priority is to help the baby's breathing, keeping his lungs well inflated. If he is on a ventilator, it will probably be adjusted to higher settings to improve his oxygenation. The doctor may decide to give more surfactant because blood in the air sacs can inactivate the surfactant already there. A restless baby who "fights" against the machine may need to be sedated.

✳ The baby may be given fluid, blood, or special medications to improve blood clotting or heart function.

✳ If a PDA is thought to be the culprit, it will most likely be treated. Most doctors wait to give indomethacin or ibuprofen, the usual treatments, until the bleeding has stopped because these medications can interfere with blood clotting. If the medication doesn't work, the PDA can be closed surgically if it's still causing problems.

(*Continued on page 206*)

In Plain Language: What Is a PDA?

PDA stands for patent (which means open) ductus arteriosus (which means arterial canal in Latin). A PDA is not an anatomical flaw. It is simply a blood vessel near the heart and lungs that was a normal, necessary part of your preemie's circulation when he was a fetus. It's meant to close shortly after birth, then disappear. But in many premature babies—some 40 percent to 60 percent of all preemies, and 65 percent of those born at less than 28 weeks of gestation—the PDA lingers. (It's not surprising; according to Mother Nature's timetable, a preemie would still need his PDA in the womb.) Most PDAs eventually close on their own, are not dangerous, and don't need to be treated, but if a PDA makes it more difficult for a baby to recover from respiratory distress syndrome or other complications of prematurity, it can be treated with medication or, rarely, with surgery.

A big change, from the womb to the world

When a baby is born, he has to leave his sheltered environment in the womb and start breathing on his own. That pivotal first breath triggers a big change in the baby's lungs, opening them up and filling them with air. As a fetus, he got oxygen from the placenta, so he didn't need to send blood to his lungs. But after birth, the baby's blood circulation must switch to a new route, with the blood traveling to the lungs to pick up oxygen. This rerouting of blood flow, among other events, involves closure of the PDA.

As the picture on page 205 shows, the ductus arteriosus is a small blood vessel connecting the pulmonary artery (the main blood vessel from the heart to the lungs) and the aorta (the big-gest artery, which carries blood from the heart to the rest of the body). Before birth, the ductus is open and most of the blood flowing from the heart into the pulmonary artery takes a detour through the PDA into the aorta, bypassing the fetus's lungs, which are not used yet for breathing. When breathing starts at birth and the lungs expand with air, blood flow to them increases. A sudden rise in the blood oxygen level, among other signals, gives the PDA the message that it's time to close.

The first phase of closing generally occurs within a baby's first few days of life. The ductus tightens and narrows so that no blood flows through it. In the second phase, which spans the next several weeks to months, the PDA is replaced by scar tissue and becomes just a thread.

In some preemies, the PDA doesn't close within days or even weeks after birth. Some PDAs remain open for many months, closing spontaneously sometime during a baby's first year of life without interfering with his health, growth, or development. In others, it tightens and closes briefly, but reopens before scarring takes place so blood begins flowing through it again. (It usually will close again later—on its own or with help from the doctors.)

What if the PDA remains open?

After delivery, when a baby begins breathing, the blood flow shifts direction through the PDA: Now it goes from the aorta backward into the pulmonary artery, adding to the blood that the lungs are getting. If the PDA is starting to tighten and narrow, allowing just a little blood to go through, the baby may not be disturbed by it at all. On the other hand, if the ductus is still large and wide open, the lungs may be burdened with too much blood, making it harder for the baby to breathe, and overloading the heart with work to pump extra blood to the rest of the body, to compensate for what's going backward through the PDA.

A large PDA can lead to such complications as pulmonary edema (a buildup of fluid in the lungs) and congestive heart failure (this scary term doesn't represent an irrevocable verdict but a treatable, if still serious, condition in which the heart shows signs of tiring from having to pump all of the blood the body needs). Some doctors think a PDA also makes a baby more likely to develop chronic lung disease and necrotizing enterocolitis (a bowel disorder called NEC for short), but others believe these two conditions occur together just by coincidence in babies who are very premature and sick. In extremely premature babies, PDAs have also been linked to a higher incidence of intraventricular and pulmonary hemorrhage in the first few days of life, possibly because of changes in blood flow to the brain and lungs. Unfortunately, studies have not shown any long-term benefits, in terms of greater survival or better developmental outcome, from closing the PDA before those problems can develop (probably because the side effects of treatment cancel the benefits).

How a PDA is suspected and diagnosed

There are several clues that raise suspicion that there is a PDA:

* A murmur on a chest exam (but sometimes a PDA is completely silent);
* An increase in the baby's heart rate, or bounding pulses in his arms, legs, or chest;
* Low blood pressure;

* Decreased urine output (if the kidneys get less blood flow they make less urine);
* Widening of the blood pressure interval (for instance from 60/40 to 70/30);
* An enlarged heart and fluid in the lungs (seen on a chest X-ray or heard on a physical exam);
* Worsening of a baby's breathing problems.

This last possibility can be a real disappointment, arising just when a preemie with RDS should be rapidly weaning from a ventilator or supplemental oxygen. Why does the weaning become so difficult? For several days after birth, while a preemie is still suffering from RDS and receiving respiratory assistance, the pressure in his lungs remains high. The high pressure in the lungs blocks some of the blood flow from a PDA (just as a clogged drain won't let too much water through), so the lungs don't get overloaded with blood. But after a few days, as the baby recovers from RDS, his lungs expand and the pressure in them falls. If there is a large PDA, a lot of blood can flow back through it into the lungs, stressing them and causing a recurrence or persistence of respiratory problems.

A PDA is generally diagnosed by a baby's neonatologist and then confirmed with an echocardiogram, a completely benign, painless test that uses ultrasound waves to get a clear picture of the structure and function of your baby's heart and surrounding blood vessels. An echocardiogram can be performed without even moving a preemie from his isolette.

How a PDA is treated

If your baby has a PDA but, thankfully, no symptoms, he does not need any intervention. The doctors will monitor him carefully to catch signs of any possible complications early. The PDA will most likely close by itself—usually within a few

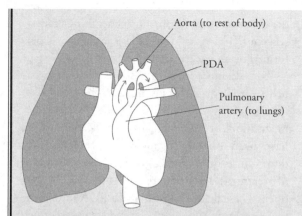

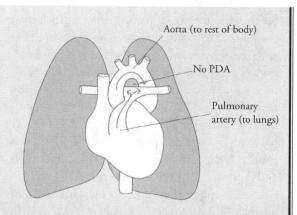

Before birth: blood flowing from the heart through the pulmonary artery is diverted into the aorta through the PDA, bypassing the lungs (not yet used for breathing).

After birth, with a closed PDA: normal circulation.

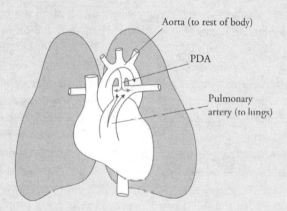

After birth, with a PDA: blood in the aorta can flow backward through the PDA into the pulmonary artery, burdening the lungs with too much blood.

weeks, but sometimes it takes months—and you'll soon forget about it and its pretentious Latin name!

Other medical problems, such as anemia and infection, can worsen a PDA or prevent its natural closure. Doctors are aware of these conditions and will try to correct them.

But if your baby's PDA looks like it is delaying his recovery from RDS or causing other complications, his doctor may decide to intervene. She will most likely prescribe indomethacin (also known as indocin) or ibuprofen (yes, as in Advil or Motrin), drugs that cause the PDA to constrict and close. They work in about two out of three babies. Both are given intravenously, usually in several doses over a couple of days. Your baby will be closely monitored for side effects, including poor blood clotting, fluid retention (a problem with indomethacin), and pulmonary hypertension (a rare problem with ibuprofen). His feedings will probably be stopped while he's being treated because the medications reduce abdominal blood flow to the intestines and a few babies have had intestinal perforations. Most of the time, though, babies do fine. Both indomethacin and ibuprofen, unfortunately, are much less effective in closing a PDA after the first two weeks of a baby's life, although doctors may still decide to give them a try.

If treatment with medication hasn't worked or isn't a good option because a preemie is too old (what an irony for a premature baby!) or can't tolerate the side effects, and the doctors believe his PDA is causing such serious problems that it should be closed immediately, the remaining option for a preemie is surgery (see page 347). To parents, the idea of surgery on their little baby can be really unbearable. Some parents mistakenly think that an operation to close a PDA is heart surgery. But a PDA ligation doesn't touch the heart muscle at all. In fact, in many hospitals the operation is performed by general, not cardiac surgeons. The risks involved are small if it is performed by an expert surgical team.

You should know that some neonatologists believe it is not worth taking even the small risks that go along with treating a PDA, with either medication or surgery. They think that PDAs have been unfairly blamed for problems they don't cause or that the potential complications of treatment are worse than letting a PDA stay open. These doctors opt to give a PDA more time to close by itself—as it often does, even much later. They cite clinical studies that failed to show a benefit from closing preemies' PDAs early, in the first few days of life. They point out that there have been no definitive studies of babies with late, symptomatic PDAs to see how they do when they are allowed to go without treatment. Perhaps those babies would be OK if left to recover on their own. New research is needed before this question can be settled.

Overall, the thing to remember when you first hear about a PDA is that it makes great sense to be optimistic, because the chance that it won't do your baby any lasting harm at all is very high.

When your baby's vital signs have stabilized, the crisis is over and you should really try to relax. Your baby will have to be gradually weaned from his higher vent settings, as his lungs heal. But thankfully, a pulmonary hemorrhage, scary as it is, is something from which most preemies recover.

Low Blood Pressure

I've always heard that high blood pressure is a problem, but why are the doctors and nurses so concerned about low blood pressure in my baby?

Premature babies normally have lower blood pressure than full-term babies because of their smaller size. That is not a problem. But because of their immaturity, their regulatory systems to keep blood pressure stable are not as effective and sudden increases or decreases in blood pressure can damage vital organs.

If blood pressure is too low (doctors call this hypotension), some parts of the body may not receive enough blood and that region's cells can be damaged. (The brain is particularly vulnerable in preemies, in part because of its fragile blood vessels, which can break and lead to an intraventricular hemorrhage, and in part because the mechanisms that should protect it from extreme changes in blood flow are still immature.) Thankfully, most of the time hypotension can be controlled and reversed without causing any harm. In rare cases when a baby's hypotension is extremely severe despite treatment, the doctors may talk to his parents about the possibility of withdrawing life support because of irreparable damage to the heart, brain, kidneys, or intestines.

Low blood pressure can have a number of different causes in preemies. If your baby weighs less than about 1,000 grams and his low blood pressure occurs on his first day or two of life, chances are that it's just due to the immaturity of his blood pressure regulatory systems, which are gradually adjusting from the womb to the outside world. This kind of hypotension tends to go away on its own within a week and is nothing to worry about. Some doctors don't even treat low blood pressure in a healthy young preemie as long as clinical signs show that he is getting enough blood flow (he's urinating enough, his heart isn't beating too fast, and acid isn't building up in his blood), feeling that it is normal for him at this stage of his life.

Another possible cause of hypotension in an otherwise healthy premature baby is dehydration, because preemies' thin skin and immature kidneys don't hold fluids in well, and because the frequent blood draws they need for lab tests can deplete them of fluids. This is easily correctable with fluid or a blood transfusion. Also, a PDA, a fetal blood vessel that can remain open in preemies, can lead to low blood pressure, which will rise as the PDA closes.

However, low blood pressure can also be a sign of serious illness in a preemie. It is found in babies who suffered from a lack of oxygen at birth (signaled by severe fetal distress during labor) or blood loss during delivery (perhaps from a placental abruption). It can occur when a preemie has severe respiratory distress syndrome (RDS), infection, or a heart malfunction. If blood pressure suddenly collapses, it may signal an acute complication, such as a pneumothorax (a tear in the lung that allows air to leak out).

If your baby is sick, his blood pressure will begin to rise on its own as he recovers. In the meantime, while doctors are treating his illness, they may also try to raise his blood pressure with a medication, such as dobutamine or dopamine, that improves the blood-pumping ability of the heart. (Dopamine also tightens blood vessels.) If these don't work well enough the doctor may try a more potent medication, epinephrine. If he thinks that your baby's blood vessels are still too loose and flabby as a consequence of his immaturity—imagine that, in a slim preemie!— he may give your baby hydrocortisone, a synthetic version of the natural hormone cortisol that's part of the blood pressure regulatory system. Hydrocortisone tightens the blood vessels, and tighter blood vessels mean higher blood pressure.

All premature babies will have their blood pressure checked frequently. The youngest and frailest are constantly monitored through an arterial catheter, which is more accurate than a blood pressure cuff and allows for immediate intervention if blood pressure becomes dangerously low. Believe it or not, no one knows the exact minimum blood pressure that is safe for a preemie. So, some neonatologists look less intently at the number and more at clinical indicators of whether a baby is getting enough blood flow. Most doctors aim to keep the mean blood pressure at or above the baby's gestational age—for example, a mean blood pressure of 24 in a 24-week preemie—a general rule supported by studies describing the range of blood pressures normally seen in premature babies. More conservative neonatologists try to keep a baby's blood pressure even higher, at 30 or more even for younger babies, believing this will improve blood flow to the brain. If a baby has pulmonary hypertension, many doctors also prefer a higher blood pressure because that can help raise the oxygen saturation level of his blood.

Leaving Hydrocortisone Behind

Hydrocortisone is just what some preemies need to overcome low blood pressure during the first few days after delivery. It is usually tapered off over a period of two to three days, but occasionally the process takes longer.

Why? Because when the body is given hydrocortisone, it typically reacts by damping down its own production of cortisol (the natural hormone that hydrocortisone mimics), as if the body knows it is getting plenty artificially and doesn't want to overshoot. Weaning a baby off hydrocortisone in small steps gives his body a chance to pick up the slack and gradually increase its production to a normal full level.

But in some preemies, the tapering off may last much longer. They may just need higher than usual levels of cortisol for their bodies to function appropriately. Or their natural cortisol production may have been suppressed more deeply and longer than usual in response to the medication. Using trial and error, the doctor lowers the amount of hydrocortisone the baby is getting and waits to see whether the baby's body responds by increasing its production of cortisol enough to keep his blood pressure up. Sometimes the process is one of stops and starts, two steps forward and one step back.

Any wrinkle like this can make parents frustrated and anxious, but you should try to be patient: Eventually your preemie will produce more cortisol on his own as his body matures. Two to four weeks usually does the trick.

If your baby is one of those whose weaning process takes several weeks, his doctors will be extra careful during the following months in the hospital and at home. That's because there's a possibility that his cortisol production will remain slightly suppressed. That's not usually a problem, but since cortisol is an essential part of the body's response to stress, helping to fight infection and injury, if your baby encounters a major stress within the first six months, such as surgery or a serious infection, he may need a so-called stress dose of hydrocortisone from his pediatrician.

To avoid getting unnecessary stress doses of hydrocortisone, some babies may be given a special test before leaving the hospital to ascertain definitively that their cortisol production has bounced back to normal levels. Your baby's doctor may recommend one, or he may feel that it's not worthwhile since a few months from now you won't even have to think about this anymore.

It all sounds very complicated to anyone who isn't a neonatologist. As a parent, you should rely on the choices your baby's doctors are making and try not to be too apprehensive. In the vast majority of cases, hypotension either goes away by itself or can be effectively treated, and its possible negative consequences prevented.

Diagnosing Pneumonia

They don't know if my baby has pneumonia. Shouldn't they be able to tell?

It's disappointing, especially to parents trying to safeguard the health of their children, to be reminded that medicine is not an exact science. To make a diagnosis, both clinical evidence and experience—the clinical eye of a good physician—are needed. But that detective process isn't always quick and smooth, and some questions may never be answered with certainty.

Pneumonia—an infection deep in the lung that impedes a baby's respiration—is particularly hard to verify in premature babies. Why? Because the symptoms of pneumonia can be the same as those of RDS: excess lung fluid (from a PDA, for example), an area of collapsed lung (from a plug of mucus), or inflammation (caused by the ventilator). In each case, a preemie will breathe faster and harder than normal and have lower oxygen levels in his blood. Even an X-ray of the baby's lungs cannot reliably distinguish pneumonia from many other common respiratory problems in preemies.

What makes pneumonia even trickier is that it can be caused by many different infectious agents: bacteria, viruses, or fungi, which can infect a preemie before birth, during delivery, or in the NICU. Depending on what kind of pneumonia is suspected, the doctors may perform different tests and cultures of a baby's respiratory secretions, nose, throat, eyes, blood, urine, or other tissues. But culture results can take up to several days for bacteria, and a week or more for viruses and fungi, and even then, a culture can be falsely negative if the infected tissue wasn't sampled (perhaps because it's too deep in the lung to reach) or falsely positive if it turns up simply harmless organisms from the upper airway that live in every baby's nose and throat.

Eventually, with patience and repeated tests, pneumonia and its cause can often be ascertained. But it may not be necessary or wise to pursue a definitive diagnosis. The most reliable cultures are obtained from deep in the lung, where the infection would be, but these may require invasive tests, even a lung biopsy, that carry some risk. And it may be too dangerous to wait that long. As soon as doctors suspect pneumonia in a preemie, they'll give him a course of broad-spectrum antibiotics to try to stop an infection before it gets worse. Usually that does the trick. If not, they'll probably search further. If a guilty microorganism is found, your baby will receive the appropriate antibiotic for as long as it is needed to eradicate the infection.

In addition to antibiotics, a premature baby with pneumonia will receive all sorts of supportive care in a NICU. He will often receive respiratory assistance, with extra oxygen or a ventilator, and his fluid and nutrient intake will be closely watched. If he's very anemic (meaning his red blood cell count is low), he may be given a blood transfusion. Red blood cells carry oxygen throughout the body, so boosting their numbers may help when oxygenation is a problem. Everything will be done to help his lungs recover. This scary complication is, unfortunately, quite common in preemies, but they have an excellent chance of overcoming it.

Catching Infections from Other Babies

The baby in the isolette next to my son's has been diagnosed with an infection. Is my son going to get it?

Nurseries know all too well that good fences make good neighbors. All hospital nurseries take precautions to prevent the transmission of infections. They follow guidelines issued by the Centers for Disease Control and Prevention, and many American hospitals have infection control departments that formulate policies based on their own circumstances and special needs. So you should feel reassured: If there were a significant risk that your baby's neighbor could spread his infection to other little patients, he would have been moved to an isolation room, or other barriers would have been put in place, until he was no longer contagious.

Infections are spread in nurseries by two main routes. The first is by contact with an infected person's skin, stool, urine, saliva, or blood. The second is by breathing in droplets shed when the infected person coughs or sneezes. To prevent the spread of infections, the NICU medical staff follows standard rules, such as washing their hands before touching a baby (with either soap and water or a gel or foam disinfectant), changing gloves between patients, and carefully handling and disposing of every instrument or object that has come in contact with blood, body fluids, or broken skin.

The transmission of most infections that preemies get—such as diarrhea, urinary tract infections, skin and wound infections, and most kinds of sepsis, pneumonia, and meningitis—can be prevented just by observing these precautions. Most preemies who have such infections as these don't need to be isolated from their baby neighbors.

Infections spread by respiratory droplets include colds, flu, and some kinds of pneumonia. To infect another person, the virus or bacteria must come in contact with his eyes, nose, or mouth. But droplets containing these microorganisms can usually be propelled in the air only a very short distance and the germs have a short life span. So, they can't reach babies in the next bed or isolette, which by regulation are spaced a certain distance apart. Nurses, however, can pick up these kinds of infection from babies, and sick staff and family members can infect babies with whom they're in very close contact. So nurses, doctors, and relatives who get close to babies with respiratory infections, or who themselves have colds, will wear a hospital mask over their nose and mouth. And even if a doting grandparent or close friend shrugs off her sore throat, it's best to ask her to wait before meeting your delicate preemie.

Infants who have infectious diseases that are more highly contagious, or resistant to conventional antibiotics, will be put in isolation rooms or in an area of the nursery separated by screens or curtains until the danger of spreading the infection is past. Often babies who are contagious are cared for by only a few members of the nursing staff who don't come in contact with unexposed babies. In that way, spread of the infection is limited.

Of course, no system is perfect, and there are occasional outbreaks of infection or inadvertent exposure of the babies in the nursery to a disease like chicken pox. When outbreaks occur, hospitals often do detective work to pinpoint the source, if possible, and do everything possible to interrupt the transmission. Babies who were exposed, but not yet infected, may be treated with preventive medications or vaccines, and sometimes quarantined until it's clear that they're not contagious.

It's natural for parents, who want to do everything to protect their preemie, to become nervous about what their baby is being exposed to in the nursery. But thanks to all of the precautions, most infections that preemies get they don't catch from their neighbors.

In Plain Language: Infections in Preemies

Babies get infected by coming in contact with a potentially dangerous germ, or microorganism. The usual infectious microorganisms in preemies are bacteria, viruses, or fungi. Many of these live harmlessly (either temporarily or permanently) on a baby's skin, in her intestines and airways, or elsewhere in her body. But sometimes a microorganism overcomes a preemie's first-line defenses. It starts to reproduce very quickly and spreads to a place it shouldn't, and an infection results. If the infection remains small and contained (a superficial skin wound, for instance), it may resolve with only a local antibiotic or no treatment at all. But other infections can be more serious and damage vital organs like the lungs (pneumonia), liver (hepatitis), kidneys (urinary tract infection), or brain (meningitis). These infections require more extensive therapy. Most serious of all is when the bloodstream is invaded by many microorganisms. In that case, vital functions like body temperature, respiration, heart rate, and blood pressure can become unstable. Doctors call this sepsis. Luckily, thanks to antibiotic therapies and attentive supportive care, the majority of infected preemies recover well.

The most immature preemies, and those in intensive care the longest, are most at risk of infection. Premature babies are particularly vulnerable to infection for several reasons:

* Their immune systems are immature and don't fight off infections well;
* Life-saving intensive care techniques, such as intubation, catheterization, surgery, and feeding with intravenous nutrition, increase a baby's risk of infection;
* The stress of being born early, and some of the medical complications of prematurity,

afford opportunities for microorganisms to flourish;
* All hospitalized patients—including preemies—are exposed to germs that may be particularly virulent or resistant to conventional antibiotics.

Diagnosis and treatment

The symptoms of infection in preemies are non-specific and can be confused with normal difficulties that preemies often have. Apnea and other breathing problems, low blood pressure, high or low blood sugar, an excess of acid in the blood, abnormal blood cell counts, jaundice, feeding problems, even seizures and temperature instability—all may indicate an infection—or not. Your baby's doctor will probably suspect infection if there's been a sudden worsening of her condition or if several new signs or symptoms show up at once.

The usual diagnostic workup for infection in preemies includes:

* Obtaining cultures of blood, urine, and often spinal fluid and other potentially infected sites, such as a baby's skin, eyes, or respiratory tract;
* X-rays of her chest or abdomen to look for signs of inflammation;
* Lab tests to make sure that an infected baby's organs are functioning appropriately and that such important substances as blood gases, electrolytes, and calcium, as well as blood cell counts, remain at normal levels. These tests of organ function are also used to gauge the severity of the infection.

Since early treatment is often crucial to reverse a preemie's symptoms, the doctor will probably start a course of broad-spectrum antibiotics while the infection is merely suspected, not proven. When the cause is finally found (culture results may take several days to weeks), a more specific antibiotic may be used. Other therapies, such as transfusions, treatment of seizures, and support of breathing and blood pressure, will be used if your baby needs them. If the infection hasn't cleared up after a few days and your baby has a central line (see page 268), the doctors may remove it for fear that it may be harboring the infection.

Sometimes, frustratingly, no guilty culprit is found to be the organism behind your baby's worsening condition, leaving parents and doctors with lingering questions as to whether a preemie's symptoms were even due to infection. This may happen if the infection is in a place that can't be easily or safely cultured, such as the lungs (you can read more about this on page 209), or simply because the available tests are not sensitive enough to detect small numbers of organisms or specific enough to distinguish an infection from inflammation due to other causes.

Infections preemies may get in the NICU

Most of the infections that preemies get while they're in the hospital are caused by microorganisms in their own body that get out of hand. But despite careful preventive measures, preemies may also be infected by other patients, the medical staff, or visitors.

Infections preemies may get at birth

Some preemies get infected around the time of birth. These so-called early-onset infections are usually caused by bacteria in the mother's amniotic fluid and birth canal. These bacteria might be harmless to the mother but infect her baby, or they can infect the mother, too. They can be transmitted to the baby during or just before labor and delivery. Bacterial infections are a major cause of premature birth, and can provoke early delivery without infecting the baby. Some research suggests that certain kinds of bacteria might cause few obvious symptoms in the newborn but increase a preemie's chance of developing chronic lung disease because of ongoing inflammation. Other microorganisms can cause life-threatening pneumonia, sepsis, or meningitis.

You may have been tested or treated during pregnancy or labor for the most notorious of these organisms, Group B strep. If you were treated for Group B strep, your baby's infection most likely was prevented. If your obstetrician suspected that you had chorioamnionitis (an infection of the membranes and amniotic fluid that often leads to premature delivery), she may have cultured your amniotic fluid, placenta, urine, and genital tract and treated you with broad-spectrum antibiotics. Treatment of chorioamnionitis certainly helps to prevent spread of the infection to the baby, but it isn't always successful.

Infections preemies may have gotten earlier in pregnancy

Sometimes an illness that a mother gets during pregnancy is transmitted to her fetus. Most common colds and flus don't harm the baby. But some infections, including syphilis and such viruses as HIV, rubella (which causes German measles), herpes, and others, can. The most serious of these so-called congenital infections result in miscarriages, premature delivery, birth defects, and problems with growth and development.

Babies who have congenital infections are often small for their gestational age. They can be severely ill with pneumonia, hepatitis, meningitis, anemia, and all the other signs of sepsis, or not show any symptoms. Some babies with congenital infections never develop symptoms yet may remain contagious for months. Others have problems that show up later, such as difficulties with vision, hearing, motor skills, or learning.

The diagnosis of a congenital infection is usually made with cultures or other lab tests (of the mother's blood or amniotic fluid, or the baby's blood, urine, or spinal fluid). Sometimes the infection is suspected because of findings on a baby's first physical exam (for example, a large liver or spleen or a skin rash), initial lab abnormalities such as low blood cell counts, or the presence of calcified areas in her liver or brain that show up on X-rays or a head ultrasound.

Effective treatments are available for some of these congenital infections (for example, syphilis or toxoplasmosis) but not all. If your baby has a congenital infection, her doctor will explain what further tests he recommends. He'll also discuss with you what can be done, and how to ensure her best possible future growth and development.

Parents, preemies, and infection

An infection is a truly scary event in a young preemie's life. If a mother or father is convinced that they were the cause of her illness, they may feel devastated. But try to remember that most of the time no one really was to blame, and feeling guilty or assigning responsibility is a waste of your precious energy. Your baby needs you to stand strong at her side now while she's going through this big trial, to help her feel comfortable, recover, and grow.

Hand Washing

I'm really concerned about hygiene in the NICU. I always wash my hands before going in, but I've seen other people, including doctors and nurses, who don't seem as careful.

You're absolutely right to be careful. Simple hand washing before handling a premature baby, using either soap and water or an antibacterial gel or foam, is the most effective way to control the spread of infection in a neonatal intensive care unit. All parents and visitors who come to the nursery to see their preemies should wash their hands to get rid of the extra load of bacteria they may have picked up from such sources of contamination as a doorknob or staircase railing, a car steering wheel, or a bus seat.

What about their shoes, their clothes, their hair? Interestingly, several studies have shown that requiring visitors to cover their clothing with a clean hospital gown or preventing family members from touching preemies does not lower the rate of infection. Nor does prohibiting all visiting in the NICU, even if the visitors include young children. You should of course avoid going to the nursery if you're sick with a cold or flu. And if you've been in contact with somebody who has a contagious illness, such as an older child with measles or chicken pox, be sure to let the doctor or charge nurse know before you visit. They'll want to make sure that you're immune to that illness; if not, you could inadvertently expose the babies to it, even if you don't have any symptoms.

The medical staff is well aware of the risk of infection in premature babies, and the necessary strategies to control it. Hand washing between patients is mandatory in all NICUs. (Just know, though, that if the medical staff uses an antibacterial gel or foam, you may not see them go over to the sink when they clean their hands.) If the doctor or nurse expects to come in contact with blood, body fluids, skin sores, or mucous membranes, like when they put in an IV or suction a baby's endotracheal tube, they will also wear gloves. Procedures that involve entering deep body spaces, such as spinal taps or placing central lines, are performed under sterile conditions. And if a doctor or nurse must work in the nursery despite having a cold, she'll wear a mask over her nose and mouth to prevent spreading any infectious droplets.

Visitors in hospital nurseries (who are mostly, like you, the parents of little patients) generally react in a responsible way, trying to comply with precautions to control infections. But people get ill at unpredictable times and can be forgetful. Thus, if you look around you in a neonatal intensive care unit, you may see somebody sneezing or blowing his nose, or a mother, coming back from pumping breast milk, who forgets to wash her hands before touching her baby. Should she wash her hands again? Probably, yes. But should you be outraged or scared by what may look to you like unforgivable carelessness? Certainly not. That sneeze may be an innocent allergy, and that mother may have washed her hands in the breast-pumping room. There may even be times when it's more important for a nurse to rapidly assist a baby rather than stopping to wash her hands before coming to his aid.

Some well-meaning parents take the hygiene issue so seriously that it becomes an obsession, leading them to scrutinize the behavior of every visitor and all of the nurses and doctors. But good hygiene shouldn't be confused with sterility. A NICU can't and shouldn't be a sterile ward, because babies need to feel the comforting, healing touch of human skin on their bodies in order to grow and develop normally. Also, premature babies need to be exposed to the microorganisms that are part of our normal environment to develop antibodies and strengthen their immune defenses against them.

If you happen to notice in your preemie's nursery a person who consistently violates common sense rules of hygiene, you should point this out to someone on the medical staff. But don't let an exaggerated fear of infection ruin your pleasure in being with your baby, holding him close to your skin, and putting the tip of your finger in his mouth to feel how strong his sucking has become. These are things your preemie needs, too, to develop happily and healthily.

Siblings' Visits

My older daughter is begging to visit her new brother in the hospital. Will we be endangering our baby's health by exposing him to his sister's germs or hurting our daughter emotionally by letting her see the baby connected to tubes and wires?

Sometimes young children, who aren't yet burdened by second thoughts and responsibilities, seem to know by instinct what the right thing is to do. This appears to be true with your daughter. Her requests raise an important point. Her baby brother was born, and she needs to get acquainted with him as soon as possible, for her sake and everybody else's in the family.

Your worries are understandable. Families find themselves torn between their desire to take their older children to the NICU and their concern over damage it might do—exposing the older siblings to the shocking sight of the new baby looking tiny and sick in a scary hospital environment, and exposing the preemie to any infectious illnesses an older child may be carrying. Some parents end up deferring a hospital meeting indefinitely, but that can be a mistake.

Several studies have found that sibling visits do not increase the rate of infection in a NICU, provided that the young visitors wash their hands and are screened for contagious illnesses by their parents and the hospital staff. Studies have also indicated that the benefits of sibling visits can be substantial.

(Continued on page 217)

How to Help Your Older Children

Everybody is familiar with the inner conflicts a child experiences when a little brother or sister is born in the most normal, happy circumstances: feelings of elation and pride are mixed with a painful sense of being dethroned by the new arrival, with whom the parents' love and attention must now be shared.

No wonder a premature birth makes things so much harder for older siblings—it takes away all the benefits and magnifies the disadvantages. There's no adorable new baby at home to cuddle, pretend-parent, or be proud of. And the adults' anxiety about the infant's health, topped by the organizational problems of a hospitalization, make older children feel excluded and sometimes even abandoned.

Just imagine that your mother and father are spending long hours in the hospital, making strange child-care arrangements for you with relatives or unfamiliar caregivers, possibly even sending you away from home. Meanwhile, because they are grappling with their own grief and disappointment over the loss of a normal delivery and healthy, full-term newborn, they aren't as available to comfort you—and at times may be so distracted that they overlook your reactions or needs altogether.

Of course, different children react differently. Some adjust more easily than others. The main thing to keep in mind is that for some older siblings this can be a time of great stress, when they need a lot of reassurance.

Understanding your children's feelings

Your children's feelings will be partly determined by how old they are. Even toddlers can sense when you are anxious or upset, and their lives are shaken by changes in your emotional state and absences. Older siblings often have one or more of the following feelings:

* They feel guilty about negative thoughts they've had or bad behavior.
* They fear that they caused the baby to come early by something they did, such as hitting you in your tummy accidentally or in anger, or wishing that the baby would die. (If this sounds strange, remember that children often engage in magical thinking.)
* They feel jealous and angry about the disruption of their cherished routine and the time you are spending on your preemie.
* They are afraid they will catch the baby's illness, just as they've heard that people catch colds, and will have to go to the hospital, too.
* They worry that the baby will die.
* They are afraid that the baby is suffering, or that he has deformities or other problems far worse than he really does.
* They find it hard to believe that there really is a new baby in the family, because he's absent and the situation is so different from what they expected.

Recognizing your children's signals of distress

Some kids show their stress, others keep it hidden. But you can look out for some typical cues. Here, too, age will play a role.

Preschoolers may regress to habits like bedwetting and thumb sucking, or may develop eating or sleeping problems. They may be irritable and disobedient, or alternatively may be excessively clingy and demanding of attention.

Older children may become inattentive at school. They also may regress to behaviors—such as bed-wetting, thumb sucking, or clinginess—that are more characteristic of a younger child. They may act indifferent toward their parents and the new baby. Try not to be offended; that may be your child's way of protecting her feelings or expressing her anxiety.

How you can help your children

How do you offer adequate reassurance, when faced with such strong feelings?

✴ **Be open and honest.** Tell your children what's going on with the baby, even if they don't know what questions to ask. (Talk about your baby by name, as you would any other member of the family.) Keep in mind that you are the best judge of the amount of information your own kids can understand and handle. For children who are two or three years old, a simple explanation that the baby needs to get bigger and stronger before coming home is usually enough, while older children may benefit from a brief description of why the baby was born so early and what his main medical problems are.

✴ **Tell them that they may see you cry or get agitated, but it's not because of something they did—in fact, having them is a solace to you.**

✴ **Whenever you can, continue their reassuring daily routines.** If you can't take them to their Mommy-and-me classes or the park, try to arrange for someone they enjoy, such as their grandfather or a beloved babysitter, to fill in.

✴ **Squeeze in an intimate, one-on-one time each day with your other children, even if it's just a short interlude of cuddling and telling them how important they are to you.** Make it a point

every once in a while to ask them how they're feeling, and to soothe their fears and worries.

✴ **Foster a bond between your older children and the new baby in the hospital.** If your hospital allows siblings' visits, take them to meet their new sister or brother in the NICU. Ask them to paint pictures, choose a family photo, and pick out a stuffed animal to put on or near the baby's bed. Create thank-you notes from the baby to his big siblings. Get photos and reports about how the baby is doing (for instance, how much weight he has gained or how his feeding has improved) specially addressed to your older children by doctors or nurses. Ask for your children's help in setting up the baby's room at home.

✴ **Involve your older children in updating your web site if you have set one up to keep family and friends informed about your preemie.** Depending on their age, they can simply help you choose a new photo to post, draw a picture, or write a report of their visit to their baby brother or sister in the hospital. Encourage them also to post their own personal news, about a good grade they got in school or a fun play date. This way they will feel that they're getting some attention, too, and will also get loving feedback from your circle of relatives and friends.

Making a sibling's visit successful

To be successful, a visit to the new baby in the hospital should be prepared for, if possible. You can show your older children pictures, describe how preemies look, and explain why they may need help breathing and eating before they catch up and become like other infants.

✴ **If your older children have sent a meaningful object of their choice—a toy, a drawing, a photo—make sure to display this gift in or** near your preemie's bed during the visit, pointing out that it keeps the baby company and reminds him of his brother or sister.

* **If the nurses give permission, encourage your children to gently touch the baby and talk to him.** Try to focus on their reactions during the visit and answer all of their questions.
* **Some nurseries have special programs for siblings,** set up by the March of Dimes or hospital staff, that are designed to help older sisters and brothers express their feelings, lessen their anxiety, and learn what goes on in a NICU through fun activities such as creative play, reading, and arts and crafts.

Even after a single quick visit to the nursery, it will be easier to tell the older children about the baby, mentioning people or things they may remember from their visit. Some kids will want to talk a lot about their experience, and others won't, at least for a while.

With your help, your older children will be able to stand strong at your side while your preemie heals and grows in the hospital. Patience and sensitivity will bear fruit for a long time, especially when the baby comes home. His brothers and sisters will have learned how to love him already. And you will know that you gave all of your children your best support.

After visiting their baby sisters or brothers in the hospital, older children had fewer behavior problems, higher self-esteem, and more of a tendency to express, rather than internalize, their feelings. They were more likely to look at caring for the baby as a shared family effort.

Considering the benefits of sibling visits and the few risks involved, most NICUs now allow it. (The one exception is during winter cold season. From around November through March, some NICUs, out of an abundance of caution, prohibit visitors under a certain age, often 8 to 12 years old. The thinking is that catching a cold or the flu can be serious for a preemie or anyone in intensive care and that young children are less reliable in reporting any signs that they may be coming down with something.) So you shouldn't be shy about inquiring about your nursery's policy or asking the staff to help you organize the visit. Most likely you'll find doctors and nurses surprisingly helpful and supportive.

Sometimes the visit may consist of only taking a brief peek at the new baby through a glass wall. Or if your preemie is stable, his older sibling may be able to touch or even hold him. For longer visits, a young child may want to draw or color,

or an older one may want to read to the baby. So if you're planning to stay for a while, consider bringing crayons and books, since your kids will need to be quiet and well-behaved for this. No matter what, the visit will be remembered by your child as a significant experience.

Besides visits, there are other useful things parents can know and do to help their kids at home. You can read about those on page 215.

Making an Isolette Feel Like Home

We can't bear the idea that our tiny baby is all alone in the hospital. A friend suggested that we decorate her isolette and make a recording of our voices that the nurses can play when we're not there.

For months you've been imagining bringing your baby home to a cozy bassinet. When you weren't holding her, she'd have been surrounded by soft blankets, teddy bears, and musical mobiles that would convey how precious and loved you wanted her to feel.

Parents like you, with nurturing spirits, feel heartbroken at the thought of their babies lying alone in the NICU, even though they know it's temporarily the best place for them to be. Like your friend, many wonder: Why not try to create a little of that personal, warm touch in the intensive care unit?

We have two reactions. One: It's a wonderful idea, and you should certainly do it. Two: It needs to be executed with care.

The reason is that although preemies need their parents and signs of love, they are easily stressed by stimulation, and stressing your baby is just the opposite of what you're trying to accomplish. As your preemie becomes older, she'll be able to handle increasing amounts of stimulation without getting overwhelmed. Often very premature and sick infants can tolerate just one kind of sensory activity at a time, whether it's being talked to, being touched, or having something to look at. Though it comes as a surprise to parents at first, the things that we intend to be pleasant, positive stimulation can be just as stressful for their preemies as negative stimulation.

So the best way to start is with a few carefully chosen additions to your baby's home away from home; you can plan to "redecorate" and introduce new elements later as you get to know her better and she gets closer to term. Before buying any object for your preemie in the NICU, make sure to ask the staff whether it is appropriate and allowed (sometimes an innocent stuffed animal can be a possible carrier of infection). Also, remember that anything you leave in the nursery can always get switched with some other baby's possessions by mistake or get lost. The following guidelines will help you choose the right kind of personalization for your preemie's environment in the NICU:

* **An isolette cover.** No premature baby benefits from being confronted constantly by bright overhead lights. (Some intensive care nurseries keep the lights dim when they're not needed; others don't.) So one of the best things you can give your baby is an isolette cover, made of thick fabric, to shield her from excessive light. Whereas some experts advocate always keeping the youngest preemies in near darkness to mimic the womb, others think that preemies of all ages need cycles of light and darkness. They say that the day-night rhythm stimulates hormones, promotes a healthy sequence of activity and rest, and helps a baby's sight and hearing to develop normally. In any case, even during the day, light should never be shining directly into a baby's eyes. You can ask your baby's doctor or nurse for advice on whether to keep a cover on your baby's isolette all the time or only at night.

Some nurseries automatically give isolette covers to every baby, others give them to parents who ask (so do!), and some don't have them at all. If your nursery doesn't, you can buy one from various suppliers (see page 591)—or, easier yet, just bring a blanket or quilt from home, drape it over your baby's isolette, and fold the sides up so the nurses can see your baby and reach the isolette's doors. Make sure the fabric is thick enough to keep out the light (it will also help absorb some of the loud hospital noises), and choose one whose pattern isn't too bold. It can even be dark, as the womb is; don't worry, your baby will still get more than enough stimulation if you or the nurses interact with her during the day or when you notice that she's awake.

* **Works of art: family photos, pictures, and mobiles.** What does a baby want to look at when she's awake? Something that's appropriate for a newborn at one gestational age can be inappropriate for another. For example, those striking, black-and-white designs that are believed to be appealing to full-term babies may be overwhelming to a preemie. In fact, experts are wary of any fixed image in an isolette. If it's stressful and a preemie can't move away from

it, she has to use up valuable energy to tune it out. What about faces? They are a preemie's favorite thing to look at, especially her parents' faces, or her own in a mirror. But even these may be better if introduced intermittently, when you or a caregiver is there and can pay attention to signs that your preemie wants more stimulation, or has had enough and needs a rest.

✳ **The special sound of your voice.** Preemies are drawn to the familiar voices of their parents, and researchers have noted distinct differences between the genuinely loving intonations of a mother's or father's speech and those of a well-intended but nonparental caregiver. On the other hand, just as preemies need to be protected from bright lights, they also need to be sheltered from sounds, which tend to bombard them in the NICU. Many parents assume that an isolette muffles noises, but the opposite is true: Loud sounds reverberate inside it. And noise has been associated with physiological signs of stress in premature babies, who are still supposed to be hearing only their mother's heartbeat and the soft, muted sounds of the womb.

So should you put a tape recording of your voices, talking and singing, in your baby's isolette or not? That depends. If you have good rapport with your baby's nurses and can count on them to observe and make sure that the tape is comforting your baby rather than disturbing her, by all means do it. However, if you notice that your baby is particularly sensitive to noise or if you think that the nurses may just play your tape indiscriminately over and over again, then your baby may be better off without it.

You may have noticed the CDs of heartbeat sounds you can buy. They are supposed to be soothing for full-term babies, but what about preemies? There's no reliable research either way. Some caregivers believe that this most familiar rhythmic sound may be calming for a preemie and may muffle the stressful other noises that bombard her in the NICU. It makes sense. But if you want to give this a try, take care. As with other recordings, the volume should be set extremely low, and you or a nurse should watch your baby's cues to see when the recording is soothing and when it becomes overstimulating, and should be turned off. If these conditions can't be met, don't feel bad: Your baby will still have the joy of hearing your own live voice and heartbeat when you are with her.

✳ **Mommy's scent.** Here's something wonderful you can do for preemies of all ages, since even the youngest preemies recognize the smell of their mother. By introducing your scent into the isolette, you can give your baby precious continuity at a time when she is experiencing so many new and different things. It's simple to do. Just take a small cloth and keep it tucked against your body for a while, perhaps overnight. Keep it against you while you're in the hospital holding your baby. Then when you go home, leave the cloth behind with her. (Just be sure to tell the nurses why it's there so they don't mistakenly remove it.) You can do this again with a clean cloth each day or as often as you like.

✳ **Teddy bears and other stuffed companions.** The truth is, your baby probably won't even notice a teddy bear that you put in her isolette. But it still can be an important addition. Just like a stuffed animal on the shelf of a full-term baby at home, one in an isolette makes a statement: This is a real *baby*, not a clinical case—a child who is cherished and given special, carefully chosen things of her own.

Some stuffed animals—like long snakes—can be extremely comfortable for a preemie to lie against, also. It may seem funny that the best choice of cuddly toy may not be a traditional bear or bunny, but a soft stuffed snake curled around your baby can help her feel contained and tucked in, a feeling that's very soothing to a preemie and one of the best ways to alleviate her stress. The snake can be a creative substitute for the rolled-up blankets that nurses often use to help premature babies stay in a comfortable, side-lying position. At other times, it may be something that her little hands can grasp and hold. Just make sure to ask whether stuffed animals are permitted in your NICU before buying one.

✶ **Beautiful baby clothes.** There's something very special about dressing your baby. Like seeing a teddy bear keeping a preemie company in her isolette, seeing a preemie in real baby clothes can warm any parent's or nurse's heart. When babies are still on radiant warming beds, they're usually kept undressed so the NICU staff can quickly see any small change in their condition. They also have to be naked when they're under phototherapy lamps for jaundice so the light can reach their bare skin. But at other times, clothing is fine. Just make sure that what you choose fits loosely and is made of a soft fabric, that you wash it once in a gentle soap before putting it on your baby, and that it's not too expensive, since clothes occasionally (though not often) are lost in the nursery. (Let the nurse know to put aside your baby's special clothes for you to wash at home rather than putting them in the collective NICU laundry.) Little hats and pairs of socks are great, and so are other outfits if they open easily in front, so your baby can be examined and have her diapers changed.

Don't worry if your baby's clothes are a little big at first; that's part of the charm and will eventually become one of your fond memories. Many web sites offer a good choice of cute preemie clothes (we've found some for you and listed them in Appendix 6, page 591).

Even though these guidelines are worth considering carefully, if there's one thing that all parents learn, it's that no two little individuals are alike. Your preemie, no matter how tiny, already has her own distinct personality, with her own likes and dislikes. Her personal preferences are far more important than any general guidelines, and as you spend time with her, you'll have the intimate joy of beginning to discover and respond to them.

Parents Asked to Leave

Sometimes when I'm visiting my baby, the nurses ask me to leave for a little while. One time it was change of shift, and another time they said there was a procedure I shouldn't watch. What's so secret that I can't be there?

When you're asked to leave your preemie's bedside, it's natural to feel upset. If a nurse or doctor is going to do a procedure, such as drawing blood or doing a spinal tap, you may be anxious about the pain your baby will suffer while you're not there to comfort him. If the doctors are making rounds, you may feel entitled to hear firsthand how your baby is doing. If it's a change of nursing shift, you may not understand how your presence could interfere. And above all, why should you lose some of the precious minutes you could be spending with your baby, instead of waiting idly in the corridor or family room?

There are some good reasons—and some debatable ones. Some nurseries ask parents and visitors to leave the room for privacy reasons during the change of nursing shift and while the doctors make rounds, when detailed information about each patient is passed on. Federal regulations require health care providers and hospitals to protect the privacy of their patients—all medical information is considered confidential—and it is especially easy to overhear intimate information about other babies and their families at those times. In teaching hospitals, there may be the idea that such a policy allows residents and medical students to express themselves more freely and accurately because they can feel more at ease asking questions and admitting their lack of knowledge without feeling embarrassed in front of parents. There are certainly two sides to this, though: You could argue that doctors-in-training should learn to speak openly and sensitively in front of parents, and that confidential information is discussed at all times of day at bedsides in the NICU, not just during rounds or change of shift, yet no one asks you to leave then.

The truth is that each hospital is responsible for deciding how to implement the federal regulations and protect patients' privacy. Policies vary from nursery to nursery. (There are even some that instead of asking parents to leave give them headsets with earphones so they can't hear what is said when another baby is being discussed.)

What about when there's a procedure to perform, either on your baby or a baby nearby? Sometimes a NICU has rules requiring parents to leave for safety reasons, since space is often tight in the NICU and during procedures, equipment and people may have to move around freely and rapidly. In addition, the medical staff may be concerned about your emotional reaction (don't take this personally; it probably applies to all parents) or that your presence could make them feel nervous, interfering with their ability to complete the procedure quickly and smoothly.

It may be that they shouldn't be so worried about that. One study looked at whether it made a difference when parents were allowed to be present while doctors or nurses performed simple medical procedures on their children in an emergency room. The researchers evaluated the amount of pain felt by the child (as signaled by his behavior and the intensity of his cry), the successful performance of the procedure, and the anxiety level of parents, doctors, and nurses.

One of the findings may be reassuring to parents who prefer not to stay with their babies during a procedure: The parents' presence didn't make a difference in reducing their children's pain. On the other hand, the performance of the medical staff wasn't impaired by the parents' presence, and there was one major benefit to staying: a much lower anxiety level in mothers and fathers. "We should encourage parents who want to be present to stay during procedures," the study's authors concluded.

Some parents will gratefully exit so as not to witness their baby in pain, while others will be reluctant to leave, feeling that even if they can't take the pain away, they can offer their baby something very important: the assurance that his parents are there to comfort him. Since it's only fair to take into account both the parents' instincts and the medical staff's nerves, don't hesitate to speak up. If your nursery has no rules requiring parents to leave, it may be your call to make. Even in nurseries with rules, there is often some flexibility built into them. More and more, nurseries are allowing greater participation by families in their baby's care. So if you feel strongly that you want to stay with your baby during a procedure, be sure to convey that to the staff; they may be able to accommodate you.

When to Circumcise

We want to have our son circumcised, but the doctor is telling us to wait. It seems that he doesn't understand how important this is to us.

The doctor may seem insensitive to your wishes, but actually he's just trying to be extremely sensitive to your son's health.

Any kind of stress—and that certainly includes a surgical procedure, even a relatively minor one like circumcision—can be destabilizing to a newborn preemie, causing changes in breathing, heart rate, and other vital functions that could lead to complications. The procedure itself will be safer later, too: the smaller the area the doctor has to work with, the more difficult the surgery is to perform. For both reasons, all elective surgery is usually postponed until premature newborns get bigger and stronger and their medical condition is stable.

In most nurseries, circumcision is done a few days before a baby boy is discharged from the hospital. Although that isn't as soon as you'd hoped, you can bet your son will be circumcised by the time he's lying on your changing table at home.

Medical Costs

We have no idea how much all of this intensive medical care is going to cost or whether we can afford it.

In the midst of your other worries, at some point, naturally, it crosses your mind: Are we going to be able to afford all of this? Thankfully, the answer is almost certainly yes. Your baby will be able to stay in the hospital as long as she needs to, getting the care she deserves—and it won't bankrupt you.

To be sure, you may get some steep bills, but private insurance companies and Medicaid usually offer excellent coverage of intensive care. And you have an ally—the social worker at your baby's hospital—who should be able to guide you in managing the financial end of this experience.

Here are the basics you should know. As you might guess, intensive care hospitalization is ex-

tremely expensive: An average day in a neonatal intensive care unit now costs around $1,000 to $2,000. (Your hospital may charge more or less than this, and rates change every year.) When your baby leaves intensive care and graduates to an intermediate care unit, the daily cost will go way down, to several hundred dollars a day, though it still won't be cheap.

But the situation is not as dire as it sounds because, first of all, if either you or your spouse is covered by insurance, the chances are that your baby is, too. (Make sure to notify your insurance carrier immediately of your baby's birth. Some plans give you 30 days after delivery to include a baby in your coverage.) Many insurance plans pick up 80 percent to 100 percent of the hospital and medical costs.

If you do not have insurance, you may be eligible for Medicaid. The social worker should be able to give you information on your state's program (Medicaid eligibility and benefits differ from state to state) and help get you enrolled. Medicaid generally picks up the entire cost of the baby's hospitalization. If you are insured, some states have government programs that may also pick up medical costs that your insurance company doesn't. (Be aware that Medicaid and private insurance plans don't always cover circumcision or the cost of transporting a baby back to his community hospital when he no longer needs intensive care in a NICU far from home.)

The social worker can also tell you about or help you contact any other government programs or private charities that may be willing to help out. Some assist families while their babies are in the hospital, others provide support for those whose babies have continuing medical needs once they get home.

If the amount that's left for you to pay—either the deductible and co-pay if you're insured, or more if you're not—is still overwhelming to you, most hospitals will be willing to work out a payment plan. Many hospitals will agree to spread payments out over a number of years. Some will also use a sliding scale based on a family's ability to pay, rather than fixed fees, or will make agreements on a case by case basis to reduce charges that aren't covered by insurance.

Undoubtedly, you're going to have other expenses besides the medical bills, and if your baby's hospitalization is long, these can really add up, too. The social worker may also be able to help you with some of these; she may have discretionary funds to give out for parking, or meal coupons, or equipment like breast pumps or car seats to lend to parents who are strapped for funds. If your baby's hospital is far from your home, she can tell you whether there is a Ronald McDonald House nearby—a nonprofit lodging where parents of sick children are welcome to stay for free—so you can save the cost of a hotel.

Since the social worker can help you negotiate so much of this, don't hesitate to contact her. She'll be glad to help alleviate your anxiety about these practical matters, so you can concentrate on your baby.

Coping Emotionally

I need help! I'm feeling so emotionally overwhelmed.

Don't think for a second that you're the only one. Most parents who deliver a very premature baby are confused and emotionally overwhelmed for weeks or months. It's not strange at all, considering the mounds of new, often frightening information you're getting, the utterly different world of the NICU you find yourself a part of, and the disruption of your life that any birth—but especially a premature birth—entails. Not only are your feelings normal, they're healthy. Acting as if nothing traumatic or stressful had happened would indicate that you're trying to

shield yourself from reality. The best way to heal is to do what you've done already: acknowledge your emotions and need for help. This is a necessary step, and there are others you can take, too, so that you and your little one can move on with your lives together.

Most likely, there's a bright future ahead for you and your baby, and his premature birth is only a temporary crisis. But at this moment things are hard. No parents can truly prepare themselves for a newborn who needs intensive medical attention and isn't at home in his bassinet. Certainly, all mothers and fathers go through an initial period of adaptation to a new baby and the new responsibilities that come with him, and some of what you're feeling may be just that. But a premature birth can add on much more:

* **Worry**—and for parents with sick babies, perhaps even terror—about whether your baby will come through this OK;
* **Regret** that you can't enjoy the intimacy with your newborn you longed for;
* **Uneasiness** at having to deal with doctors and nurses whom you are completely entrusting with your baby's well-being;
* **Guilt** that you let down your baby and perhaps your partner;
* **Confusion** as to why this happened;
* **Sadness** that your baby is being deprived of a normal life's beginning;
* **Anger** that it happened, undeservedly, to you and your child;
* **Shock** that your baby and family are the actors in this weird, unexpected drama;
* **Helplessness** at not being able to turn back the clock and make it all come out differently.
* **A sense of spinning** through wild extremes, from joy, excitement, awe, and hope for the future to dread, fear, bitterness, and even numbness.

(Continued on page 226)

Who Can Help You with Your Emotions?

Helping yourself: In the privacy of your home you can let your emotions unravel in ways you may not feel like doing when you are surrounded by people in the NICU. Spend some time listening to your favorite music. If tears come, give yourself permission to cry freely. Sobbing, yelling, even expressing your anger by punching a pillow can be liberating. If you feel you're not ready to talk to anyone else about all this right now, try first talking to yourself by keeping a diary. Jotting down some notes every night after visiting your baby or calling the NICU could help you put into words—and balance—your greatest hopes and worst fears. (And, believe it or not, you are going to want to remember many of the details of this experience, which will always be one of the most important and meaningful of your life.) Any kind of creative or artistic expression may be of great comfort to you at this time. You can start now, even if you've never tried this kind of activity before. Some parents have written poems about their babies' time in the NICU; others have made sketches or painted pictures. Some mothers and fathers go home and while thinking of their baby play or improvise on a musical instrument. No matter whether you're experienced or a novice, art can be a safety valve that eases your pain and brings a measure of peace to your mind. Take the time to exercise (outdoors, especially—the release from the unnatural confinement of the NICU can be exhilarating). Walking, swimming, gardening, yoga, any kind of physical activity will help calm your emotions and clear your mind. (Did you know that exercise is a very powerful antidepressant, as potent as prescription medications?) As much as possible, try to eat right and get enough rest. A healthy lifestyle helps control stress and negative emotions.

Help from your partner: While you explore your emotions, if you have a spouse or partner, remember that there's probably at least one other person who wants and needs to share all of this with you. Chances are, there's no one closer to what you're experiencing than the other parent of your baby. In fact, studies have shown that both mothers and fathers of premature or ill newborns find each other to be their best source of support and help during the first weeks their babies spend in a NICU. To cultivate that mutual support, it's important to share with your partner the details of your baby's daily events and your reactions to even the tiniest triumphs and setbacks. Without that fine-tuning, there's a risk of building up misunderstandings that in the future may cause you pain. Even if your partner cannot express his or her emotions now, you should make the effort to keep your feelings open. The love you both nurture for your infant can give you the strength to overcome a crisis that would be tough on even the happiest couples—and perhaps to emerge with an even stronger relationship.

Help from your family and friends: Probably there are other people with whom you're intimate who can share your baby's daily ups and downs with you, and to whom you can express your deepest feelings. Whether it's your mother, father, sibling, or best friend, they most likely want to help in any way they can. If they hang back, it may be that they're afraid of intruding, in case you don't want them to be involved now. In fact, they may be feeling some of the same emotions you are but don't feel they have permission to say so. Even if you aren't ready to reach out to a lot of friends and family members, it can help to choose at least one or two people to talk to freely and involve as much as you can. Invite them to come visit your baby and give them a tour of the NICU. You'll be helping those close to you by letting them help you, and you won't have to carry this tremendous burden alone.

Help within the NICU: Because having a baby in intensive care is known to be an unfamiliar and difficult experience, all NICUs have staff and resources to support parents. Some are common, others are unique to each hospital. Be sure to ask what's available to you. Your NICU may have a March of Dimes family support specialist, a trained professional who is there to support and comfort you in ways you need. The specialist can give you written information and help you make records and keepsakes; put you in contact with other NICU parents and support groups; and suggest and facilitate ways for your family members and other children to understand what is happening or get closer to your premature baby. A social worker connected with your NICU can do many of those things, too, and is the right person to ask about financial and practical problems that concern you, such as the cost of your baby's medical care, health insurance issues, financial aid that may be available, and transportation and accommodations (which can be costly if you live far from the hospital). Both social workers and family support specialists are trained in helping parents who are grieving and fearful about this unexpected outcome of their pregnancy, and may be able to help you express and understand your emotions.

Help from other parents, in person or online: Support groups usually consist of parents of babies now in the hospital like you, or "graduate" parents who make themselves available for talking and listening to mothers and fathers of hospitalized premature babies. Current parents can share your joys, fears, and uncertainty, and make you feel less isolated. Graduate parents can give you the insight of somebody who's been there. They can explain things to you in plain, understandable, nonmedical language. Most of all, as living proofs, they'll comfort you that there's a happy life coming after the NICU. You, too, can look forward to that. Support from other parents is also readily available online, where you can join one of many blogs (such as the March of Dimes Prematurity Campaign's forum called Share) or start your own (you'll be amazed how many hits—and eventual online friends—you'll get). It's easy to log on when you have a moment at home, and many NICUs have computers available in the hospital for parents. Reading the conversations, it won't take you long to find parents who have something—or a lot—in common with you. When you share your baby's story and your feelings, and become part of the online community of parents of premature babies, your online friends can be your private, cherished source of support for many weeks or months to come. They're there just when you need them, going through what you are.

Help from mental health therapists and physicians: For some parents of preemies who feel they need emotional support, the best choice may be seeking help right away from a mental health therapist. If you are already seeing one, you might want to add some extra sessions. If you need to find a specialist, look for a psychologist, psychiatrist, or social worker with experience and expertise in counseling families through medical crises. Some NICUs have therapists on staff to whom the social worker can refer you. A psychologist can offer you various types of psychotherapy, including short-term kinds of talk therapy that are effective. A psychiatrist can diagnose and treat anxiety or depression, if you are suffering from either, with both psychotherapy and drugs. In particular, postpartum depression is very common in mothers of preemies—and very treatable—and can be exacerbated by having a baby in the hospital. If you have trouble sleeping, like so many parents of premature babies who are worried, a psychiatrist or your family doctor can prescribe an effective sleep medication. (And of course, consider reducing your caffeine intake.)

Help from religious advisers: A hospital chaplain (a minister, rabbi, or priest who visits and counsels families and patients in the hospital) or your own religious adviser can discuss with you all of the spiritual issues related to your experience, and in particular the meaning of this experience for your baby and family. Don't exclude the possibility of talking to a hospital chaplain whose faith may be different from yours, because his compassion, knowledge of the issues that illness raises in a family, and willingness to address ethical questions and profound concerns may help you find some of the peace of mind that you're looking for.

The list of upsetting feelings can be so long—those are just some of them. But when at least part of your emotional burden is spelled out, it may feel less heavy.

Don't feel that you're being disloyal to your baby, your partner and family, yourself, or, if you are religious, to God by not being hopeful and optimistic all the time. Recognizing and acknowledging fear and dread—and for many people, praying for strength—may be the most helpful way to handle these painful emotions. Unexpressed, they can fester and undermine the joyful, comforting feelings that being with your baby will also arouse.

Ultimately you will heal emotionally and regain your inner strength, with time and the help of good social and psychological support from your family, friends, advisers, and the new relationships you develop in the NICU. In the box starting on page 224, you can find advice on how to help yourself and get help from others.

While the stress and emotional pain you're experiencing right now is normal and understandable, you should be aware that mothers of preemies are at higher risk for postpartum depression. If you feel so bad that you are thinking about hurting yourself, please talk immediately to someone close to you and seek help. If nobody is around, call 911. It's an emergency.

Chances are that in a brief time you'll feel much more in control. You will never forget what you're going through now, but you can learn how to accept and make sense of what happened. This upsetting period in the beginning of your baby's life can also be an occasion for personal growth, individually and as a couple. Many people feel they come out of it as better, more mature people and more understanding parents.

MULTIPLES

Babies in Different Hospitals

One of our twins is in a hospital near home, but the other one was taken to a bigger hospital an hour away. I don't know how we're going to handle the logistics.

You always knew that having twins was going to double both the rewards and trouble of parenting. But who could imagine you'd have to take care of two newborns in two different cities at the same time! If you have enough time in your day to travel back and forth between hospitals, you could, of course, spend some morning hours with one twin and afternoon or evening hours with the other. But many parents find it too difficult to juggle daily double hospital visits with their other obligations.

The first thing to do may be difficult at first, but it's important: Allow yourself to accept that it's OK for you not to see both of your twins every single day. Even if you skip a few days, the attention and intimacy they get from you in these early weeks is plenty to help them recover and grow, so long as it's gentle, sensitive, and loving when you're together.

Here are some other possible solutions to your problem:

* **Split up the visits with your spouse or partner,** each of you spending some time each day with one of your babies, but alternating so you both get to spend some time with each.
* **Together with your partner, spend one day,** or a few days, with one baby, and the next day or few days with the other. This will give you and your partner some time together, which can be important in maintaining your relationship.
* **Ask a grandparent, friend, or someone else close to you to step in** and help you by visiting one of your preemies when you can't. You may think you are burdening them, but more likely they are eager to find a way to help you. Who wouldn't be honored to be chosen for the task that requires more trust than any other?
* **Try to have your other twin transferred to the larger hospital, too.** Particularly if you have

significant transportation problems, and if your twins are expected to remain in separate hospitals for several weeks or more, you may want to investigate this possibility. Stumbling blocks you may encounter could include the lack of an available bed for your relatively well baby, and the expense of transporting your twin if your insurance doesn't pay for non-medical moves.

* **Visit your sicker baby more often, for now.** You may even want to consider staying at a hotel near the distant hospital for a few days, while your sicker twin is most unstable. Remember that responding to one of your twin's needs is not playing favorites—it will even out over time, and there will be plenty of times in the future when you'll be doing the same for your other twin. (Instead of a traditional hotel, many parents choose to stay at a Ronald McDonald House near their baby's hospital. These nonprofit lodgings are located near many children's hospitals around the country and offer parents a private room, meals, and sometimes other services, such as a shuttle to the hospital or support sessions with other families. Visitors are asked to donate a small amount, but if you can't afford to pay, you can stay for free. If you're interested in staying at a Ronald McDonald House, ask the social worker or nurses at your baby's hospital for a referral to the nearest one.)
* **Recognize that if your sicker twin is on a lot of pain medication or heavily sedated** (as is often true for a few days after surgery, for instance), he really won't be aware of what's going on and who's there. This is a time when your other twin may appreciate your presence more. (But don't feel bad if you still need to be with your sicker twin for your own emotional needs or peace of mind. During a critical illness, that's how most parents feel.)

Fortunately, this particular logistical hardship doesn't usually last for more than a few weeks. Either your sicker baby will soon catch up with his sibling and be able to join him in the same hospital, or your other twin will be discharged home. You may still find it difficult to divide your time between your babies! But leaving behind worries about transportation, traffic jams, parking places, and travel expenses to two hospitals can only make things easier.

Keeping Twins Near Each Other

I've seen pictures of twins sharing the same bed in the hospital. Why can't our twin daughters even share the same room? I don't want them to be separated.

Most nurseries try their best to put multiples near each other, since it's easier and nicer for their families, but it isn't always possible when the babies first arrive in the NICU. They may have to be separated initially if one sibling is sicker than the other, since some nurseries have designated areas or rooms for babies who need the most acute care. (The training of the nurses who work there, the nurse-to-baby ratio, and the equipment and layout may all be different.) Even if that's not an issue, it may not be possible to give siblings the same nurse, and they may have nurses who are stationed far apart from each other. (Nursing assignments are carefully juggled so that no nurse is too overloaded to provide good care to all of her patients.) Sometimes twins are separated at first simply because there aren't two free bed spaces next to each other when they arrive. Some parents feel more strongly about this issue than others, so you should certainly mention to the nurses that it's important to you. Most likely they'll arrange for your twins to be close together as soon as possible.

"Cobedding" multiples—putting them in the same bed so they can feel each other's presence as they did in the womb—has been common for many years in some Scandinavian countries. In the United States, the practice of cobedding is more recent because there was little research on its benefits and risks and many medical professionals had concerns. It is now becoming more common, and in many hospitals is standard practice once twins are stable enough to be sleeping in open cribs. (Most isolettes and radiant warmer beds aren't big enough for two.)

Certainly to parents of multiples it seems natural that their babies, who have been lifelong companions, would be a much-needed comfort to each other in a new, harsh world. And there have been a few inspiring stories of premature twins who were struggling—with apnea and bradycardia or poor oxygen saturation—until they were put in the same bed, where they snuggled into each other and quickly became more stable.

The results of small clinical studies thus far have not been as dramatic, with some showing benefits—such as slightly reduced apnea, increased weight gain, or decreased stress—and others not. But they also haven't uncovered any harms. (Neonatologists had been worried about potential risks, fearing that a doctor, nurse, or technician could mix the babies up and compromise their treatment, or that such close contact would increase the likelihood that they would pass infections from one to another, or that they would need different amounts of heat to keep from getting too hot or too cold. Right now, there is no evidence of these problems.)

Remember that precautions need to be taken. For your babies' safety, if either has an infection, is on a ventilator, or has an umbilical catheter or chest tube (which could be accidentally dislodged by a little neighbor's kick, pull, or bump), they will probably have to wait. But don't hesitate to ask the nurses if, and when, your baby girls can be finally reunited.

IN DEPTH

How to Make Your Baby Feel Loved in the NICU (or Developmental Care)

Dear Mommy and Daddy,

I know I came out sooner than you expected, and I understand that you had to put me in the hospital nursery until I mature and grow. But I'm still your little baby, and I wish you could do something to make me feel a little better here. Can't you think of something?

Love you,
Your New Arrival

How do you give your newborn baby the feeling of being loved when she is surrounded by beeping machines, secluded behind plastic walls, and subjected to occasionally painful, though necessary, medical procedures? That's a tough question, and parents of premature babies worry about it tremendously. Some write it off as an impossible task—but they shouldn't.

There *are* things you can do. Many are recommended by proponents of a field spanning neonatology and psychology called developmental care, which over the past few decades has influenced the way preemies in the NICU are taken care of by doctors, nurses, mothers, and fathers. If you want, you can begin putting some of these ideas into practice yourself right away.

Don't think that you're going to read anything truly surprising, or without the ring of common sense. Developmental care is based on a simple but extremely important idea: that premature babies, who were still supposed to be floating in the womb in peaceful synchrony with their mothers' bodies, need to be protected from becoming overloaded and stressed in the hospital environment. By softening the discrepancy between what a baby experiences in the womb and in a loud, bright, bustling intensive care nursery and by paying attention to her signals (how she tells you what makes her feel good and what is upsetting to her), you can help protect her while she's in the hospital and maybe even affect her medical outcome—as well as making her feel cared for.

Isn't this what any good parent would do by instinct?

The Science Behind Developmental Care

The goal of developmental care is to provide a premature baby with appropriate amounts and kinds of stimulation, as nature intended, and to protect her when possible from things that overwhelm her immature senses.

Whether it's something obviously unpleasant, like a loud noise, or something seemingly innocent, like a vivid mobile or a painless touch during a diaper change, the immature nervous systems of preemies aren't adept yet at screening out sensory input and get easily overloaded.

All of us have physical reactions to stress, adults included. A preemie usually will make one or more characteristic movements—some that all parents would recognize, such as crying or frowning, and others that may be different from those of full-term infants, like splaying fingers or yawning. As a premature baby feels increasingly out of control, the stress may lead to changes in her breathing, heart rate, or blood pressure that can become medically destabilizing.

As scientists learn more about the effect of early life experiences on the wiring of the brain, many also wonder whether taking preemies out of the womb and placing them in the starkly different environment of the NICU, at a time when the brain is developing so rapidly, may even alter the architecture of their brains.

One thing researchers have noticed is that as premature babies grow into toddlers and school-age children, they have a higher incidence of subtle problems like learning disabilities, attention deficit disorder, excitability, and anxiety than other children. There could be many reasons for this, including prenatal conditions and problems in the home environment.

But consider what is happening in brain formation while many premature babies are in the NICU. During the second and third trimesters of pregnancy, the brain's billions of neurons migrate through the cortex to specific locations. Then they develop interconnections, or synapses. There are too many synapses for all to survive, so over the next weeks, months, and years they get gradually pruned down. It is thought that connections that are strengthened through stimulation and life experiences will be preserved, while those that aren't used will wither away. If you believe (as most scientists do) that Mother Nature knows

best and that the womb is the optimal environment for a fetus, you can't help but wonder about the effect of those early days in the technological environment of the NICU.

What does the research say about whether developmental care might help? A systematic review of dozens of clinical research studies on developmental care concluded that it has positive medical effects. Premature babies who received developmental care were found to make a quicker transition to bottle feeding or breastfeeding, have better growth in the short term, spend less time on ventilators, and have shorter hospital stays. At 24 months corrected age (or 24 months after their due date, see page 412) they have improved neurodevelopmental outcomes.

But the reviewers also pointed out flaws in some of the studies that raise questions about the validity of their findings, and many experts believe that the jury is still out. Developmental care specialists, in turn, argue that for many reasons their multifaceted method cannot be tested as rigidly as a medication or distinct procedure. Thus it may be some time before we know for sure how effective developmental care is in improving a preemie's medical outcome. But certainly it can help your baby realize that she isn't alone and her feelings aren't being ignored. Someone is by her side, looking out for her, responding to her signals, and soothing her. That in itself is enough. If there are other benefits, so much the better.

Lower the Lights and Reduce the Noise

OK. How do you make a NICU more like a womb? A NICU is a NICU, and preemies need its special care. But small changes like dimming the lights and making it less noisy can bring back for the babies some comforts of their mothers' wombs.

Bright light can be arousing to preemies, contributing to sensory overload, and in some babies can cause oxygen desaturation, rapid heart rate, and lost calories. Moreover, when bright light shines in their eyes all the time, it is harder for preemies to come to an alert state when they're awake, and to experience regular, daily cycles of waking and sleeping—both of which are considered important for a baby's development.

Developmental care suggests keeping the youngest premature babies in darkness as much as possible, introducing day-night light cycles only for older preemies. It recommends:

* Dimming the overhead lights;
* Covering isolettes with thick blankets or special covers to shut out light (if your NICU doesn't provide one, you can bring a pretty one from home);
* Using lower, more focused bedside lights when a baby needs care and turning them off promptly when she doesn't;
* If your baby is on an open warming bed, or is awake when you take her out of the incubator, shelter her eyes from direct light.

You should know that not all specialists in brain development agree; some recommend using dim lights and isolette covers only at night even for young preemies, saying that daytime light, as long as it isn't glaring, is actually a powerful positive influence on development. They point out that in the womb, everything from the mother's blood pressure to her heart rate and body temperature creates a day-night rhythm for the fetus. Until this question is studied rigorously, nurseries and parents will have to come to their own conclusions.

Experts are unanimous, though, that noise should be kept to a minimum around every isolette. Loud sounds lead premature babies to a state of arousal that interferes with sleep, depletes energy, and wastes calories. Sudden noises may cause oxygen desaturation, crying, and changes in pressure in the brain. It's easy for adults, who are more adept at tuning out sounds, to underestimate the amount of noise a preemie is exposed to. Although isolettes may look like quiet havens, sounds inside them are often amplified. The minor act of placing a bottle on top of an isolette measures 108 decibels, and shutting one of the portholes measures 111; by comparison a lawn mower typically measures around 100.

So, developmental care's guidelines are to:

* Speak calmly in an even tone of voice so as not to startle your baby (if you just whisper, your young preemie might not be able to hear you yet);
* Avoid playing loud music in the nursery;
* Shut isolette cabinets and portholes gently;
* Avoid tapping fingers or placing bottles on an isolette;
* Use an isolette cover, which will help dampen noise as well as light.

Many parents wonder whether they should make a tape recording of their voices to put in their baby's isolette. This can be good for some babies in some situations, but for young or easily agitated babies, the sweetest sound may be the sound of silence.

Family in the NICU

The most important thing you can do to make your baby feel loved is to be with her. Developmental care specialists insist that parents and families should be at the center of the NICU, allowed at their baby's bedside twenty-four hours a day, and treated by the medical staff not as guests but as the primary caregivers for their babies. You may hear this concept called family-centered care.

Developmental theorists believe that nature has adapted babies to need two other environments, besides the womb, to support their development: their parents' bodies and a family group. Since in their first weeks or months, many preemies don't get the so-called on-parent-body phase that full-term newborns bask in at home, a pivotal part of developmental care is kangaroo care, in which a preemie is held against her parent's naked chest, skin-to-skin. A leading developmental care theorist calls this the "mother bed," although fathers do it, too! (You can read about how to do kangaroo care on page 249.)

Nurseries that encourage family-centered care are often designed to offer a home away from home around a baby's bed, with a comfortable chair nearby and a folder or mailbox that the nurses and parents can use to leave notes for each other. You may be encouraged to import some of the warmth of home by hanging family photos and siblings' drawings and bringing in special clothes or blankets. Mothers are always supported, practically and emotionally, in their decision to breastfeed their preemie, which takes real time and commitment.

Of course, in our society most parents have jobs, older children, or other obligations that make spending all day in the NICU impossible. And mothers or fathers should not get so tired or stressed that they can't take care of themselves, physically and psychologically. If you want, you can build shifts for your baby by calling on a small, consistent group of grandparents, aunts and uncles, and close friends. You can also ask whether your hospital has volunteers who act as "cuddlers," tenderly holding the baby they're assigned to for an hour or so a day.

Your preemie isn't the only one who will benefit if you immerse yourselves in her care. You will, too. After the loss involved in a premature birth, it's tremendously affirming to start caring for your baby and to realize that your relationship may actually be stronger and deeper because it started earlier than you expected.

Following Your Baby's Cues

According to developmental care theory, a premature baby is engaged in a valiant struggle to adapt the unexpected hospital environment to her needs. She is actively trying to regulate the amount and kind of stimulation she gets, in order to avoid sensory overload and to continue down the normal developmental path she was embarked on in the womb. To help her, we should follow her lead by simply following her cues.

Preemies have different needs: Each is at a different stage of development, has a different degree of medical stability, and her own distinctive personality. If you want to express your love to your baby and stimulate her at the right times and in the right ways, you have to listen to her signals. You'll find a list and illustrations on page 234 of the typical gestures and expressions a preemie makes when she's stressed, or in the process of calming herself, or feeling calm and content. Keep them handy! Over time your baby's nervous system will mature and become less fragile. For now though, she needs especially sensitive care to help her remain as calm and comfortable as possible.

How to Handle Your Baby

Once you begin observing your baby's cues, you're ready to give her developmentally appropriate care. Of course, don't expect to play and kid around with her yet. In fact, one of the most important parental roles at this point is shielding your tiny baby from too much stimulation, not offering it. Parents learn not to be offended if their preemie wants just small, rather than bold, demonstrations of love from them.

Try to follow these guidelines when you can:

✳ When you approach your baby, be quiet or speak softly. Don't tap on the incubator or place objects on top of it.

* If your baby is peacefully asleep, don't wake her. She has a tremendous need for sleep, which promotes brain development. Watch to see when she awakens on her own, and then begin to interact with her. What if you're rarely able to visit your baby and are there for only a short, precious time? You could wake her just enough to move her gently from her bed to your arms, where she can quickly fall asleep again.

* It's a good idea to start with just one kind of stimulation at a time, such as talking or singing gently to her, or delicately touching her, or holding her in your arms, or letting her eyes gaze for a while at your face. The younger your baby's gestational age, the more easily she can become overwhelmed, so the briefer and gentler any stimulation should be. Watch for her signals. When she gets a little older and is looking calm and content, you can start offering her two kinds of stimulation at the same time.

* The sense of touch is the first sense to develop in a baby. If the nurses say your preemie is too young or too sick to hold in your arms, try just giving her one of your fingers to grasp in her hand. As soon as you get permission from the nurses, you can gently put your hand or finger on her skin. Avoid any stroking or rubbing, which are too arousing.

* When you're holding your preemie in your arms, keep her arms and legs firmly but gently contained and her neck supported. As soon as the nurses say it's OK, start doing kangaroo care, which will give you and your baby great joy.

* Even if your baby has to stay in her warming bed or you don't have time one day to do kangaroo care, you can calm her and let her feel your presence by giving her what developmental care calls a "hand womb": Give her your finger to grasp, and place your other arm behind her body, cradling her feet, bottom, and back and cupping her head in your hand. Another way to snuggle her is to cup one of your hands around her head and the other around her knees, helping her to keep them flexed and tucked closer to her chest in a relaxed way. Whenever she wants to move out of these gentle hand cradles, let her, and help her with support and containment again as she settles down. She will feel safe and protected.

How to Comfort Your Baby

While a full-term baby is mature enough to accept various kinds of stimulation and stay calm, tuning things out when they're becoming disturbing to her, a premature baby is less able to shut out stimuli and to calm herself down after being disturbed.

If your baby's cues say that she's stressed, you can help to calm her:

* Premature babies like to lie on their stomachs best. It makes them feel secure and in control of their movements, in contrast to lying on their backs with their arms and legs splayed out (think how a baby animal doesn't like to expose his tummy). So if your baby is on her back, try putting her on her stomach. She may also like lying on her side if you support her all around with your arms and hands (as described above) or with a nest of rolled-up blankets.

* Preemies also get a feeling of control and security by being contained within boundaries, so wrapping your baby tightly in a blanket may help to calm her. (But don't keep her swaddled too tightly all the time. She should be able to move as she did in the womb.)

(Continued on page 236)

What Your Baby Is Telling You—How to Read Her Cues

Babies express themselves through their behavior. By learning to recognize and respond to your preemie's cues, signaling when she needs comfort from too much stimulation or when she is ready for more, you'll make her feel more competent and cared for, and maybe even help her long-term development. Please keep in mind that the following list of preemie signals is not complete, and that some of them may have a different meaning for your baby that you'll soon discover as you spend time with her.

* Relaxed arms, legs, and facial expression;
* Even skin color;
* Smooth movements;
* Stable breathing;
* Limbs and head tucked to the abdomen;
* Looking around;
* Alert and cooing or almost smiling.

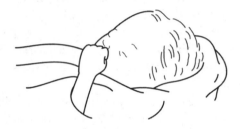

A self-calming gesture.

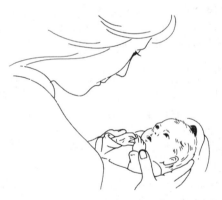

A calm and alert baby, focusing on her mother's face.

Adapted with permission of Children's Hospital Oakland, CA

Signals that often mean "I feel content." When you see these, you can assume that your baby is comfortable and likes whatever sensory input she's getting. Keep it up! You can even try to introduce a little more stimulation at times like these, when she's at her most open.

Signals that often mean "I am soothing myself." These signals indicate that your baby is feeling somewhat overloaded but is trying to calm herself down. It's good to encourage this kind of self-regulation by gently helping her make these movements or not interfering if her self-soothing is working. But don't ratchet up the stimulation now, either.

* Putting hands on face;
* Sucking on fingers or hands or searching for them (you can help her find them);
* Clasping hands together;
* Grasping something;

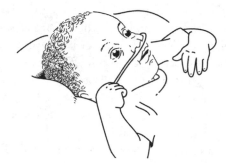

A hyperalert baby with a wide-eyed, staring gaze.

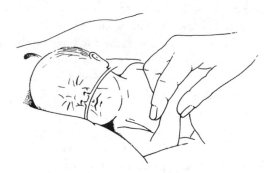

Grimacing and frowning.

Adapted with permission of Children's Hospital Oakland, CA

✳ Tucking into corners of the isolette or other boundaries.

Signals that often mean "I feel stressed, please help." When you see these, your baby needs some kind of change or rest. Try limiting the stimulation she's getting and soothing her with some of the comfort techniques described on page 233. Remember that preemies can often take only one kind of stimulation at a time; for example, being held or being talked to, but not both.

✳ Yawning;
✳ Faster breathing;
✳ Pale, blotchy, or blushed skin;
✳ Frowning or grimacing;
✳ Grunting or spitting up;
✳ Flailing arms or legs or spreading fingers apart;
✳ Jerking or twitching movements;
✳ Arching back and neck;
✳ Crying and fussing;
✳ Staring with glassy eyes and furrowed brow;
✳ Averting gaze; floating or shutting eyes;
✳ Suddenly falling asleep;
✳ Face and limbs becoming limp and flaccid (a sign of exhaustion, different from comfortable relaxation.)

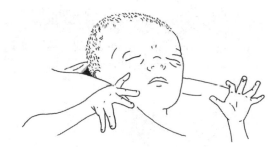

Finger splaying, a possible sign of stress.

If you're ever not sure about what you're seeing, ask a nurse to take a look at your baby with you. Soon, with time and attention, you'll be the number one expert at reading your baby, and the nurses will be asking you!

✳ Sucking can be wonderfully soothing to your preemie. Even if she's too young to breast-feed or bottle feed, you can let her suck on a tiny pacifier (ask your nurse for one) or the tip of your pinky. Not only will you help to calm her, but you'll give her good practice for the nutritive kind of sucking she will master soon.

✳ If your baby is undergoing a painful procedure, giving her a pacifier to suck on—especially one dipped in sugar water—may soothe her and even reduce her pain.

Be Sensitive to Transitions

Preemies are particularly vulnerable to stress during transitions: for example, at the start of any caregiving cluster, when a nurse shifts from one activity to another, or when she finishes her tasks and leaves a baby alone. Too often, caregiving tasks in an intensive care nursery are done impersonally and quickly, without taking the baby's needs for soothing into account. (One researcher documented that nurses spent only a minute or so near a preemie's isolette after completing their tasks, although babies would initiate signs of distress for up to five minutes after the caregiving activities—often after the nurse had left.)

Using developmental care practices, nurses prepare a baby for an intervention and help her recover afterward. The nurse approaches a preemie calmly, talking to her soothingly before any activity begins and while it is taking place. All the while, the nurse watches to make sure the baby is doing well and stops to give her a rest when she seems to need it. Parents are also encouraged to be part of all caregiving (from simple diaper changes to painful events like drawing blood), since their intuition can tell them when their baby needs soothing.

Afterward, the nurse stays at the bedside until she's sure the baby is calm again. When a parent is there, calming and comforting their baby after an intervention is a perfect job for them. So whenever possible, try to be in the nursery while your baby is getting her bath and feedings, and plan to stay for a while afterward. You'll be encouraged to hold her, letting her feel your loving arms around her as she drifts peacefully and contentedly back to sleep.

This is just a sampling of some of the important facets of developmental care for your premature baby that you can learn to do yourself, with the support of the NICU staff. Unfortunately, as long as she's in the NICU, you can't shield her from experiencing some unpleasant and painful things. Although it's not the sheltered cosseting you wanted to give her at home, adopting any pieces of this sensitive approach can make your relationship with your baby more fulfilling—and help make your little one feel loved.

CHAPTER 5

SETTLING DOWN
IN THE HOSPITAL

· · · · · · · · · · · ·

Making the NICU the best possible home away from home for you and your baby.

· · · · · · · · · · · ·

PARENTS' STORIES:
SETTLING DOWN IN THE HOSPITAL*

It sounds like a contradiction in terms. But, yes, premature babies and their families do settle down in the hospital nursery. To the compelling rhythm of their daily weight gain, the bigger babies—the "feeders and growers"—are marching toward going home soon. Experience makes the medical gadgetry less intrusive and disturbing to parents of the preemies who still need to be carefully watched. Parents discover how to get closer to their babies, despite the high-tech, impersonal ambience.

My baby girl, Chloe, was born at 27 weeks, under two pounds. When she was just a week old, and still being given oxygen, a nurse asked me if I wanted to "kangaroo" her. Blurred images of jumping Australian animals with pouches came to mind. How could that relate to us? Well, I found out. The nurse got a screen to give me privacy and told me to unbutton my shirt. Then she had me sit on a rocking chair and handed me Chloe, with only her diaper and a wool hat on. "Put her against your naked skin and hold her upright, her head between your breasts," the nurse said. "I'll cover her back with this blanket. She'll sleep peacefully listening to your heartbeat." So we sat there together for more than an hour. And we have been doing it every day for the last three weeks. For me, it's heaven. I long for it so much that every day I wake up and rush to the hospital. Chloe seems to thrive on it, too; the nurses say she looks so peaceful, and she's never had an apnea in my arms. Now she's learning how to nipple, and

---

* *Parents' Stories* describes events and feelings that really happened or that could happen. Every situation is unique of course, and you may relate to some parents' experiences and reactions more than to others.

steadily putting on weight. Maybe it doesn't have to do with kangaroo care. But I like to think she's getting better partly because of me. I feel that I'm breathing my life into her when I hold her so close. We have a private nest in the middle of the hospital nursery.

After the frantic quality of the first days, time in the hospital relaxes into a more reassuring routine, which can last just a few days, or many weeks for the babies who still have a lot of maturing to do. In the process, the parents learn a lot about prematurity, and keep busy doing things for and with their babies. Their behavior is controlled, but underneath, anxiety still looms. It may take only a spark to ignite it again.

"There's still a few minutes to go before the nine o'clock feeding," I tell myself with relief while I wait for the elevator. Every tile under my feet looks familiar; I'm a veteran NICU father by now. It's been a month since our twin boys Simon and Zachary were born, eleven weeks before term, and I've come to visit them every single day. We've had an intense time here, with setbacks and improvements. Simon got pneumonia and went back on a ventilator. He's off the vent now but still smaller than his brother. "Zac has such an appetite," I mumble with a smile, preparing to see him awake and eager for his bottle. How strange, he's not here, I must have taken a wrong turn. But I know the baby girl on the left: This is the right spot. While looking at the empty space where my son's isolette has always been, I'm starting to feel dizzy. Now something must have happened to Zac. I'm rushing to the nursing station, ready to shout "Where is my baby!?" when one of the doctors approaches me. "Are you happy that Zachary graduated to the step-down unit?" she asks. "Your wife was so excited about it on the phone. And it probably won't be long before Simon joins his brother." What is she talking about? The step-down unit. Where preemies go when they don't need as many doctors or nurses around. The good news came this morning, a few minutes after I left the house. I never imagined. I'm still breathless, but I can feel my tension slowly deflating, like air from a punctured tire. Let's go see how Zac is doing in his new place. Or should I first visit Simon, and hold him for a while? Gee, when you have twins, you really have to juggle.

Social relationships are not always easy to resume after the premature birth of a child. A birth is supposed to be a happy event. But when a newborn has to stay in the hospital for weeks, people often don't know the appropriate way to react. Perceiving that awkwardness, parents ask themselves: How much do I have to tell about my baby? Is there a correct formula I should know?

"You look painfully thin, my dear! I can't believe you just had a baby!" My wife is embarrassed, and I'm annoyed that she has to respond to that comment for what seems like the hundredth time. "I didn't have much time to put on weight, since my pregnancy lasted barely six months," she utters, startling the older woman. "But our daughter Emily is doing great," I step in, trying to rescue my wife. "Would you like a drink?" It is true that Emily is much better now, but her fight to survive in her first few days has taken a heavy toll on us. While I lead my wife to our table, holding her hand, I can feel how nervous she is. This wedding party is our first social engagement since Emily's birth, almost two months ago. "What kills me is that I have to tell our story over and over again," my wife says. "But you don't have to," I object. "Why do you assume that everyone knew your due date? Besides, people don't know anything about premature babies, so they can't understand what you're talking about." Somebody is approaching us: it's Mary, my second cousin, with a tall, handsome boy at her side. "I just wanted to introduce you to my nephew Matthew. He was a preemie. And look at him now!" she says. Mary is eager to know all about Emily;

she's nice and engaging. So I have to start recalling, beginning from day one, the delivery. My wife, sipping a drink, nods and gives me glances of approval. This time it's my turn to be the storyteller.

Some parents manage to deal with impossibly rigid schedules, trying to reconcile their daily chores with caring for their baby in the hospital. But in striving for perfection, they may overlook something important—and come to realize that flexibility is the key.

I've always been very organized. So when our third child, Phil, was born a month and a half ago at 28 weeks of gestation, it didn't take me long to work out a daily schedule to accommodate visits to him in the hospital with taking care of my two older sons, who are in school, and my other million engagements. I don't have a minute to spare. But it is such a joy to watch Phil's progress. I get to stay with him for two feedings. At noon he nipples from a bottle (that I give him!), while the three o'clock feeding comes quickly through gavage to keep him from getting too tired. Then I have to put him right away in his bed and kiss him good-bye: it's time for me to go. Today, though, things went differently. A nurse I hadn't met before was assigned to Phil. When she saw me standing up right after the gavage, she asked: "Are you going already? Your baby just ate; can't you hold him for a little longer?" "I'm afraid that's not possible . . ." I began to say. But then I looked at Phil, well-fed and fully asleep in my lap, a satisfied expression on his round little face. To him, a meal is a meal, coming from a bottle or a tube in his stomach. The good part is getting full and relaxed and napping in the cocoon of my arms. How could I be so blind and interrupt this moment of bliss? That was it. I blew my schedule. I was late to pick up my kids. We had fast food instead of a healthy meal. I'm afraid we'll have to get accustomed to a little disruption, from now on.

Most parents spend a rather isolated time in the hospital nursery even though they're surrounded by other families, nurses, and doctors. They are too focused on their babies to be able to develop other relationships. Even if they would like to reach out, they may not have the time or sheer energy to do it. Others are luckier.

Here she comes, Liz, silent and swift, a figure in black slacks and a crisp white shirt. Her eyes are focused on her son's isolette to make sure nothing has changed since she left him yesterday. I know her anxiety, because it's also mine. "He's awake, he's been kicking the air for a while," I whisper, and she gratefully smiles back in return. Liz is my friend here in the step-down unit, where our premature sons are now out of danger but still learning the basics of being a newborn. When she's not here, I check on her son from a distance, without intruding, and I know she does the same with mine. What makes me feel we're friends? Lots of smiles, silent words, understanding nods at each other while we're holding our babies in our rocking chairs, like stranded sailors waving at each other from nearby islands, the sound of the waves covering their voices. Every morning we forecast our future from our babies' last numbers. "How many apneas?" "How much weight did he gain yesterday?" We had a few longer conversations in the corridor, rushing back from pumping our breast milk; both eager to talk but also wary of losing too much time chatting. Precious minutes belonging to our babies. Who will go home first? Let's make sure we exchange phone numbers. I had an image, a fantasy of our sons playing together one day, but I'm not telling her. We must live in the moment. These are things we can say only with our eyes.

Once they've settled down in the hospital with their premature babies, some parents finally allow themselves to take a break. For others, it's hard to accept that they may need it. But taking a short leave from the NICU—at least one or two days without visiting—is a fundamental sign of healing, a necessary step in the slow process of returning to normality. Things can be seen with more clarity, often with a more ample—and appropriate—dose of optimism, from a distance.

On this early summer morning, everything is too bright on the little beach facing the bay; the lush green all around, a deep smell of honeysuckle, the sunshine on the water, as still as my heart is. I haven't been really outdoors for many weeks now, not since our baby was born prematurely. I've grown accustomed to the features of his world, the hospital nursery: gray and white colors, plexiglass and steel, plastic, metal, and coarse bleached cotton. Last night he fed at my breast without getting too tired. Then he fell asleep in my arms, lulled by the rocking motion of the chair and by my whispers of gratitude and love. "You should leave," said the nurse. "We have plenty of your milk to give him, for tonight and tomorrow. And don't worry. He's breastfeeding so well, he won't forget how to do it." My husband and I had a deal. A single day at the beach, far away from the hospital. I'm a city person who functions well surrounded by concrete, but I had forgotten how beautiful it could be out here. Inside, I'm really quiet. And empty: I miss our baby. But I know at last that the tempest is behind us. Soon we'll be able to take our baby into this brightly colored world.

THE DOCTOR'S PERSPECTIVE: SETTLING DOWN IN THE HOSPITAL *

Some babies and their families never settle down in the hospital. They're grown and on their way home long before the nursery becomes a familiar setting. Others stay longer and eventually become—though it's hard for you to believe now—kind of comfortable here. You have your routine, and you know ours. We form an enclave, the staff and the long-term parents: waiting, sharing a knowledge and togetherness in this strange, intense environment.

Physical Exam and Laboratory Assessment

We'll continue to watch your baby's breathing, circulation, nutrition, and activity level and tailor our medical support to her changing needs. Sometimes new conditions will develop—a new heart murmur, for example, is commonly heard or a hernia appears. We'll investigate and handle these if they arise. Although these new problems often provoke a lot of anxiety in parents (even the slightest problem, after all you've been through, can trigger fears of catastrophe), doctors know that they're rarely life-threatening, and simply part of the routine ups and downs of a growing premature baby. As time goes by, we'll be able to give you more information about what your preemie's future medical condition is likely to be and how that might affect your family.

The passage of time brings another parameter of health to the forefront—how well your baby is growing. Doctors are particularly interested in growth because it's the engine for the near-miraculous, self-healing ability of a preemie's body. Healthy new tissue can grow and repair a previous injury to the brain, the lungs, or the

* The Doctor's Perspective describes how your doctor may be thinking about your preemie's condition, and what she may be considering as she makes medical decisions. All of the medical terms and conditions mentioned here are described in more detail elsewhere in this book. Check the index.

intestine. And growth goes hand in hand with development. Your baby's new and more mature tissues can function in ever more sophisticated ways, so her body will become more adept at regulating its vital functions itself. As she grows and matures, she'll need our medical help less and less, and eventually she'll graduate from our hands to yours.

We'll monitor your preemie's growth by weighing her daily and measuring her head circumference weekly. (Babies who are more than a few months old may be weighed less frequently, because small, daily fluctuations become less important. Babies with large intraventricular hemorrhages will have their head circumferences measured more frequently, to evaluate changes in ventricular size, as well as brain growth.) Because a baby's length changes too slowly to be a good reflection of her immediate nutritional status and is hard to measure accurately, we won't be following her length as closely. We may also check her nutritional status with lab tests that measure the protein and minerals she has available to make muscle and bone, some vitamin levels, and her red blood cell count to see if she's becoming anemic. These tests are particularly important in babies who are fed intravenously with TPN and may need further nutritional supplementation.

Nearly all babies lose weight in the first ten days or so after birth—from fluid shifts, and until the mother's milk supply and baby's feeding behavior are well established. Doctors also don't expect babies who are acutely ill to grow well—they're using almost all the calories we can give them to fight their illness. But after that, while your preemie is convalescing, we'd like to see her gain on average 15 to 30 grams a day. (Thirty grams is an ounce, so that's about a third of a pound a week.) If she's gaining faster than that, we may worry that she's retaining fluid rather than actually growing, or that we're giving her too much food. If she's gaining more slowly, we'll

probably try to increase her calories or cut down on her energy expenditure, maybe by limiting the number of meals she takes by mouth (sucking requires a lot more energy than being gavage-fed) or by keeping her in an isolette a while longer so that she doesn't have to generate so much of her own heat.

If your preemie was born at less than about 30 weeks of gestation, weighed less than 1,500 grams at birth, or was unstable or sick, we'll ask an ophthalmologist when she's approximately a month old to examine her eyes. He'll do a detailed examination of her retina to see if she's developing any signs of retinopathy of prematurity (ROP), a disorder affecting the way the blood vessels grow at the back of a preemie's eye. Neonatologists don't have the expertise to do this kind of an exam, so we'll be relying on the ophthalmologist to tell us the results, determine how frequently your baby should get follow-up eye exams (usually every one to two weeks until approximately her due date), and choose any appropriate therapy. We wouldn't be surprised if she has some mild ROP, as that's extremely common in the youngest preemies and doesn't require any treatment. But if her retinopathy is more severe, she may need a procedure to stop it from progressing. As long as your baby has any ROP, we'll keep her in a medical center where she has easy access to a pediatric ophthalmologist, so she doesn't have to be transported back and forth frequently for eye exams.

When she's close to term, we may also get an ultrasound or MRI of her brain to help decide what kinds of follow-up services to recommend after she's discharged. We'll be looking for any signs of brain injury that may increase her risk of developmental problems. But always, we'll keep in mind that there's so much we can't know from a brain scan: There could be invisible areas of damage and healing; it shows us only what the brain looks like, not how well it's working; and it has no way of assessing the resilience and strength of a child and her family. I remind myself not to trust these brain scans to predict the future, and just use them when they can help mobilize resources for one of my little patients.

All preemies will get a hearing test before they're discharged. We usually wait until a preemie is at least 32 weeks adjusted age, and try to do it after a good meal, because the test is more accurate in older babies who are quiet and relaxed. If the test is abnormal the first time, we don't worry much; there are a lot of falsely abnormal screening tests. We'll just repeat it in a week or two. Often the second test will show us that the baby's hearing is normal.

Common Issues and Decisions

Breathing: For babies with respiratory problems who are in the hospital a long time, the weeks they spend on the ventilator or on oxygen can seem interminable to their parents, and apnea of prematurity may seem to go on forever. In reality, your baby's time frame may be absolutely typical of babies her age and size. That's one of the things we'll be evaluating—whether she's showing the usual breathing immaturities (in which case, time, good nutrition, and nurturing will be almost all she needs) or whether her respiratory patterns indicate that we should be looking for other diagnoses or escalating our therapy.

We'll be assessing whether or not she's developing chronic lung disease (BPD) based on how comfortable and independent her breathing is becoming, how much oxygen she needs, and how her lungs look on chest X-rays. Officially a diagnosis of BPD isn't made unless a baby has required supplemental oxygen for at least four weeks, and it's not considered significant unless she's still needing extra oxygen when she's older than 36 weeks adjusted age, but doctors often know sooner if a baby has some lung damage. Babies with mild BPD may just need some

oxygen or a little CPAP for support until they recover on their own. Others may do better on medications, such as diuretics to get rid of excess fluid in their lungs, or bronchodilators to open up their airways (especially if they wheeze or sound "tight"). Babies with severe BPD who are on very high ventilator settings and are still not breathing well may improve with a short course of steroids, weaning to lower settings that are less damaging to their lungs or even coming off the ventilator altogether. Since nearly all of these treatments have some side effects, we may want to give a baby a brief trial of a therapy to see how well she responds before making it a regular part of her regimen. Even if we decide that your baby does have some chronic lung disease, this is by no means a sentence of doom. Only preemies with the most severe lung damage have long-lasting serious problems. I look at a baby with mild or moderate BPD as apt to be with me longer, requiring some more attention and care, but with a bright and open future. And I hope her parents see that, too.

Even if your baby is being given caffeine for apnea of prematurity, she's probably still having some A's and B's (apnea and bradycardia)—most preemies do. We don't worry about apnea of prematurity if most of a preemie's bradycardias are mild (meaning her heart rate stays above 60 beats a minute), her apneas usually resolve with just some mild stimulation, and she's averaging fewer than 10 to 12 episodes a day.

But if your baby's apnea is worse that that, we'll consider whether something else may be exacerbating it. Some preemies are very sensitive, and react to noise, light, or handling by having A's and B's. If there's a quieter spot in the nursery, we may ask the nurses to move her there and to limit stimulation as much as possible. If her apnea has suddenly worsened, we'll worry that it could be from an infection and may check for that with blood tests, cultures, a chest X-ray, or other tests. Some babies need more oxygen and have more apnea when they're anemic, so we may see whether giving her a blood transfusion helps. And if the A's and B's occur mostly when she's feeding, pacing her so that she has more time to breathe between sucks, or thickening her milk or formula so that she has better control of her swallowing, may help. We may decide to do a formal X-ray swallow study to help us know what would work best for her.

Feeding: Speaking of feeding, another developmental process that can seem interminable to parents, particularly if their preemie is having difficulty with it, is "working up on feeds." This is the feeding journey that ends when your baby's intestines can digest all the food she needs to thrive and her brain is giving her all the right signals to take it in. This sometimes long process can be nearly as frustrating to doctors and nurses as it is to you, but we've learned from experience that patience pays off. There comes a time for most babies, after they reach some more advanced level of maturity, when the problems—whether diarrhea, constipation, bloating, reflux, or poor nippling—just, seemingly miraculously, resolve. In the meantime, we'll be adjusting the content of your baby's feeds, their timing, and the amount she's getting, deciding when to challenge her with more and when to back down. The reason we don't just push on with more and more feeds, regardless, is our concern that she could develop NEC, or aspiration pneumonia, or a general dislike of eating if feedings are advanced recklessly. The reason we don't stop pushing her feedings at all is that as long as she needs TPN or gavage feedings she's tied to the hospital. And parenteral nutrition simply can't nourish her as well as her own gastrointestinal tract is meant to do. We know that practice helps babies learn to nipple-feed better and better but not pressing too hard, and keeping feeding time pleasant, is im-

portant for her to desire and enjoy eating in the future. So it's a balancing act—one of the many that we do with preemies until they take over their own vital functions.

Anemia: All preemies gradually become anemic, with their red blood cell count dropping to its lowest point at about two months after birth, then slowly rising again to normal. Many preemies show no symptoms, not seeming to mind being anemic. If your baby is active and growing well, doesn't need increased respiratory support or have worsening apnea, and doesn't have an excessively fast heart rate, we'll probably decide that she's tolerating her anemia just fine. But if she has symptoms, or we think her blood counts are likely to drop further before her body can make enough on its own (which might happen, for example, if she's less than six weeks old, getting a lot of blood tests, or having surgery), then we'll be deciding whether to correct her anemia sooner, rather than waiting for it to resolve on its own later. It can be a difficult decision because many of the symptoms of anemia can be seen in perfectly normal, non-anemic preemies. And there's no magic number marking the best red blood cell count for a preemie to have, or one that's dangerously low.

If we decide that treatment is warranted, we'll be choosing between giving your baby a blood transfusion or a medication called erythropoietin (epo for short). As usual there are risks and benefits to weigh. A blood transfusion works immediately, but it carries some small risks and can postpone the time when your baby's own body takes over the job of making lots of new red blood cells. Epo usually involves one to three shots a week, takes a couple of weeks to work, and has to be given with iron supplements, which can be hard to digest.

If your baby needs blood soon, we'll probably opt for the transfusion. We might also choose the transfusion if she's gotten blood in the past, and we know that the blood she'd get now would come from the same donor as before. (This could happen if your hospital has a policy to dedicate a donor's blood pack to a specific baby, giving that donor's blood only to her until it runs out.) In that case, the transfusion carries no extra risk of infection. But if we think she might continue to need more blood even after the dedicated blood pack has run out, and she can wait a little while for her anemia to be corrected, we'll probably begin her on erythropoietin. That way she'll need fewer transfusions in the long run.

Infection: Many preemies who are in the hospital for more than a few weeks will end up being evaluated and treated for an infection (although far fewer of them will actually have one). There may be blood and urine tests, perhaps a chest X-ray or spinal tap, cultures of other areas that may be infected, and some IV antibiotics. We wish we could be more discriminating about who gets evaluated, eliminating some of those false alarms that make trouble for preemies and basket cases of their parents! Unfortunately, we're not very good at determining who does and doesn't need to be treated for an infection, because the symptoms are often the same as those that all preemies may show intermittently—for instance, apnea, a temporary need for more respiratory support, feeding intolerance, or mild metabolic abnormalities. Preemies have immature immune systems and don't fight infections well. So we're often loath to just wait and see whether a baby's symptoms develop into anything serious or not, for fear that severe complications might occur while we wait. Occasionally the diagnostic tests are inconclusive, and your baby's doctor has to decide, based on his experience and knowledge of your baby, whether her symptoms are truly due to an infection or not. Most of the time, if your baby does have an infection, treatment works and she'll recover from it completely.

Timing of back-transfer: If your baby is in a hospital far from home, there will come a time when she no longer needs state-of-the-art neonatal care. She'll be able to return to a hospital closer to home, where she can grow and mature until she's ready to go home with you. We consider a baby ready for such a "back-transfer," as we call it, only when she's stable and no longer needs complicated reevaluations (including eye exams for ROP) or changes in therapy. This is a time for celebration—a graduation as momentous as high school! Many parents are anxious about this transition, afraid that their baby is too fragile to travel or won't be cared for as well in a local hospital. But you can be sure that doctors and nurses take the responsibility for their little charges very seriously, and would never transfer her if it were unsafe, or to a hospital that couldn't adequately take care of her. Some hospitals can handle more complex patients than others. For example, some nurseries accept preemies on oxygen (knowing that they can evaluate any problems and wean a baby to room air safely), while others do not. The medical staff planning your baby's back-transfer is aware of what kinds of patients your community hospital can handle. And your baby's doctor will discuss her medical condition with the physician and nurses there so that all important information is passed on.

There are a lot of benefits to moving to a hospital closer to home. It's true that you'll be leaving a place and people you've become familiar with, and perhaps attached to. But this is a move closer to normalcy. You won't have to travel as far to see your baby, so you can spend more time with her, with your family or friends, and on daily tasks. You'll be able to relax in the knowledge that your baby has reached a comfortable level of stability. Your baby may be calmer—in the nursery of a community hospital there's usually less hustle and bustle than in a neonatal intensive care unit. Her own pediatrician or family doctor can start getting to know her by taking care of her medical needs in his own hospital. And your baby's former intensive care bed can be made available to another sick baby who may desperately need it.

Family Issues

Let's talk about some of the temptations that parents who have babies in the hospital for a long time may fall into. Some are counterproductive and best to watch out for and avoid if you can.

It's tempting to compare the progress that your baby is making with other babies in the nursery, particularly if you're making friends with other parents. Don't. There are always unique features that make your baby's path different from any other's. Some babies tend to take little gradual steps forward, while others seem stuck for a while but then surprise everyone with a great leap of progress. Every baby can have a triumph or a setback, and it takes longer to get over some kinds of medical conditions than others. It's no better or worse to have trouble with breathing than digestion—or anything else.

Try not to compare yourself to other parents, either. Parents are people with individual needs and temperaments who will cope differently at various times in their baby's hospitalization. Remember that there is no such thing as "the" experience of having a premature baby. There is only your experience . . . and yours . . . and yours.

Try to avoid the temptation to see a lack of visible progress as failure. Your baby's doctor will tell you if medical treatment really isn't working, and you should certainly take that seriously. But usually it's just that growth and development take time. Your baby's internal unfolding schedule of maturation is directing the time frame of his recovery much more than the doctors are. The doctor will periodically try to move things

forward. If your baby doesn't tolerate, say, an extubation from the ventilator or an increase in his feedings, it's not a setback. It probably just means we've moved too fast. Patience is a virtue for all parents—but especially for parents of preemies!

If you're in the hospital long enough, and learn the medical jargon, you'll be tempted to judge how your baby is doing by focusing on numbers: the amount of oxygen she's getting, her vent settings, her oxygen saturations, how many apneas she's had, her blood counts, etc. It's not surprising that this happens—numbers are objective measures in plain view, and the doctors and nurses use them to monitor your baby's condition and help plan her treatment.

But numbers can be misleading. The experience that doctors and nurses have with thousands of babies allows them to put these pieces of information in context, while parents can be sent into a tailspin by normal up and down variations. Some abnormal numbers indicate true improvement or worsening, but others are just ebbs and flows around a plateau, or even false readings. Some dips and spikes are unimportant for one baby but crucial for another.

Although it can be very informative for parents to have doctors and nurses interpret the significance of what they're measuring, it's not helpful for you to focus too much on the changing, or unchanging, numbers—what is helpful is for you to gather the kind of knowledge that parents are best at, like how peaceful or uncomfortable or interactive your baby is and what makes him feel good or bad. The involvement he needs from you is a tender touch and loving voice, not more measurements and spinning dials.

And finally, you may take your time at the hospital to extremes—either putting everything else in your life on hold or feeling like there's no point in coming to the hospital because there's nothing you can do. It's tempting to relegate everything else to secondary importance until this momentous time has passed. And, for a while, everything else will be less important. But then other responsibilities, pleasures, and bonds should reassert their rightful place. Despite the difficulties, you should try to maintain some of your normal daily activities. Leave the hospital for a while—and don't feel guilty about it. You can be a better parent if you're more balanced and refreshed. Try not to let important relationships languish. It's not just your baby who needs you, but your spouse or partner and other children—and they can support parts of you that are vital for your own strength and health. By bolstering yourself, you can bring to your baby's world in the NICU the strength and depth that will enrich your time together, now and in the future.

On the other hand, it may be tempting to stay away from the nursery to escape sad conversations and feelings of loss, or to avoid meetings with strangers and the discomfort of a harsh environment. You absolutely do need breaks and time away, but don't ever think that your presence doesn't count. Even if you feel powerless, you can do something great—give your baby a mommy or daddy to touch him in a way that none of the nurses or doctors do, to whisper to him that you love him and are there with him, to show him he's not alone. That's what you'll be doing for the rest of his childhood; you might as well start settling into it now.

Getting Acquainted with: Apnea and Bradycardia

Although it will be a few years before your preemie learns the ABC's, she may already be an expert in a different kind of A's and B's—the NICU variety.

The expression "A's and B's" is shorthand for episodes of apnea (a pause in breathing) and bradycardia (a slow heart rate), two of the most common problems of premature babies. These episodes frighten parents, and keep nurses busy attending to all of the beeping alarms. But doctors worry about them only if they're unusually severe or if they appear to be a sign of some underlying illness. Most of the time they aren't; all they mean is that your preemie's control of her breathing is still immature. It's not that surprising when you consider that she wasn't supposed to be breathing air yet at all.

It's normal for preemies to do something called periodic breathing; they take some rapid breaths and then pause for five or ten seconds before taking the next one. Only when a pause lasts for at least 20 seconds, or is accompanied by a slow heart rate or change in the baby's skin color, is it considered apnea. Bradycardia—or a "brady"—is defined as the slowing of a baby's heart rate from its usual range of 120 to 160 beats per minute to a rate of fewer than 100 beats per minute. (A preemie's heart beats about twice as fast as a typical adult's.) In most cases, it's a result of apnea.

What causes apnea in premature babies?

The complex system that regulates everyone's breathing and heart rate is not yet fully developed in preemies. Sometimes the immature respiratory center in your preemie's brain may forget to send a signal to breathe, so breathing movements stop. Other times her brain may remember to send the signal to breathe and her chest will move as it should, but the muscles that are supposed to keep her upper airway open become lax, so airflow to the lungs stops.

The failure to send the signal to breathe can be brought on by deep sleep or, strangely enough, a lack of oxygen. Sedative medications can make it worse. And if a baby breathes quickly for a while, her body may overcompensate with an overly long pause for a few moments afterward.

Apnea may be triggered by stress from common procedures, such as suctioning mucus from the baby's airways, or from a change in temperature, as when she's placed on a cold scale to be weighed. Pain or sheer fatigue can cause it, as can too much stimulation of her immature senses (loud noises, for instance). Apnea can even happen in response to seemingly normal actions like feeding, having a bowel movement, stretching, or excessive bending of the neck.

A's and B's also increase in the 48 hours after a baby is given vaccines or anesthesia. So to be safe, some hospitals won't give a preemie vaccines right before discharge if she has had A's or B's within the past few weeks. (It's no problem; your baby's doctor will be sure to schedule them earlier and keep her on a monitor, or her pediatrician will do the honors after more time has passed.)

To make things more complicated, apnea and bradycardia can also occur as a symptom of other illnesses, including respiratory distress syndrome (RDS), intraventricular hemorrhage, seizures, infection, and necrotizing enterocolitis (NEC). If your baby's A's and B's follow an unusual pattern—starting very suddenly later on, for example, or growing increasingly severe—then her doctor will investigate the possibility of an underlying medical condition, which will need to be treated for the apnea to disappear. But this is less common than simple apnea of prematurity alone.

Who gets apnea of prematurity?

A lot of preemies: 80 percent of those born before 30 weeks of gestation, one third of those born between 30 and 34 weeks, and 7 percent of those born at 34 to 35 weeks.

How apnea of prematurity is treated

Sometimes, if it's very mild, apnea of prematurity isn't treated at all. When a baby's apnea or bradycardia alarm goes off, her nurse will watch to make sure that she starts breathing again on her own. If she doesn't, the nurse will stimulate her with a gentle tap or rub, which usually does the trick.

Some babies have more frequent or severe episodes of apnea, when they need more vigorous stimulation or extra oxygen. Once these babies are pink and breathing again, they're fine, but their doctors will probably want to treat them with medication to help prevent such episodes from recurring. Very young preemies, who are more prone to apnea, are often put on medication early, even before they have severe episodes of apnea, as a preventive measure.

The most common medication for apnea of prematurity is caffeine. Although it's a startling thought that your newborn is being given a double espresso, hold the cup, caffeine is very effective at stimulating respiration, which is just what your baby needs. Researchers recently discovered that treating apnea of prematurity with caffeine has other positive effects as well, reducing the risk of persistent breathing problems (called bronchopulmonary dysplasia) and long-term developmental problems. It almost never gives preemies the jitters or prevents them from sleeping. (If your baby has a too rapid heart rate or is irritable, or has some other symptom that could be due to too much caffeine, her doctor can reduce the dose, although it's rarely necessary.) Babies on caffeine do tend to grow a little more slowly for a while, but they soon catch up if they're given more calories. Once your baby's apnea of prematurity goes away, the medication will be stopped and she'll lose her caffeine privileges until you give her the OK later on.

There are other, nonmedical ways to make apnea and bradys less frequent. One is to reduce their triggers, such as sudden changes in temperature and overstimulation. Also, studies have shown that premature babies have less apnea when they lie prone (on their stomachs); that's one reason you'll see most preemies sleeping on their stomachs in the NICU. (This concerns some parents who are aware that there's a greater chance of sudden infant death syndrome in full-term newborns who sleep on their stomachs, but this isn't a worry for preemies on monitors in a NICU.)

Pulsating or rotating beds may reduce apnea temporarily and are used in some NICUs. To avoid too much neck flexion and obstruction of babies' airways, nurses carefully position preemies in their isolettes. You'll learn to make sure that your baby's chin doesn't fall forward when you are feeding or just holding her in your arms. Your baby's nurse can show you how. And one recent study found that the smell of a few drops of vanilla on a cloth in a preemie's isolette reduced apnea. Ask your baby's doctor if you can spice things up for your baby this way!

If your baby is not responding to these measures, she can also be treated with additional respiratory support—CPAP or "high flow" air or oxygen—which works on two fronts: The flow of gas in her nostrils and throat stimulates her to breathe, and the extra pressure helps keep her airways open. If a baby's apnea is very severe, she may be put on a ventilator temporarily, which will give her the extra breaths she isn't taking herself. Once the serious episodes have subsided, the doctors will take her off the vent.

The course that apnea of prematurity takes

Apnea of prematurity tends to take a predictable course. It usually starts within the first few days of life. Some babies have two or three episodes a day, and some have more than a dozen—but over time, as their bodies mature, their apnea becomes milder, occurring less frequently and requiring less intervention to stimulate them to breathe again. It almost always disappears by two to four weeks before a baby's due date, although occasionally it can persist for a couple of weeks after. A general rule of thumb is that the earlier a preemie was born, the later her apnea of prematurity tends to go away.

If you're wondering whether your baby's apnea really will disappear soon, we can tell you this: Many parents have the same doubts, and almost all of them are pleasantly surprised when their baby's apnea goes away on schedule. Chances are you'll be pleasantly surprised, too, but if your preemie turns out to be one of the few who need more time, don't worry. Her homecoming will probably be delayed only a week or two.

A parent's concerns

Several concerns are foremost in a mother's or father's mind when their baby has apnea. One is: Could one of these episodes be life-threatening? If your baby has simple apnea of prematurity, the chances of her having a life-threatening episode are minuscule. She has monitors to alert the nurse when her vital signs are weakening. The monitors are set to give the nurses plenty of time to respond before she is in distress. The nurses know just how to stimulate her, or even resuscitate her, if necessary.

Another frequently expressed concern is: Can A's and B's cause long-term damage? Mild or occasional apnea or bradycardia, even when followed by desatting (oxygen desaturation), is believed to pose no danger. Babies can safely tolerate low amounts of oxygen for short periods of time. But if apnea is more severe, with frequent, deep desats, a baby's risk of developing retinopathy of prematurity or pulmonary hypertension does increase. Whenever a premature baby's heart rate remains below 50 or 60 for more than a few seconds, blood flow to her organs may be inadequate, increasing her risk of NEC and other organ damage.

A's and B's may also be harmful to babies who are recovering from surgery and need good oxygen and blood flow to their wounds. But even then, as long as the baby's oxygen levels and heart rate rise again quickly and the deep A's and B's are infrequent, there's little chance of a problem.

Finally, parents often wonder: Will apnea of prematurity increase my baby's risk of sudden infant death syndrome? This isn't something you need to worry about. Apnea of prematurity is not related to SIDS. It goes away as your baby matures, and when it is gone, it is completely and totally behind you.

QUESTIONS AND ANSWERS

Kangaroo Care

I've read about kangaroo care, and my instinct tells me it's the right thing to do. But I haven't seen another mother doing it yet, and I don't know how to get started.

If your baby had been born at term as expected, holding her is something you wouldn't have given much thought to. It would have been the most natural thing in the world.

For most full-term babies, much of early infancy is spent snuggled against their parents' bodies—feeding in their mothers' arms, falling asleep on their fathers' chests, and being held close up against them throughout the day, crooked inside an elbow or over a shoulder.

But when your baby is born prematurely, you don't have many opportunities to do what comes naturally. Maybe that explains the appeal and benefits of kangaroo care, which means nothing more than holding your naked preemie (usually clad in just a diaper) against your own naked, warm chest. With a blanket draped over your baby's back to keep him warm, you can sit that way for hours at a time, quiet or talking, still or rocking, and, at times of greatest peacefulness even falling asleep together.

Encouraging parents to hold their baby skin-to-skin in the NICU is one of the most important recommendations made by developmental care experts (see page 229). In part, this is because kangaroo care is the gentlest kind of touch stimulation, known to benefit a baby's growth and development. In addition, by reestablishing a physical connection, it restores the natural dependence of the baby on his parents for care and well-being. You shouldn't be shy about asking your doctor or nurse to help you start doing kangaroo care. If your baby is ready for it, there's no reason to hesitate.

What are the medical and long-term effects of kangaroo care? We don't know the whole answer to that question yet, but so far, research results are very encouraging. Studies have consistently shown that up against the heat of their parents' bodies, these preemies maintain their body temperature as well as or better than in an incubator. Babies held skin-to-skin during breastfeeding are more likely to be nursing one month after hospital discharge, and their mothers produce more milk. Researchers speculate that skin-to-skin contact helps stimulate lactation. Some studies have found that while preemies are being held skin-to-skin they cry less, have less apnea, higher levels of oxygen saturation, longer periods of restful sleep, and a reduced response to pain. They also gain weight more rapidly and are more alert than preemies who don't get kangaroo care.

Kangaroo care helps parents, too. Researchers observed that mothers who did kangaroo care with their preemies were less depressed and more sensitive to their babies' needs. Holding your premature baby skin-to-skin seems to reduce some of the stress of the hospitalization, and deepens the bond between you and your child. It's common for parents to say that kangaroo care has a profound impact on them, giving them the feeling that they're being the kind of parent to their baby that nature intended.

A few recent studies indicate that kangaroo care may also be beneficial to babies in the long run. Preemies who had been held skin-to-skin had longer attention spans, gazed more at their mothers, and could handle more stimulation at three, six, and twelve months of age. Some experts aren't surprised that skin-to-skin holding may enhance a preemie's long-term development because it offers something that all babies are biologically programmed to expect: parental nurturing and physical contact during infancy. Other experts, skeptical about long-term effects, recommend skin-to-skin holding simply because it is a way to make a preemie happier, to smooth out the wrinkles in her day. Still others believe that nakedness is nice, but that extended physical contact with you, clothed or not, is what's important. So, if you're uncomfortable doing skin-to-skin holding in the nursery, perhaps for modesty or privacy reasons, and would rather hold your baby clothed, that's fine, too. Your baby will love it.

By the way, real kangaroos do know something about prematurity. The baby kangaroos they give birth to about once a year are only partially developed, so they hop into their mother's warm pouch and continue their development there for months. The human version of kangaroo care originated a few decades ago in a crisis at a hospital in Bogotá, Colombia. Its intensive care nursery was so poorly equipped and had such a high infection rate that it started a new program, discharging even the tiniest premature babies within hours or days after birth, to be held and cared for by their mothers at home, kangaroo-style. In the first few years, the results were stunning: The number of neonatal deaths significantly decreased, as did the number of abandoned infants.

Since then, the practice of kangaroo care, done voluntarily by mothers and fathers in intensive care nurseries, has spread around the world. Kangaroo care is so easy and natural that you'll be an expert after your first try.

Here's how to get started:

* **Ask the doctor or nurse if your baby is stable enough for kangaroo care.** Practices vary; some nurseries prefer that a baby be breathing on her own, or with just supplemental oxygen, while others encourage it even for babies on ventilators.
* **Wear a shirt that opens in front.** If you don't have one, just ask the nurse for a hospital gown, and put it on without any other clothing on your chest.
* **Find a comfortable chair.** Some nurseries now have special recliners for kangaroo care, but a

regular rocking chair is great, too. If you don't see one near your baby's bed, don't hesitate to ask where you can find one.

* **Ask a nurse to place your baby comfortably on your chest.** First you or the nurse should undress your baby down to her diaper. Then open your shirt or gown (if you want more privacy, ask if your nursery has a portable screen—most do), and have the nurse place your baby upright on your chest, between your breasts, with her cheek resting comfortably on your skin. Help her get into a comfortable position if she squirms a little. Cover your baby's back with your shirt or gown and with a light blanket. The nurse will periodically take your baby's temperature to make sure she stays warm enough. If she gets too warm from the heat your body gives her, you can remove the blanket. (Don't worry if your preemie has a little apnea or bradycardia or needs to have her oxygen turned up a bit when she is moved from her bed to your arms. There's nothing wrong with needing some extra support during the transition—and it will be well worth it.)

* **Now . . . relax!** That's what's most important. You can try talking or singing to your baby for a while, letting her enjoy the pleasurable sound of your voice, and then letting her rest while you rock, recline, read a book, or fall asleep yourself. You can stay together as long as you like and the nurse agrees. Some parents and babies do kangaroo care for just a half hour a day, while others stretch it out as long as possible—to four or five hours or longer. Once you get started, you'll probably understand why. These are precious moments for a parent and child.

* **And if you have twins, you can try it with two at once.** For shared kangaroo care, ask the nurse to place one of your babies on each of your breasts, so they are lying face to face.

Amazingly, in a couple of published case studies, each of the mother's breasts adapted separately in temperature, warming up or cooling down to meet the heating needs of each twin. What could be better than basking warmly (but not too warmly) together?

Breastfeeding a Preemie

My baby was born very premature. When will he be able to nurse from my breast?

Though it may be hard for you to imagine now, in just a few weeks your young preemie probably will begin his breastfeeding lessons. In the past, breastfeeding was considered too tiring and stressful for preemies, because babies have to suck more forcefully to get milk from the breast than from a bottle. Preemies were usually allowed to nurse only after they first learned how to nipple from a bottle without distress.

Now that approach has changed. Evidence has shown that many preemies can begin breastfeeding several weeks earlier than they can safely drink from a bottle (as early as 28 to 30 weeks, rather than 32 to 34 weeks). Some studies have found less oxygen desaturation, less bradycardia, warmer skin temperatures, and better coordination of sucking and breathing when preemies nursed at the breast than when they drank from a bottle at the same age.

The reason is simple. A baby can regulate the milk flow from the breast with his sucking bursts; when he pauses to breathe, milk stops flowing. A bottle with an artificial nipple, though, delivers milk partly through gravity, so in order not to choke or gag, a baby has to learn how to stop the milk flow with his tongue or by clenching his jaws, while swallowing and breathing in the meantime. It's a complex technique that requires more mature coordination.

Your baby will have to wait until he is off a

ventilator, and probably off CPAP too, but he can start breastfeeding even if he's still getting supplemental oxygen through a nasal cannula, provided that he's breathing at a normal rate. (Babies who are breathing faster than 70 to 80 times a minute don't have enough time between breaths to suck and swallow safely.) A nurse will stay close by to make sure your baby's oxygen saturation remains high before, during, and after his first breastfeeding tries.

Even if breastfeeding is easier than bottle feeding, the path to peaceful nursing in their mothers' arms can still be laborious for preemies born at a young gestational age. Establishing a generous milk supply with an electric pump will help, and should be a top priority for you. If your baby's hard work doesn't yield much, she won't feel as compelled to keep trying; your sweet milk is her reward for her strenuous feeding efforts. (For the same reason, an ample milk supply is crucial when a baby is switching between bottle feeding and breastfeeding.)

You may also find the following suggestions helpful:

* **Kangaroo care.** This is the perfect preparation for breastfeeding for a very young baby. When the doctor thinks he's stable enough, even if he's still on a ventilator, your preemie can learn to recognize your smell and feel the pleasant contact of your warm skin on his. If he's not on a ventilator, he may start to lick and nuzzle your nipple, and perhaps begin practicing sucking. (Since this stimulation may induce a strong letdown reflex with a sudden pouring of milk from your nipple, which may be dangerous for a baby who cannot yet coordinate breathing and swallowing, it's safer to pump and empty your breasts before kangarooing.) Gradually, as your baby matures, he will start to latch on and actually breastfeed. Kangaroo care can also help preemies keep warm during their early breastfeeding sessions. Kangaroo care is very easy to do (you can read about it on page 249).

* **Introducing the smell and taste of breast milk.** To help a young preemie develop a sucking reflex, you can introduce him to your milk earlier than he's able to drink it. With his doctor's permission, a few times a day put a drop of milk on your baby's lips. He will love its smell and taste; later he'll associate those pleasurable sensations with his feedings.

* **Nutritive and nonnutritive sucking.** A baby born very prematurely, who has had an endotracheal tube in his mouth and been fed with parenteral nutrition or by gavage for more than a month or so, may have difficulty associating sucking with the pleasant feeling of having his hunger satiated. To prepare him, it can be helpful to let him suck while he's being gavage fed, either by giving him a tiny pacifier, or better yet, letting him suck at your breast. (Since your baby is not ready to coordinate sucking and swallowing yet, you should pump first.)

* **Breastfeeding positions.** Sit comfortably in a chair and lay your baby on his side across your lap, tummy-to-tummy, surrounding him with the arm on the side of the breast you want him to latch on to first and using the other hand to position your breast. Then, bring your baby up to your breast so his mouth is on your nipple, making sure that you are supporting his head and shoulders and that they are straight. (It's more difficult for him to swallow when his head is turned to one side.) This is also the most natural way to begin breastfeeding while doing kangaroo care.

* **Helping your baby latch on.** Sometimes a small baby can't latch on to his mother's nipple because it's too large for his mouth. If this happens, you can help your preemie by shaping your nipple between your thumb and

first two fingers. Or you can try using nipple shields: No matter what size or shape your nipples are, these will make it easier for your preemie to latch on and nurse more easily. A nipple shield lengthens and flattens the nipple, allowing the milk to flow out with less suction so that your baby needs less strength and coordination. Most preemies continue to benefit from nipple shields for several weeks after they've gone home, until they can breastfeed effortlessly.

* **Pumping after breastfeeding sessions.** Until your baby is fully mature and an excellent feeder, it's a good idea to pump after he finishes nursing. Not only will you make sure your breasts are completely empty, which will improve your milk supply, but he'll get the benefit of any of the rich, slower-flowing hind-milk he may have left behind. Don't be afraid to offer that milk to him in a bottle after his breastfeeding session—as long as he keeps practicing breastfeeding, he *will* become good at it, and those last nutritious drops of your milk will help him grow bigger and stronger, bringing that day ever closer.

* **Frequency of breastfeeding.** Young preemies are usually introduced to breastfeeding progressively. The timing of breastfeeding should be based on your baby's feeding cues, starting when he looks ready, awake, and alert. (Soon enough, with the help of your nurse, you will learn how to read his signals.) The frequency of your baby's breastfeeding will also depend on your availability. Short, multiple feedings are better than a single longer session, if you can be with your baby in the hospital at different times during the day. For several days and weeks, most preemies alternate breastfeeding with gavage or bottle feedings of breast milk—or special preemie formula, if their mother's milk supply cannot satisfy all of their needs. (Don't feel bad if this happens to you;

it's a very common situation. Just feel proud of every drop of breast milk you are able to give your baby.) Before you take your baby home, you may be asked to room in for 24 hours to be sure your preemie has the stamina to breastfeed well around the clock.

* **Getting help with breastfeeding.** Even if your baby is not on supplemental oxygen, you'll need the assistance of a nurse or lactation specialist during your early breastfeeding sessions to make sure your baby doesn't show any sign of distress, such as color change, apnea or bradycardia, oxygen desaturation, or a drop in temperature. Another major concern for any first-time mother is whether her baby is actually feeding. If you can't feel when your letdown reflex occurs, don't worry: Some mothers eventually become aware of it, but many never do. In the beginning, the nurse will check to see if your baby's sucking pattern has changed (indicating that he's getting milk) and if he's swallowing. Sometimes your letdown reflex can be too strong for your inexperienced preemie, who may choke on too much milk; the nurse will help you not to panic and will show you how to handle the situation. Your baby's nurses or a lactation specialist will work with you and your preemie to develop comfortable and effective ways to nurse. Soon, you and your baby will be left alone to breastfeed in quiet.

* **Assessing whether your baby is getting enough milk.** Every breastfeeding mother worries about this, but especially mothers of preemies. Try not to worry: you can be sure that your baby's doctor and nurses will be watching him carefully. Your preemie's behavior (whether he's fussy or satisfied), how many wet diapers he has, and his daily weight gain will make it clear whether he's taking in enough milk. Your baby may even be weighed before and after a breastfeeding session to

determine just how much milk he took in. If you feel your breasts soften during the feeding, it means that milk is being removed. Your baby is doing that!

Nipple Confusion

Will my baby have nipple confusion if the nurses give her bottles when I'm not in the nursery to breastfeed?

A premature baby won't be discharged from the hospital until she's steadily gaining weight and taking all of her feedings herself from the breast or bottle. Since a baby has to eat every few hours, there may be feedings at night and other times when her mother is not around. Some doctors and nurses, afraid of creating "nipple confusion" between a bottle's artificial nipple and the breast, will avoid giving a bottle to a preemie who has just started to breastfeed and will feed her by gavage, instead, when her mother is not there. Others, however, think it's more important for a baby to practice feeding on her own, and believe that if nipple confusion occurs at all it is minor and fleeting. They point out that most breastfed babies at home get bottle feedings at times from their father or other caregivers, and the bottle doesn't cause them to forget their perfect technique.

Concern about nipple confusion stems from the different techniques needed for sucking from a breast and a bottle. Breastfeeding requires vigorous, forceful sucking, and as soon as the baby stops sucking, so does the flow of milk. With a bottle, the milk flows out continuously and more rapidly, so the baby doesn't have to suck as hard, but she does have to learn how to stop or block the flow of milk when she's ready to take a breath or swallow.

If you feel strongly one way or the other, let the nurses know how you prefer your baby to be fed in your absence. If you agree to your baby's being bottle fed, a reasonable compromise may be to wait to give her a bottle until after she learns to breastfeed well. That way, breastfeeding is primary for her. Finger-feeding is another compromise; it involves feeding a baby through a gavage tube taped to a caretaker's little finger, which the infant sucks together with the tube. This method avoids any nipple confusion, while giving a baby the satisfaction of sucking while being fed. Since finger-feeding is more time-consuming than giving a bottle, the nurses may not be able to do it. But when the father is visiting the nursery, doing kangaroo care together with finger-feeding is the closest approximation to breastfeeding a dad can have.

You may want to keep in mind that if you opt to forgo bottle feeding in favor of gavage when you're not there, you may be asked to room-in with your baby in the nursery for 24 to 48 hours before she goes home. That's so the medical staff can observe your baby when you nurse her exclusively, to be sure she continues to grow well and doesn't get tired from the extra effort when she is taking in all the nourishment she needs on her own.

Milk Supply

Every time I pump in the nursery I get frustrated, seeing how much milk some mothers can express. My milk supply, instead, seems to be getting less and less.

When beginning breastfeeding, some mothers have to clear more hurdles than others. One of the most disappointing—and one that can turn into a real obsession—is a mother's realization that her milk supply is diminishing or insufficient.

But a mother of a preemie who is expressing her milk should be prepared for this; it frequently happens, and it's usually not her fault. True, some women are able to express large quantities of milk without extraordinary effort. Seeing them carrying bottle after bottle from the pumping room can make mothers with a more scanty milk supply feel inadequate. But they really shouldn't. Studies show that the majority of mothers of preemies can't keep up with their growing baby's nutritional needs, so their breast milk eventually needs to be supplemented with donor milk or preterm formula. Some of the conditions that lead to preterm delivery, such as maternal anemia, diabetes, or infertility, can reduce the volume of a mother's milk supply. Also, an electric pump can't equal a nursing baby in stimulating a mother's breast, for both mechanical and emotional reasons. Breastfeeding a baby is a highly emotional experience—for many women, a good letdown reflex appears only after their baby starts to nurse at their breast—and the stress and emotional turmoil following a premature birth are unfortunate companions for a mother who chooses to nurse.

Thus, some mothers, especially those who have been exclusively pumping for several weeks, find that despite the time and energy they've invested in pumping, their milk supply isn't increasing as fast as their infant's demands. For most women who pump, there is a lactation cycle, which can last days or months, during which their milk supply first increases, then gradually diminishes until it reaches zero. Sometimes the cycle can be restarted after that point, and sometimes not.

Here are some useful tips to reinforce a dwindling milk supply:

* **Drink more, eat well, get more rest.** Keep a bottle of water handy for before and after you pump, and remember to drink at least six to eight big glasses of water, milk, or other liquids a day. Breastfeeding also requires adding about 600 calories to your normal diet. Allow your-

self to nap frequently, and try to get as much help as you can with your older children and family chores. Your preemie in the hospital needs you to visit him, but it is equally important that you go home, relax, and rest.

* **Don't start birth control pills again right away.** The hormones in birth control pills and also in Depo-Provera (a contraceptive given by injection every three months) have been found to reduce breast milk production. Birth control pills that do not contain estrogen are thought not to interfere with milk supply as long as they're started no sooner than four to six weeks after delivery, but some women report that their volume of milk is reduced. So if you've recently restarted birth control pills, you might want to try a different contraceptive method.

* **Don't smoke.** If you're a smoker, you're surely tired of hearing people tell you not to smoke. But if you can stop while you're breastfeeding, it may have a significant effect on your milk supply. Research has shown that the amount of milk produced by mothers of premature babies who smoke is substantially less than the amount produced by those who don't.

* **Massage your breasts before pumping.** Start by placing warm washcloths on your breasts for relaxation, and then take a few minutes to massage your nipples and the surrounding areolas in a circular motion, gradually increasing the pressure. Massage can help your milk flow more easily through the ducts and relieve engorgement. Tactile stimulation can also increase the release of the hormone prolactin in your bloodstream, possibly boosting your milk production.

* **Do kangaroo care.** Skin-to-skin contact with their babies has been shown to increase mothers' milk supply.

* **Look at your baby's picture, listen to his voice, smell his scent.** When you're at home,

The Possibility of Later-Onset Lactation

Not all mothers are ready to start pumping within a few hours of their preemie's birth, as breastfeeding experts suggest. Sometimes mothers are sick themselves. Often they are worried about their babies, and so distraught that expressing milk may seem completely out of place. But when the initial crisis is over and their preemie's condition has stabilized, they may regret that they haven't started their lactation.

Hope is not lost, though. Breast tissue and mammary glands don't immediately switch back to their prepregnancy state. Hormones that bring back menstruation and inhibit the ability to breastfeed take a while to return. The window during which lactation can be reinstated varies from a few days to a few weeks, so you may still be in time.

The best way to find out if you can achieve later-onset lactation is to consult your obstetrician and a breastfeeding expert. (For a referral, call La Leche League or International Lactation Consultant Association; see page 591.) The methods they suggest will probably be a combination of those advised to increase a scarce milk supply (explained in more detail above):

* Frequent pumping and breast massage;
* Diet;
* Rest;
* Increased fluid intake;
* Medications.

Milk production cannot be guaranteed, and even if you get your breasts going, it may be just for a short time. But if you want to try, it's certainly worth the effort.

---

a picture of your baby, a tape recording of his voice, or his odor on a recently worn T-shirt or gown can put you in the right mood to sit down, relax, and express your milk. Just hearing an infant crying (not necessarily your own!) or stroking their face with their baby's clothing can stimulate the letdown reflex in many mothers. Remember, though, if these mementos of your baby make you feel very sad and emotional, pumping may be more difficult rather than easier.

* **Pump more often.** Sometimes pumping every two hours or so for a few days can help increase a mother's milk supply. According to breastfeeding experts, the key is to pump more frequently, not for a longer time: if you do it 10 or 12 times a day, 10 minutes per breast will be enough. If you're not double pumping yet, you should try it.

* **Have your pump checked.** More often than you think, electric pumps (even of the same brand) can differ in sucking strength or may need to be adjusted. If you notice that your breast yields more milk with the pump you're using in the hospital than the one at home, send your pump back to the pharmacy or supplier and ask for it to be replaced.

* **Inquire about medications and herbal remedies.** There are medications (metoclopramide and reserpine) that your obstetrician can pre-

scribe to stimulate your milk production. Since babies can be sensitive to drugs in mother's milk, your doctor may need to consult with your preemie's neonatologist. There are also several herbal preparations—brewer's yeast, fenugreek, herbal tea mixtures—sold in health food stores, that may increase a mother's milk supply but you should never take them before asking your baby's doctor. Some of these remedies contain essential oils, such as fennel or anise, that may appear in your breast milk and cause your baby to have feeding difficulties, vomiting, or lethargy. A premature baby is at greater risk for complications from these substances than a full-term newborn. If you do try a medication or herbal remedy, you should know in about three days whether it's working for you.

✳ **Consider a Supplemental Nursing System (SNS).** This low-tech, effective device may increase your milk production when your baby is trying to latch on but not yet good at sucking from your nipple. It consists of a container filled with your expressed breast milk, donor milk, or formula, which you hang around your neck with a cord (see illustration). Attached to the bag is a thin tube that is taped to your breast, the tip placed against your nipple. The goal is to have your baby suck your nipple and the tube at the same time; he'll get milk at the right flow and volume, learning that he can get nutrition and satisfy his hunger from your breast. While your baby practices the art of breastfeeding, your breast will be stimulated by his sucking, possibly increasing your milk production. You can purchase a Medela Supplemental Nursing System online or at your pharmacy. Consider buying the long-term SNS, not the disposable one, which can be used for only 24 hours.

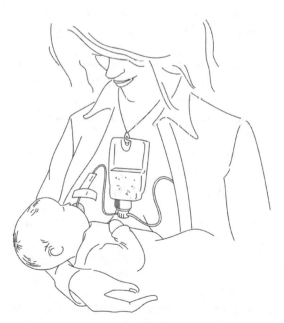

A supplemental nursing system can help nourish a preemie, while at the same time stimulating a mother's lactation.

Keep a positive attitude, hoping for the best, because worrying is only going to diminish your milk. If these tips don't work, don't feel guilty, and be grateful that your preemie can also thrive on donor breast milk or preterm formula. All studies point out the benefits of even partial breastfeeding, and particularly stress the importance of feeding a preemie colostrum, the rich, dense milk a mother expresses during the first few days after delivery. So be proud that you've given some of your precious breast milk to your baby. Your breastfeeding experience is a success regardless of its length.

Learning to Bottle Feed

I'm so frustrated! My baby has already taken a few bottles, but the nurses keep on feeding him with the tube. Doesn't he need more practice? How is he going to get it right?

No wonder you're so eager to leave gavage feedings behind. Being ready to drink from a bottle is a major step forward in your baby's physical and psychological development. But feeding by mouth is a difficult task for a premature baby, who until 32 to 34 weeks of gestation may not be neurologically mature enough to focus his attention and behavior as much as bottle feeding demands, or to coordinate sucking with swallowing and breathing. A younger baby simply may not be strong enough yet. (Try sucking on a bottle yourself for a few minutes, and see how much work it is!) So the path to getting all of his nutrition from a bottle can be longer than you think for your baby, and he may sometimes seem to be taking two steps forward and one back.

Chances are that your baby's nurses aren't being lazy or inattentive to his needs. On the contrary, they are probably doing just what feeding experts recommend for preemies who are learning to bottle feed: putting quality above quantity, watching his cues, and offering him a bottle only when he shows he's interested. Successful feeding for a young preemie isn't a matter of making him drink as much milk as possible (a too enthusiastic nurse or parent can force milk from a bottle into his mouth but that is likely to make him less, rather than more, keen on bottle feeding.) Rather, practice works best when he's ready and receptive to take a bottle, which means giving him all the time he needs to mature, develop his skills, and learn how to enjoy sucking and satisfying his hunger at the same time. Eating should become a pleasure for him, too, after all!

One or two bottle feeding sessions a day may be all a premature baby can handle at first, while all of his other meals are still given to him by gavage. It's a good start! While your baby is still learning, try not to be too anxious or impatient. Gradually you'll see the number of times a day he's ready to try bottle feeding increase. Your nurses will be happy to explain how your baby signals that he's ready for feeding (or not) and to teach you the best and safest techniques for holding him, feeding him, burping him, and getting enjoyment out of giving him nutrition. These are some of the things they might point out to you.

"I am ready to learn to feed" cues

When your baby shows these signs, it means he's mature and stable enough to try nipple feeding. Before each scheduled feeding time, your baby's nurse will check to see that all of these cues are present, and if they are, your baby will get a bottle feeding lesson. If not, he'll be fed by gavage.

* Your baby can keep calm and alert for at least five to ten minutes at a time.
* When you touch or stroke his lip, he quickly opens his mouth and drops and curls his tongue, ready to receive the nipple, and searches for it.
* When he's offered a pacifier or the tip of your pinky, he immediately sucks on them. (Nonnutritive sucking is such great preparation for feeding young preemies that each feeding may begin with about a minute of pacifier time, as the nurse evaluates your baby's tone, breathing, and general alertness.)
* He has good muscle tone, so he's able to keep his body flexed and his arms and hands pulled in toward the midline (showing he has enough energy for nipple feeding).
* His breathing is quiet and regular, and his oxygen saturation is over about 93 percent.

A few hours later, when it's mealtime again, the nurse will recheck his feeding-readiness cues and will continue to do that on a set schedule (usually every three hours).

"I am hungry" cues in older preemies

An older preemie, who is able to show his hunger, may be fed on demand when he shows the following cues:

* He's swiping his mouth or putting his hand to his mouth.
* He's sucking on his fingers, fists, or a pacifier.
* He's very alert, or restless, fussy, and crying.
* He's rooting (moving his lips and opening his mouth toward something touching his face).

Positioning

The best position for your baby's first feedings is side-lying—turned on his side on your lap with his face toward you, his body wrapped in a blanket with his arms and hands free, his head and chest supported and elevated to a semiupright position by a rolled blanket, pillow, or the curve of your arm, and your hand on his back so you can feel the rhythm and depth of his breathing.

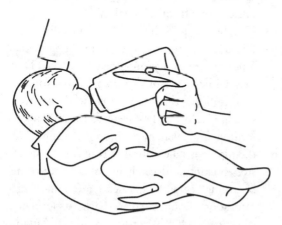

In the "sidelying" feeding position, the baby lies on his side on the lap of the feeder, with his head and chest semi-elevated and supported by the adult's arm (a pillow or a rolled blanket can be used for extra support). A hand placed on the baby's back helps to monitor his breathing.

Ask the nurse to show you how to position him even more precisely (for example, with his arms forward and his trunk straight, not rounded) so that his suck will be strongest. Swaddling him in a blanket helps him keep centered and calm so he can concentrate on feeding.

Choice of nipple

Premature babies are fed with a slow-flow nipple. This kind of nipple releases milk at a slower rate than a regular one, so it is better suited to the smaller mouth and less coordinated suck-swallow-and-breathe reflex of a preemie. A slow-flow nipple releases milk at a speed that's closer to that of milk flowing from a mother's breast, so if your baby is being both breastfed and bottle fed, his sucking and swallowing experiences will be more similar. Taking in too much milk too quickly increases a preemie's likelihood of spilling and dribbling milk out of his mouth instead of swallowing it, as well as his risk of aspiration, oxygen desaturation, apnea, and bradycardia.

"I can feed well" cues

These are the signs of an ace bottle feeder, which your baby eventually will be! They give you a sense of what you are aiming for.

* Once your baby starts feeding, his sucking quickly becomes smooth and rhythmical.
* His steady, strong sucking is well-coordinated with swallowing. You can tell he's comfortable by his calm and relaxed face. His eyes, which may be open or partly closed, shift back and forth, following the sucking and swallowing pulse.
* He doesn't spill any milk from his mouth.
* His breathing, oxygenation, and vital signs are stable, even during an occasional burst of sucking.

* He maintains good muscle tone and body flexion, showing he is alert and has enough energy for feeding.
* If he is not swaddled tightly, he tends to bring his hands toward the bottle.

Things you should avoid

These things are tempting to do, as a way to get a preemie to take more milk from a bottle, but not a good idea:

* Pressing on your baby's cheeks to encourage sucking, or pushing under his chin to help him swallow. (These maneuvers increase the flow of milk out of the nipple, and he may not be able to handle that. Also, forcing him to suck and swallow when he doesn't want to can make feeding an unpleasant experience and actually lengthen the time it takes him to get to full nipple feedings.)
* Pressing the nipple on your baby's tongue to release more milk. (Because he isn't controlling the flow with his sucking, this could lead to aspiration.)
* Twisting or jiggling the bottle to stimulate sucking when he pauses. (You should let him resume sucking when he's ready. He may need to breathe or rest.)
* Pressing your baby's palm to trick him into opening his mouth if he loses interest in feeding.
* Moving your baby a lot during feeding. Your baby can lose precious energy adapting to each change, and too much movement can increase reflux and make him vomit.

"I need a break" cues

Feeding is wonderful, but it's hard work for a preemie. These signs will tell you that your baby is tired and needs a rest.

* You can hear and feel your baby taking shorter, faster breaths (this is called "staccato breathing," a musical term for a short, pointed sound), or he stops breathing for more than three seconds at a time.
* His tongue slides off the nipple, making a clicking sound.
* He starts sucking too fast, gulping and making gurgling or yelping sounds in his throat. (Taking too much milk without enough time to breathe can lead to apnea and bradycardia or aspiration.)
* He sounds congested, or his nose gets stuffy. (This can indicate reflux up into his nose; he may need his nose suctioned out.)
* He gags, coughs, chokes, hiccups, or thrusts his tongue out.
* He shows he's distressed by raising his eyebrows, blinking or widening his eyes, arching his back, becoming restless, pulling away from the nipple, waving his arms, or swiping at the bottle.
* His face turns pale, ruddy, or bluish.
* He shows he's tired by drooling milk out of his mouth and becoming limp (because he's losing muscle tone from exhaustion).
* He falls asleep in the middle of a feeding.
* His oxygen saturation level drops more than 5 percent, or he has an apnea or brady. (These may be late cues of distress or exhaustion, or may indicate that he simply needs pacing— several breaks of a few seconds throughout the feeding in which he is brought upright and the nipple is taken out of his mouth so he can stop sucking and catch his breath. Once he's breathing regularly, his heart rate and oxygen saturation should increase back to normal. If the apnea or brady persists, gently rubbing his back can help.)

As soon as you notice one of these cues, gently stop the feeding. Give your baby time to reorganize his breathing and get his energy back. Feeding can be resumed after a brief rest, suspended for this meal, or continued by gavage. Your nurse will make this decision at your side. Remember that it is quality, not quantity that counts. By putting your baby in the driver's seat and letting him decide how much milk he can tolerate and enjoy from a bottle, you are helping him develop excellent feeding skills. Studies have shown that premature babies who are nipple-fed based on their behavior and readiness rather than a predetermined schedule move on to full oral feedings sooner.

Making gavage feeding into practice time

If your baby is still getting some gavage feedings, it may help to pair them with behaviors like sucking and holding. During gavage feedings, giving a baby a pacifier, holding him on your lap, and even placing a drop of milk on his tongue or dipping the pacifier in milk can help him associate the pleasant feelings of sucking, tasting, and smelling with having his hunger satisfied. Feeling your body against his while the tube feeding comfortably fills him up is a precious bonding experience that is preparing him (and you!) for the future pleasures you will share during feedings.

Helping a baby who's having a hard time feeding

Sometimes a preemie is ready to eat, but once the feeding gets started, he becomes disorganized or unstable. Here are some things to try that may help him focus and become calm enough to eat well:

* Stop feeding your baby and offer him a pacifier to suck on for a few minutes. Not having to concentrate on the feel and taste of milk,

or the task of coordinating swallowing with breathing, may help him settle down.
* Reduce the sensory stimulation he's experiencing (pull the curtains around his bed, turn off the lights, stop rocking) to help him focus on feeding only.
* Swaddle him with his arms in a midline position inside the blanket (to help center him and get him focused on his mouth).
* Ask the doctor whether giving him extra oxygen during his nipple feeding attempts is worth a try. (Preemies tend to suck for a longer time before taking a breath than term babies, so their oxygen levels can drop during feedings. If a baby is short of breath, he'll be less willing or able to suck and swallow.)

If he's having trouble with desats, apneas, and bradys during feeds, try pacing him (see the description under "I need a break" cues on page 260).

Burping

Not all newborns need to burp at every feeding, and preemies are no different. Some babies burp on their own during a feeding when they need to, but many don't. Just as you look at your baby's cues for feeding, you should also follow his lead on burping. If you notice he's getting restless when he's nippling, try burping him. You'll immediately find out if some extra air in his stomach was bothering him. You can take advantage of one of your baby's natural pauses to burp him, or if he doesn't stop on his own, give him a burp when he's about halfway through his feeding and again when he's finished, unless he's peacefully asleep.

Burping techniques are similar for breastfed and bottle fed preemies, although an infant who drinks from a bottle may need to burp more often. Holding him upright against your shoulder, facing toward you, and gently rubbing his back should do the trick. Be forewarned: even a kind pat on the back can be too much for a preemie (it may agitate him or even make him throw up what he just ate). Another good burping technique is to sit your baby upright on your lap facing away from you, head leaning slightly forward, with his chest, neck and chin supported with one of your hands (leaving your other hand free to rub his back). Or you can lay him on your lap, belly down, with his head resting on one of your thighs, his stomach on the other, and his back ready to be stroked. By far the most creative burping technique some nurses use on preemies is called "hula burping." You can try it, too: At the end of a feeding session, hold your baby standing up and gently sway his hips around in a circle like a hula dancer! Over time, you'll find which techniques you and your baby like best.

Afterglow

The moments after your baby has fed can be some of the most intimate and loving that you'll share together. Try to arrange your schedule so you don't have to rush off after a feeding. Hold your baby tenderly, letting him feel your warm closeness as he gradually drifts back to sleep. For him, there can be no greater joy.

Day by day, even feeding by feeding, you'll see your baby progress, gradually taking less time and more milk or formula at each session. There will be some ups and downs: some sleepy or uncoordinated days, when feeding doesn't go as well as you expected; some spitting up or episodes of feeding intolerance (most preemies go through that); some more gavage feedings to save precious energy; possibly some adjustments in what he's eating to help with reflux, improve his feeding technique, or ensure the best possible growth. But you'll have lots of rewards along the way, too. You'll enjoy a new time of closeness and tender interaction, when you can give your baby nourishment and he can thrive on the satisfaction of

actively taking it in. Feeding is finally becoming a total pleasure for your baby, as it will become a great source of joy for you too.

Baby Is Not Gaining Enough Weight

My baby isn't gaining weight as fast as the doctors think she should. They tell me not to worry but are adding things to her formula. Should I be concerned?

How to help a premature infant grow well outside of her mother's womb is one of the biggest issues in neonatal medicine. It's easy to understand why. Good growth is a sign of good nutrition, and good nutrition is crucial for a preemie's recovery and well-being in the short run, as well as for her lifelong health and development. But because most preemies take a while to begin feeding properly and they don't all grow at the same pace, doctors have to figure out each little patient's nutritional needs and adjust her diet to meet them.

In your daughter's case, the doctor is probably supplementing her formula with extra nutrients based on his knowledge of your baby's age, health, blood tests, previous growth rate, and activity level. It's commonly done, and no cause for worry. There are many reasons why a baby's diet may need to be supplemented. Preemies who are using a lot of energy drinking from a bottle or breast rather than being gavage fed, who have to keep up their body temperature because they are outside an isolette, who breathe faster and harder than other babies, who are fighting a medical complication such as an infection, or who are just particularly lively may all need more calories to sustain and speed their growth. Babies on special formulas because they've had feeding intolerance or whose X-rays or blood tests show that their bones aren't as hard and thick as they should be may also need additional nutrients. Breast milk is often supplemented to raise its calorie level and to give preemies more calcium and phosphorus. You can ask the doctor to explain what your baby is being given, and why.

Weight is a highly charged issue for parents of premature babies, who have to get used to the idea that their infant's birth weight is a fraction of a full-term newborn's. Then, like term babies, most preemies lose from 5 percent to 15 percent of their weight in the first week or so, and it may take up to three weeks for them to regain their already meager weight at birth. Once a baby has regained her birth weight, doctors want her to gain 15 to 30 grams a day—the same growth rate she would have had in the womb—and gear much of their treatment to making sure that happens. It's not surprising, then, that parents of preemies await the rite of the daily weighing with eagerness and apprehension.

But the scale doesn't tell the whole story. Babies may gain or lose mere water weight (usually from changes in fluid intake, medications like diuretics, or conditions that affect the kidneys, heart, or lungs). Being weighed on one scale one day and another the next can deceptively change a baby's weight. And a preemie's weight may change dramatically when medical equipment, such as IVs, arm boards, or CPAP prongs, are put on or taken off—or even when she has a large bowel movement!

Real growth is sustained over time and is most accurately reflected in increases in a baby's length and head circumference. In the hospital nursery, head circumference is measured at least once a week. A normal steady increase, ideally about one centimeter a week, indicates that the baby's brain is growing as it should. Body length is more difficult to measure accurately but it can be done using a special measuring board. A premature baby's length should also increase by about one centimeter a week.

Good nutrition is not only a matter of the total number of calories. To detect particular nutritional shortages, doctors check blood and urine tests. For instance, one reason for poor growth is a deficiency of sodium or bicarbonate, too much of which can be lost in the urine by a preemie's immature kidneys. Low levels of calcium and phosphorus together with a high level of alkaline phosphatase may indicate a shortage of the minerals needed to make strong bones. Scarcities of protein, salts, and other minerals, such as iron and zinc, can also cause slow growth. Many of these problems can be corrected by changing or supplementing a baby's nutrition.

Sometimes a premature baby's weight gain stalls because she's suffering from an illness, such as pneumonia, sepsis, or NEC. Fighting a disease can increase a baby's need for calories, but it also may put her at greater risk for feeding intolerance, so her doctors might decide not to enrich her diet right now, or to add some intravenous nutrition until she recovers. As she heals, her growth should catch up, too.

If a preemie isn't growing as well as she should—and even if she is, in order to give her the best known nutrition—her diet may be supplemented in several ways:

* **Breast milk may be supplemented with human milk fortifier.** Proteins, fats, and carbohydrates are the body's main building blocks. According to experts, the best kinds are those contained in breast milk, which are slightly different from those in formula. Although breast milk from a mother who has delivered prematurely has more nutrients than milk from a mother of a term baby, it still isn't sufficient for the tremendous growth requirements of a very small baby. To make up for that, human milk fortifier is added. It contains extra calories (in the form of protein, fat, and carbohydrate) and addi-

tional vitamins and minerals (such as calcium, phosphorus, sodium, iron, copper, and zinc). When a preemie is tolerating her fortified feedings fully, even more iron and vitamins are given, and sometimes a separate protein powder is added as well. (Donor breast milk in particular often needs more protein.) The resulting diet is the best nutrition available for a small preemie, giving her the advantages of breast milk (which helps her fight infections and is better digested and tolerated than formula) together with the extra nutrients she needs for bone mineralization and growth.

* **Breast milk can also be supplemented with preterm formula.** When more calories are needed than can be provided by human milk fortifier alone, preterm formula can be added to breast milk, too. Whereas fortifiers raise the calorie count of breast milk to 22 to 24 calories per ounce, with the addition of preterm formula, the calorie count can be raised as high as 30 calories per ounce, while still giving a preemie just the right balance of nutrients.

* **Preterm formula can be supplemented with multivitamins.** Special formulas for premature babies are designed to be as similar as possible to breast milk without its shortages. The proteins, carbohydrates, and fats of preterm formulas are more easily digested by a preemie's immature digestive system than those in formulas for full-term babies. They also contain higher concentrations of vitamins and minerals.

If a baby on preterm formula is eating less than about 5 ounces a day, she may still need multivitamin supplements to meet the recommended daily requirements. Some of the vitamins that are particularly important for preemies are folic acid (a B vitamin), which helps combat anemia; vitamin D, which helps strengthen bones; vitamin K, which helps

prevent bleeding; and vitamins A and E (both antioxidants, which help prevent the tissue damage that is involved in many complications of prematurity, including bronchopulmonary dysplasia, retinopathy of prematurity, and brain injury). These vitamins, together with minerals like iron (which is added by the manufacturer to some infant formulas), can be considered a premature baby's best nutritional allies. Doctors usually supplement them automatically, without monitoring blood levels, if they know a preemie isn't getting enough.

* **Preterm formula or breast milk can be supplemented with probiotics.** If a preemie is having trouble digesting and absorbing all the nutrients he needs, doctors may add probiotics (good bacteria) to his feedings. Probiotics can help a preemie absorb nutrients better, and protect him against NEC (an inflammatory disorder of the intestines). Babies who recently received more than a couple of days of antibiotics may also be given probiotics, because antibiotics can kill good bacteria as well as bad ones. Some nurseries give all very premature babies probiotics.

Some preemies need even more calories than standard preterm formula or fortified breast milk provides. One solution is simply to increase the amount of food they're given. Or, for babies whose fluid intake must be restricted because of their medical conditions, it is possible to create a very concentrated feeding by mixing preterm formula with less water than usual. (Be sure not to do this at home unless you're instructed to do so by your baby's doctor. If not done judiciously, it can overload a baby's system and make her dehydrated and sick.) Occasionally, special additional carbohydrates, protein, and fats are added to preterm formula or breast milk to increase its caloric content.

A Preemie's Caloric Needs

Ideally, a premature baby should grow as much as she would have in the womb: about 15 to 30 grams a day. To grow that well, most preemies need to get about 110 to 120 calories a day for each 1,000 grams of their current body weight; they need about 70 calories so as not to lose weight. But babies' energy requirements vary a lot and may be higher or lower depending on their metabolism, activity level, and health (since fighting an illness can require more calories).

Most preterm formulas contain 24 calories per ounce, transitional formulas for older preemies usually contain 22, and formulas for term babies 20. Breast milk is usually considered to have about 20 calories per ounce (the exact number will vary from as few as 16 to as many as 34 depending on the mother's recent diet, how soon after delivery it is, and other factors; calories in pasteurized donor breast milk are often a little lower) but when breast milk is fed to preterm babies in the hospital nursery, it is usually supplemented with milk fortifiers to reach an estimated 24 calories per ounce (see page 264).

Knowing that, you can make a rough calculation of how much milk your baby should get. Let's say she weighs 1,000 grams. Her daily caloric requirement is about 120 calories. If she's eating 24-calorie (that's 24 calories per ounce) formula or breast milk, she should take five ounces of milk a day.

Because concentrated formula is more difficult to digest and some babies don't tolerate it initially, doctors usually increase the caloric content of a baby's feeding gradually, over a week or so. (Babies on very concentrated formulas tend to get constipated and need yet another nutritional supplement—prune juice!)

Some babies don't tolerate even unfortified breast milk or regular preterm formula. This may be because they've had NEC or another intestinal problem that has left them with difficulty digesting and absorbing nutrients. Or they may be allergic to the proteins in cow's milk (which are the base of most infant formulas) or have difficulty digesting lactose, the sugar in milk. Both an allergy to cow's milk protein and lactose-intolerance tend to run in families. (Babies with these problems usually do well with breast milk but not formula.)

Thanks to the many modified formulas available today—lactose-free, those with different kinds and concentrations of proteins and fat, and elemental (meaning predigested)—babies with most kinds of feeding intolerance can be nourished successfully. Since these formulas may lack some of the nutrients in preterm formula, however, preemies on nonstandard formulas may need further nutritional supplementation. A preemie with severe feeding intolerance might even need a little supplemental intravenous nutrition for a while until his tolerance improves.

There are some other common conditions in preemies that often require dietary supplements to insure good growth. Preemies on diuretics lose a lot of essential salts in their urine, so many of them will be given supplements of potassium, sodium, and chloride.

(Continued on page 270)

In Plain Language: What Is Necrotizing Enterocolitis?

If premature births could be prevented, very few babies would suffer from NEC. Necrotizing enterocolitis is an intestinal disease of the newborn that almost exclusively affects preemies. Even in intensive care nurseries, NEC is not very common: only about 6 percent of premature babies with a birth weight less than 1,500 grams and 8 percent with a birth weight less than 1,000 grams get it. (The younger they are, the higher their risk, as with many scourges of prematurity.)

Still, since NEC is dangerous and not always easy to diagnose, parents of preemies often hear it mentioned as a possible complication. Many times this ends up being only a NEC scare with a happy ending, to everyone's relief. But if your baby is, in fact, diagnosed with NEC, you shouldn't panic. Although serious, this illness can be overcome in the majority of cases with medical treatment or, if necessary, with surgery. It is a trial, but it can be endured.

Why NEC can be so serious

NEC is an inflammation that damages the lining of the intestine. It may affect only a small portion or large areas of either the small intestine or the colon (the large intestine), and when severe it may cause the bowel to tear, or "perforate." Most often the inflamed area heals and recovers perfectly well, but sometimes a part of the intestine is so damaged that it will not function and needs to be surgically removed. NEC is sometimes accompanied by an infection of the gastrointestinal tract or bloodstream, but even without an infection, all of the baby's vital organs may become unbalanced, posing a serious threat to his life. Fortunately, the vast majority of babies with NEC survive the illness.

The uncertain origin of NEC

Of all the complications of prematurity, NEC is one of the least understood. Medical researchers still don't know for sure what causes it, and why some preemies develop it and others don't. It's believed that an injury to the immature intestinal tract, caused by a lack of blood flow and oxygen or an infection, starts the chain reaction leading to NEC. The damaged intestinal tissue can then be invaded by bacteria that normally live peacefully in the gut without causing problems. When they become too numerous, though, they contribute to the inflammation and damage characteristic of NEC.

What might cause imperfect blood circulation in a baby's intestine, starting this process? Possibilities are problems during delivery, such as a placental abruption or very low fetal heart rate; maternal cocaine use (because exposure to cocaine in the womb can disrupt a fetus's circulation); a period of time when a baby's blood pressure was very low (caused by sepsis or a large PDA, perhaps); or treatment with medication to close a PDA (PDA-closing medications cause blood vessels to narrow, so reduce blood flow). The usual episodes of apnea and bradycardia that preemies have don't seem to be linked to the development of NEC (although it's not clear whether particularly severe A's and B's are). In the past a prime suspect in the origin of NEC was poor intestinal blood flow from an umbilical catheter, but this has now been dismissed. There have been some reports of preemies getting NEC after a blood transfusion, so the role of transfusion as a possible cause of NEC is currently being investigated.

Occasionally cases of NEC in hospital nurseries happen in clusters, possibly indicating that they are linked to an infectious strain of bacteria or virus. But if another preemie in the nursery has NEC you shouldn't get anxious because it's rare for a baby to be contagious.

So far, doctors have found only a few ways to help preemies avoid getting NEC. Steroids given before delivery, which make a preemie's intestines mature faster, help prevent it, as does feeding breast milk rather than formula, and supplementing a preemie's feedings with probiotics ("good bacteria"). Some studies, though not all, have found that a slow, rather than very rapid, increase in the quantity of milk or formula a preemie is fed each day lessens the risk of getting NEC; therefore, most neonatologists are cautious when they increase the amount of food a preemie is given.

Oral feedings: Risky or beneficial?

Feeding is associated with the development of NEC (although babies who have never been fed can get it, too). For this reason, when doctors know that the blood flow in a preemie's intestinal tract is acutely compromised (by very low blood pressure, for example, or while he's being treated with indomethacin for a PDA), they will usually stop feeding him.

Doctors used to think that NEC could be triggered by lingering, undigested residuals of milk in the bowel, something that is common in preemies because of their immature digestive system. But postponing oral feedings until preemies are older and more mature doesn't prevent NEC. On the contrary, neonatologists today believe that preemies should be cautiously introduced to tiny amounts of milk as soon as possible because the process of digestion itself can stimulate the stomach and intestine to mature faster and make it less likely for NEC to occur.

For this purpose, the best first nutrition a preemie can get is breast milk. Breast milk has powerful protective qualities against NEC. If a young premature baby can't get her own mother's milk, pasteurized donor breast milk is the next best choice. Human milk has unique components that help the intestine mature and change the environment within it, promoting the growth of "good bacteria" (which help digestion) and preventing the overgrowth of other bacteria (which can initiate the inflammation of NEC).

If your premature baby is formula fed, though, you can take heart. Recent medical research suggests that supplementing formula feedings with probiotics (good bacteria, such as *Lactobacillus* and *Bifidobacterium*) can reduce a preemie's risk of getting NEC. In some studies, even babies fed breast milk were less likely to get NEC when probiotics were added. Good bacteria have always been part of the human diet, as essential active ingredients in healthy foods like yogurt, cheese, and wine. Added to preterm formula they—like breast milk—may help populate a preemie's gut with healthy bacteria that promote digestion and counteract the overgrowth of other more dangerous microorganisms. Some doctors are still waiting for the results of bigger clinical trials to confirm the benefits and safety of probiotics, and to establish what kind and dose of probiotics is best. Other neonatologists are already introducing them in the diet of preemies who are most at risk for NEC. At the moment, it's not clear how much preemies who are fed exclusively with their mother's breast milk will benefit. You can ask your baby's doctors what their thinking is on probiotics, and what the latest research is showing.

How NEC develops, and how it shows up

The earlier a baby is born, the longer the time before he is no longer at risk for getting NEC. The average age of onset is about three weeks of age. Sometimes NEC seems to come out of the blue, particularly if a preemie is feeding and growing and seemingly doing well.

NEC can be puzzling when it comes to diagnosis, too. Its early signs can be mild and mimic those of an infection or instability due simply to prematurity: more frequent apnea and bradys, temperature instability, a change in blood sugar levels, increased acid in the blood. Other signs may point to a problem with digestion but are often the same as those caused by innocent feeding intolerance from gut immaturity: the presence of milk residuals in the stomach, a slightly distended belly, vomiting, diarrhea, or invisible blood in stools, picked up on what is called a guaiac (pronounced "GWY-ak") test.

But babies who are developing NEC can worsen quickly. They may have an acute respiratory crisis with severe apnea and bradycardia, pass visibly bloody stools, develop a very distended and tender abdomen, and show signs of sepsis, with lethargy, low blood pressure, and abnormalities in blood chemistry and clotting. Advanced NEC can show up suddenly also, with no early warning.

Full-blown NEC is detectable by X-ray: doctors see pneumatosis, meaning tiny bubbles of intestinal gas inside the damaged bowel wall. An X-ray can also show whether air has leaked out of the bowel through a tear or perforation, a condition that requires surgery. Once a baby is diagnosed with NEC, he may get an abdominal X-ray as often as every 12 to 24 hours to detect a perforation as early as possible and to determine when the pneumatosis resolves—a milestone in recovery.

Although an X-ray can confirm a diagnosis of NEC, X-ray findings can also be vague and not definitive. In that case, NEC is diagnosed using a combination of X-ray findings, observation of the baby, and blood tests, which in NEC may show low levels of sodium, white blood cells, and platelets and too much acid in the blood.

How NEC is treated

Doctors are always on the alert for the first signs and symptoms of NEC because early intervention is the key to giving your baby the best chance to fight this illness and recover from it well. When they suspect NEC, doctors give a baby's bowel a rest by stopping his feedings, giving him only intravenous nutrition for a while, and inserting a tube in his stomach (passing through the nose or the mouth) to remove extra gas and secretions. They also take an X-ray of his abdomen, do blood and urine cultures to detect infection, monitor all of his vital signs for the slightest deterioration, and start a course of broad-spectrum antibiotics. The nurse will measure the circumference of the baby's belly frequently, to monitor how well the intestines are passing gas and emptying. His blood counts, blood chemistries, and X-rays will be repeated periodically until they're back to normal.

Antibiotics are usually continued for 7 to 14 days to treat infection and stop the progression of the illness. If the baby's breathing worsens, he may need to be put on a ventilator. His blood pressure will be sustained with fluids and medication if needed, and if his blood counts are low, he may get one or more blood transfusions (red blood cells for anemia and platelets or plasma to correct the blood clotting problems that can accompany severe NEC). Some babies may also get IVIG (intravenous immunoglobulin—an infusion of antibodies—to help fight infection) if their white blood cell count falls very low. Babies with NEC generally will have a surgical consultation, but the majority do not end up needing surgery.

A baby with NEC will be fed intravenously with parenteral nutrition until his intestines heal. Most neonatologists wait until a baby's vital signs have stabilized and the pockets of gas in the bowel wall have been gone for five days or more before gradually resuming oral feedings. His feedings will be advanced slowly and cautiously, usually over at least 7 to 10 days, until he no longer needs intravenous nutrition. Formula fed babies will initially get a predigested formula (which is easier on the intestines than regular preemie formula) or donor breast milk. Breast fed babies will resume their mother's breast milk.

When medical therapy alone is successful, NEC usually lasts from two to three weeks from its first onset to full recovery—quite a long haul. But the critical stage of the illness is often over much sooner, and many babies are stable after a couple of days. Your baby's doctor can tell you when the crisis stage is past so you can relax.

If despite all therapies, the infant's condition deteriorates or if X-rays reveal perforation of the bowel or areas of damaged intestines that aren't recovering, then surgical treatment is needed. The insertion of a peritoneal drain, a simple procedure performed at the bedside under local anesthesia, often allows a baby to overcome the acute stage of NEC and to heal. A peritoneal drain is a soft plastic tube placed in the abdomen through which infected secretions and gas can escape. When peritoneal drainage isn't enough, an operation to remove any torn or dead bowel and to clean out any infected areas is done. If your baby needs either of these surgical procedures for NEC, you can read about them on page 356.

After NEC, in the short and long run

Most of the time, once a premature baby recovers from NEC there are no further flare-ups or serious difficulties. But occasionally the healing process leaves scars in his belly or intestines that cause complications later. The most common result of scarring is a stricture, or narrowing, of a small area of the bowel. A stricture, if it's mild, may be completely unnoticeable. If it's tighter, it can block the movement of gas and stool and cause cramps, abdominal distention, vomiting, constipation, or intermittent bleeding. If a baby is having feeding difficulties after NEC, the presence of a stricture or other obstruction can be diagnosed with special X-rays using dye (either swallowed or given as an enema) to outline the shape of the intestines. If a stricture is found, usually it can be easily corrected with a simple and safe surgical procedure.

Occasionally, scarring can obstruct the flow of bile into the intestine, causing jaundice. This often resolves on its own over time.

The most serious long-term consequence of NEC is called short-bowel syndrome, which occurs when very extensive portions of the intestine are damaged and must be removed. Be assured that it occurs only rarely. The loss of large amounts of the intestine leads to a lack of digestive capacity, with malabsorption of nutrients and water, undernutrition, and risk of dehydration, electrolyte (blood chemistry) abnormalities, and frequent infections. Sparse oral feedings may need to be combined with intravenous nutrition for months or years, and a child's liver function and growth and development may be compromised.

If your baby has this complication, try to be optimistic, keeping in mind that many infants with short bowel syndrome eventually overcome it and make the transition to total oral feedings. This is possible because of the amazing capacity of the remaining portion of intestine to adapt and increase its digestive and absorptive properties. Studies show that this process starts within just 48 hours after removal of large parts of the bowel, and that resuming small quantities of oral feedings is crucial to stimulate the adaptation. There have been cases of babies left with less than 20 centimeters of small intestine who were able to leave TPN behind, and whose intestines were found to be fully adapted by three to four years of age. If a child's intestine isn't adapting quickly or completely enough, sometimes bowel lengthening surgery can be performed later to add precious amounts of intestinal capacity.

Premature babies who had NEC are at a slightly higher risk for developmental delays for reasons that aren't yet clearly understood. Medical researchers are studying the effects that acute inflammation can have on a preemie's developing brain cells, perhaps contributing to a brain injury. Attentive follow-up and early intervention,

if needed, are of utmost importance to give an infant the best chance to develop to the best of his potential. Preventing long-lasting growth delays is also crucial to ensuring normal intellectual development in preemies. The good news is that doctors are becoming better at avoiding malnutrition during and after NEC with parenteral nutrition and appropriate vitamin and mineral supplements. That, together with the wonderful ability of the human bowel to regenerate itself, gives your baby a great opportunity to grow after NEC into a happy, thriving child.

And babies with reflux often have cereal added to their milk to help their feedings stay down. (Cereal, too, can cause constipation that may require the gentle help of a little prune juice.)

Many parents might be thinking now that to be able to feed their preemie, they need a Ph.D. in biochemistry. But be reassured: Most feeding supplements are given for just several weeks, and few infants need them once they're discharged from the hospital. Some special diets—like more concentrated formula, milk thickened with rice cereal, or for the youngest breastfed preemies, fortifier added to pumped breast milk—may continue for a long time, but they are easy to deal with at home.

For now, trust the creativity of your baby's doctor, who with the help of the NICU's dietician will try new regimens until the right menu is found: the one allowing a baby to eat, digest, fight her illnesses, and grow. What other chef has such a challenging but rewarding task?

Scalp IV

This morning I had the worst surprise. I found my baby with an IV in her head. It looks awful, and I'm afraid it will injure her brain.

It looks like medical aggression of the worst kind. Not satisfied with having pierced your daughter's feet, ankles, hands, and arms already, the doctors have stuck in yet another needle—this time in her scalp. Looking at it, your heart sinks and you think, this time they've gone too far. You don't understand why they would do such a seemingly dangerous thing to your baby.

Well. Some medical procedures look painful and invasive but in reality are quite benign. A scalp IV belongs in that category. As you already know, intravenous catheters are required to deliver the fluids, nutrients, or medications that your baby needs to recover and thrive. The simplest and safest IVs to use are those in the small veins lying close to the surface of the skin. If your preemie has been in the hospital for a while, the superficial veins in her arms and legs may have housed quite a few catheters, and need a chance to rest and recover from any inflammation.

There's another place left that has safe, superficial veins, though: the scalp. A scalp IV is usually easy to insert, and like all IVs, painless for the baby once it's in. It has the advantages of being readily visible for the nurses to check, and less likely to be knocked out than a catheter in a hand or foot. Since the catheter runs very superficially just under the skin, it doesn't pose any risk to the

Central Lines

A central line is a catheter that lies in a large, deep blood vessel close to, or sometimes within, the heart. Central lines are used if a premature baby may need an IV for more than a few weeks (for instance, if he's not expected to be able to eat for a while or if long-term antibiotics are required for an infection), if he needs medications that would be irritating to smaller blood vessels, or simply because there aren't many suitable peripheral veins left in which to place catheters. Because large, deep veins aren't as fragile as superficial ones, central lines can usually be left in place for as long as they're needed (think how many needle sticks this will save your baby) and more concentrated substances can be delivered through them.

There are two types of central lines: cuffed and uncuffed. Uncuffed lines (called PICCs, for percutaneously inserted central catheters) are tiny, flexible catheters that are usually inserted in the NICU by a neonatologist or nurse practitioner. The pain medications and sedatives given in the NICU are adequate to keep a baby comfortable and still throughout the placement. Cuffed catheters (the most common are called Broviacs) are somewhat larger and stiffer, with a cuff to hold them in place under the skin. The insertion of a cuffed line is a more complex procedure, requiring minor surgery under anesthesia

or deep sedation, but once it is in place, it lasts longer.

Sometimes the neonatologist or nurse practitioner has difficulty getting the catheter where it needs to go. In that case, a surgeon may be asked to help place a central (or even a peripheral) IV line in the NICU using a "cut-down" technique, which involves making a small incision in the skin so that a vein can be seen and held as a catheter is placed directly into it.

After the doctors put in a central line, they'll take an X-ray to make sure it's in a good, safe place. If the line is uncuffed, they may recheck its placement with an X-ray every couple of weeks or so because it can loosen and move a bit over time.

Because all central lines are foreign objects that dwell deep inside the body, they carry a higher risk of serious infection than peripheral IVs. (If your baby happens to get a line infection, the doctors will treat him with antibiotics and may remove the catheter.) There is also a very small risk that the line could poke through the vessel it's in, causing bleeding or delivering its fluid into the surrounding tissues, which could then become irritated or damaged. But balancing these risks are enormous benefits: Central lines are essential tools to give your baby what she needs to heal and grow.

brain, which is securely protected by the thick bones of the skull and several layers of tough membranes.

Despite their many advantages, scalp IVs are

somewhat lacking in the looks department! The doctor or nurse may have shaved off a patch of your baby's hair where the catheter was inserted, and he may now be wearing cotton pads and an eccentric-looking little cap to keep the IV from being dislodged. Soon you may find it cute (some doctors and nurses swear they do), but the main reason most nurseries use scalp IVs only when necessary is the initial reaction of shock they often cause in parents. Just remember that the IV is temporary, and under your baby's future hair there will be no evidence that it was ever there.

A Baby's Positioning and SIDS

Why do the nurses put my baby down on her stomach when that's been proven to increase the chances of SIDS?

Here's a bit of history that will help you understand: When the American Academy of Pediatrics wrote the original recommendations for the Back to Sleep campaign, which strongly advocated putting healthy, full-term babies to sleep on their backs or sides to reduce the risk of sudden infant death syndrome (SIDS), they excluded preemies with breathing problems.

The American Academy of Pediatrics 1992 guidelines said: "For premature infants with respiratory distress, for infants with symptoms of gastroesophageal reflux, or with certain upper airway anomalies, and perhaps for some others, prone may well be the position of choice." Prone means tummy-down.

There are good reasons for this. When young preemies lie on their stomachs, they're able to breathe more easily and less rapidly, and the oxygen level in their blood increases. Preemies sleep better on their stomachs, with more quiet sleep, an important sign of maturation and brain development. Moreover, lying on their backs too much can create certain postural problems for premature babies later on. (For example, when young preemies lie on their backs, they tend to have their legs splayed out, frog-like, simply because they don't have the muscle tone to adopt other positions. So as older infants and toddlers, they're more likely to have problems with turned-out hips or ankles and feet.) And preemies seem to like being on their stomachs, which lowers their stress levels, conserving their precious energy and keeping them more stable.

The only problem is that some parents, seeing their babies tummy-down in the intensive care nursery, erroneously assume it's safe to continue this practice at home.

(Continued on page 276)

Why Is My Baby's Chest Indented?

One reason preemies breathe better on their stomachs is that gravity and the support from the bed keeps their chests from sucking in too deeply, so their lungs stay inflated better. Preemies have very flexible chest walls because the cartilage in their ribcage isn't very firm yet. So when they inhale, particularly if they're breathing hard, their chests may suck in deeply, caving in at the middle. Some parents even worry that their babies have strange, permanently indented chests. They don't; it's just temporary!

Getting Acquainted with: Reflux

As any parent knows, being a baby means spitting up now and then after a good meal of breast milk or formula. Doctors call this gastroesophageal reflux—reflux for short—and most of the time it's perfectly normal, causing no problems. In fact, all full-term babies have some reflux, and their parents usually don't do much about it, except for spending a lot of money on laundry detergent!

But there are some babies who have reflux that is especially severe, causing them to spit up or throw up more than usual, or to have other symptoms because of it. For them, treatment may become important.

Until recently, treatment of reflux was widespread in intensive care nurseries, because doctors believed that in these tiny patients reflux often caused apnea, bradys, and oxygen desaturation during or after meals, and contributed to chronic lung disease and slower weight gain. But research has not supported a causal connection between episodes of reflux and these symptoms in most preemies, and medical practice is changing. In fact, in preemies, reflux is more apt to follow an episode of apnea and bradycardia than to cause it.

Some neonatologists continue to treat reflux, believing that it still causes symptoms in some individual babies. Since all medications, so valuable when needed, also carry risks of their own, there are tests that can be done to establish whether reflux really is the problem for your baby. There are also simple changes in your baby's feeding or sleeping position that you may see the doctors and nurses try because they reduce reflux in some preemies.

Happily, with time (for babies' upper intestinal tracts to mature and become better coordinated) and treatment when it's necessary, reflux is almost always a temporary problem, not one of the more serious, threatening complications of prematurity.

What is reflux?

The best way to understand reflux is to picture what is supposed to happen when we swallow food. First it travels down the long tube that connects the mouth to the stomach, called the esophagus. At the bottom of the esophagus, there's a little "gate" that opens to let food pass into the stomach: a muscle called the lower esophageal sphincter. After the sphincter lets food go through to the stomach, it closes again so the food can't go back up.

Your stomach is like a blender: it mashes up the food, mixing it with acid. When the blending is finished, another gate, a muscle at the bottom of the stomach, opens and lets the food move on to the small intestine.

OK. What if babies have reflux? They swallow their food, which travels normally down their esophagus and into their stomach. But while their stomachs are churning away, the lower esophageal sphincter reopens, letting some of the food escape back up the esophagus. Sometimes, but not always, it even goes all the way out of the mouth.

If the food that is regurgitated doesn't contain much acid, it's called nonacid reflux, which is what babies usually have during feedings and for an hour afterward (because food mixes with the stomach acid and neutralizes it). If the regurgitated food contains a lot of acid, it's called acid reflux, which typically occurs an hour or more after feedings when the stomach is emptier.

When is reflux a problem?

Virtually all babies (and, in fact, all adults, too) have some reflux. Research shows that healthy infants have about 24 episodes of reflux in a 24-hour day, and half of them spit up two or more feedings a day in their first few months of life. (Only 1 percent are still vomiting by the time they're a year old.)

So reflux is only characterized as problematic when someone has too much of it or it causes other complications. Adults complain when they have reflux that is bad enough to be painful and cause heartburn, a burning sensation when food mixed with stomach acid irritates their esophagus.

When is reflux a problem in preemies? When it is severe enough to cause one of the following symptoms: irritation of a baby's esophagus leading to bleeding or pain during feeding; slower weight gain because frequent vomiting or refusal to eat deprives the baby of precious calories; aspiration pneumonia caused by inhaling regurgitated breast milk or formula into the lungs; apnea, bradycardia, or oxygen desaturation during or after meals; chronic lung disease or airway inflammation. Preemies with BPD especially may have trouble with reflux because they're more prone to oxygen desaturations and need more calories to grow, and their harder breathing can make reflux more severe.

Keep in mind that all of these symptoms can also occur independently of reflux for other reasons. So if your baby's doctor suspects that reflux may be causing her problems, before starting treatment he may want to confirm this possibility with diagnostic tests.

One test is called a pH probe. A small tube is placed through your baby's nose and down into her esophagus. The tip of the tube has a sensor that can detect acid, so it knows when there is acid reflux from the stomach. It is usually left in place for 24 hours, recording all episodes of

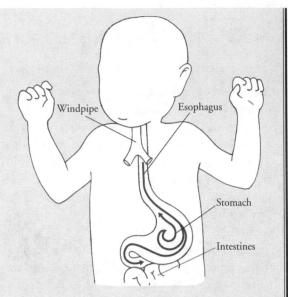

With GE reflux, food from the stomach can escape back up into the esophagus, reach the throat, and sometimes enter the windpipe.

acid reflux on a computer. The test tells doctors whether an unusual amount of acid reflux has occurred. With additional special technology, it can also tell whether the timing of reflux episodes corresponded to your baby's bradycardia or other symptoms.

Another test, called impedance monitoring, can be done at the same time as a pH probe to detect nonacid reflux. Your baby will get a second small probe that measures pressure changes in the esophagus—normal ones from swallowing, and others associated with episodes of reflux. Taken together, the pH probe and impedance monitoring can provide a picture of both acid and nonacid reflux.

The doctor may also request a special X-ray called an upper GI (for gastrointestinal) study. Your baby will be fed a liquid dye that shows up on X-rays and a radiologist will watch as it travels down her esophagus, through her stomach, and into her small intestine. With an upper GI, the doctors can get an idea of how quickly and completely her stomach empties and make sure she doesn't have any blockages, kinks, or narrowings in her stomach or upper intestinal tract that might be causing the reflux or making it worse. If she has a reflux episode during the study, they can also see how high in her esophagus the dye goes and whether she aspirates any into her lungs (an indication of how severe the reflux is).

Treatment of reflux in preemies

If there's no anatomic abnormality, reflux will almost always go away on its own eventually. Nevertheless, for now your baby may need some relief from its symptoms if they're causing her problems.

Her doctor and nurses will first try some simple adjustments that help some babies: feeding her smaller amounts more frequently, thickening her milk or formula with cereal, burping her more often during feedings, feeding her continuously using a pump, waiting longer between feedings, or switching to a predigested formula. They will raise the head of her bed and make sure she is lying stomach-down or on her side during and after meals, since on her back, reflux is worse, and it is easier for refluxed food to get into her airway or lungs and cause choking or breathing problems. (Whether the left or right side is better is still being studied; a recent trial indicated that lying on the right side, which empties the stomach fastest, may be best for an hour after meals, and the left side may be best after that, since it minimizes the reflux of what is left behind. You can ask your baby's doctors and nurses about the latest findings.)

Caffeine, which is used to treat apnea of prematurity, can make reflux worse. So if the doctor thinks your baby's apnea is mild, he may try stopping caffeine to see if her reflux improves.

If these measures don't work, your baby may be given medication for her reflux. Two kinds are commonly used. One kind, such as Reglan, improves the mobility of the stomach and intestine so food spends less time in the stomach, making a quicker getaway down into the small intestine. The other (usually Pepcid or Prevacid) reduces the production of stomach acid so when reflux does occur, it's less irritating to the esophagus. (Antacids increase a preemie's risk of infection, so your baby will be watched carefully for any signs. Reglan can cause abnormal body movements, but it's very rare to see this side effect in preemies.)

If medication doesn't help and a baby's symptoms are severe, doctors may try passing her feeding tube beyond her stomach into her intestine so the food can't reflux up the esophagus as easily. This can work well, but it's hard to keep the tube in the right place for long.

Finally, if these temporizing measures fail and complications from the reflux are serious, surgery will be considered. This is rare, so don't expend energy worrying about it now. There's more on the operation for reflux, called a fundoplication, on pages 364–366.

How long will reflux be a problem?

Just as the rest of your preemie's movements and bodily systems are pretty uncoordinated right now, so is her upper gastrointestinal tract. Her reflux will probably get a lot better by around six months of age, and disappear by the time she's one or two.

It's possible that your baby will have a slightly longer hospital stay because of her reflux and will need to keep taking medication after she goes home. Fortunately, most preemies with reflux tend to eat, grow, and thrive as well as their peers.

There are some suggestions for dealing with reflux at home on page 403. They may be helpful at first, but chances are you won't need them for long.

It isn't! While premature babies are in intensive care, they are being constantly observed and monitored, so any problems with their vital signs will be noticed and responded to immediately. At home it's a different situation, and laying your baby on her back is extremely important, to reduce the risk of SIDS. In fact, putting a preemie "Back to Sleep" at home is even *more* crucial than for a full-term baby, because preemies are at higher risk for SIDS.

To model for parents what they should do, many experts in the medical community want hospitals to put preemies to sleep on their backs starting at least one week before they leave the hospital (your baby's nurses may start doing this even sooner, once she's breathing comfortably and can remain calm when she's lying on her back), and the AAP guidelines now omit the exception for preemies. At that point, you can whisper to your baby that being "Back to Sleep" means she'll soon be Home to Sleep, too.

Skin Care

My baby has such delicate skin, and to bathe her they're using plain old Dove soap! Couldn't they come up with something better for preemies?

When it comes to skin care, a minimalist approach fits premature babies best: the fewer and simpler products that are used, the better. That's because a young preemie's skin is so thin and sensitive that it can be hurt by rough handling or rubbing and will absorb many of the substances that are put on it. Exposure to strong chemicals (including perfumes) at this very early age can cause irritation and may possibly contribute to future development of skin allergies.

So most NICUs opt for a light use of the most common baby soaps (such as Baby Magic) or adult soaps with a neutral pH and no perfumes or dyes (like Dove or Neutrogena) to bathe the babies. Some nurseries have tried special antimicrobial or disinfectant soaps to fight skin infections. However, these products contain chemicals that can build up to toxic levels if preemies absorb too much through their skin, so they'll be used very sparingly—to sterilize your baby's skin before putting in an intravenous line, for example. The goal is to maintain good hygiene with a minimum of intervention.

Since any soap can irritate a preemie's skin, bathing isn't usually done more than two or three times a week. The tiniest preemies, born under 26 weeks of gestation, may get just a sponge bath in plain water at body temperature with no soap at all. Bigger preemies have the fun of getting dipped in a basin of warm soapy water. Research hasn't shown that the use of soap rather than just water reduces the germs on a premature baby's skin or her risk of infection.

Washing can also aggravate the dryness of a preemie's skin, which because of the immaturity of its sweat glands is short of water and natural oils. When skin is dry, simple contact with clothes or bedding can cause irritation and injury, and germs can invade more easily. You might think that a moisturizer or emollient would help, but several studies of premature babies who were treated with an oil-in-water moisturizing lotion found that although they had less dehydration and fewer skin lesions they also had more infections, perhaps because the lotion helped certain kinds of germs to flourish.

Once your baby is mature enough to go home or just a short time afterward, her pediatrician will probably tell you that her skin is ready to handle the same mild baby soaps and shampoos as a term baby, from such classics as Johnson's to a panoply of newer organic, ecofriendly options. But for now her delicate skin will get only the purest and simplest kind of care.

Tiny Babies with Big Diaper Rashes

What infant doesn't get a diaper rash at least once? Preemies, with no reason to be exempt, get them, too. A diaper rash starts because a baby's skin is easily irritated by exposure to urine and stool, and commonly progresses from a simple skin irritation to a mild infection. A diaper rash caused by yeast can spread quickly and look scary: a bright red chafing with red bumps that may extend from the diaper area up the belly or down the thighs. Sometimes a baby will have a yeast infection in his mouth at the same time.

Preemies are at a slightly greater disadvantage than term babies in the fight against diaper rash because their skin is especially sensitive and their immune systems not as mature. In addition, their bowel movements are more irregular and thus harder to predict, and since they sleep a lot and don't vigorously broadcast their need for a diaper change, they may go longer with a dirty diaper. (Nurses don't want to wake preemies unnecessarily, so they check their diapers every few hours at scheduled care times.) Also, some preemies develop loose stools when their milk or formula is fortified, and diarrhea is especially irritating.

In the NICU diaper changes are scheduled around feeding times (usually every three hours) and whenever else the nurses see (or smell!) that they're needed. Dry washcloths, or ones moistened with water only, are used to clean preemies' little bottoms. Avoiding soaps and prepackaged baby wipes, which can deplete a baby's skin of its natural acid barrier, and keeping the diaper area as dry as possible are the best preventive measures.

What is done when a rash or irritation develops? A preemie's skin can be protected and allowed to heal by applying a thick layer of barrier cream, such as any of the common white ointments for the diaper area. At each diaper change, he is cleaned without removing the whole layer of cream, and more is added on, generously. A yeast infection can be treated with an antifungal cream or powder that's applied several times a day, before the barrier cream. If a baby has thrush (white spots in his mouth caused by a yeast infection), he'll be given an antifungal liquid to take orally. If you're breastfeeding, the doctor may also give you some antifungal cream to rub on your nipples between feedings so that you don't catch your baby's infection. Steroid creams, which calm inflammation and are sometimes used to treat diaper rashes in older babies, can be dangerous if used too much on preemies because their thin skin can absorb too much of the medicine, so they are generally avoided.

If a rash is really severe, with bleeding, the nurses may decide it's worth the extra mess to let your baby go without diapers at all for a while. That way, moisture isn't trapped on the skin to irritate it. They may even put your baby's bare bottom in the air under a heating lamp to thoroughly dry his skin. (He'll look like a sunbathing beauty who doesn't want a diaper tan line!) But don't worry; although a bad diaper rash looks awful, with proper care and attention it will soon be gone.

Antibiotics

I always try to avoid antibiotics when I have a cold or the flu. Now my daughter has been put on them for several weeks. I wonder about the consequences.

Your attitude toward antibiotics is wise. As you probably know, they may encourage the growth of resistant organisms (meaning germs that have become accustomed to antibiotics and are therefore difficult or impossible to fight). It is a problem in our society as a whole. Doctors are well aware of the risk and know not to prescribe antibiotics lightly.

The first question you should ask is whether your daughter's antibiotics are to prevent her from getting an infection or to treat one. The chance of a preemie developing a bacterial or fungal infection in the NICU is so high (about 40 percent of babies born under 28 weeks of gestation get one) that some neonatologists use antibiotics as a preventive measure. For instance, it is the policy in some NICUs to give antibiotics to all extremely premature babies who have a central intravenous line, to lower their risk of getting a bloodstream infection. Medical practice differs, however, depending on the rate of certain kinds of infections in a particular NICU and the judgment of the neonatologists working there, and on whether the benefits of preventive antibiotics outweigh their risks. You should feel free to ask your baby's doctor about the policy in your NICU and the reasons for it.

The value of preventive antibiotics is controversial for preemies, but if your baby has been diagnosed with an infection, antibiotics are the cornerstone of treatment. Preemies in particular have immature infection-fighting abilities and need the extra help that medicine provides. Your daughter's treatment may seem long to you, but her doctors must believe it is needed to completely eradicate the infection.

In an individual patient, antibiotics don't generally breed resistant organisms unless the same medication is taken intermittently over extended periods of time. While your preemie is in the hospital, any germ she's infected with will be tested to see which antibiotics are effective against it. If it's resistant to some, the doctors will choose another that works better.

Most antibiotics can be used safely in preemies. Their side effects are generally well known (most commonly, changes in kidney or liver function, loss of salts and minerals, changes in blood counts, and hearing problems). Doctors will monitor your baby for these effects and stop the medication or reduce its dosage if complications develop or safe blood levels are exceeded. With close monitoring, it's rare for any long-term damage from antibiotic treatment to occur.

Antibiotics may also temporarily alter the kinds of organisms that live peacefully within a baby's body. Since these organisms help with digestion and fight off other germs, some babies on antibiotics will get diarrhea or other infections. Allergies to antibiotics are almost never seen in preemies, so you don't need to worry about that.

Other infection-fighting therapies, such as an intravenous infusion of antibodies (like IVIG) to boost a baby's natural antibody levels, or treatment with medications to stimulate the production of infection-fighting white blood cells, may be used in special cases, such as for some viral infections or when a baby's blood counts are especially low. But antibiotics remain the primary life-saving weapons to fight premature babies' infections.

They aren't perfect, but they'll help keep your baby safe during this especially vulnerable time.

If Your Baby Is Put in Isolation

You've probably heard—and doctors are well aware—that some bacteria circulating in hospitals today have become resistant to common antibiotics. Among the most prevalent are certain strains of staphylococcus, or staph, that are resistant to penicillin and its modern relatives, methacillin and oxacillin. These strains are called MRSA (for methacillin resistant staphyloccus aureus) or ORSA (for oxicillin resistant staphylococcus aureus), two different names for the same thing. We'll use the term MRSA in our explanation that follows, but you can substitute ORSA if that's the name your doctors use.

A baby who has MRSA may be sick or may be perfectly fine and simply colonized, meaning the bacteria are living peacefully in him without causing problems. (Being colonized might sound like something out of a sci-fi film, but it couldn't be more normal. Researchers recently discovered that there are more bacteria than human cells populating all of our bodies.) Most colonized babies will never become sick from the MRSA they carry, although some will. MRSA can be more virulent than other kinds of staph infections, but fortunately it can usually be treated successfully with less common and more powerful, but still readily available, antibiotics.

When a premature baby is diagnosed with an antibiotic-resistant infection or is infected with any illness that is highly contagious, such as some viruses, his incubator may be moved to a separate room, isolated from all of his fellow little patients to try to prevent the spread of the germ. Nurses and doctors will wear gloves and gowns, and perhaps even masks over their noses and mouths, when they come into your baby's room to care for him. A glaring sign reading "Contact Precautions" may go up on his door.

It is very upsetting for parents who are already worried about their baby's illness to see him treated as a threat to others. The isolation is even more difficult to understand once the acute stage of the infection is over and concerns about your preemie's health subside. Why can't your baby come out of isolation now that he's doing fine? Must you still, after having had contact with him, avoid the other preemies and their parents? When is this going to end? And who is to blame for your child's illness: a nurse or a doctor? Perhaps even you?

Isolation can be a long haul, lasting a few days to several weeks or more, often beyond the time a baby's own health is threatened. That's because colonization can persist even after the infection has subsided. As long as a baby is colonized, he is able to spread the germ to others, who could become ill from it.

Most NICUs will want to see that your baby is free of the resistant or highly contagious germ before discontinuing contact precautions and taking him out of isolation. Usually this means testing him several times, a few days to a few weeks apart, to be certain the bacteria or virus is gone and he can no longer pass it to anyone else.

Since you have been touching and caring for your baby during the isolation, you and your other family members might have become colonized, as well. It's even possible that you had the bacteria or virus, unbeknownst to you, before your baby got sick. MRSA, for example, is now quite common in the general population. (But as you can imagine, it is not a welcome guest in a NICU, and once it's detected, doctors must do what they can to contain it or keep it out.) Try not to blame anyone—yourself or your baby's medical team—unjustifiably. It usually isn't possible to know who had a bacteria or virus first once it has been passed around, since many people can be healthy carriers.

It can be difficult—and sometimes impossible—to completely eradicate colonization with MRSA or other bacteria or viruses once the organism has gained a foothold. To do so, it may be necessary to treat not only your baby but your entire family

for a much longer time with different, powerful antibiotics—and this doesn't always work. Some doctors will consider trying (only after having asked for and obtained your opinion and consent), but others will advise against it, preferring just to keep your baby in isolation until he's ready to go home.

Once your baby is discharged from the hospital—healthier, with a more mature immune system, and no longer surrounded by preemies who can't adequately fight infection—there are usually no more precautions that need to be taken. Then you can finally start forgetting this disturbing part of your NICU experience.

Abnormal Thyroid Test

The health department said my baby's newborn thyroid test was abnormal. The doctors are checking it again. Is that serious?

Most probably your baby's abnormal test is just a temporary consequence of her immaturity, and nothing is really wrong with her thyroid. Transiently low thyroid levels are extremely common in preemies, occurring in all 23- to 25-weekers, more than a third of 26- to 29-weekers, and about 10 percent to 15 percent of 30- to 33-weekers. By the time a baby reaches about 34 weeks, thyroid levels tend to become normal spontaneously, without treatment. Chances are there's no need for you to worry.

Nevertheless, your baby's doctors will do another screening (and perhaps a third when she's four to six weeks old if her birth weight was less than 1,500 grams) to make sure that she doesn't have true hypothyroidism, which is more severe and long-lasting. Since adequate levels of thyroid hormone are important for the development of the brain, as well as skin, bones, and other tissues, a baby who is diagnosed with true hypothyroid-

ism will be given thyroid hormone replacement therapy immediately (in liquid or pill form) to prevent delays in her neurological development and growth. The sooner it's given, the better it works. But this problem is very rare.

To promote early diagnosis and prevent the worst consequence of a lack of thyroid hormone—mental retardation—a mass population screening was started in 1975, administered by each state's health department. Today, all newborns get a routine blood test for hypothyroidism within their first week of life in a program that, like immunizations, is considered one of the most successful efforts of preventive medicine. It has allowed thousands of kids to grow up completely normal by detecting their hypothyroidism early enough. Early blood screening is particularly important for preemies because many symptoms of hypothyroidism—such as an inability to keep up body temperature, poor feeding, constipation, prolonged jaundice, puffiness, and lethargy—are subtle and easily confused with common conditions of prematurity.

The temporary low thyroid readings that are often found in premature babies, however, are caused by factors that soon disappear.

(Continued on page 282)

False Alarms on Newborn Screens

Just like all newborns, your baby will be screened automatically for various medical conditions, such as hypothyroidism, PKU (phenylketonuria), sickle cell anemia, galactosemia, and others. (The diseases screened for vary by state.) Each test is potentially beneficial, but for a newborn preemie, it's also another opportunity for a false result. What causes inaccuracies in these tests? Here are some of the more common causes:

* Intravenous feedings with total parenteral nutrition can falsely elevate some substances in the blood;
* Not feeding the baby may mask some metabolism problems;
* Steroids given to the mother before the birth can temporarily alter the newborn's hormone levels;
* Stress the baby experiences after birth can temporarily alter hormone levels;
* Blood transfusions can mask genetic problems or blood diseases;
* Minor errors, such as collecting too much or too little blood for the test, collecting it too soon after birth, or even allowing the screen to sit for a few days in a hot mailbox, can affect the test's accuracy;
* Plain old immaturity, something every preemie has, can make almost any level abnormal.

Even if a preemie had a normal thyroid screen at birth, if she weighed less than 1,500 grams when she was born the test will be repeated when she's four to six weeks old because of a very small risk that she may have had a falsely normal test result. It is just a precaution, nothing you should worry about. Also, premature babies who had a blood transfusion before their first newborn screen will have the screen repeated four to six months after their last transfusion when all of the transfused blood is out of their system. The purpose is to detect and treat, as soon as possible, a blood disorder (such as sickle cell anemia) that may have been missed on the first screening test. You and your baby's pediatrician will get a reminder to do this from the state lab when it processes her newborn screen.

In general, if there's any suspicion of a false result on a newborn screen or if the original testing conditions weren't optimal, the solution is to repeat it (or if a quicker answer is needed, to order tests through the hospital's laboratory) when a preemie is older, healthier, eating, and several months after his last blood transfusion. Doctors are aware of this and will do it automatically if it's needed.

The most common, not surprisingly, is simple immaturity. The hypothalamus—the part of the brain that regulates the secretion of many hormones—operates at a lower level until it is fully mature. Sickness in a premature baby—whether RDS, lack of oxygen, infection, or hypoglycemia—can also cause an abnormal thyroid reading. These preemies aren't really hypothyroid, and their seeming disorder disappears by itself without treatment in a few weeks as they recover from their other medical problems.

There are other, less likely causes for a preemie to be hypothyroid. If a pregnant woman has a thyroid disorder, her illness or the medication she's taking to treat it can pass to her fetus during pregnancy. Its effects may linger for a while, show up as an abnormality of a newborn's thyroid screen, perhaps even cause some symptoms in her baby, and then go away. Iodine, found in antiseptics in many hospitals, can alter the functioning of the thyroid gland. When these antiseptics, such as Betadine, are used on the umbilical cord or to disinfect the skin before blood drawing or surgery, a preemie's immature skin can absorb too much iodine. But doctors are aware of this risk, and use iodine-containing products sparingly, if at all, in preemies.

It's hard not to feel threatened by any irregular test your baby may have, as you may fear a lifelong chronic condition. For premature infants, though, it is much more likely that your anxiety will be as fleeting as your baby's abnormal thyroid test.

How Much Time to Spend with Your Baby

I'm really torn about how much time my husband and I should spend with our daughter in the hospital. We both have jobs and an older son to take care of.

In all the research on premature babies there's none that can offer a simple answer to the question: How much time should parents spend in the NICU?

Yet even the most devoted parents of preemies grapple with this question, explicitly or implicitly, every day their baby is in the hospital. Some, like you, must strike a balance among conflicting obligations. Others live far from the hospital. Some just wonder how hard to push themselves against the natural limits of physical and emotional fatigue.

Most parents have an intuitive sense that their preemies need them during these stressful, difficult days, weeks, or months in the hospital—and they're right. There is plenty of evidence that being held, touched, and talked to by an affectionate caregiver are important spurs to any infant's emotional and cognitive development. It is known that some babies and children who are deprived of loving care for a long time can suffer from a disorder called failure to thrive: They don't grow normally, no matter how much they eat. And some children develop what psychologists call attachment disorder; having had no early experience of being comforted by one or a few, special caregivers, these children never develop the capacity to form trusting, affectionate relationships or to comfort themselves.

So it's critical that your baby get plenty of love as she grows. But plenty doesn't mean that you have to envelop her in your presence 24 hours a day while she's in the hospital. That would be wonderful, but isn't realistic for most parents. Fortunately, most preemies are hospitalized for only a few weeks or months, at a stage when nature didn't intend them to be attuned to receiving affectionate touches and loving gazes at all, but rather developing by themselves in the womb.

We sought advice from some professionals who think about these kinds of issues, and almost all delivered essentially the same message: Do all you can to maximize your time with your baby, but don't feel guilty or worry about the times you can't be there.

One expert in the field of developmental care, which studies the effect of the NICU experience on premature babies, says this: Your baby benefits from the time that you give. If you are free and can be with her all the time, and you're enjoying it, do it. (Just take care of yourself, you'll get tired.) If it's a real struggle for you to be there six hours a day, but you can be there for four hours, do that. If you can only get there for one hour a day, your baby will enjoy that hour. In a couple of years, will you be able to tell the difference? Probably not.

One reason, he explains, is that the normal attachment process between baby and parent takes place throughout the first year or two of life. When a preemie is hospitalized for only a few months, any disruption in the process is fleeting, and can easily be mended once the baby gets home.

A similar response comes from a psychologist who does research on attachment problems in adopted children who spent the first months or years of their lives in orphanages. He explains that babies who were deprived of a loving caregiver only before six months of age seem to recover completely. In fact, he suggests that if you can get only limited time off from your work and have the choice of taking it while your preemie is still in the hospital or after she gets home, you should seriously consider waiting.

A few other pieces of advice:

* **Using your time in the hospital well is as important as how much time you spend there.** A developmental care researcher recalls two mothers, one who lived far from the hospital and could only visit her preemie on weekends but lavished devoted attention on her baby while she was there, and another who

came daily but always with some girlfriends to whom she paid more attention than her baby. The first baby showed no signs of attachment problems later, while the second one did.

* **Time your visits so you're with your preemie for as many feedings as possible.** These are times when you can really interact, whether you simply give your baby the feel of your arms around her while she is gavaged or you give her your breast or a bottle.

* **Hold your baby as much as possible while you're with her and consider holding her skin-to-skin.** Many studies have found that parents who have early and ongoing physical contact with their babies—whether it starts with just the feel of a tiny, soft hand or snuggling up close—are likely to be more involved in caring for them later on, and loving touch is known to foster a baby's growth and development. You can read about the benefits of what's called kangaroo care, an intimate way of being with your preemie, on page 249.

* **If you are concerned that you and your partner can't visit your baby enough, enlist help.** A grandparent, aunt, uncle, godmother, or close friend whom you trust to be sensitive and responsive to your baby can help provide her with the human warmth she needs until she gets home. Some NICUs even have cuddlers (volunteers who spend time in the nursery holding babies whose parents can't be with them). Since it's best for your baby to become familiar with the people caring for her, encourage whomever you choose to visit her regularly. And let the nurses know whether you want them to consider your baby if a cuddler is available.

* **If you are spending a lot of your time at the hospital, take some breaks.** These aren't just for your sake, but for your preemie's, too. You aren't hurting her by taking care of yourself;

you're renewing your energy so you can be a better parent.

* **Don't feel guilty.** Whatever you're doing, it's the best you can. Preemies have intuition, too, and your baby knows that.

Whether to Go Back to Work

I always took for granted that I could be a mother and a working woman, but that was before having a premature baby. I don't know if I should go back to work as planned.

For some mothers, the choice is clear: they need to keep working for financial reasons, or want to because their career is so important to them. For other mothers, deciding whether to stay at home with their baby or go back to work can be agonizingly difficult.

It's not just mothers of premature babies who have these feelings. Leaving your newborn, even if she's big and healthy, is a difficult choice, no matter how much you cherish your career. Having a preemie, though, does involve some special considerations. When a preemie leaves the hospital, she may still be more difficult to care for than a term newborn (for instance, she may be fussier, have more feeding difficulties, or be on a cardio-respiratory monitor for weeks or months). That makes it harder for her parents to entrust her to a babysitter or to find daycare that can accommodate her needs. Some parents, who have to deal with the consequences of a medical complication, find their choices drastically limited. For instance, daycare is not advisable in the first year for a baby with BPD because she's more apt to get sick from infections (see page 413).

While it's impossible to give you advice about such a decision, which depends on your child's and family's circumstances and your personal priorities, there are a few things you may want to consider.

* **You may be eligible for a leave of absence from your job with the assurance that you can return to work after your leave is over.** The Family and Medical Leave Act requires employers with 50 or more employees to offer 12 weeks of unpaid leave related to pregnancy problems or childbirth. (If you're lucky enough to work for a company that offers some paid maternity leave, it may or may not count as part of the 12 weeks.) You are eligible if you have been working for your employer for 12 months, have worked at least 1,250 hours during the last year, and work in a location where your company has at least 50 employees. (Companies can claim exceptions for their highest-paid key employees.)

* **To ease the financial sting, you may also be eligible for disability payments for the first few weeks you don't work after your baby is born.** Ask about your employer's programs. Under state-run disability programs (only a few states have them), new mothers typically collect disability pay for six weeks after a vaginal delivery and eight weeks after a C-section.

* **If you will be taking just a temporary leave of absence from your job, you may find it more satisfying for you and your baby to postpone your leave until your baby comes home from the hospital.** Although it is hard to return to work when your baby is still small and fragile in the hospital nursery, you can be sure that she's well cared for there by her doctors and nurses. Moreover, young preemies who are still at an earlier stage of development don't need much stimulation. Taking time off after your baby is discharged instead will give you more leeway to get her home schedule well-organized and settled, and to find the best kind of child care for her before you go back to work. By the time she's home, your baby will be even more responsive and ready to get intimately acquainted with you.

✳ **For a working mother's complicated schedule to run smoothly, few surprises or extra burdens should disrupt her daily routine.** One thing to take into account is whether, because of your baby's medical needs, there will be more than the average number of bumps in the road. Consider how able and willing your partner is to pitch in when an unforeseen situation arises with your baby's health, and how flexible your schedule needs to be.

✳ **Remember that there are many good recipes for a happy family life and career, and what works well for another woman may not be best for you.** It may help ease your mind to know that researchers have been unable to establish whether children who are in daycare or at home with a baby-sitter are better or worse off than those who are at home with their mothers. Good quality child care—no matter who gives it—is what's most important.

✳ **Because there is often no single right answer to this question, it's rare for mothers to stop wondering and reevaluating, whatever decision they make.** Many shift gears later, and go through various phases in their lives as their feelings and child's needs change.

Parents Feeling Depressed

Now that I'm home from the hospital, I spend hours just sitting next to our daughter's empty bassinet, crying. Is this postpartum depression?

The baby blues can hit any mother a few days after delivery. Many new mothers may feel happy one moment, then suddenly find themselves crying by their baby's bassinet, as you do, even when the baby is in it!

Most new mothers—and a few fathers to a lesser degree—experience some blues in the first week or two after their baby's birth. In addition to causing floods of tears, the baby blues can make you feel anxious, fatigued, unable to concentrate or make decisions, and easily irritated. Loss of appetite and difficulty falling asleep are also common. In mothers, these mood swings are partly due to hormonal changes. But stress also plays an important role, as parents realize the full extent of their new responsibilities and make adjustments to settle into their parental roles. Sleepless nights don't help, either.

Most cultures recognize that some emotional and practical upheaval will occur after delivery and try to provide for that. British midwives talk about the ten-day weepies. In China, new mothers are never left alone in the first month and families are constantly helped in their daily chores. In the United States and many European countries, it's traditional for grandparents to visit for extended periods of time after a baby is born if they don't live nearby.

For parents of preemies, the huge stress of having a premature baby heightens and complicates the normal reactions after birth, sometimes causing emotional upheaval to be more serious and last longer. Several studies have found that in the month after delivery, parents of preemies are significantly more depressed and anxious than parents of term babies. One study reported that by a month after delivery, 13 percent of mothers whose babies weighed 1,500 grams or less suffered from serious psychological distress, compared with just 1 percent of mothers of babies born at term. Besides depression and anxiety, they were more apt to feel hostile, guilty, and incompetent at parenting and to isolate themselves socially. Less severe signs of psychological stress were found in up to one-third of the mothers. Such emotional reactions are more frequent in mothers whose preemies are at high risk for medical complications, but even mothers of big, relatively healthy preemies may experience them.

Another study found that 85 percent of mothers and 65 percent of fathers of extremely premature babies experienced crisis reactions in the week after delivery, consisting of disbelief, anger, guilt, sadness, and sometimes uncontrollable crying. An early delivery is itself so scary that even many parents of healthy preemies react with shock and anxiety. No wonder. While a preemie is in the hospital nursery, his parents suffer from worry about him, being separated from him, fear of what the future might bring, and the difficult struggle to adapt to an intimidating environment.

Although you may continue to feel worried and stressed during your baby's hospitalization (riding what many parents have described as the rollercoaster of a preemie's first weeks), your feelings of crisis should soon subside. Mothers of premature infants begin to regain their emotional balance in the first weeks and months after birth, and by the end of the baby's first year, their psychological distress, on average, has been found to be similar to those of mothers of term babies. (When premature children continue to be at high risk for long-term health problems, their mothers understandably are more likely to report moderate symptoms of depression and anxiety for longer. In one study, 24 percent were still depressed after two years, compared with 10 percent of term mothers. But by the end of the child's third year of life, almost all mothers of preemies have adapted well to their situation, showing a strong attachment to their children and satisfaction with their parenting experience.)

While most parents of preemies find that they're gradually adjusting to their situation, some mothers go on to develop a real postpartum depression. The risk factors for postpartum depression are a family history of it, severe premenstrual syndrome (PMS), or a previous psychiatric illness. It can evolve from the baby blues or strike at any time in the first year. Because stress also plays a large role in its development, fathers can get postpartum depression, too.

A deep sense of anxiety or depressed mood

that persists longer than a few weeks and is severe and debilitating is what distinguishes significant postpartum depression from normal baby (or preemie) blues. Feelings of helplessness or hopelessness, loss of self-esteem with guilt and self-accusation, poor appetite, and an inability to sleep, even when you are tired, are some of the common symptoms of depression. In addition, postpartum depression may be signaled by reactions such as:

* extreme irritability, with explosions of hostility and anger;
* feeling confused, with a progressive inability to organize even easy things (such as making a shopping list);
* unnatural agitation and excitement;
* violent thoughts or actions directed toward yourself, your family, or your baby;
* recurring suicidal thoughts.

In some parents, the depression passes on its own in a few months; in others, if untreated, the changes in personality and behavior can last for years.

What can you do if you think you may be experiencing a postpartum depression? First of all, you should accept that any emotional reactions you're having are a normal consequence of what you're going through and not feel guilty or shameful about them. Second, you should try to talk about your discomfort to the people who love you (your partner, your family, your friends). Many people find solace by seeking out religious counselors—hospital chaplains or their priest or rabbi—who can offer spiritual guidance. If your friends and family or your religion do not accept postpartum depression as a serious illness that needs to be treated, please seek the advice of a physician or mental health professional (a psychiatrist, psychologist, or social worker) immediately, before you get into danger—and even if you have a good personal support system, talk to a professional after about a month, or sooner if your symptoms are severe, to make sure you get counseling, antidepressant medications, or hormonal supplements if you need them.

Here's something encouraging for you to know. While parents of preemies suffer more from stress reactions, and particularly from depression, during their baby's hospitalization, by about a month after their baby has come home, parents of preemies actually handle day-to-day stress and overwork better than parents of term infants of the same age. This may be because they adjust faster to the reality of their baby's needs (perhaps having imagined them to be greater than they actually are), while parents of term infants find that their newborns need more care and attention then they'd expected. Also, despite the pain of separation, a preemie's stay in the hospital has one positive effect: Mothers have more time to recover physically, and have usually recouped their strength by the time their babies come home.

So take heart: parents of preemies do regain their emotional balance, as other new parents do, just a little more slowly sometimes, depending on their children's health. In fact, although it may seem like small consolation now, once your baby comes home, this painful experience is likely to make you appreciate him and the happiness he brings you even more.

Your Baby Is Still on a Ventilator

My daughter is still on a ventilator, and even though the doctor tells me that she's making good progress, there have been several times when he lowered her vent settings and then had to raise them again. The way it's going, I'm afraid she'll never be able to breathe on her own.

It almost never happens that babies need to be on ventilators for the rest of their lives, and it's rare for a preemie to be on one for longer than a few months. Especially since your baby's doctor feels that she is making good progress (and even if her progress were to stall or backtrack for a while), there's no reason to believe she'll be any different. So you shouldn't worry about that.

That's the rational answer. On an emotional level, we empathize with your fear. All parents wait for that moment when their baby is free of the ventilator, reassuring them that she can accomplish the vital act of breathing independently. No matter how long your baby has been on a ventilator, it can be extremely frustrating—even agonizing—when the doctor is trying to wean her from it and it's not going smoothly.

You should certainly talk to your baby's doctor and tell him about your anxieties. Most parents have a few fears which the doctors aren't even aware of and often can dispel quite quickly. In this situation, they will probably tell you that weaning from the ventilator often involves taking two steps forward and one step back. There are times when it might involve taking one step forward and one step back, or sometimes, unfortunately, even two steps back. One thing that's universally true: it always takes longer than parents want.

If your baby seems to be having trouble coming off the ventilator, there could be many reasons why. Your baby's doctor can tell you whether any of the following common reasons apply to her.

* **Simple prematurity.** Some babies who are extremely young and small just need more time. The reason is that a very tiny baby's lungs haven't yet developed enough to breathe efficiently, and her chest wall and respiratory muscles are still weak. When she breathes, her chest wall may be sucked in deeply, compressing and deflating her lungs too much. Without enough of the old air left in them, her lungs can't remain open and ready to expand

for the new air to come in, and it may take more strength than she has to keep breathing deeply and regularly. Many babies have to reach an adjusted age of 26 weeks gestation or more before they overcome this problem. Very young babies also may need a few weeks for their respiratory drive to mature if apnea is keeping them on the vent.

* **Lung damage.** Unfortunately, those valuable lifesavers—ventilators and extra oxygen—are double-edged swords. At high levels, they can interfere with lung development and cause some lung damage themselves. Babies who develop lung damage from the ventilator and oxygen need time to heal. Once your baby's oxygen and vent settings are not so high, as long as she's getting good nutrition to grow new lung tissue, the healing will outstrip any injury they're causing. (In general, oxygen concentration is considered high when it's more than about 60 percent. It's more complicated to determine what counts as a high vent setting, since that varies with the size and age of the baby. You can ask your baby's doctor to help you understand how much respiratory support your baby is getting.) Sometimes the doctor can push the weaning from the vent along by giving a baby steroids; but since steroids can have serious side effects, no one wants to use them unless it's absolutely necessary. If the doctor tells you that your baby has BPD (lung damage that persists for more than a month or so), you can read about it on page 293—but many preemies' lungs will heal before then.

* **Problems in the airways.** Airways are the pathways through which air travels on its way into and out of the lungs. Starting at the nose and mouth, and including the throat, trachea, and large and small bronchi branching deeply into the lungs, they conduct air to the areas of the lungs where oxygen is taken in and carbon dioxide is moved out of the body. A problem in the airways can make a ventilator necessary, even though the rest of your baby's lungs work just fine. There are a few possible airway problems, including malacia, in which the airways are too soft and floppy, collapsing rather than remaining open as a baby breathes (most preemies simply need extra time for their cartilage to stiffen up); an obstruction inside the airways, such as swelling or scar tissue from the endotracheal tube (if the baby is still small, she may grow out of this as her airways get bigger and the obstruction becomes relatively smaller, or it might be removed surgically); and, least common, an anatomical abnormality that compresses the airways from the outside, such as a cyst or abnormal blood vessel (which may be able to be surgically corrected or outgrown). The doctor can check for these problems by doing a bronchoscopy, which you can read about on page 291, or an X-ray called an upper GI study, described on page 274.

* **A new wrinkle in the baby's health.** Sometimes just when a baby is breathing better and her ventilator settings are steadily going down, something happens to weaken her medical condition—an infection, surgery, aspiration of some vomit, a PDA, or some other complication. In that case, the doctors must fix the problem—and start the weaning process again.

We know it's easier said than done, but the most important advice we have for you is to try to be patient. Weaning a baby from a ventilator is really a matter of trial and error; doctors don't have an exact way to tell when a baby's lungs are ready to function on their own. It's not really a setback when your baby's ventilator settings are lowered then raised again—it's just that the doctor was guessing that your baby was ready, and it turned out to be a little too early. She'll come off the vent in her own good time—showing us parents once again that children will determine their own schedule, thank you!

Steroids

My baby is having a lot of trouble breathing, so the doctor has talked to us about trying steroids. Isn't that dangerous?

You're right that steroids are powerful drugs with serious side effects. You can be assured that the decision to give them to preemies is never taken lightly. As with any drug, it's always a matter of weighing the risks and the benefits—and in this case, because the risks are especially momentous, your baby's doctor is probably encouraging you to be a partner in the decision. We'll tell you a little about both the pros and the cons so you'll have an idea of the kinds of things you'll want to take into consideration.

Just so there's no misunderstanding, you should know that your doctor is talking about a different kind of steroid from the drugs used by athletes to enhance their performance. (Although he *is* hoping to enhance your baby's breathing performance.) Your baby probably has severe BPD or is beginning to develop it, and has been on a ventilator for a while. With steroids, the doctor is hoping to dampen your baby's immune response, thereby cutting down on inflammation— the body's reaction to an injury, germ, or irritant. This can be a big boon to a preemie on a ventilator. Since the ventilator always causes at least some injury to the lungs, it's very common for a preemie's lungs to become inflamed. The same is true for his trachea and vocal cords, which tend to be irritated by the endotracheal tube. They may swell, secrete a lot of mucus, and over time become scarred. This inflammation in the lungs and airways makes it harder for a baby to breathe, sometimes causing him to need extremely high ventilator settings or keeping him

dependent on the ventilator for many weeks or months.

Preemies with BPD are thought to have an even stronger than usual inflammatory response, possibly from being exposed to bacteria in the womb (because their mother had an infection like chorioamnionitis, for example), because their immune system is not well regulated (usually due to immaturity), or because a strong inflammatory response is just in their genetic makeup.

That's why steroids often work quickly and dramatically: A baby's need for oxygen may go way down within a day or two, and he starts weaning from the vent. Not every preemie with breathing problems responds to steroids, but in general, they've been found to lower the incidence of BPD, reduce ventilator settings, and lead to earlier extubation from the vent. Giving steroids to preemies right before they're extubated (when their lungs are believed to be ready to breathe on their own) also minimizes the chance that they'll land right back on the vent simply because of swelling in their airways. And steroids have even saved some babies' lives.

Certainly you want your baby to come off the vent as soon as possible—and to soon be snuggling in your arms—but what about the risks? One major short-term risk is that a baby's immune response will be suppressed so much that he'll be more prone to getting infections. Another is that a small number of preemies—from 2 percent to 20 percent in various research studies—develop a tear in their intestine that requires urgent surgery to repair. Babies on steroids often have a jump in blood sugar or blood pressure, but doctors will watch carefully for these problems to catch and treat them before they become serious. It's also common for a baby to grow more slowly while he's getting steroids, and although he will catch up later, it's not clear whether this period of slow growth has any lasting effects on the baby's health.

What is of gravest concern, though, is that

steroids have been identified as a factor in some of the serious developmental problems that some preemies later have. For example, in one study of preemies treated with the steroid dexamethasone, the babies' chances of survival increased, but 40 percent later had major disabilities (cerebral palsy and mental retardation), compared with 20 percent of those who did not receive dexamethasone. Researchers say the results make sense: It's known that steroids interfere with brain development in animals, and one study reported that on MRI scans, premature babies who were treated with dexamethasone had substantially smaller brains.

It's important to understand that we are talking here about a specific steroid, dexamethasone, that is typically given to preemies intravenously for a few weeks to improve their BPD. Other steroids, used in other ways for other purposes, may not carry the same risks. For instance, you may have gotten steroids before your preemie's birth to boost the maturity of his lungs. This one-day or two-day treatment with a different steroid, beclomethasone, is known to be extremely safe. A shorter course of dexamethasone—only three doses—given to some babies just before they come off a ventilator to keep their airways from swelling, is also thought to be safe, although the long-term effects have not been studied. The same goes for hydrocortisone, a steroid that is often used to raise preemies' blood pressure. It is believed to be safer than dexamethasone, but more long-term research is needed.

When side effects are of particular concern, as they are, say, for babies with severe BPD who may benefit from being on steroids for many weeks, steroids can be inhaled rather than taken intravenously. The hope is that they'll suppress inflammation in a baby's lungs without affecting the rest of his body. But steroids given this way aren't as powerful and may take a week or two rather than a day or two to work. They don't seem to increase a preemie's risk of infection but may slow his growth, just as intravenous steroids do. Long-term studies haven't been done to tell us definitively whether they are safer than steroids taken intravenously.

Also keep in mind that research is ongoing to find ways to reduce the risks of giving steroids to preemies with BPD. Many doctors believe there are probably safe ways to give them—perhaps different kinds of steroids, lower doses, or different timing of treatment. Or the key may be identifying those few babies who need them the most. Severe BPD itself can cause developmental problems, so treating only babies who would otherwise go on to develop severe BPD with steroids could, on balance, improve rather than worsen their long-term development, as well as save some of their lives. Perhaps by the time you are reading this, more will be known, so don't hesitate to ask your doctor about this.

If you do decide to try steroids, the doctor will watch closely to see how your baby responds. If she thinks your baby is not benefiting from them, she'll stop them within a matter of days. If your baby does get a lot better on steroids, the question will be when to take him off. The doctor may stop them after a few days, pleased that they helped lower the ventilator settings and oxygen to safer levels, or she may taper them off slowly over a longer time. A shorter course of steroids will cut down on side effects but may not provide as many benefits.

It's hard to imagine a more excruciating dilemma for parents whose baby is struggling to breathe and survive. When providing a potentially life-saving medication also means possibly hurting your baby's chances of developing normally, what can one do or think? Above all, it's important for you to know that there is no clear right or wrong answer. For many parents, this is a time of reaching deep down inside themselves, of reflecting on their most profound values.

(*Continued on page 292*)

Bronchoscopy: A Peek Inside Your Baby's Lungs

Say that your baby is really having trouble weaning off the ventilator—not just by your measure, since all parents get understandably anxious and think a normal time frame for weaning is way too long. If your baby has come off and gone back on the vent three or four times, has tried steroids, the doctor is hearing sounds that could indicate an obstruction of the upper airways, or some areas of his lungs aren't clearing up on X-rays, and the reasons aren't apparent, then it's time to find out why things aren't going according to plan.

One way to do that is with a procedure called a bronchoscopy. A long tube or "scope" with a fiberoptic viewer on it is passed through the vocal cords, down the trachea, and into the bronchi (the large airways of the lungs). The specialist who does the procedure simply looks around to see what's going on that may be making breathing more difficult. She may also take cultures of lung fluid and samples of the cells in the airways.

Some of the things your baby's doctor might be wondering: Is there scar tissue from the endotracheal tube, or some other mass or cyst that's causing an obstruction? Is there a condition called malacia in which the baby's airways are soft and collapsing, and need time for the cartilage to stiffen up to hold them open whenever he takes a breath? Is there an infection so deep in the lungs that it didn't get cultured through normal sampling? Is there inflammation from reflux, caused by aspiration of milk or formula? A bronchoscopy can often answer those questions and provide information needed to guide future treatment.

There are two kinds of bronchoscopies: flexible and rigid. A flexible bronchoscopy, usually done by a pulmonologist (a lung doctor), is often the first choice because it can be done right in the nursery with the baby lightly sedated but awake. It usually takes about 30 minutes and isn't very comfortable, but your baby will be given some local anesthetic—a little spray in the back of his throat—and intravenous sedation to make sure it isn't painful. If your baby is on a ventilator and his endotracheal tube is big enough, he may not even need to be extubated; the bronchoscope will be passed right through it and he'll breathe around it. One of the reasons this technique is preferred is that the pulmonologist can see the baby's airways at work as he breathes and can tell whether or not there's malacia.

If the endotracheal tube is too small for the scope to fit through, or if the baby isn't stable enough to be extubated during the procedure or to breathe well around the scope, then a rigid bronchoscopy can be done. This procedure is usually performed by a surgeon in an operating room with the baby under general anesthesia. Your baby can be ventilated through this bigger scope and kept physiologically stable for the duration of the procedure. The doctor won't be able to diagnose malacia (since a baby's airways aren't moving naturally while he's under general anesthesia), but she can look deep inside the airways for inflammation or obstruction and collect samples of fluid and cells to culture for infection. During a rigid bronchoscopy, if an obstruction is found the surgeon is sometimes able to remove it right then and there.

A bronchoscopy of either kind can cause some discomfort afterwards, but not for very long. Sensitive babies may need sedative medication for a few hours, but others are fine as soon as it's over, or just need a little Tylenol. And when the scope sheds light on your baby's lungs, it also sheds valuable light on what steps to take next in his treatment.

Some parents feel that their child's life is worth preserving at all costs; others feel that it is more important to protect their child from a serious risk of major disabilities. If you are uncertain—as so many parents are—you may want to talk to your most trusted advisers, or the hospital social worker or chaplain, to help you come to a decision with which you can feel at peace, whatever outcome it brings. And feeling at peace with a heartfelt decision is exactly what loving parents should do.

ET Tube Accidentally Pulled Out

My baby is always trying to pull out his ventilator tube, and yesterday he finally succeeded. Is there any possibility he's going to hurt himself?

Very little. You'd be surprised how common it is for babies to pull out their own endotracheal, or ET, tubes or for the tubes to slip out accidentally. Accidental extubations (the technical term for removal of the tube from the windpipe) can happen simply because the tape near the baby's mouth that holds the tube in place gets wet from saliva and comes loose. Or in some of the younger babies, just because the windpipe is tiny, and there's a very small distance between the right and the wrong position. Bigger, stronger babies who are able to turn their heads or pull on the tube when it's bothering them—a mature act of coordination for a preemie!—are the ones who are most likely to extubate themselves.

Although there are some risks from accidental extubations, and the NICU staff tries hard to prevent them, the chance that they'll cause a significant problem is very small. In an intensive care unit, nurses are always within a few steps of every bed. If there is a decline in a baby's heart rate or oxygen levels, an alarm will sound and within seconds a nurse will start giving him puffs of air or oxygen. (An oxygen bag or puffer is usually kept at every bedside for this purpose.) This will nearly always keep the baby breathing well enough until his tube is reinserted. The reinsertion itself is sometimes accompanied by complications like bradycardia, but that rarely lasts more than a few seconds—not long enough to be damaging.

If your baby was eating, his feedings may be stopped for a few hours as he resettles himself. A chest X-ray may be taken to make sure the tube is back in the right position. The worst part of the episode, usually, is that it's a bit uncomfortable for the baby when his tube is reinserted if there's no time for the doctors to give him a little pain medication beforehand. Some babies may develop hoarseness or swelling around their vocal cords, from repeated intubations. These are almost always temporary.

If your baby pulls out his endotracheal tube more than a few times, his doctor may try inserting it through his nose rather than his mouth. This can be done only on bigger preemies (the nostrils of littler ones are too small for the tube), and the procedure is a little harder and slower, but the tube will be more stable. The doctor may also consider restraining a baby's movements, prescribing sedatives, or using measures such as swaddling, nesting, or cutting down on exciting stimuli such as light, sounds, and touch, since a calm baby is less likely to extubate himself.

(*Continued on page 298*)

In Plain Language: What Is BPD?

When a premature baby who had respiratory distress syndrome at birth is still on a ventilator several weeks later, doctors usually suspect he has developed chronic lung disease, or BPD (bronchopulmonary dysplasia). This means that the very life-saving assistance he has required—supplemental oxygen and mechanical ventilation—has damaged his delicate lungs and impaired their natural development or healing. BPD is a catch-22: a baby is dependent on respiratory assistance, but this assistance is exactly what prevents his lungs from recovering.

The medical answer to this dilemma is a slow process of gradual weaning from respiratory aids, along with good nutrition, possibly medication, and a lot of care and attention to help the baby's lungs grow and heal.

Thankfully, many cases of BPD resolve in just a few more weeks. But it can take longer. Some babies go home on supplemental oxygen. Parents should know, though, that the most severe forms of BPD are rare. The majority of premature babies recover from it, in time, without serious long-term consequences.

What babies are at risk for BPD

Without neonatal intensive care, BPD wouldn't even exist. It's a mixed blessing: BPD occurs because preemies who were born too young to breathe on their own are now surviving.

The earlier a preemie is born, the more immature his lungs and the higher his risk is for BPD. Besides immature lungs, any other medical condition that causes preemies to require mechanical ventilation and supplemental oxygen at high levels or for longer than a few days (such as pneumonia or prolonged apnea) increases their risk of developing BPD.

Researchers now believe that some babies are genetically more susceptible to BPD than others—the same way some adults are more prone to, say, obesity or high blood pressure than their friends. Also thought to be at greater risk are preemies who were exposed to bacteria in the womb (because their mother had an infection such as chorioamnionitis, for example): They may have a stronger than usual inflammatory response—the body's defense mechanism against infection and injury—and get more swelling and irritation in their lungs when they're on a ventilator or supplemental oxygen.

Therapies that can speed up the development of the lungs and make respiratory distress syndrome less serious (such as steroids administered to an expectant mother before a premature delivery, surfactant, and good intravenous nutrition) have helped lower the risk of BPD. Giving vitamin A shots to very young preemies and treating apnea with caffeine have also been shown to help. Doctors have also become better at limiting damage to the lungs by carefully monitoring preemies' oxygen levels and minimizing the settings of the ventilator (overstretching the lungs, in particular, seems to be harmful, and the initial use of a high-frequency ventilator in some instances may be helpful). But the high rate of BPD in the youngest infants (around 40 percent or more for those weighing less than 1,000 grams at birth) is the price they pay for a very good chance of surviving RDS and the other complications of prematurity. It's a reason for worrying, but also for rejoicing.

What can happen in a preemie's lungs

Initially, a preemie who is born before his lungs are mature has RDS (respiratory distress syndrome), which injures his lungs by causing inflammation. The inflammation makes breathing even more difficult, so oxygen and a ventilator are often needed to support the baby's respiration.

Meanwhile, lung cells near the injury try to repair the damage by quickly multiplying and differentiating. But the normal development of the lung and the healing process are disturbed by the force of the ventilator and the extra oxygen the baby is getting. (A preemie's fragile tissues aren't able to withstand a lot of stretching and strong pressure from the ventilator, as it pushes air into the lungs. And oxygen is particularly toxic to the immature lungs of preemies, because they're deficient in the natural antioxidants that protect the body from the damaging effects of oxygen's free radicals.)

In some babies with BPD, the normal development of the lungs abruptly comes to a halt. Later, their lungs grow bigger but with fewer air sacs than usual and less branching of the airways. Thus there is less surface area in the lungs to absorb the oxygen the baby needs. In other preemies, usually ones who were born older, the problem is more one of damage: As new lung cells grow and become injured, patches of useless scar tissue form throughout the lungs, disrupting their normal functioning. This is also why BPD is called dysplasia, meaning abnormal tissue growth.

How and when BPD is diagnosed

If after the first week of life a preemie's need for respiratory support is increasing instead of going down, he may be developing BPD. A chest X-ray will show haziness or scarring in his lungs. The diagnosis is confirmed if he's still on oxygen by four weeks after birth or by 36 weeks after conception, when his lungs are expected to be mature enough for him to breathe on his own. (The latter criterion—oxygen at 36 weeks after conception—is more accurate for babies born at less than 30 weeks gestation and is better at predicting which babies will go on to have long-term respiratory problems.) Babies with BPD tend to breathe faster and harder than normal. They may become short of breath or wheeze from too much fluid seeping into their lungs, because their airways have become soft and collapsible, or from a tightening of their airways, similar to asthma.

Like any illness, a baby's BPD can be mild, moderate, or severe, depending on how bad his symptoms are and how much respiratory support he needs. If a preemie is still on a ventilator or CPAP, or still needs more than 30 percent oxygen by the time he's eight weeks old or 36 weeks corrected age (whichever comes later), then most neonatologists would consider him to have severe BPD.

What preemies need to overcome BPD

For their lungs to heal, preemies with BPD need attentive, supportive care in the hospital nursery. Although each of the following therapies is used to treat BPD, not all babies benefit equally from them, and some have more risky side effects than others. Your baby's doctor will recommend treatments she thinks will help, and you should feel free to ask questions and participate in decisions about which ones to use:

✳ **Nutrition.** Preemies with BPD need to eat more than other babies because they use up more energy breathing, and the extra calories and nutrients are crucial for building healthy new lung tissue. Along with keeping damage to a minimum, nutrition is the key to overcoming BPD. Good nutrition is sometimes difficult to achieve, though. If a baby's fluid intake needs to be restricted, his breast milk or formula may be densely concentrated, making it harder to digest. Intravenous nutrition, which most preemies need for a while, is not as wholesome as breast milk or formula. And sometimes starting to nipple feed is difficult and frustrating for a preemie with BPD, because a baby who has been on a ventilator for a long time may not have had a chance to practice sucking and may associate touch around his mouth with negative sensations from the endotracheal tube. For all of these reasons, preemies with BPD are often smaller than other premature babies and may continue to get tube feedings to bolster the calories they take in themselves. But as they recover from BPD, they can experience remarkable catch-up growth.

* **Pulmonary hygiene.** Suctioning can help prevent obstruction of a baby's airways by mucus and secretions and keep small areas of his lungs from collapsing.

* **Fluid management.** It's common for fluid to build up in the lungs of preemies with BPD, which can interfere with their breathing. So doctors may restrict the amount of fluid a preemie gets intravenously or in his feedings.

* **Medications.** Diuretics (medicines that increase urination) can reduce fluid in the lungs, bronchodilators can open the airways, and steroids can reduce inflammation, easing weaning from oxygen or the ventilator.

* **Treatment of exacerbating conditions**

  - If your baby has a PDA, his doctors will consider whether closing it might help decrease excess fluid in his lungs.

  - If he has pneumonia or any other infection, it will be treated to reduce reliance on a ventilator or oxygen.

  - If your baby has anemia, correcting it could improve his blood's ability to deliver oxygen throughout his body.

  - If he has pulmonary hypertension (high blood pressure in his lungs), his doctors will try to bring it down by temporarily keeping his oxygen saturation levels higher and maybe giving him medication. Reducing blood pressure in the lungs will ease some of his heart's workload, keeping it healthier.

  - If malacia (meaning the lung's airways are too soft and collapsing) is contributing to your baby's breathing problems, his doctors may avoid bronchodilators because they could make his airways even floppier. Your baby may need CPAP or high flow oxygen for some months, while he outgrows the problem.

  - The medical staff will try to prevent reflux and aspiration since they can increase airway tightening and lung inflammation.

* **Developmental Care.** Some preemies with BPD are very sensitive to overstimulation, and are easily stressed by bright lights, noises, and touch. Reducing overstimulation may be especially helpful for babies with BPD because stress can lead to oxygen desaturation, airway tightening, and higher blood pressure in the lungs—all of which can worsen BPD. You'll find suggestions for reducing stress in NICU—guidelines for developmental care—on page 229.

The usual course that BPD takes

Caring for a baby with BPD is a patient process of trial and error whose goal is to keep a preemie stable while gradually weaning him from the ventilator and oxygen. The doctor finds the right pace for reducing respiratory support by closely monitoring blood gases, oxygen levels, and the baby's comfort. The time frame will vary, depending on the severity of a baby's lung injuries. It most often takes several weeks but can stretch to months. Rarely, a baby with BPD will need supplemental oxygen for several years.

Most preemies with BPD are able to inflate their lungs by themselves before they can maintain good oxygenation, so they come off the ventilator first and oxygen later. Some are treated with CPAP or high flow oxygen through a nasal cannula for a while to help keep their airways open as they make the transition from the ventilator to breathing on their own.

At various times in the process, the doctors may decide to try different kinds of ventilators, or switch modes on the same ventilator, to find what works best for your baby. It's not always easy to predict, and finding the best way to support a baby with BPD is often a matter of trial and error. Also, the best solution can vary over time as a preemie grows or circumstances change (if he gets an infection or needs surgery, for example).

One thing you may notice is that the doctors are satisfied if your baby's oxygen saturation level is somewhere between 85 percent and 95 percent. Don't be surprised, even if it goes against your instincts, which are to push for 100 percent. Aiming lower avoids exposing him unnecessarily to excessive vent settings and oxygen, which can be damaging. Once your baby recovers enough to breathe room air, you'll see that his oxygen saturation levels will gradually rise naturally on their own until they're close to 100 percent.

On the other hand, if your baby has severe BPD, the doctors might decide that he needs higher oxygen saturation levels—in the mid to high 90's. That's because babies with severe BPD can develop high blood pressure in their lungs (called pulmonary hypertension). Pumping against high pressure puts a strain on the heart, which can be very serious or even fatal if it's not corrected. Often, simply raising a baby's oxygen saturation levels lowers the blood pressure in his lungs and protects his heart. (The trade-off is that the extra oxygen may make his BPD worse.)

A baby who has pulmonary hypertension may also be treated with medications like sildenafil or nitric oxide, which can lower blood pressure in the lungs. A baby can continue taking sildenafil at home—it's an oral medication—but there are no long-term studies yet to say how safe it is. To check for signs of cor pulmonale—this particular kind of heart strain—preemies with severe BPD are usually monitored every month or so with an ultrasound of their heart or an EKG. Fortunately, despite their BPD, most preemies' hearts remain healthy.

Since intubated babies can't eat by mouth and must be kept from moving too much so that they don't accidentally dislodge the endotracheal tube, prolonged intubation threatens a preemie's ability to grow and develop normally. There is a surgical procedure called a tracheostomy, in which a breathing tube is inserted directly into the trachea, which will allow a baby to move more freely, interact with his environment, and use his mouth, tongue, and face to express himself. You can read more about it on page 362. A tracheostomy is usually considered if a baby is approaching his due date and it looks like he'll still need a ventilator for at least a few months more. It can be temporary, though, and doesn't prevent a baby from eventually coming off a vent.

Fortunately, most babies with BPD get well quickly enough to go home shortly after their due date breathing completely on their own. But even babies who are still on oxygen are usually able to go home with their families. By the end of their second year of life, and often well before then, nearly every baby with BPD leaves supplemental oxygen behind.

Some parents have to be especially strong before arriving at that happy ending because a few families, whose babies have severe BPD go through very hard times in the hospital. Parenting a baby with severe BPD in the NICU can be difficult, and at especially bad moments things may feel like they are spiraling out of control. Please don't be scared: you're going to overcome these moments. But you may feel better if you know that certain patterns of behavior are typical of babies with BPD, and they'll be outgrown as your baby's breathing improves.

Some babies with BPD have sudden episodes when their oxygen saturation and heart rate suddenly plummet (they "desat and brady") and they don't respond right away when a nurse gives them more oxygen and extra breaths. These episodes (sometimes called BPD spells) are thought to be caused by an abrupt increase in blood pressure in the lungs or a sudden narrowing of the airways. If this has ever happened to your baby, you know how terrifying it can be. Occasionally a baby who has come off the ventilator will have to go back on because of a bad BPD spell. Unfortunately, until a baby's BPD improves considerably, these frightening episodes may occasionally recur. When they finally end and are behind you, the relief and comfort is enormous. (You're not alone if it takes some time for you to really believe it and relax.)

Another challenge for babies with the most severe BPD is that they can become so agitated by their struggles to breathe that they become oversensitive and react negatively to even the gentlest stimulation. Their parents' attempts to soothe and console them (even by simply holding them) may stress them more. Some severely affected babies have episodes of frantic restlessness followed by periods of exhaustion. Depleted of energy, they may become lethargic, sleeping a lot or appearing depressed and unresponsive, even in their mothers' or fathers' presence. There's noth-

ing more frustrating or painful for a parent than being unable to comfort and interact with your child. It's normal to feel devastated, resigned, and angry when you can't seem to make any difference in your child's life. But the answer is not to disconnect from your baby: just imagine that you've been put on hold for a while by a disturbance on the line. Try to remain strong, go often to see him in the hospital, stand by him. Slowly you'll notice a two-way communication developing. You'll see that your love will be acknowledged by your baby and amplified.

How babies do after BPD, in the long run

Despite the fact that babies who get BPD are often the youngest and sickest preemies, about 80 percent of them survive and recover. A baby's prognosis will vary a lot depending on whether his BPD is mild or severe.

If your baby has mild BPD, chances are that he'll be breathing completely on his own by the time he goes home.

For those with more severe BPD, the first year or two of life can be more difficult, but families should take heart, because things are likely to improve. Babies with moderate BPD may go home on oxygen but usually come off within a few months. You'll find some guidelines for caring for your baby at home on page 383. They're important to keep in mind because preemies with BPD (and especially severe BPD) are more likely to get respiratory viruses and ear infections in their infancy. Respiratory infections may become serious, and a baby might need to be rehospitalized. Parents should be aware of this possibility, and seek medical attention if their baby starts to have more difficulty breathing.

Preemies who had BPD are also more susceptible to coughing and wheezing during childhood, and shouldn't be exposed to cigarette smoke or other airborne irritants, such as chemicals in home cleansers. Most commonly these symptoms gradually subside and by young adulthood are often mild or gone. Children who had BPD may have smaller lung capacity, too, with less ability to exercise strenuously. But this usually doesn't prevent them from running, playing, and living normal, active lives—and many probably don't even notice it.

BPD is frequently accompanied by other complications of prematurity. It can prolong a baby's hospital course and slow his weight gain and body and brain growth at a crucial time. Still, the majority of preemies with BPD go on to develop normally, although some will have developmental delays. (Lasting delays are seen mostly in preemies with severe BPD who were on a ventilator for longer than two months in the NICU.)

When there are lasting developmental problems after BPD, they may be motor problems (disorders like cerebral palsy, involving uncoordinated or abnormal movements) or cognitive problems (including mental retardation or learning difficulties), although these long term de-velopmental problems are more closely related to whether a child, in addition to BPD, had an intraventricular hemorrhage or periventricular leukomalacia. Also keep in mind that cognitive ability is greatly influenced by environmental factors (such as the parents' educational level, socio-economic status, and attentiveness to the child). This means that parents who provide a nurturing and stimulating environment can improve their baby's chances.

To be the best parents of a child who is recovering from BPD, you'll need to acknowledge the huge emotional load you carry: the trauma of a premature birth, prolonged anxiety from a long and complicated hospitalization, and possibly, worry about what the future may bring. If your baby is still recovering when he goes home with you, practical problems may add to your distress, making it difficult to resume a normal lifestyle for a while. Be sure to get any help you may need, emotional or physical, because the support you get will put your baby's interests on top, too. Gradually you will heal together, as your baby thrives on your love and attention and you thrive on his.

Every once in a while, some good comes from an unplanned extubation. The doctors may discover that your baby can breathe on his own better than they expected, and he may be allowed to stay off the ventilator. Also, babies who are reintubated get the benefit of a cleaner endotracheal tube, and sometimes a larger one that may provide better airflow, sooner than the doctors might have made the switch otherwise.

By the way, some neonatal nurses claim they can tell a lot about a preemie's personality from the start, and they'd say you've got a feisty little guy on your hands. Over the next few months and years, you'll find out whether they're right!

Hoarse Voice

I was so eager to hear my baby's voice, but now that she's off the ventilator, she sounds as hoarse as Louis Armstrong.

Imagine that great American jazz musician and your teensy preemie having something in common! Actually, it's typical for babies who have been on ventilators to have hoarse or weak cries when they come off; their vocal cords get slightly irritated and swollen by the endotracheal tube, and it usually takes several days for them to return to normal. Preemies who have been intubated for a long time (several weeks or more) may not recover their full vocal powers for a couple of weeks.

There's a very small chance of more damage to the vocal cords, so if your baby's voice doesn't sound normal after a couple of weeks, her doctor will investigate whether the vocal cords are moving as they should be. But given how unlikely that is, you really shouldn't worry about it now. Instead, try just to relax and wait for your baby to demonstrate her first full-volume clear cries. Eventually you may look back wistfully on this brief period when her fussing was still easy on your ears.

High Blood Pressure

My baby has high blood pressure. Why would a little baby have that, and how serious is it?

Most people associate high blood pressure with middle-aged men and women who are getting a little chubby around the waist. But this condition affects skinny preemies, too—though for different reasons.

Just as in adults, blood pressure fluctuates, so your baby's medical team won't get concerned about an abnormal reading here and there. Hypertension doesn't tend to cause problems unless it's extreme or goes on for a long time—many weeks or months—so it's rarely an urgent issue. (The exception is a very young preemie in the first week or so of life who could have an intraventricular hemorrhage if her blood pressure gets too high.) Over time, however, high blood pressure can damage blood vessels and organs, such as the kidney, heart, and eye, so your baby's doctors will want to monitor it and, if it remains consistently high, treat it. The doctors will also try to determine the reason for the elevation and attempt to fix that underlying condition if they can. Even if a cause can't be found

(which happens fairly often), the good news is that blood pressure can be lowered very effectively with medications. Most of the time it will then gradually go away on its own over several months.

You should know that what counts as high blood pressure in a preemie is very different from what counts as high blood pressure in an adult, so don't be surprised if the numbers sound low to you. The numbers that are considered normal increase as a child gets older, so your baby's doctor may have to look at a chart to determine whether your preemie's readings are elevated for her age and size. Even then, the doctor may need to use her judgment because norms for the smallest and youngest preemies aren't well worked out yet.

What might cause blood pressure to be too high in a baby in the NICU? The most common reason is simply agitation or discomfort. Most often, the hypertension will go away when the baby calms down; in that case, the doctors won't even consider the high blood pressure readings to be significant. If they persist even when she's quiet, though, it may be that she needs more pain medication—or if she's being weaned from a pain medication she's received for a long time, that her dose shouldn't be lowered quite as rapidly.

Babies with persistently high blood pressure will get a kidney ultrasound because the kidney, believe it or not, plays a major role in regulating blood pressure. The doctors will make sure that the kidneys have formed normally and are draining properly. They may also check for a kidney infection; if your baby has one, treating it with antibiotics may solve the problem. Sometimes in babies who have had umbilical artery catheters, a small blood clot or area of inflammation forms in the artery leading to the kidney and causes hypertension. This is treated by removing the catheter, if it's still in place, and giving the baby medication to treat the high blood pressure while her body takes care of eliminating the clot or easing the inflammation all by itself. It usually takes several weeks to resolve. (Additional therapy to remove a clot is rarely necessary.)

Severe hydrocephalus (a buildup of fluid in the brain that can occur in preemies after an intraventricular hemorrhage) can cause high blood pressure, but once the extra fluid is removed, the problem should disappear. If a baby is taking steroids, they can elevate her blood pressure; the solution may be to lower the dose, or just treat the hypertension until she comes off steroids. And babies who have severe BPD can get high blood pressure. In this case, the hypertension lasts longer, but as the BPD gets better it should gradually go away.

Not infrequently, after considering all of these possibilities, doctors still have trouble figuring out the cause of the hypertension. But fortunately, serious persistent causes are rare in preemies. So try not to be too concerned. Chances are that your baby's blood pressure will soon be back down and you won't have to worry about it again until she's middle-aged and chubby around the waist.

Eye Exam

My baby's going to have her eye test tomorrow, and I couldn't be more anxious about it. I know vision problems are very common in preemies.

Many people associate prematurity with vision problems. Even though it's true that this is a possible complication of a premature birth, it's probably less common than you think.

The eye condition that affects premature babies is called retinopathy of prematurity, or ROP for short. It's explained in detail on page 301, but you don't need to read that unless your baby's eye exam tomorrow reveals that she has it.

Here's all you need to know right now. Fortunately, these days most preemies who get ROP

have a mild form that goes away completely on its own. There was a tragic epidemic of ROP in premature babies in the 1950s, which is probably why the problem became so well known. But that was a long time ago, and it was caused by giving preemies high concentrations of oxygen without regard to how much they actually needed—a practice that has long since been abandoned. Now that neonatologists know that excessive oxygen can damage a preemie's retinas, premature babies are given only as much oxygen as they need to keep their blood oxygen saturation (which is continuously monitored) within an acceptable range.

The eye exam, done by an ophthalmologist at your baby's bedside, will be quick and cause only mild discomfort. About an hour before, your baby will be given eye drops to enlarge her pupils so the back of her eyes will be more visible. Just before the exam starts, most ophthalmologists give another set of anesthetic drops so she won't feel pain. (Some nurseries use other soothing techniques, also, to help babies get through the exam comfortably. Don't hesitate to ask in advance whether your baby can have a pacifier dipped in sugar water or one of the other special comfort aids for preemies that are described on pages 118–120.)

Your baby's eyelids will be held open with a clip and the corners of her eye pressed gently with a small flat rod (which looks a lot worse than it feels) because that's the safest and most accurate way to do the exam. Some babies don't seem to mind, while others make it clear that they don't like having their eyelids held open or having someone shine a bright light at them. The ophthalmologist will look all the way into the back of your baby's eyes, using a medical instrument called an indirect ophthalmoscope, to see whether her retina's blood vessels are growing normally. After it's over, the ophthalmologist can tell your baby's doctor the results immediately.

(*Continued on page 306*)

In Plain Language: What Is Retinopathy of Prematurity?

Once a premature baby's eyes open—usually by 26 weeks of gestation—she can see, though very fuzzily. Over the next several weeks, she'll gradually become able to focus on objects around her, and eventually you'll notice her staring with fascination at your beloved face. It will take until a couple of months past her due date for her to begin looking around and enjoying the sights. Her visual abilities will mature as she does. So it should come as no surprise that inside, her eyes are still developing, too.

Beginning at around 16 weeks of gestation, the retina (the lining inside the back of the eye that senses light and forms images) starts to develop a network of blood vessels. This intricate web initially forms near the center of the retina, at the very back of the eye, as blood vessels grow outward from the optic nerve. Gradually the blood vessels spread toward the periphery of the retina, eventually covering its surface. By around the time of a full-term birth, their growth is complete.

These blood vessels, which supply the retina with oxygen, sometimes don't grow as planned after a premature birth. They are supposed to spread from areas of high oxygen (in other words, where they already are), into areas of low oxygen (where they haven't formed yet). But once the baby is born, the signals directing blood vessel growth can become confused or disrupted by the extra oxygen she is getting (even oxygen from the air), episodes of low oxygen (because of RDS or apnea, for example), and numerous other differences between the womb and the world. Errant signals may initially halt blood vessel growth or even lead to new growth that is dangerous, with vessels growing in the wrong direction, away from the retinal surface rather than along it and toward

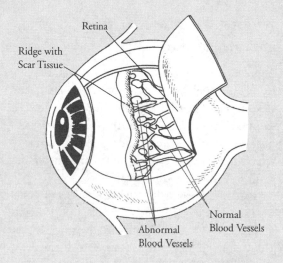

In ROP, new abnormal blood vessels grow at the edge of the normal blood vessels supplying the retina and can form a ridge of scar tissue that may pull on the retina and damage it.

Adapted with permission from *Understanding Retinopathy of Prematurity*. IRIS Medical Instruments, Inc., a subsidiary of IRIDEX Corporation 1996

its edges. These abnormal vessels can slow or stop the development of normal ones, sometimes leading to distortion of the retina or even causing the retina to lift away and detach from the back wall of the eye.

The possibility of vision problems arouses great fear, and many parents feel terrified and distraught when doctors diagnose ROP in their baby. But the wonderful fact is that most cases of ROP—roughly 90 percent, by some estimates—cure themselves spontaneously. Within a few months, milder cases of ROP resolve as the retinal blood vessels resume a normal growth pattern and complete their development, leaving most babies with good vision. An additional group of babies will need treatment but can avoid serious damage with its help. In most cases, even babies with severe ROP will end up with useful—and often even good—vision.

Why some babies get ROP and others don't

A great many premature babies never develop ROP. As usual, it's the youngest, smallest, and sickest preemies who are at greatest risk. ROP is so uncommon in babies born after 32 weeks of gestation that it is not even standard practice to screen these preemies for it unless they had a difficult or complicated medical course.

Preemies born at less than 28 weeks of gestation are the ones who are mainly at risk. Roughly 45 percent of babies with a birth weight between 1,000 and 1,250 grams, 75 percent of those between 750 and 1,000 grams, and 90 percent of those less than 750 grams develop some ROP. While these numbers sound high, keep in mind that the vast majority of these babies will outgrow the condition with minimal or no harm done by the time they're three or four months past their due date.

Doctors still don't know the exact cause of retinopathy of prematurity. They learned the hard way, from an ROP epidemic in the 1950s, that too much oxygen is one major factor. At that time, premature babies were often given oxygen whether or not they had breathing problems, and after a while it became apparent that those who were given high concentrations of oxygen were developing ROP in especially large numbers. Research suggests that preemies who are on high levels of supplemental oxygen for a prolonged period of time, and possibly those who have a lot of wide swings in their blood oxygen levels—from very low to very high—are particularly prone to ROP. Today, doctors are able to measure oxygen levels in the blood more precisely and give babies only as much oxygen as they need. The risk of

ROP is kept as low as possible without harming the baby's medical stability.

Although some research has suggested that bright or fluorescent lights in the NICU may contribute to the development of retinopathy of prematurity, reducing light exposure in clinical trials (in one large study, by having preemies wear goggles for at least their first month of life) doesn't seem to decrease the incidence of ROP.

Other possible risk factors that need further study include intrauterine growth restriction and chronic inadequate oxygen during pregnancy; poor weight gain after birth; intraventricular hemorrhage; apnea; anemia; blood transfusions; infection; use of medications such as indomethacin, erythropoietin, or steroids; respiratory distress syndrome; high levels of carbon dioxide in the blood; seizures; and vitamin deficiencies. It's not clear yet whether these factors have an independent effect on ROP or whether they're just another indication that smaller, sicker babies are at greater risk.

Twins, triplets, and other multiples are no more likely to develop ROP than single babies born at the same gestational age and weight. Boys and girls seem to be at equal risk, but black babies are at less risk than babies from other racial groups. Some research indicates that preemies who receive surfactant after birth are less likely to develop ROP. There's also some evidence, although it's not considered conclusive, that treatment of vitamin E deficiency may be helpful, and vitamins are routinely given to preemies in the NICU.

Diagnosis: The eye exam

Most NICUs have regular screening programs for ROP: All babies who fall under a certain gestational age or birth weight—usually 30 weeks and 1,500 grams—as well as older and bigger babies who have needed a lot of breathing support or had other medical complications—get routine eye exams before they leave the hospital. The timing varies, but the first exam is typically scheduled about four to six weeks after delivery.

The timing of the next, follow-up exam may be anywhere from a few days to a few weeks later, depending on a baby's risk for ROP or if she has it, its severity. Once the blood vessels in her retina have finished growing, she won't need any more exams for ROP. (Later on, all preemies, whether they had ROP or not, will get at least one eye exam in their first year of life to check for nearsightedness, lazy eye, and crossed eyes, problems that are more common in preemies, especially those who had ROP, than in term babies.)

How ROP is classified

When ROP occurs, it is usually in both eyes, but it may be more severe in one eye than the other. If your baby's ophthalmologist does see some sign of retinopathy on the exam, he'll describe it using four criteria:

The stage of the ROP conveys how mild or severe it is. It describes the condition of the retina at the border between where the blood vessels have already grown (called the vascularized retina) and where they are still trying to go (called the avascular—meaning lacking blood vessels—retina). Although retinopathy of prematurity is a progressive disease—it starts at Stage 1 and may keep going through Stages 4 or 5—it doesn't always progress, and may stop at any earlier stage and disappear entirely. Here are the official definitions of the various stages of ROP:

* **No ROP—Stage 0.** The blood vessels are growing normally so far, but they have not yet completed their development to cover the whole retina.

* **Mild—Stage 1.** When ROP is only at Stage 1, the eye doctor sees a white demarcation line where blood vessel growth has temporarily halted, separating the normally developed retina (the vascularized retina) from the undeveloped retina (the avascular retina).
* **Mild—Stage 2.** The demarcation line has been replaced by a ridge of tissue.
* **Moderate to severe—Stage 3.** The ridge has gotten bigger, and new abnormal blood vessels have formed, extending upward away from the surface of the retina toward the front of the eye. (When these are just starting to form, they are often referred to as "popcorn" because of the way they look: round and discrete. If the ROP keeps progressing, these popcorn merge together and attach to the ridge, becoming Stage 3.)
* **Severe—Stage 4.** There is pulling on the retina due to the abnormal blood vessels, causing it to partially detach. Since some of the retina is still attached, vision remains possible. Surgery to reattach the retina is usually recommended.
* **Severe—Stage 5.** There is pulling on the retina due to the abnormal blood vessels, causing it to totally detach. A baby with a complete retinal detachment cannot see at all or sees light only. Surgery to reattach the retina can sometimes restore some vision.

The zone or location of the ROP indicates where it is happening in the eye. Zone III (where the blood vessels form last, around the edges of the retina) is of least concern, followed by Zone II (the section next closest in), followed by Zone I (in the center of the retina, where the vessels first start to form and the clearest "bull's eye" vision is located).

The extent of the ROP describes how large an area is involved. It's measured in the number of hours on an imaginary clock. If you picture the baby's eye as the face of a clock, and there is retinopathy between, say, 12:00 and 4:00, then the extent of the baby's ROP is four clock hours.

The presence of "plus disease" means that the blood vessels in the center of the retina, near the optic nerve, are especially dilated and tortuous, wiggly rather than straight. Plus disease indicates that the ROP is severe and is expected to progress rapidly, with a high risk of retinal detachment.

APROP (Aggressive Posterior ROP) is a severe form of ROP that involves extensive plus disease and doesn't progress through the usual stages. It often leads to retinal detachment.

Doctors can convey a lot about a baby's ROP using this shorthand classification. For example, ROP that is Stage 3, Zone I with plus disease is severe enough to require treatment, while ROP that is Stage 1, Zone III will almost always disappear on its own.

Every baby with ROP must have carefully timed follow-up exams until the ROP disappears. Even if your baby has already been discharged from the hospital, it's extremely important not to miss these follow-up appointments, since early treatment can make all the difference for your baby's eyesight.

Modern tools to fight ROP: Laser therapy and cryotherapy

Since most cases of ROP cure themselves spontaneously, there is good reason to hope that the need for treatment will never arise for your baby. In deciding whether to treat your baby or just follow his eyes closely, the ophthalmologist will consider how severe the ROP is, how close it is to the central portion of the retina that's most important for vision, and how likely it is to progress. Most ophthalmologists recommend treating ROP

in Zone I (which is near the center of the retina) at any stage of severity if there is plus disease (so, likely to progress rapidly), but simply following it closely if there's no plus disease and the ROP is only Stage 1 or 2 (mild). When ROP is in Zone II, ophthalmologists usually treat it only if it has progressed to Stage 2 or 3 *and* there's plus disease. And ROP in Zone III is very rarely treated.

We're very lucky today. Forty years ago, no treatment for ROP was available. Then a procedure called cryotherapy was developed, which involved freezing the undeveloped, peripheral retina to make the abnormal blood vessels shrink. In a large research trial, cryotherapy cut the risk that severe ROP would progress to retinal detachment in half, from 43 percent to 21 percent, establishing cryotherapy as the first effective eye treatment for ROP.

More recently, another large study helped determine the best time to treat severe ROP, this time using laser treatment, which has been used for over two decades to treat eye disorders in adults and is now state-of-the-art for babies, too. Today most babies have the benefit of receiving this more modern treatment, which is at least as effective as cryotherapy and far less uncomfortable for the baby. It works in a similar way: tiny patches of the undeveloped peripheral retina are targeted, helping to arrest the growth of abnormal blood vessels and scar tissue and reducing the chance of retinal detachment and blindness from ROP.

Laser therapy is often performed right in the nursery. With the same type of instrument the ophthalmologist uses to examine your baby's eyes, he can deliver a laser beam through the pupil directly to the retina. Your baby will get pain medication (which will also keep her relaxed and quiet) and maybe another medication to keep her from moving at all during the procedure. Babies who are placed on a ventilator just for the treatment can usually come off it as soon as it's over.

If your baby needs surgery

In a few babies, the retinopathy of prematurity keeps progressing, even after laser therapy. If it reaches Stage 4 or Stage 5, the eye doctor generally recommends surgery to reattach the retina. There are two surgical options, which are discussed on page 360. (If your baby has APROP her treatment may vary, since treatment for it is still evolving and some promising new approaches are being studied.)

With surgery, too, early treatment is the key to the best possible outcome for your baby. So please forgive the repetition, but once your baby is diagnosed with ROP, don't miss those follow-up exams. It's even a good idea to ask your baby's nurse or doctor when the next eye exam is scheduled so that you can help keep track of the date in case your baby is transferred to another medical team or to another hospital.

What you can expect in the long run

The long-term effect of ROP on a baby's vision depends on whether the illness caused permanent injury to the eye.

The body's response to mild ROP is a testament to self-healing. If the ROP regresses and disappears without treatment, the eye most often grows and develops normally. Thus babies who had Stage 1 or 2, and even many with Stage 3 retinopathy of prematurity that didn't require treatment, usually have normal, or nearly normal, vision, or can see well with glasses. By the time your baby is 6 to 12 months old, if no serious problem from her ROP has been identified, you'll be able to relax—there probably won't be one.

Babies who had Stage 3 retinopathy of prematurity that did require laser treatment can also have good or very useful vision, although most will need glasses for various degrees of nearsightedness.

In more than 90 percent of all cases, ROP never reaches Stage 4 or Stage 5, involving partial or complete detachment of the retina. But even if it does, if the retina is only partially detached, depending on where the detachment is, there's a chance that a baby will have useful vision after surgery. After complete detachment of the retina, although some vision may be recovered through surgery, it's likely that the baby's ability to see with the affected eye will be very severely impaired.

In general, babies who had retinopathy of prematurity are more likely to be nearsighted than other preemies. Strabismus (crossed eyes) and amblyopia (lazy eye) are also more common in premature babies who had ROP. Since both problems are usually treatable—with eye muscle surgery for strabismus and eye patches and glasses for amblyopia—all premature babies who had ROP are followed carefully during their first few years of life.

In a very small number of cases, complications may show up later. Glaucoma and late-onset retinal detachment have been reported in a few teenagers or young adults who had ROP as babies. (Luckily, the prognosis is far better than when retinal detachments occur in infants.) For this reason, all children who had severe ROP should continue to have retinal exams annually throughout adolescence and young adulthood.

Retinopathy of prematurity has long been one of the most feared complications of a premature birth. But just remember, even if your baby develops it, the odds that she will emerge with good vision are high.

Some nurseries—especially smaller ones without a pediatric ophthalmologist on staff—are using a new technique for the eye exam, in which a nurse or neonatologist takes digital photographs of the baby's retina. A special camera system analyzes the retina's appearance and sends the images and data to a pediatric ophthalmologist who can read them from a distance. In detecting moderate or severe ROP that needs treatment, digital photography appears to be just as effective as a traditional eye exam and can save a baby from having to travel to another hospital to be examined. There's one drawback: The photographic technique doesn't visualize the periphery of the retina quite as well, so it can miss some mild ROP or be less reliable in telling when a baby's retina is fully mature (when the risk period for ROP is over). But what's most important is knowing whether or not your baby needs treatment.

After the exam, don't be surprised if your baby has a big tummy for a few hours or doesn't tolerate her next feeding. That is a fleeting result of the medicine in the dilating drops, which can slow down the movement of gas and food in a baby's gut. She may also have more A's and B's and desats if she doesn't like to be stimulated. The drops will make her very sensitive to light, so she may be more comfortable if you keep her isolette covered with a blanket for a few hours afterward.

Your daughter will probably have more than one eye exam, since premature babies get follow-up exams until the blood vessels in their eyes have finished growing (usually around their due date), or to monitor their ROP if they have it. The timing of your baby's follow-up exams will depend on her risk for ROP or its severity. Most of the time, preemies in the NICU are examined every one to two weeks, beginning four to six weeks after birth.

After your daughter's retina is mature and the ophthalmologist tells you she's no longer at risk for ROP, she'll be scheduled for a follow-up exam when she's around six months of age. This later exam is to make sure she's not developing some other less serious kinds of eye problems that preemies can get, primarily crossed eyes or lazy eye. All preemies are at increased risk of these, but especially those who had ROP. Fortunately, therapy for these conditions is very effective if they're found and treated early.

Just remember, if your baby was born after 28 weeks of gestation the chances of her having problems from ROP are small, and even in younger, sicker babies, who are most likely to develop ROP, the majority end up with good vision. So try to put this particular problem out of your mind for now. The chances are that you're worrying unnecessarily.

Hearing Exam

My baby failed his first hearing test. We're devastated, but the doctor says there's a good chance his hearing will be normal. How can that be?

It's definitely too soon for you to worry. You can't imagine how many false scares there are on preemies' first hearing tests—lots of them. Parents are understandably terrified by the results, only to find out later that their baby has perfectly normal hearing.

The hearing tests done on newborns are actually hearing screens, designed to be overly inclusive so they don't miss any babies with hearing problems. It's only if a baby has difficulty in a later, more definitive hearing test that he'll be diagnosed with a true hearing impairment—far fewer than the number who fail the newborn screens.

Here are some of the reasons that a preemie may falsely fail his hearing screen:

* The room may have been too noisy;
* Ear wax (or if the test was performed within a few days after delivery, amniotic fluid or

vernix) may have been blocking the baby's ear canal;

* The baby may have been crying, fussy, or wiggly;
* The baby may have had an ear infection or some other medical problem, like jaundice, that temporarily affected his hearing;
* The baby may have an immature, narrow ear canal that is too small for accurate testing;
* The baby's brain may still be immature (not a surprise, in a preemie!).

If you notice that your baby startles in response to sudden loud noises and sometimes seems to be listening to the sound of your voice, then a severe hearing problem is unlikely, although he could still have a milder impairment. Even if you don't notice these things, that's not necessarily a bad sign. Because a preemie's hearing may not be fully developed yet (see page 151), what may seem like a loud sound to you may not be to your baby. And even if he is disturbed or stressed by a noise, his reaction might not be immediately clear to you, because preemies don't always react to sounds the same way full-term babies do. For instance, instead of startling, he may lose muscle tone or close his eyes.

In any case, your baby will get his hearing tested again in a few days or weeks, either in the nursery if he's still in the hospital or as an outpatient if he's gone home. If he passes, you can relax. But even if his screen is abnormal a second time, he may still be just fine. One study found that around a quarter of preemies in the NICU temporarily had increased fluid in their middle ear that did cause mild hearing problems, but they were just transient. Most of these resolved on their own within a few weeks when the excess fluid went away. Your baby will be scheduled for a definitive hearing test when he's around three months of age and you'll know more then.

Organizations like the National Institutes of Health and the American Academy of Pediatrics advocate (and most states now mandate) that all newborn babies get screened for hearing loss, because early detection and intervention, ideally before six months of age, is crucial for a child to learn how to understand and use spoken language. Preterm babies are usually screened in a slightly different way than healthy term newborns because they're more prone to a particular kind of hearing loss, caused by damage to the nerves that are responsible for sensing and processing sounds.

The main risk factors for hearing problems in a preemie are:

* birth weight under 1,500 grams;
* occurrence of an intraventricular hemorrhage;
* the presence of a viral infection at birth;
* meningitis;
* extended use of certain medications;
* very high bilirubin levels;
* lack of oxygen around the time of birth or need for respiratory support in the NICU;
* abnormalities of the ear, head, or neck.

While these factors increase a preemie's risk, still only about two out of 100 premature babies will have a significant hearing impairment.

A preemie's hearing screen, usually done right in the nursery in his own bed, only takes about 15 minutes, doesn't hurt at all, and is harmless. Called an ABR (for auditory brain response), it involves giving him a set of earphones and placing a few little electrodes attached to pads on his head, with paste to hold them on. Alternatively, a small probe may be placed in his ear. Clicking sounds are delivered into the baby's ears and his brain waves are recorded. The recording is either interpreted by a computer or reviewed by an audiologist (a specialist in hearing problems), who compares it with a normal pattern.

When a baby does turn out to have a hearing problem, you can be sure it will be followed carefully, since early detection and treatment is a tremendous advantage. At the appropriate time, usually around three to six months corrected age, the baby may get a hearing aid, and he and his family will start working with a communication specialist. Later, if his hearing loss is severe and caused by nerve damage, he may get a cochlear implant. The success of cochlear implants is quite astounding: 80 percent of children have their hearing ability substantially restored. But try not to think about all of this yet, since it's still unlikely you'll have to.

Anemia

My baby's doctor wants to give her shots three times a week so she won't get anemic. Is that worth it? Will it work?

Your baby's doctor is probably talking about giving her erythropoietin (or "epo"), a hormone that stimulates the production of red blood cells. All infants become anemic (meaning they develop a shortage of red blood cells) in their first two to three months of life because a newborn's natural secretion of epo temporarily falls, causing a slowdown in the creation of new red blood cells. She gradually becomes more anemic until her red blood cells reach a low enough level to switch the secretion of erythropoietin back on.

It's a natural cycle that doesn't cause any problems in most full-term newborns and a lot of preemies. Your baby's doctor will monitor her hemoglobin (the substance in red blood cells that carries oxygen) and hematocrit (the concentration of red blood cells in her blood) to make sure they don't fall too low—and may also check something called a reticulocyte count (a measure of newly made red blood cells) to see that she starts producing new red blood cells when she should.

But the natural cycle is more pronounced and lasts longer in preemies (especially younger ones,

with birth weights under about 1,500 grams). That's because small preemies grow very rapidly and need to make a lot more blood to keep up with their increasing body size. At the same time, their red blood cells are depleted by frequent blood draws, and their levels of erythropoietin are lower than in term babies. In fact, this early anemia is so universal that it has been dubbed anemia of prematurity.

In some premature infants, the anemia becomes serious enough to affect their medical condition. Since red blood cells transport the oxygen that the body's organs and tissues need to function and grow, anemia may prolong a baby's reliance on supplemental oxygen and may aggravate cardiac problems since the heart has to work harder to distribute oxygen. Very anemic preemies also tend to be less energetic, eat less and gain less weight, and may have more apnea. Sick babies are most likely to have trouble when they're anemic.

In the past, blood transfusions were the only answer. Even today, a premature baby who suddenly develops anemia and is sick will need one or more blood transfusions, the only fast-acting effective treatment. But blood carries a small risk of infection. Thanks to bioengineering, babies like yours now have the option of getting laboratory-produced erythropoietin to try to prevent severe anemia of prematurity in advance.

The medication is given to a baby one to three times a week, intravenously or as a shot, for about six weeks or until she reaches 36 weeks of gestation. Epo takes a week or two to work, and has been shown to reduce the need for future blood transfusions. While it's painful to think of your tiny baby getting shots, this one doesn't hurt much at all. So far there are no known serious risks or side effects, although epo hasn't been available long enough to see how the babies who got it are faring in adulthood. There is a question whether it might increase the risk of the eye disease called ROP (retinopathy of prematurity), but studies thus far have not found a definitive link.

Since production of red blood cells requires iron, a preemie who goes on epo also needs to take iron supplements, which are usually given orally or may be put in your baby's intravenous nutrition (TPN). Since iron can upset the stomach, it may worsen feeding intolerance, so babies aren't usually started on epo until they are stable and tolerating most of their breast milk or formula feedings. Some babies who take iron have dark green or black stools and may get a little constipated. Don't be scared: the color might be weird, but it's harmless. The doctor will make sure your baby has adequate levels of protein and vitamins when he's on epo, too.

Which is better for your baby, epo or a blood transfusion? There are pros and cons to both. One thing your doctor will consider is whether your baby has already had a transfusion and could get more blood from the same donor. In that case, without exposure to a new blood donor, the risks would be so low that a transfusion might be preferable. On the other hand, if a transfusion would mean exposing your baby to a new blood donor, the balance might tilt toward epo. Either way, you can feel confident that your baby will be getting an effective treatment for her anemia.

Heart Murmur

The doctor told me they just discovered my baby has a heart murmur. Not something serious again! How could they not have found it before?

Your baby is in good company. It's not uncommon for preemies to have a heart murmur suddenly appear at a few weeks of age, and it usually indicates something that's harmless or merely needs to be followed for a while. Heart murmurs that arise from serious problems usually show up within the first week of life. If your baby happens

to have had an echocardiogram (perhaps because the doctors were checking to see if she had a PDA) and you already know that her heart is normally formed, there is even less reason to worry. If your baby hasn't had an "echo" yet, she might get one now, or the doctors may wait for a few days or weeks to see whether the murmur persists. (Harmless ones can come and go, whereas serious murmurs last.)

Anything new that comes up at this point, just when you were beginning to be more optimistic that your baby was out of the woods, can feel like a terrible blow. But most of the time, late-appearing heart murmurs in preemies are due to something called peripheral pulmonic stenosis (PPS). That's a fancy name for nothing of consequence; it means that the blood flow through some small and sharply bent blood vessels to the lungs is turbulent, causing a swishing sound. Doctors don't know why it suddenly appears in some premature babies who are a few weeks old (perhaps the vessels change shape or position as the baby grows), but preemies just grow out of it, and it doesn't cause any problems.

Other possible reasons for the murmur are less common. One is a PDA (a fetal blood vessel that failed to close) that the doctors haven't noticed before, either because it hasn't caused any symptoms or didn't show up on an earlier echocardiogram. (A PDA can partially close and then reopen. There's a full description of PDAs on page 203.)

If a PDA is the cause of your baby's murmur, it may in a sense be good news. If your baby is doing well, the PDA isn't affecting her much, so the doctors may not even treat it. They'll probably just watch to see if it closes by itself or causes any problems in the future. On the other hand, if your baby is still on a ventilator, the doctors might think that her PDA is a contributing cause. If a PDA is making it more difficult for a preemie to recover from respiratory distress syndrome, after it's fixed she could get better. And you might have the red flag raised by the murmur to thank.

Other possible causes of a late heart murmur are a little hole in the heart, which often closes on its own, or a tight or leaky valve, which is almost always noticed earlier if it's a serious problem. For either of these it's the same situation as for a PDA: If your baby is doing well, she probably won't even be treated. If she's been having difficulties, this discovery may be the key to her treatment and recovery.

Finally, the murmur could be caused by other, usually innocent things (for example, anemia, a tiny extra blood vessel, or just the way your baby's heart is positioned in her chest) or by something the doctors may never discover because it won't cause your baby any problems. Consider it the special sound of your preemie's heart.

Hernia

I thought men got hernias from lifting things that were too heavy. Why in the world does my preemie have one?

Hernias are very common in premature babies—not surprisingly, if you consider how they occur. An inguinal (meaning in the groin area) hernia forms when a loop of intestine—or occasionally, in girls, an ovary—slides down into the groin from the abdomen through a canal that's open in the fetus but normally closes during the last few weeks of gestation. Because premature babies are born when that canal is usually still open or only partially closed, a rise in pressure inside their abdomen from crying, straining to have a bowel movement, or just breathing hard can cause a hernia. On average, 15 in 100 preemies develop a hernia, compared with only one in 100 term infants. The likelihood is greatest for those preemies who were younger and smaller when they were born or who have chronic lung disease. Premature babies who have a VP shunt are also

more likely to develop a hernia because of the accumulation of fluid and increased pressure the shunt creates in their abdomen. And, in general, preemie boys are more likely to get a hernia than girls.

An inguinal hernia usually shows up as a swelling in the groin, extending down into the scrotum in boys and into the labia in girls. It may be on only one side or on both. It will get bigger and smaller at times, depending on whether your baby is crying or calm, for instance, and as the size of the intestine in it changes. It may even disappear temporarily, but once a hernia forms, it won't go away completely unless it is repaired surgically.

Your baby's doctors and nurses will watch his hernia closely to make sure it remains soft and pliable. If the intestine goes back and forth from his groin (where you can see it) to his abdomen (where you can't) by itself or when you gently press on it (doctors call this reducing a hernia), that's a good sign.

But if the hernia becomes hard, purple, or the loop of the intestine can't be pressed back into his abdomen, the doctors will worry that the intestine is trapped, or incarcerated. An incarcerated hernia is an emergency because it can quickly lead to some dangerous complications. One is a reduction in blood flow to that part of intestine or any other organs in the hernia sac, such as the testicle or the ovary, which could permanently damage them. An intestinal obstruction or life-threatening infection can also occur.

To avoid the risk of incarceration, your baby will need surgery fairly soon. But you shouldn't worry too much about that. A hernia repair is a very straightforward and safe procedure (see page 370). Since so many preemies get hernias, it is the most common surgery performed on small babies. And such frequent practice makes for excellent surgical results.

Because premature babies who have a hernia on one side are also likely to develop one on the other, your baby's surgeon may recommend doing

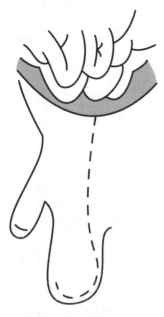

A canal between the abdomen and the groin normally closes in the last weeks of gestation.

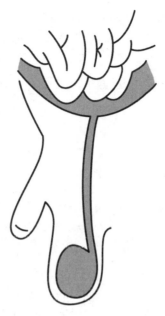

Hydrocele: a narrow passage remains open, allowing fluid to seep from the abdomen into the groin.

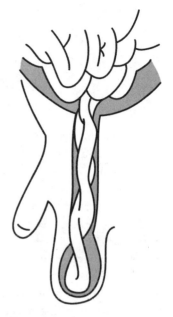

Hernia: a large canal remains open, allowing a loop of intestine to slide down into the groin.

a laparoscopic evaluation of the other side of his groin during the surgery (looking at it with a fiberoptic scope inserted through a tiny hole in the skin). Should your baby need a repair on the other side, too, it can be done right away, saving him—and you—the burden of having to go through surgery again in the future. (Also, if your baby is going to be circumcised, it can be done easily when he's under anesthesia for the hernia repair.)

Most premature infants who have a hernia are operated on just before they are discharged from the hospital nursery, when they are bigger and stronger. But an incarcerated hernia requires urgent surgery—within 24 to 48 hours if a baby hasn't developed complications from it and the surgeon is finally able, perhaps with the help of some light sedation, to reduce the hernia—or right away if there are complications and the hernia remains trapped. After one episode of in-

carceration, there is a high risk that it will happen again until the hernia is repaired.

Fortunately, only a very few premature babies develop complications from an inguinal hernia. For most, it is just another small bump—literally—along the road to their recovery.

Fractures

My baby has a rib fracture. How do I know the nurses haven't been handling him too roughly?

Parents often marvel at the ease with which nurses handle their tiny patients—deftly turning them without catching floppy arms and legs on the bedding or dislodging tubes and lines. Preemies are less fragile than they seem and a nurse's experience makes it very unlikely that she'll ever hurt a baby. So something else is to blame.

Hydrocele: A Related Condition

Hydrocele means water (hydro) in a cavity (cele). It is a collection of fluid in the scrotum around one or both testicles and makes a boy's scrotum look swollen or asymmetric. A hydrocele forms the same way a hernia does: Fluid seeps into the scrotum from the abdomen through a canal that's open in the fetus but normally closes in the last trimester of pregnancy. If the canal remains wide open, then loops of intestine can slide from the abdomen into the scrotum, creating an inguinal hernia. If just a narrow passage remains open, loops of intestine can't pass through but fluid can, creating a hydrocele.

Doctors can distinguish a hydrocele from a hernia by its shape or by shining a light on the scrotum and noting that the clear fluid inside makes it translucent. Unlike hernias, hydroceles usually can't be reduced, meaning the fluid can't be pushed back into the abdomen.

In most baby boys, hydroceles resolve on their own in the first 6 to 18 months of life. If your son has a hydrocele and it is getting smaller or staying the same size, it probably won't need to be repaired. Chances are, the canal between his abdomen and scrotum has closed and his body will gradually absorb the fluid that's left over. But if a hydrocele grows in size or periodically gets bigger or smaller, especially after a boy is 18 months old, it means that there's still a connection between his abdomen and scrotum that, at this late date, is unlikely to close by itself. Doctors then worry that a small channel might enlarge over time, causing a true hernia to develop (see page 310).

The surgical procedure to repair a hydrocele—the same as for a hernia—is extremely safe. Most children with hydroceles have their surgery as outpatients when they're about two years old, and are ready to go home just a few hours afterward.

A rib fracture, usually discovered by chance on a chest X-ray, can occur if a preemie's bones have become soft because of insufficient vitamins and minerals in his diet. Since ribs are the thinnest bones of the body, they're usually the first to weaken and can be fractured inadvertently by a movement that would normally be safe.

When severe, this nutritional deficiency is called rickets. It results in thinner, less dense bones that break easily, but thankfully, even if a preemie has rickets, once his nutrition improves he should recover from it completely, with strong straight bones and no long-term consequences.

Rickets and fractures are rare now in the intensive care nursery, usually affecting only preemies who are struggling with another serious illness so they couldn't be fed for a long time and have had to rely solely on intravenous nutrition. Normally, doctors are able to catch a nutritional shortage early when bone demineralization is just mild, and correct a baby's diet accordingly: they'll give him more calcium, phosphorus, and vitamin D in his milk or formula if he's being fed, or add them in greater quantities to his intravenous nutrition. One way doctors assess a preemie's nutrition is through blood tests. Among the warning signs are abnormal levels of minerals and other substances in his blood, such as calcium and phosphorous, PTH (a hormone that regulates calcium metabolism), and alkaline phosphatase (a measure of bone growth or loss).

The most effective way to prevent bone demineralization is to feed a baby and leave intravenous nutrition behind as soon as possible because nutrients are best absorbed through the intestine. A significant deficiency of vitamins and minerals usually doesn't occur unless a preemie is exclusively fed with intravenous nutrition (TPN) for more than a month. Preemies who are restricted in the amount of calories or protein they're given and are on medications that cause them to lose too much calcium and phosphorus are at particular risk. (For example, lasix, a potent diuretic used in preemies with chronic lung disease, causes calcium to be lost in the urine. If a baby who has bone demineralization is on lasix, his doctor may try stopping it.)

Babies who spend many weeks in a hospital nursery also may not get enough vitamin D, which is essential for incorporating calcium into bone and is normally made by the skin when it's exposed to sunlight.

Since breast milk is low in vitamin D and has less protein and minerals than a rapidly growing preemie needs, most preemies fed breast milk will have liquid or powdered milk fortifier added to their gavage or bottle feedings and will be given multivitamins. (Even parents of preemies who are nursing fully at the breast and ready to go home may be advised to give their baby several bottles a day of pumped, fortified breast milk for 6 to 12 months. Several studies have found that premature boys especially have better growth and bone mineralization if they continue to get nutrient-enriched milk or preterm formula after discharge.) A preemie who is fully bottle fed with a commercial preterm formula will get enough vitamins and minerals to make healthy bones

without the addition of fortifiers but may still need some extra vitamin D for a while.

In intriguing recent research, preemies who were given gentle physical therapy for just fifteen minutes a day, five days a week, had improved bone mineralization and growth. Although the study was too small to be conclusive and included only healthy preemies who were being fed already, past studies have come to similar conclusions. It makes sense, doesn't it, that if exercise helps *your* bone density, it would help your baby's, too? You can ask the doctor whether a few minutes a day with a physical therapist—sessions of simple, slow, passive movement exercises, designed to cause a minimum of stress—might be appropriate for your baby to try.

The good news for your baby is that his rib fracture should heal fairly quickly—in a few weeks once he's getting the dietary supplements he needs. Usually, Tylenol and gentle handling seem to keep a baby comfortable. Rib fractures don't need casts or splints; you'll just have to be especially careful for a couple of weeks when you move or hold him.

Since rickets can almost always be successfully overcome, you can think of your son's accident in the nursery as a helpful warning, leading him to get the right nutrition so he'll grow up with strong, healthy bones.

Feeding Difficulties

Every time I visit my baby in the hospital I get upset. Her doctors say she's not feeding well, so they don't know when she'll be able to go home. Yet she looks so good to me!

How could you not feel frustrated? Feeding problems—and often not even true problems, just the slow and irregular way that some young preemies gradually become adept at feeding—commonly drive parents crazy with impatience and worry. It's difficult to understand how something as basic as eating can take so long and be so hard.

When a preemie finally overcomes her serious health problems and her parents' major fears fade away, the rest of the hospital stay can become a long haul. Nothing much seems to happen. Weeks go by, and other preemies are jubilantly taken home, while your baby seems to be stuck in a swamp of feeding difficulties. Maybe she is not interested in taking the nipple or rejects it once feeding has started; she spits up milk or lets it drool out of her mouth; has apneas, bradys, or oxygen desats during feedings; chokes, gags, or looks distressed while she's eating; or simply falls asleep in the middle of drinking her bottle. Then, at her next mealtime, she may feed better, really confusing you. Some parents find themselves blaming the nurses for their baby's ups and downs or mistrusting the information they get about their baby's feedings when they're not there. A preemie's eating behavior can be so erratic that it sometimes seems the doctors and nurses are talking about several different babies rather than your one-and-only.

In the box on the following page, you'll find information about possible reasons your daughter might be having trouble overcoming all of her feeding hurdles and what the doctors and therapists in the hospital might do to try to pinpoint her problems and treat them. You will be kept updated about her progress and any plans for diagnostic tests or new therapies. You may be taught by a nurse, speech therapist, or lactation consultant a special way to feed your baby so that you can play the main role in feeding her whenever you can.

As you know firsthand, learning how to eat isn't a smooth, easy process for all preemies and it can be emotionally highly charged for their families. The urge to feed one's newborn baby is a natural and strong parental instinct, and mothers and fathers who feel they're failing at it may be filled with despair. But it's important to realize that progress in feeding can take long weeks, and sometimes months, for many premature babies. Doctors and nurses know that even the tiniest incremental steps of development and maturation add up, eventually leading to success. You should try to remember that, too, so you can keep your experiences with your preemie in perspective. In the meantime, you can support your baby by learning how to recognize and follow her cues (see page 234), making her feeding attempts as pleasurable and easy as possible. This will go a long way toward ensuring that eating is something she'll enjoy at all stages of her development.

If your baby's doctors are telling you that she might benefit from a g-tube (a gastrostomy tube, through which she could be fed directly into her stomach), try not to dismiss the idea out of hand. Of course, you're still hoping she can avoid one, but maybe you should reconsider. A g-tube is just a temporary tool to help give a baby the nutrition she needs to grow well without the stress of trying to feed her all of her meals by mouth. A baby with a g-tube usually continues to practice feeding from a bottle but in a calmer, less pressured situation—which is often the key to faster improvement. With good nutrition guaranteed, her parents often can relax, too, letting them focus more on other important developmental steps rather than obsessing about meals and weight gain.

The surgery to insert a g-tube is simple, and recovery is quick—usually just a few days—so if a baby's feeding problems are the only reason she is still in the hospital, she could be sent home soon afterward. (Don't worry, you'll be taught everything you need to know about caring for a baby with a g-tube before she's discharged.) Believe it or not, many families who initially thought a g-tube was the worst outcome they could imagine later say they wish their preemie

(*Continued on page 317*)

Feeding Therapies and Tests

Becoming a good feeder is like any other developmental milestone: Some babies get there sooner and more easily than others. Certain premature babies are at greatest risk for feeding difficulties and are likely to need some extra help when it comes to nippling:

* The youngest preemies, born at 26 weeks of gestation or less, tend to be a little less coordinated than babies who spent more time in the womb. Also, they're often more sensitive and less adaptable in handling the new, varied sensations involved in feeding by mouth.

* Babies with respiratory difficulties need more energy and time just for breathing, and that can interfere with good nippling. If a preemie had an endotracheal tube in his mouth for many months connecting him to a ventilator, he may also have developed some oral aversion (dislike of stimulation in and around his mouth) or may have some unusual reactions when his face or mouth is touched.

* Occasionally a baby will be on a ventilator or CPAP long enough to miss the normal developmental time frame when babies start nippling and will lose some of his innate ability to suck on a breast or bottle. And although breastfeeding is easier in some ways than bottle feeding for a preemie, by the time he is ready to be put to her breast his mother's milk supply may have dwindled or stopped altogether.

Trying to prevent feeding problems, doctors frequently recommend that preemies born at 26 weeks or less be evaluated early on, when they're still being fed by gavage or during their earliest nipple feeding attempts, by a speech therapist or occupational therapist. (These professionals are actually experts on all oral-motor skills, not just language or job training, as their titles suggest.) The same evaluation is recommended for older preemies who are already nippling but have feeding problems that aren't improving as easily or quickly as expected. Addressing difficulties before they become deep-rooted problems or habits, and helping a premature baby's oral-motor skills develop appropriately, will go a long way toward making it easier for him to nipple now, as well as toward helping him accept solid food, avoid speech delays, and enjoy eating throughout all stages of his infancy and childhood.

The therapist will evaluate your baby before, during, and after a nipple feeding session, checking on his alertness and muscle tone, his facial expression, the way he breathes, the shape of his jaw, and the movements of his mouth, tongue, and chin. Normal sucking and swallowing involves coordinating many muscles and nerves so milk doesn't pool in a baby's mouth, drip down his chin, or slip into his windpipe. The therapist will watch for any lack of coordination or muscle weakness, listen for sounds that could indicate that reflux or narrowed airways might be interfering with good nippling, and feel your baby's chest or back as he eats for the rhythm and depth of his breathing. She'll note if there are times when his equilibrium is disrupted and get a general sense of how comfortable or distressing the process of eating is for him.

After evaluating your baby, the therapist will make some recommendations. For example, she may suggest a series of feeding "exercises" that allow him to practice with small quantities of milk only once or twice a day at first, perhaps starting with extremely slow flow rates (the speed of milk flow can be regulated using a special bottle with an adjustable nipple control), or that he be given more oxygen during feedings, be held in a different position, or be "paced" during his feedings (this involves suspending the feeding for a minute or so at set intervals by taking the nipple out of his mouth and sitting him upright to let him catch his breath and get organized). The therapist will teach you and the nurses what to do when you feed your baby and will periodically come to the nursery to feed him herself, helping him practice and reevaluating his progress. She'll also decide when it is safe to advance his feedings (by increasing the amount of milk he's given, the speed with which it's flowing, or the frequency with which he's nipple fed). Always she'll want to avoid breathing difficulties, aspiration, or causing your baby any distress. The overall goal of feeding therapy is not only to help your baby improve and maintain his oral-motor skills so he can become a better feeder right now, but also to make sure that his experiences with feeding are pleasant and nurturing. Babies want more of the things they enjoy, and feeding is a rich, social experience that contributes to good long-term development.

Sometimes the therapist or doctor might order some special tests to evaluate a baby's nippling ability or to search for problems that could be interfering with his eating. A modified barium swallow study, performed by a speech therapist, is a series of X-rays taken while the baby is drinking milk or formula that contains barium, a liquid that shows up clearly on an X-ray, provid-

ing an image of the inside of the baby's mouth, throat, esophagus, and stomach. (The barium won't harm him and will pass out of his body in his stools.) A swallow study allows the speech therapist to see exactly where the milk goes, and when, as the baby swallows it. She can see if it pools in his cheeks or in the back of his throat, if it goes up his nose, or if he aspirates any down his windpipe. She can see how his tongue and palate move, and can change the baby's position to see whether this helps. Often the therapist will thicken the milk to varying degrees to see whether thicker liquid is easier for the baby to manipulate and swallow. (Some NICUs do a swallow study on every preemie born at less than about 26 weeks because so many of these young preemies are likely to need thickened feeds to prevent them from aspirating when they're first learning to eat.)

Another kind of test is called a FEES (for fiberoptic endoscopic evaluation of swallowing). This test, also done by a speech therapist, involves inserting a thin fiberoptic tube in one of the baby's nostrils through which the therapist can directly view the baby's nose, mouth, and throat as he's eating. A FEES may be done if the doctor and therapist think it's possible that the structure or anatomy of a baby's mouth or upper airway may be playing a role in his feeding problems or if an X-ray swallow study didn't provide enough information.

If a baby is refusing to take a bottle, pushes the nipple out of his mouth as if eating is painful or unpleasant, or is having a problem with vomiting or bradycardia while he eats or right afterward, the doctor may decide to test him for reflux. Virtually all babies have some reflux, but if it's especially severe, it can make eating uncomfortable and difficult. Reflux can be diagnosed with a simpler kind of X-ray swallow study or a pH probe (see page 274). It can be treated effectively with medication or, if needed, with surgery.

Very occasionally the therapist and doctor may recommend that a baby get a gastrostomy or g-tube (a stable feeding tube that allows a baby to be fed directly into his stomach). With a g-tube, an infant can get the nutrition he

needs and soon be sent home—the best place for him to develop well—while his parents and therapist continue to work gently and lovingly, at his own pace, on his oral-motor skills and acceptance of eating.

---

had gotten one sooner, because after it was in, parents and baby both enjoyed their time together more without the ever-present anxiety and conflict of meal times. To them, the g-tube turned out to be a great relief, as well as a shortcut to the happy homecoming of their growing, thriving baby.

Another Kind of Jaundice

My baby is jaundiced, but she's not being treated with phototherapy like before. The doctor says this is a different kind of jaundice. What does he mean?

There's another form of jaundice that's different from the kind that nearly all newborns get in their first week of life. Notice that your baby's skin color is somewhat different from when she had jaundice before: Rather than the yellowish-orange of regular newborn jaundice, now she's more of a yellowish-green. It's not most people's favorite color, but luckily, it's not often a long-lasting problem.

As you can read on page 179, jaundice is caused by a buildup of bilirubin (a yellow substance produced when red blood cells are broken down, as they naturally are in everybody). The initial underlying problem for infants, especially preemies, is that the liver is too immature at first to convert bilirubin into a disposable form which can be excreted in the stools. The phototherapy lights help by temporarily taking over the liver's job, converting the bilirubin into a form that the body can excrete.

In your daughter's case, though, there's more going on than plain immaturity. She has what's called direct, or conjugated, hyperbilirubinemia (another name for jaundice), meaning that her liver has done its job of converting the bilirubin into a disposable form, but despite that, something—a different problem in the liver or elsewhere—is holding up her body from getting rid of it.

If your daughter is still being fed with total parenteral nutrition (or TPN, the intravenous solution that preemies get until they are ready to digest breast milk or formula), then it's a good bet that's the reason for her jaundice. TPN can damage the liver over time, so by some estimates, roughly half of the newborns who need it for more than a couple of weeks develop some mild liver complications. But fortunately, damage from TPN in preemies is almost always temporary. Once a baby is being fed only breast milk or formula and no longer needs TPN, the liver gradually recovers. It does better at moving the bilirubin into the intestines, from which it is excreted, and the baby's jaundice gradually goes away.

In the meantime, your baby's doctor may give her some medication to speed the flow of bile out of her liver, may alter the composition of her TPN slightly and try "cycling" it (turning it off for several hours a day to give her liver a rest), or if her jaundice is mild and she's expected to come off TPN soon, he may simply wait. Direct hyperbilirubinemia doesn't seem to make babies uncomfortable (it can cause itching in adults) and won't cause other medical problems unless it goes on for months or more. Since babies with direct hyperbilirubinemia don't absorb fats or fat-soluble vitamins well, your daughter may also be given extra doses of vitamins A, D, E, and K. When she is ready to eat, if she's not getting breast milk she may be put on a special formula, containing a kind of fat that is absorbed more easily. (She'll switch to a regular formula as soon as she has recovered.)

The doctors may do some blood tests and X-rays to rule out other possible reasons for her jaundice that are less common. For example, direct hyperbilirubinemia is sometimes found in babies who had an infection that damaged their liver. It can be a sign of a urinary tract infection, a metabolic problem, or hypothyroidism. Occasionally a preemie who had the intestinal disease called NEC gets scarring that can partially block the flow of bile into her intestines. And rarely, it can be due to a congenital problem with the bile ducts. Your baby's doctor will tell you about further tests and treatments he would recommend if she appears to have any of these problems.

But if your baby's tests come back normal, her doctors will probably attribute her problem to TPN. Their aim, then, will be to get her off TPN as soon as possible—something they try hard to do, anyway. As soon as she can take in enough nourishment with regular feedings, the TPN will be discontinued. By a week or two afterward, you should notice with relief that her jaundice is getting better, and within a few months, it should be completely gone.

Relations with Nurses

My mood in the NICU can be so influenced by who my baby's nurse is that day. Some I like, but there is one I just can't stand, and I don't know what to do about it.

Relationships with neonatal nurses are emotionally charged for many parents of preemies, and often result in strong attachments and equally strong dislikes. At such a demanding time, when you're so anxious about your baby, you need to feel comfortable with all of the medical staff. But normal differences in human temperament always make some relationships easier than others. And in this case, things are complicated by the fact that parents and nurses have not chosen each other yet find themselves joined by—and sometimes at odds over—weighty concerns about the needs and well-being of the same baby.

Parents are particularly vulnerable after their child's premature birth. Just when they're struggling to understand what the early birth means for them and their child, they find that a NICU nurse has taken over their parental duties and pleasures. This is a real sore spot for parents of preemies. Being unable to fulfill their parental role has been consistently identified in clinical studies as a major source of parents' stress in the neonatal intensive care unit.

Parents feel incompetent and frustrated because they are unable to make their baby feel better, disturbed by being separated from him, and afraid of interacting with him because he appears so fragile. Each of these powerful feelings runs headlong into the nurse-parent relationship. Who's attending to the premature baby's needs instead of his parents? The nurse. Who spends the most time with the baby? The nurse. Who grants permission to touch, hold, change, bathe, and feed their own baby? The nurse, of course. It's natural that parents could become jealous, bitter, or passively resigned and gradually develop a sense of impotence, even if the nurses are trying to involve them as much as possible. In one study, 15 percent of parents interviewed in the NICU reported difficult relationships with the staff.

This is especially likely for parents whose preemies have to stay in the hospital nursery for several months. Sometimes the nurses who are regularly assigned to these babies become very attached to them, expressing their affection by holding them and with smiles, coos, playfulness, and gifts. Nurses who spend so much time with a baby may feel that they know his moods, needs, and ways of responding better than his parents do, particularly if his parents are not able to spend long hours in the nursery. While parents may be happy to see how much love and attention their preemie gets, which can only be good for the baby's development, they may resent how much of their parental role and authority has been usurped by the NICU staff. Not surprisingly, these feelings can engender conflict.

Most nurses are aware that parents might be jealous of them, but feel they're in a bind themselves. Some parents like the nurses to treat their children as if they were their own, others don't. What's the answer?

Psychologists talk about a need for role negotiation in the nurse-parent relationship. They mean that parents and nurses should try to understand their own responsibilities, concerns, and feelings toward the baby, and what they each expect from the other. Ideally this should be a work in progress throughout a preemie's hospitalization as the nurses gradually help parents take over what is rightfully theirs: responsibility for their baby's care.

Indeed, according to the principles of family-centered care, which are a main tenet in today's NICUs (see pages 231–232), you, and not the nurses, are at the very center of your baby's care. True, you can't give your preemie all of the special medical care he needs right now, and you can't be in total charge of him yet, so you need to rely on the expertise of the NICU staff. But your baby's nurses are specifically trained to involve you, to always consider you, and to treat you as an equal partner. Becoming more aware of how crucial your role is as a parent to your preemie in the hospital can be reassuring enough to ease some of your insecurities or self-defense mechanisms and

improve communication with your baby's nurses. That alone may help smooth some wrinkles in your relationship. The goal is to develop team spirit with all of your baby's nurses so they can give your preemie, and you, the best kind of care and support in the hospital.

Mutual understanding is the key. Even though neonatal nursing training gives tremendous importance to empathy, communication skills, and methods to involve parents in their baby's care and to provide them with practical and emotional support, anyone who works in a NICU can lose her sensitivity about what premature babies, with their shockingly small size and tubes and lines running everywhere, look like to their parents. So nurses have to remind themselves to acknowledge parents' difficulties, help them express their concerns, and be reassuring whenever possible. And parents have to learn not to interpret a nurse's matter-of-factness as callousness. It's not surprising, given different people's personal preferences, that some kinds of parents may be easier or harder for particular nurses to deal with and vice versa.

Many parents, at the beginning, need to be encouraged by the staff to become more involved with their babies. Some assume a completely passive role, expecting the nurses to provide their child with everything he needs: touch, holding, attention, and stimulation as well as medical care. Feeling uncomfortable in the NICU and uneasy about what to do, some parents show up only for infrequent quick visits, not spending enough time with their preemie to get to know him and understand his needs. As a result, the nurses, who can be very protective of the babies in their care, might disapprove of a family's behavior. Even if this criticism isn't expressed openly, it can show subtly and interfere with the relationship.

The nurse needs to recognize that passive or even absent parents are rarely uninvolved or uncaring, but may be scared, intimidated by the intensive care environment, fearful of being confronted with a reality that's too different from what they expected for their baby, or simply unaware of their babies' problems and needs. As a parent, trying to be open about your anxieties and your uncertainty about your role as a parent of a hospitalized preemie may smooth your relationship with the nurses and help you find ways to participate in your baby's care.

Other mothers and fathers ask for responsibilities or take them, with or without permission. Outspoken parents may want things done to their children only their way, sparking struggles and competition between them and the medical staff. Nurses feel that these parents are apt to judge everything they do in a critical light, taking them to task if, say, they're a few minutes late in giving a medication or a feeding.

Nurses have a duty to realize that difficult, controlling parents are often trying to establish their parental role in the only way they consider effective in the foreign environment of the hospital nursery. But if this sounds like you, try to relax your vigilance. Keep in mind that there are different nursing styles and that most little slips in schedule or varied ways of doing things won't harm your baby in the least. Sometimes a nurse won't be able to accommodate your request because of nursery rules and protocols (usually adopted for the safety of the babies, to cut down on errors and allow the unit to run smoothly). Moreover, because nurses often have tight busy schedules, there are constraints on the amount of time they can spend with each baby. You may end up having to settle for competence and consideration, and give up a little bit on the absolutely ideal nursing situation that you envision.

Thankfully, most nurseries can provide some continuity in assignments so parents can get to know and trust at least several familiar faces and styles. But nonetheless, the organizational constraints of a busy NICU often mean that dozens of different nurses are assigned to take care of one baby. When parents are faced with a nurse who's new to them—and a new relationship to develop—of course some tensions and insecurities on the part of the nurse or the parents may arise and need to be worked out. It can be a hard task for parents to deal with unfamiliarity and change over and over again. As much as you can, try not to let tiredness and disappointment simply because of the nurse's newness get in the way of your openness and good feelings toward her, or your assessment of her abilities. Instead, recognize what an effort this is for you and applaud yourself for doing it gracefully.

Of course, there might be times when, because of a nurse's temperament and needs, inexperience, fatigue, or momentary distraction—or your own stress—a situation or relationship will be handled poorly or misjudged. Most nurses say that if they make a mistake, they are open to admitting it and apologizing for it, but when they feel constantly under scrutiny or criticized by a parent, they can lose the professional emotional distance they need to do the best job they are trained to do.

It's nice to know that even with all of these common difficulties, the bright spots shine through. Parents' positive experiences with the NICU staff outnumber negative ones by far. According to research, the majority of families find neonatal nurses to be their best allies, a more compassionate, reliable, and understandable source of information than the doctors, and a major source of support in the experience of parenting a hospitalized preemie.

One of us will never forget how a motherly NICU nurse taught her with unmatchable patience to bottle feed her baby. Another nurse encouraged her to bathe her baby, in a basin no bigger than a man's shoe. If such a tiny sick baby could be bathed by his mother's inexperienced, trembling hands, it surely meant that better times could be expected. And they did come.

Memories like these are hard to forget, by parents and nurses alike. True friendship may develop, keeping nurses, parents, and preemies in touch for years after discharge. In the NICU, we heard nurses proudly telling anecdotes about the wonderful happy outcomes of former preemies they had been following from infancy through adolescence. But establishing a personal friendship isn't needed to form a positive relationship with your baby's nurses. A mutually respectful, warm partnership, with trust in each other's competence and good will, is all you need to fulfill your baby's, and your, best interest.

What if you are having persistent problems that no matter how hard you try just don't improve? There are times when you may conclude that you don't trust a nurse's professional skills, don't find her compassionate enough, or feel that she unfairly doesn't trust you or like you very much. Perhaps she has an uncanny ability to come up with comments that make you feel bad. This happened to a mother we know. Getting to the nursery and finding that a particular nurse was assigned to her baby became so upsetting to her that several times she considered talking to a supervisor. She was surprised and disturbed by the intensity of her emotional reactions, which interfered with the pleasure of being with her baby. Eventually, she decided not to do anything about it, mainly because she was afraid of damaging the quality of her son's care.

But this is a fear that you should never, ever have. Even if you speak up about someone on the medical staff, your baby won't ever be neglected because of something you say. Neonatal nurses and doctors tend to keep their feelings about parents very separate from their feelings about the babies. In fact, even if you've been labeled a troublemaker, you can take comfort in knowing that many nurses are most protective of the babies whose parents they see as not acting "appropriately."

If you're concerned about a serious offense (a lack of professional skills, for instance, noncompliance with principles of hygiene, or gross insolence, etc.), you should definitely express your complaints to the nursing supervisor or attending physician. But most often what upsets parents is something subtler or personal that may be hard to express. Mentioning what's bothering you can still be helpful. Somebody who has seen many such situations may help you better understand a nurse's behavior and perhaps make sense of what's happening. There probably won't be changes in your baby's nursing assignments since organizing the nurses' day and night shifts in a busy nursery is too daunting a task to let parental preferences become a consideration. But if what you report about a nurse fits a recurring pattern, it could lead to better awareness by the supervisors of their staff and maybe some constructive changes.

Trying to understand other people's feelings and motivations, and being open about one's own usually improves human relationships in the nursery, as elsewhere. You might try that. And later, when you're in a calmer frame of mind, take a moment to revive the images of your baby's nurses. There will be those who loved your baby or who gave her the best possible care, and who deserve to be remembered.

Changing Doctors

Do the doctors have to change so often? Just when we start to feel comfortable with one, we have to move on to another.

It's hard when the doctor you've come to trust, whom you've counted on to help you and your baby make it through this difficult experience, is leaving. Naturally, you feel like you're being deserted. Of course you question the merits of a system that rotates doctors in and out of the nursery rather than allowing them to establish lasting,

He Says "Potato," She Says "Potahto"

A confusing thing can happen when your baby's doctor changes: The old doctor and the new doctor may give you different interpretations of the same medical "fact." One may tell you that a certain test result indicates a problem while the other says the result is normal and nothing to worry about. One doctor may recommend a treatment that the other says is probably useless. One may be very concerned that your baby is behaving this way or that while the other shrugs his shoulders and seems uninterested.

When you try to figure out who's right and who's wrong, you'll usually learn something else instead: That medical diagnoses and treatment plans are rarely black or white. Two equally competent doctors can differ in their interpretations and advice.

Disconcerting? Yes, highly. But one way to think about this is that it's an opportunity to discover more about your baby and the many aspects of her condition. If you want to learn more, ask the doctor to explain what's black or white and what's gray. And don't hesitate to tell the doctor about your own parental instincts and observations. Chances are that you'll develop a good working partnership.

close relationships with babies and their families from birth until hospital discharge.

It's true that the system has some disadvantages, especially the hard transition it means for you. But its advantages are very real also, even if they're less immediately apparent. In an intensive care nursery, the days of the attending physicians are long, and often the nights are, too. The work is not just physically but emotionally draining: most doctors truly care about their patients, especially the ones they've worked with for a long time and have come to know well. Although they will never take your baby's ups and downs as hard as you do, they can't help but find sad conversations with parents, and their inability to prevent inevitable difficulties for some babies, to be wrenching experiences. Working in such an intense environment, after more than a few weeks it's unavoidable that a doctor's energy would start

to flag and his judgment perhaps suffer. To prevent this from happening, to keep every doctor's performance high, it's considered vital that all neonatologists take frequent breaks so they can come back to the nursery fresh.

If you're in a teaching hospital, your doctor may also have to rotate out of the nursery because these institutions (which typically offer state-of-the-art medical care) expect their doctors to do medical research as well as take care of patients. It's not easy on you, but it's part of the doctor's job and is intended to benefit the patients and families who receive neonatal care over the long run.

When you have moments of frustration after a changeover, as you probably will (like when you realize that the new doctor doesn't know something you think is important about your baby and you feel like shouting, "How could you not know that about my child?"), here's one other, hidden advantage of the rotating system to keep in mind: a fresh pair of eyes and point of view can be surprisingly valuable. Every doctor, even your favorite one, can get settled into a certain medical routine and way of thinking for each patient. A new doctor's willingness to say, "Why don't we try this?" may turn the tide for a baby who is having problems or enable a healthy baby to do just a little better than she is already doing now.

Cysts in the Brain

The doctor said our baby has some little cysts in her brain, and could have some brain damage. What does this mean for her and us?

When the blood flow or oxygen supply becomes insufficient in an area of the brain, some of its tissue may be damaged. This can happen to a preemie before birth (because of pregnancy complications), around the time of delivery (especially if there is fetal distress during labor and a baby has to be resuscitated), or after birth (because of many medical problems of prematurity). Several weeks after the damage occurs, the resulting brain injury may show up on a head ultrasound or MRI scan as some tiny cysts—a scarred area—or eventually as just some extra fluid where the injured brain tissue had been.

Like most abnormal features on a baby's head ultrasound, brain cysts are worrisome findings, leading doctors to recommend close follow-up for a preemie and her family. They indicate some brain damage and carry the possibility of future impairments. It's the kind of news that can shake a parent deeply. But nobody at this stage can predict just what will happen to your baby. And despite the uncertainty that you'll have to live with for some time, there are reasons to keep your hopes high.

Cysts in some areas of the brain may have no

future effects. For instance, some small single cysts (called choroid plexus cysts or subarachnoid cysts) inside the ventricles are usually insignificant, reflecting very small bleeds that are resolving or other processes that shouldn't cause any problems. More than one cyst, or cysts in more significant areas, most commonly in the white matter of the brain surrounding the ventricles (called PVL, short for periventricular leukomalacia), are more threatening, but even they may not impede normal development.

Remember that a single head ultrasound, particularly if it is done fewer than six weeks after delivery, is not always conclusive. Several head ultrasounds or another kind of study, such as an MRI scan, may be needed to confirm the diagnosis and better identify the site and extent of a brain injury. (An MRI scan is slightly more accurate at detecting smaller cysts and some other types of brain injury.) Though repeated tests and scans can create a lot of anxiety for parents, sometimes a suspected injury is revealed to be just a bad scare.

You've probably been told that you may not know for many months or more how this will affect your daughter. That's true, but how your daughter is doing now and in the near future is important, too. Premature babies who suffered from serious brain damage usually show signs of it in their first months of life; the most common consequences of PVL are problems with movement, which may initially show up as weakness and low muscle tone in their legs and trunk, later progressing to high tone and stiffness. More severely affected babies may have problems eating. If your baby still looks fine on a developmental evaluation at a year of age, there's a good chance that she will have only mild consequences from her brain injury, if any at all. Following your baby closely in the future will enable doctors to pick up problems early and manage them with appropriate expert intervention.

(Continued on page 328)

In Plain Language: PVL and other Kinds of Brain Injury in Preemies

If you've been told your baby has a brain injury, you may be dealing with unimaginably complex feelings. Your days may be interwoven with love and fear, hope and (if you are so inclined) prayer, moments of optimism that buoy you but alternate with waves of pessimism and despair. Before this diagnosis, you were hoping that the worst was over; now you're wondering whether what's before you and your baby will be even more difficult.

For now, if you are in this situation, neither you nor the doctors know what the extent of your baby's lasting injuries will be. It's difficult to come to terms with the uncertainty, to find a balance between realism and hope. Some basic information on brain injury in preemies may help, so you know what you're dealing with and when you're likely to know more than you do today.

Is there a cure for brain injury?

There is no medical treatment that is known to regenerate damaged brain tissue. But a newborn's brain is still developing. If the damage isn't extensive, if it involves only a small area or is present on just one side of the brain, then other parts of the brain may be able to take over the function of the injured tissue, in effect healing itself.

The extent of recovery can be surprising, even to doctors. Children with the same kind of brain injury can have completely different developmental outcomes, in part because of different genetic predispositions and the quality of stimulation they receive in their environment, but also because there is so much about the brain that doctors just can't see, no matter what imaging techniques they use. Brain experts have observed that the brain is much more than the sum of its parts. Its workings involve the way those parts are connected, and that is much harder to measure.

What babies are at risk for a brain injury?

Although there are many intertwined factors that can lead to brain injury in preemies and they are only partially understood, researchers believe that these play a role:

* **Younger, smaller premature babies** are at greater risk because nearly all of the bodily systems that protect them from injury or infection are more immature. Their nutrition and growth are also more apt to be compromised in the weeks after delivery, interfering with brain development and healing.
* **Low blood pressure** can lead to a disruption in blood flow to the brain.
* **Infection** and the substances the body produces in response to it, can damage brain cells, and also can cause blood flow disturbances that indirectly injure the brain. Thus preemies who had an infection or NEC (necrotizing enterocolitis) in the NICU are at risk, as are babies whose mothers had chorioamnionitis (an infection in the amniotic fluid) around the time of delivery or certain other infections during pregnancy.
* **Nutritional shortages**, especially if they go on for many weeks (as may happen when a preemie can't be fed for a long time), can stunt brain development.

✴ **A Grade III or Grade IV intraventricular hemorrhage** is accompanied by a lack of blood flow and oxygen to nearby areas of the brain, and swelling of the ventricles from hydrocephalus after an IVH can also damage the area around the ventricles.

✴ **Various breathing complications of prematurity that require a ventilator,** especially if they are severe or long-lasting, increase the risk of brain damage because they're accompanied by abnormal levels of oxygen, carbon dioxide, and blood flow to the brain.

✴ **Getting less oxygen, nutrients, or blood flow than a fetus needs in the womb** can cause brain injury. Examples are some babies who were born small for their gestational age, some who suffered from cord accidents or placental tears before birth, and some who had to be resuscitated because of complications around the time of delivery, with more than ten minutes passing before their heartbeat and breathing recovered.

✴ **Identical twins** are more likely to have brain injury because they often share placental blood vessels through which blood flow can become disrupted. Unidentified conditions early in pregnancy that lead to twinning, and problems that can occur as the embryo splits, also increase the risk of brain injury.

How brain injuries are diagnosed

A head ultrasound is performed during the first week or two of life on almost every preemie born at less than 32 weeks of gestation to find out whether there's been any bleeding in an inner part of the brain. (You can read about intraventricular hemorrhages, or IVHs as they're called, on page 190.) That first head ultrasound, though, usually can't detect whether a baby's brain tissue has suffered permanent damage. Early signs of brain injury can be subtle and difficult to recognize on an ultrasound, looking like just a slightly bright area around the ventricles. Over time, that brightness may disappear, perhaps indicating that the damage was minor, the brain recovered from it, or it was a mistaken diagnosis. Or it may develop into little cysts, which are equivalent to scars in other parts of the body. Another ultrasound or an MRI scan of the brain done several weeks later is more definitive because it takes from two to six weeks for small cysts to develop and become visible. Later some cysts may fuse together, forming larger areas in which brain tissue has been lost.

These cysts are called PVL (periventricular leukomalacia) when they occur in the white matter of the brain near the ventricles. PVL is found in about 3 percent to 4 percent of premature babies and is considered mild if there are just one or two tiny cysts in one small area. If there are bundles of larger cysts, or cysts on both sides of the brain, it's more severe. Babies with PVL are at high risk for future disabilities, particularly if the PVL is severe.

Sometimes damage similar to PVL shows up in other parts of the white or gray matter of the brain—the cerebellum or basal ganglia, for example. It, too, carries a high risk of future disabilities.

A few other kinds of brain injury can also be seen in preemies. The most common is subtle but widespread abnormalities in the texture of the brain. This doesn't show up well on a head ultrasound but can sometimes be seen on an MRI scan. New studies show that a majority of premature babies born before 32 weeks of gestation have some brain tissue abnormalities when they're in the NICU, perhaps because the maturation of the delicate, developing brain cells is disrupted by a premature birth. But thankfully, many of these injuries turn out to be self-healing or to have only mild developmental consequences.

Finally, a premature baby's brain may look normal but smaller than it should be on an ultrasound or MRI scan. This brain atrophy, as it is called, may arise from a lack of brain growth—perhaps because there was a long period of inadequate nutrition or oxygen—or from early damage to some developing cells that were supposed to have multiplied and spread. Sometimes the small size reflects just a temporary slowdown, and good growth will resume later; other times it is permanent. Recent research suggests that many children who were born prematurely have specific brain areas that are smaller than those of children born at term, and that this is associated with the learning and behavioral problems that are common in preemies.

One important thing to keep in mind is that PVL and other brain injuries are discovered by doctors on X-rays; they may not be reflected in a baby's behavior or neurological exam, now or in the future. A premature baby who is behaving absolutely normally at hospital discharge is much less likely to develop a serious, disabling impairment later.

What symptoms of brain damage would show up early? Signs that are concerning in the first weeks include seizures, and floppiness or weakness in a baby's trunk, legs, or arms. Over the next several months, developmental delays can appear (although some may not be evident until much later). Babies with PVL will most often show the early signs of cerebral palsy (poor muscle control and tone, such as when a baby can't hold her head up, her legs or arms are stiff, or she can't nipple feed well after she is expected to). Some babies with cognitive problems, as are common with brain atrophy and more extensive or diffuse injury, might show early symptoms like little interaction with their environment, being overly sleepy and lethargic—or the opposite, being irritable and easily upset by stimulation.

What you can expect in the long run

In general, when a brain injury is severe a baby will show signs within the first six months of motor or cognitive delays, or much less frequently, of deafness or blindness. Milder disabilities may take up to a year or more to become evident. Many times in preemies, the consequences only show up when a child begins school, as learning or behavior problems—or they have no consequences at all. You can be sure that your baby's doctors will keep a close eye on her development, to pick up the first signs of the slightest delay. That's because early childhood intervention and therapy are essential to help a baby with a brain injury to minimize, and possibly even overcome, a developmental delay. They will ask you to tell them about anything unusual that you notice, too.

If your baby has been diagnosed with PVL, there's a high risk of a later developmental deficit, but the severity of the consequences depends on the size and location of the cysts. Children with large cysts on both sides of the brain have more severe disabilities, while cysts that are tiny and on one side only have a much more hopeful prognosis, probably because healthy parts of the brain are available to take over the function of the damaged areas.

Overall, about 75 percent of babies with PVL will have some developmental disabilities. The majority will have cerebral palsy, and some will have cognitive or sensory problems, but often these disabilities will be mild.

Cerebral palsy is a condition in which a person has difficulty controlling her voluntary movements. In preemies the legs are most commonly affected because the nerves controlling leg movements pass closest to the ventricles. When PVL is more extensive, the nerves controlling the arms or even the face may be affected. There are many degrees of cerebral palsy, from very mild and nondisabling (which may be hardly noticeable in a child) to more moderate (in which a child may need braces to walk) or severe (in which a child may be in a wheelchair and have difficulty talking or eating).

Cognitive delays are less common results of PVL. About 45 percent of children with PVL have normal intelligence, and another 15 percent are classified as low-normal. The 40 percent diagnosed with mental retardation may be anywhere from mildly to severely affected. Mental retardation is most likely in those preemies whose head ultrasounds show enlarged ventricles with global loss of brain tissue. Studies have found that special education programs and early individual intervention may reduce the risk of mental retardation in some children (see page 492). Children with PVL who have normal intelligence have a higher risk of learning disabilities, but if detected early, these can be treated very successfully.

Less commonly, some children with PVL have seizure disorders, and much rarer still are visual impairments or deafness.

The precise outcome of other types of brain injuries in preemies is less well known. Research indicates that preemies with smaller than normal brains and those who had more subtle and diffuse injury tend to have problems with thinking, learning, or behavior, such as lower IQs, speech delays, learning disabilities, attention deficit disorder, and some characteristics of autism.

But doctors are still puzzled by the fact that findings on a baby's head ultrasound and MRI scan don't accurately predict how a child will ultimately do. Follow-up studies have found mild cognitive, learning, behavioral and social difficulties in up to 50 percent of preemies when they reach school age, yet only a small percentage had a brain injury diagnosed on a head ultrasound when they were infants. On the other hand, some children who had visible brain injuries and were considered at high risk for developmental disabilities grew up miraculously unscathed.

The information and statistics about brain injuries can be devastating for parents to learn. How can you make sense of all this without withering? For one thing, remember that the risk of disability represents the average outcomes of large groups of children, not the individual, unique clinical and developmental profile of your baby, which may be much better than average. Also, don't forget the view of the glass as half-full: many of the children who have been diagnosed with a brain injury will be normal or have only a mild impairment that does not prevent them from leading full, happy lives.

Moreover, there's good news emerging from recent large studies. Premature babies who have been followed from birth to eight years are showing that cognitive and verbal tests sometimes improve significantly over time, particularly with early intervention—another example of the ability of the brain to repair itself. The need for special assistance in class or special education also decreases dramatically through adolescence. Since these long-term follow-up studies reflect outcomes of former preemies who were born up to twenty years ago, there's a good chance that the outcomes of babies born now, like yours, will be even better because of the constant improvement in neonatal intensive care and developmental interventions.

Finally, knowing about risks means empowering yourself. You can put yourself in the best position to help your child since there's so much that can be done to assist her. The amazing ability of a child to compensate for problems, together with her parents' good faith and strength, make the most formidable team.

Doctors can't make exact predictions about the consequences of a brain lesion in a premature baby. But they are finding increasing proof of the amazing ability of a developing brain to recover from injury at least partially, and the power of a stimulating environment to help that recovery happen. You can read more about brain injury and recovery on page 324. In the meantime, keep in mind that most of the time even when a preemie does have an impairment resulting from brain damage, it won't prevent her from leading a rich and fulfilling life.

Moving to Intermediate Care

My baby was just moved to the intermediate care nursery. Everyone assumed I'd be happy about it, but to tell you the truth it makes me nervous. Is he going to get all the attention he needs?

Be assured that your baby is going to be exactly where he needs to be now: in a less hectic, calmer place where he can feed and grow peacefully and where you'll also feel more at home. Most parents find the intermediate nursery far more pleasant and comfortable than the NICU. In the step-down unit, as the intermediate care nursery is also called, you and your son will be able to enjoy more of each other without the distractions of so many doctors and nurses rushing around you, removed from the tension that fills the air in an emergency or when a newborn first arrives in the NICU.

If you feel nervous about your preemie's new accommodations, that's understandable. You've been through a crisis, and you're still emotionally vulnerable. The change of environment can exacerbate fears and anxieties that were calmed while your baby was watched so closely in intensive care. You may feel abandoned by the NICU nurses or doctors and miss their guidance and company if they don't rotate through the step-

down unit. After all, they were so involved with your baby that some of them seemed like part of your extended family.

But your baby will still have doctors who do rounds and check on him frequently, as before. True, there are fewer nurses per baby in an intermediate care nursery, but their number is designed to guarantee appropriate individual attention and care for each baby. Don't worry: the nurses can jump to provide emergency stabilizing treatment if they have to. But you're going to see it only if your baby needs it, which is something that day by day will become less and less likely. You should really be thrilled about that!

The quality of medical assistance is the same as in intensive care, but the intermediate nurses' focus is tailored to your preemie's ever-developing needs, which are somewhat different now. The nurses will help him with feeding, assist him in regulating his body temperature, position, and movements, and help train you to recognize his signals and take over some important care-giving tasks. In fact, the intermediate unit is where many babies can relax and enjoy new pleasures, such as kangaroo care, long periods of quiet time, warm baths, and infant massage, that they may not have been ready for before. With the change in focus from urgent medical priorities to developmental ones, you'll be able to see your baby much more as a normal baby, rather than as a sick one. And that's wonderful.

In a matter of days, you're going to feel more comfortable in the intermediate care nursery. Try to picture this change of location in the hospital as a step toward another transition you'll soon be making: going home with your baby. Take the step-down unit as a useful rehearsal. Here you can savor the idea of being alone with your baby but with the support and reassurance you may still need at your fingertips.

Preemie Massage

Someone told me that massage is supposed to be beneficial to preemies. Isn't that kind of odd and maybe even dangerous for a fragile premature baby?

The word massage, for many people, brings to mind brawny massage therapists who knead out the kinks in aching backs. But preemie massage has little to do with the vigorous kind of manipulation that adults occasionally enjoy. It's better described as an organized touch technique—a way of giving your baby some extra nurturing touch, which scientists now believe plays a powerful role in normal development.

There is some intriguing evidence that massage may be beneficial to preemies. In one clinical trial, a group of healthy premature babies, all of whom weighed less than 1,500 grams, got 15-minute massages three times a day for ten days. They ate the same amount as other babies but gained almost 50 percent more weight on average. The massaged babies were also more alert and active, and left the hospital six days earlier. Other studies have also reported greater weight gain, less time in the hospital, and slightly better scores on developmental tests for massaged preemies. But research experts question the reliability of these findings, pointing out various problems in the research methods and saying that more study is needed before we'll know whether massage is worth doing.

What we know now is that there are some good reasons to believe massage won't hurt a preemie if correctly done, and might even help. Touch is the most fundamental sense in a newborn preemie. It is the first sense to develop in a fetus, and since a preemie's eyesight and hearing aren't yet fully developed, and skin is the largest sensory organ, touch is the main way he experiences the world. It's no wonder that nature has wired all parents with an instinctive urge to calm their babies using touch; without ever having to be told, new parents stroke and pat their babies to soothe and comfort them.

Doctors have known for a long time that infants and children who aren't held, touched, played with, and fondly attended to can have stunted growth, regardless of how much they eat. There's even a name for this: psychosocial failure to thrive. Research in animals and humans suggests it may relate to the ability of touch and physical activity to increase levels of growth-stimulating hormones. Animal studies have even revealed that there is a growth gene that needs to be turned on by touch before it will work. Besides making us feel loved and soothing our nerves, the right sort of touch can enhance growth, cognitive, and emotional development when experienced early enough in life.

Of course, loving touch comes in many different forms: simply cradling your baby in your arms; holding him skin-to-skin against your bare chest; or if he is not yet stable enough to be picked up, letting him grasp one of your fingers as you wrap your other arm behind his head and back. You don't have to massage your baby for him to feel your touch. But if you want to try it and your baby's doctor agrees, by all means do.

Please read the following tips before you begin to make sure your massages are safe, pleasurable, and most likely to benefit your baby:

✳ **Don't start massaging your baby until you get an OK from your baby's doctor.** While massage is perfectly safe for preemies who are old enough and medically stable, it may not be for young or sick ones. Since a young preemie's skin is fragile, we recommend that you wait until your baby is at least 30 weeks adjusted gestational age before starting. Babies in the research trial mentioned above weren't massaged until they were an average of 31 weeks and off oxygen and IV feedings.

* **When the right time comes, don't hesitate to begin.** Some massage proponents believe that for massage to promote weight gain it may need to be started when a preemie is still less than 1,500 grams. But even if it doesn't make a difference in your baby's weight, she'll still enjoy the benefits of your loving touch.

* **Ask the doctor whether your baby's leads, attached to the cardiorespiratory monitor, need to stay on during the massage.** The doctor will consider how stable your baby is and how long the massage will last in deciding whether it's safe or not.

* **Choose a time for the massage when your baby isn't likely to be hungry but not just after he's eaten**—perhaps an hour or so after feeding time.

* **You may take all of your baby's clothes off for the massage if he is going to be staying in his isolette or warming bed.** Some people even take the diaper off, but be prepared for things to get a bit messy if you do! It's very common for a baby to urinate as his muscles relax during a massage. If he's in an open bassinet, you might ask the doctor if it's OK for him to wear only a hat during the massage, or you might massage him under a loose shirt or gown.

* **Wash your hands thoroughly before beginning the massage and then warm them by rubbing them together vigorously.** To protect your baby's delicate skin, make sure your nails are short, and that you aren't wearing any dangling or protruding jewelry on your hands or wrists.

* **A preemie's skin is so soft and smooth** that your hands may glide easily even without any massage oil or lubricant. It's safest to avoid them if you can, and certainly if you are doing regular massages, because oils and moisturizing lotions may increase the risk of infection. If you would like to use one once in a while, ask the doctor first, and avoid any product that contains perfumes or dyes (see page 273).

* **Place your hands on your baby and talk to him** for a moment to let him know you're there before you start massaging. Once you start massaging, don't talk too much, in case it's too much stimulation for your baby. Let him focus on your touch.

* **For the massage itself, use a gentle but firm touch rather than a light stroking one.** Preemies don't respond well to a light stroking touch, presumably because it tickles them and isn't soothing. Apply moderate pressure but try not to pull on the skin.

* **You can try a routine similar to the one used in research studies:** For the first five minutes with your baby lying tummy-down in his isolette, put your hands through the portholes and stroke him starting at the top of his head and moving down to his neck, shoulders, back, waist, legs, feet, arms, and hands; then turn him over so he's lying on his back and for the next five minutes flex his arms and legs very gently, holding each flex for about ten seconds; finally, turn him back over for another five-minute stroking period similar to the first.

* **If your baby starts to cry or show signs of stress during the massage, stop and comfort him.** You might try placing your hands gently but firmly over him without moving them for a minute or so. Once he seems calm and comfortable, you can keep going. But if he again becomes unhappy, you should stop the massage. He knows best when he's had enough, and maybe he wants to be left alone right now. (Don't we all sometimes feel that way?) You can try it again some other time.

✳ **After you've finished massaging your baby,** you might want to hold him snugly for a while, perhaps rocking him, so both of you can enjoy the pleasure and intimacy of the moment.

Transfer to a Hospital Closer to Home

They just told us that our baby is ready to go back to the hospital where he was born. How could he possibly be strong enough to travel 30 miles?

It's natural for you to feel anxious, both about the travel and the adequacy of care in a smaller, community hospital nursery. But what the doctors are telling you is that your little tyke is now stronger than you think. After all you've been through, it's going to take a while before you can believe it. But your baby has made it through the most arduous part of his journey, during which he needed state-of-the-art neonatal care. He's now medically stable, less vulnerable, and ready to take on some new experiences, including a trip that will bring him closer to the arms of his loving family.

The most important thing to realize is that your baby's doctors would never let him go on a trip or to a nursery that wasn't safe. Your baby will probably travel in an ambulance that's like a mobile intensive care unit with his isolette, monitors, and if he needs them oxygen, intravenous equipment, and drugs. He will be accompanied by at least one specialist in neonatal care, usually a neonatal nurse, who can provide emergency medical care if need be. (If you want to travel with your son, too, you can ask his doctor. The answer will depend on the hospital's policies and whether there is enough room in the ambulance.)

Your baby's doctors will know what kind of patients his new hospital nursery can give good care to. Feel free to ask them to go over this with you. For instance, if your baby needs follow-up eye exams for retinopathy of prematurity, ask if there's a specialist to do them. You can also make an appointment to tour the nursery and meet the staff who'll be taking care of your baby. Ask specific questions to get reassurance on the following points: Are they able to provide care for the conditions your baby has? Have they done it before? Under what circumstances would your baby be sent back to his current hospital?

Most parents can't really relax until their baby has been in the new nursery for a few days and they've witnessed for themselves that all of his needs are being met. Just as parents of older children often lose sight of how much their kids have grown because they see them every day, it often takes a move like this for parents of a preemie to realize just how far their baby has come.

If your baby was born at the hospital he's moved to, he'll probably be greeted with open arms by the doctors or nurses who helped care for him the day he was born. If he wasn't born there, he'll still be received warmly by a staff who feel he's part of their community and are eager to care for him.

Many parents underestimate the advantages of being in a smaller, quieter nursery that's near home. Your preemie will probably see more of you and maybe his siblings or grandparents, since it won't take as long to reach him. His pediatrician can start establishing a relationship with him and help you get familiar with any local specialists or support services you may need. The nursery itself will probably be a lot calmer than you're used to, and that's good: it means more precious quiet time for your baby and more individual attention from the nurses for him and you.

Every now and then, a baby will lose weight for a few days after back-transport (as the move to a hospital closer to home is called), or need a little more supplemental oxygen, or tolerate his feedings less well. It doesn't mean that the new nursery isn't taking good care of him; it's just that your baby needs some time to get settled into his new home.

If none of this eases your fears and you believe your son is better off staying where he is, it may help to raise your concerns with his doctor. The hospital can't move your baby without your permission, and you may convince the doctor of the wisdom of keeping him a little longer. But most likely, the doctor will try to convince you of the many good reasons for the move to take place, including your baby's own needs and the need to open intensive care beds for sicker babies, as your son once was. Just remember that the doctor cares about your baby's well-being, too, and whatever other factors she's balancing, she's not going to do something that would hurt him.

On the other hand, even if you and your baby's doctor are convinced of the advantages of finishing his hospitalization in a nursery closer to home, you may need to check with your insurance company first. Some insurance plans will not pay for the cost of the ambulance transport (necessary for preemies, who are traveling in isolettes and connected to monitors) if your baby's current nursery can provide all the medical services he needs. The NICU social worker can advise and help you with this.

After the move, your baby may still remain under the comforting watchful eye of his current doctors if your NICU has a follow-up clinic. Many clinics see their NICU "graduates" every few months for a few years. Even if there's no clinic, you can call your baby's old doctor if you're worried about something important. Neonatologists tend to be caring and protective of the babies they've cared for, so even when you move, you don't have to say a final good-bye.

Vaccinations

My older son got his first vaccinations when he was two months old. Is a preemie scheduled according to his birth date or his due date?

This is one time when you don't have to pull out that mental calculator and start figuring out your baby's corrected age. The American Academy of Pediatrics generally recommends that preemies receive immunizations on the same schedule following their birth dates as full-term babies, no matter how early they were born.

That means your baby would get his first series of immunizations two months after birth: the DTP vaccine (diphtheria, tetanus, and pertussis, which is another word for whooping cough), polio vaccine, and Hemophilus influenzae b (Hib) vaccine. Hemophilus influenzae b bacteria can cause various kinds of serious infections, such as meningitis.

Since many adults have lost their pertussis immunity over the years, this might be a good time for you to get a booster, too. (Booster immunizations for pertussis are recommended every ten years.) Whooping cough has made a big comeback in the general population and although it isn't usually dangerous in healthy adults, it is annoying and painful. Until your preemie completes his second or third set of vaccinations he won't be immune to it, so you could pass it to him if you get it. And pertussis lasts for months—wouldn't it be the worst timing to get it when your preemie is still in the NICU?

For a long time, neonatologists and pediatricians were concerned about giving immunizations to preemies who were still very young and small. They wondered whether preemies' immune systems were mature enough for the vaccines to produce adequate, lasting levels of immunity. There's been a lot of research on this, and those doubts have largely been dispelled. One exception, though, is the Hepatitis B vaccine. The first dose is usually given to term newborns on their first day or two of life, but preemies get it later, at 30 days of age, when the vaccine is more likely to be effective. (If a preemie is healthy and stable enough to go home earlier than that, he'll get the vaccine at the time of his discharge from the hospital.) Also, if your baby was treated at some point with IVIG (intravenous immunoglobulin) for an infection, all his vaccinations will be postponed for a few months because his body's response to vaccines will be dulled for a while.

The American Academy of Pediatrics recommends immunizing all infants against Rotavirus (a virus that can cause severe diarrhea and vomiting, especially in premature babies) with three doses of vaccine, beginning at two months of age. But although your baby should get Rotavirus shots eventually, the first dose won't be given to him until he's discharged from the NICU. The reason is that the Rotavirus vaccine contains pieces of weakened but live virus that are completely safe for the baby who gets it and for children and adults with normal immune systems, but possibly not for other unvaccinated preemies in the nursery whose immune systems are immature. (The virus can be shed in a vaccinated baby's stool and inadvertently passed around by nurses or parents after changing diapers.)

One temporary side effect of the first DPT, polio, and Hib shots is that a premature baby may suffer from an increase in apnea and bradycardia, or a return of A's and B's even if he hasn't had them for a while, for 48 hours afterwards. As a result, doctors do not give these vaccines less than 48 hours before a preemie is sent home, and keep him on a cardiorespiratory monitor (or put him back on one) until 48 hours have passed. If your preemie is sick when he's due for his immunizations, the doctor may decide to postpone them briefly until he's well. You may notice that

your preemie is fussy for 12 to 24 hours after his shots, and some babies get a mild fever. A little Tylenol usually helps with that.

After your preemie comes home, it's also recommended that he and everyone living in the house with him get a yearly flu vaccine, beginning when he's six months old. That's because preemies are at high risk of getting a severe case or complications from any respiratory infection, and the flu is a particularly nasty bug.

Rumors about the dangers of vaccines and their possible link with autism and developmental delays have led some parents to refuse immunization for their babies. But multiple large and well-done studies have shown that these fears are unfounded and that autism is not more common in children who received vaccinations. You should know that millions of lives have been saved and serious disabilities avoided thanks to the vaccines all children are offered today. You can keep your premature baby safest by making sure he gets the immunizations he needs.

MULTIPLES

Breastfeeding Twins

The nurses convinced me to pump breast milk for my twins. It's OK now while the nurses are tube feeding them, but isn't it going to be too hard for me to breastfeed two babies?

According to many mothers who have successfully breastfed premature twins (you can get in touch with some of them through La Leche League—see page 591—or your hospital's lactation counselor), it may not be an easy or tidy business in the beginning. But if you can just hold fast, after the first demanding weeks double nursing will deliver double the rewards for you and your babies. Maybe we can help with some

Timing of Vaccinations for Multiples

If you have premature twins, triplets, or more in the NICU, they may not all get their first shots on the same day (one might be sicker than another or they might be discharged from the hospital at different times). But once your babies are home, you're going to be looking for ways to save time when you can. Since the timing of vaccinations is somewhat flexible, if you remember to ask your neonatologist and pediatrician early enough they can probably work out a way to put all of your babies on the same schedule for your convenience. Often it's just a matter of thinking to plan in advance.

---

of your concerns and explain why breastfeeding twins may be the best choice for many mothers:

* **Quality.** The benefits of breast milk for premature babies are still unparalleled, even by the latest preterm formulas. Among its many benefits (see page 139), a diet of human milk helps protect your babies from infections— and having two babies sick at the same time is double-trouble!

* **Quantity.** A mother's breasts can make enough milk to allow healthy twins (or even triplets) to grow and thrive during their first months of life. Nature manages this feat by the simple mechanism of supply and demand: there's no more powerful stimulation for plentiful production of breast milk than twins nursing, even more so when they're sucking at the same time, one at each breast. (That's why now, while your twins are still gavage fed, you should try to express your milk by double pumping. There are more tips for establishing and boosting your milk supply on page 251.)

* **Time and money.** Time is something very precious to mothers of twins. Nursing twins, especially simultaneously, takes a lot less time than washing bottles, preparing formula, and then feeding each baby, one after the other, many times a day. You'll also save money, about $3,000 a year, the average cost of formula for two babies.

* **Partial breastfeeding if your milk supply is low.** If you have enough breast milk to feed both babies, that's great. If not, dividing the available milk between babies, and supplementing it with formula (an option called partial breastfeeding) will provide both of them with the benefits of nursing.

On the other hand, you might discuss with the doctors the possibility of providing breast milk for only one of your babies for a while. Since breast milk is easier to digest than preterm formula and it provides more protection against infections, you may decide to give breast milk only to your smaller, sicker twin, if your supply is limited. Although it's a tough decision you would prefer not to make, it's still better than stopping breastfeeding altogether. And for now, until your milk supply increases—or indefinitely—your other, stronger twin should grow well on formula.

Try not to feel guilty if you end up feeding your stronger twin formula. Remember that providing breast milk is not the only way to show parental love. Kangaroo care can be an excellent substitute for the intimate contact of breastfeeding, making both of your babies feel that you're utterly there for them, and it may even stimulate your breasts to produce more milk. Some mothers do it with both twins at the same time, holding them face to face, one on each breast. It will take the nurse an extra couple of minutes to help you get set up, but once you're ready, you'll discover how exhilarating it is being so close to both your babies. A few small studies on shared kangaroo care have confirmed that twins—and even triplets—can maintain a warm, steady body temperature, and everyone enjoys the peaceful bonding experience.

* **Beginning to breastfeed.** It is never easy to start nursing in the NICU. Chances are you've got a couple of sleepy preemies who are still learning to coordinate sucking, breathing, and swallowing, or who have been feeding from a bottle already and may need just a little time to sort out any nipple confusion they might encounter. Add on a disturbing lack of privacy, time, and help—since not all of the medical staff may be equally supportive of your nursing efforts—and some justified stress, and the list of difficulties is complete.

One strategy some mothers suggest is to introduce the breast to one baby before the other to avoid getting too frustrated with two inexpert babies at the same time. This may happen quite naturally in the hospital nursery if one of your preemies is ready to begin nursing before the other. (One twin may have been healthier or simply matured a little faster.) After nursing, you pump milk for the other twin. At

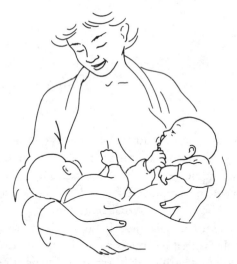

A mother nursing her twins together.

the next feeding, you start with the pumping (pump just enough for one baby without fully emptying your breasts), then continue with breastfeeding the baby who's learning to nurse so that over the course of the day, both twins will get some of the foremilk and some of the hindmilk. (The breast milk that comes out first has different nutritional qualities from the milk that comes out last.)

By the time the other twin is ready to be introduced to the art of nursing, the first will probably have become sufficiently acquainted with it that you feel more confident. (You're likely to be more confident in your baby's ability to breastfeed after just a few feeding "lessons.")

* **Breastfeeding twins simultaneously.** When both babies nurse well, it can be done, and mothers talk about it as an exhilarating, tender experience. It's not easy to be discreet, though. Since you have both arms full of babies, you can't easily juggle things around to shield yourself from people's eyes. So this is something you may want to try first where you have some privacy.

Breastfeeding Triplets?

Yes, it is possible to nurse an entire family of babies! Nevertheless, it is a very demanding enterprise, requiring a mother who can count on a lot of help and support, self-confidence, a good dose of stubbornness, and total dedication.

The first requirement to ensure the success of this breastfeeding feat is to establish a generous milk supply. Since the vast majority of triplets are born prematurely, a mother can achieve that only by getting used to pumping her breast milk often and consistently, starting right after delivery.

But having enough breast milk to satisfy three babies—completely or partially—is just the beginning. Be prepared, for the first few months, to just eat, drink, and sleep in your time off from breastfeeding your premature triplets. The problems you will face are mainly those already mentioned for twins but with a bonus baby added in. And while simultaneously nursing two babies can be very helpful to you, too, it is never the end of the story.

La Leche League or support groups for parents of multiples (see page 591) can put you in touch with mothers who have successfully nursed triplets. All of their personal testimonies stress the importance of having round-the-clock help at the beginning: someone who can assist you during the day and at night, can bring you the babies, make sure they're all fed (overlooking one is easier than you think!), change them, put them back to sleep, and help provide you with the healthy food your body needs to feed a trio of newborns.

In time, things are likely to become more organized and easier to manage, but you'll still need a lot of assistance with the babies, as well as with any older children you may have and with household chores. So although one mother can breastfeed triplets, it may take a village to help her do it!

There are many benefits to simultaneously breastfeeding twins—like being less sleep deprived. Nursing your twins together will halve the total feeding time, which in a day can add up to several precious hours.

* **Breastfeeding twins one at a time.** If you find simultaneous breastfeeding a little weird, don't force it on yourself. To avoid the emergency situation of both babies waking up at the same time and screaming to be fed, you can wake one of them a little early and nurse him first. In time, you'll know which of your babies is calmer and can wait for a few minutes, entertaining himself.

* **One twin feeding better than the other.** The most frequent obstacle for both simultaneous and one-at-a-time breastfeeding is having to deal with one good breastfeeder and one slower, less efficient one. You may not immediately notice any difference in your babies' sucking patterns, so you may just assume that when they stop nursing they are both satisfied. But one twin may not be satiated, just tired or needing to be burped, and should be

kept at the breast for longer. The imbalance may show up after a few days with one twin's slower growth. To fix that, you may want to breastfeed this baby longer and give him occasional extra bottles of breast milk that you've pumped after your breastfeeding sessions. This hindmilk (which comes out after a few minutes) is richer in calories and should help your smaller baby catch up on his growth.

Lots of practical and emotional help—from friends and family, and particularly from an understanding partner or spouse—can make an enormous difference in a mother's experience of breastfeeding twins. Eventually the turmoil and confusion of the first weeks will evolve into a reassuring routine, pleasurable and relaxing, as well as efficient.

Nonetheless, successful breastfeeding doesn't depend on your goodwill alone. So if you have to give up your plans to breastfeed, don't torment yourself. What's most satisfying is watching your twins grow, no matter how you feed them.

How to Divide Your Time

Who needs me more, our smaller and sicker twin, who is still on a ventilator, or our healthier baby, who really seems to love being held?

That's a tough one—and it's the kind of dilemma you'll soon get used to. For years beyond your babies' hospitalization, you're going to be juggling and balancing your children's different needs, trying not to feel guilty for short-changing one or the other and wishing you could split yourself into two equal pieces.

Unfortunately, that isn't possible, and right now you have two babies who both need you. So you do have to make some choices. While we can't make that easy by giving you a definitive answer, we can offer you some advice that may help.

* **Don't keep your distance from your sick twin.** Many parents hold back emotionally when they have a newborn preemie who's sick. They may be afraid of falling in love with their baby and then losing him. They may be having trouble adjusting to the shock of having a baby who isn't the perfectly healthy newborn they always imagined. They may be trying to shield themselves from the pain they feel when they're with their baby and see him struggling. All of these feelings are normal, but they don't last. When they're gone and pure love has taken their place, you won't want to be left with regrets that you weren't there for your baby when he needed you.

* **Keep in mind that even though your sick twin seems less responsive, he still benefits from being with you.** Your baby needs to be in an intensive care nursery to get well, but being in that environment isn't easy for him. A sick baby needs a lot of quiet rest and gets easily overloaded by stimulation, so the bright lights, loud noises, and medical rather than loving touches can be very stressful to him. His parents can soothe him better than anyone else. If the nurses say your baby is stable enough to pick up, you can hold him in your arms or even skin-to-skin against your warm chest. (See kangaroo care, page 249.) If he's not ready to be held yet, you can soothe him in other ways: by letting him grasp your little finger, by making a "hand womb" around his body (see page 233), by massaging him if his skin is not too fragile (make sure to ask the nurses first and see page 329); and by talking and singing to him in the voice he recognizes so well from his days inside the womb. Until

he's older and more stable, try just one form of interaction at a time.

∗ **Don't assume your healthier twin is less needy because she's stronger.** With your sicker baby, who needs a lot of peace and quiet, a little time with you goes a long way. If your healthier twin thrives on being held, it may mean that she can benefit from longer periods of interaction and more stimulation (using all of the same techniques mentioned above). If you decide that's the case, and give your healthy baby more time right now, don't feel guilty. The important thing is to follow your intuition and give each baby what's right for now, even if it's lopsided. You have years ahead of you to even things out.

∗ **Stretch the amount of time you have by setting priorities.** For the moment, it's appropriate to neglect your housework, your errands, and your friends (they'll understand). Let others do the cooking, or eat pizza and takeout food. If possible, ask your partner to spend time with the babies in the hospital, too. And remember that somebody close to you—a grandparent, uncle, aunt, or friend—may be happy to accompany you to the nursery, providing you with an extra pair of loving arms to hold one of your babies, or to take turns visiting them when you can't. Don't feel guilty asking for this special kind of help. Just make sure that the person you choose has time to visit the hospital consistently, so they and your babies can get intimately acquainted and thrive on each other's presence.

∗ **Don't think there's a magic formula—a "right" amount of time—for a parent to spend with a preemie each day.** There isn't, as long as you visit both of your babies consistently, and try to respond to their different needs, trusting your instincts and feelings day by day. More than quantity, the quality of your presence is important. Preemies, like all babies, know when their parents love them. That's what counts.

IN DEPTH

The Father of a Preemie

Every father, of course, has his own personal way of coping with an event as stressful as a premature birth. But fathers of preemies have some things in common: pain and a sense of loss because the birth and your newborn baby weren't what you had planned and dreamed; concern that your wife or partner needs emotional and practical help, as does your newborn in the hospital and any older children you may have at home; insecurity about what the future might hold for your baby; tension from the need to balance competing demands from different parts of your life; and a strong desire to handle this family crisis as well as possible. What's the best way to support your family and meet your own needs and responsibilities? What should you expect of yourself? Do you have a special role as the father of a preemie?

A Father's Personal Experience

One father we know, a friend whose triplets were born extremely premature, agreed to share his experience with us. He is an army officer who has been decorated for heroism in battle. He told us that he had never been as afraid as when his babies were in the NICU. We think his words may help other fathers make sense of what they are going through. He said: "Those days in the NICU are still the hardest of my life. I would relive the toughest moments in Iraq every day to never have to experience the NICU and see my girls struggle like that again. Rest assured, the NICU is combat. It is not *like* combat, it *is* com-

bat. The difference is that in combat people are shooting at you, while in the NICU the bullets are the roller coaster of your own emotions. In combat, you're worried for the lives of the soldiers you trained. In the NICU, the soldiers are the children you created."

Typical Emotional Reactions

The premature birth of a baby is experienced by most parents as a fearful and dangerous event, and like any powerful threat, it sets off a "fight or flight" response. This is a reaction, essential to survival, that humans share with animals. In this state of alarm, all energies are completely focused on overcoming or fleeing from the danger, so feelings of fatigue, pain, or anguish may not sink in. If you exhibited almost superhuman strength in the rushed beginning of your baby's life—going without sleep for many hours; shuttling between hospital, home, and work; dealing with countless decisions and arrangements—it's because the fight or flight response was keeping you going. Because men are often raised to keep their emotions in check, the shocking moment of a premature delivery and the following hours or days of emergency may be, paradoxically, the easiest to handle for a father.

Later, though, as the initial emergency subsides and you begin to realize the full extent of what's happened, strong emotions may surface. Psychologists interviewing fathers and mothers after premature deliveries have documented high levels of anxiety, grief, and fear in addition to such positive emotions as amazement, hope, and love. So if you feel overwhelmed with anxiety and contradictory emotions, that's to be expected.

Fortunately the anxiety generally resolves as the baby recovers and grows. But many parents of preemies have said that for the rest of their lives they have occasional flashbacks of panic brought on by something as simple as a cold their baby catches or a beeping smoke detector that sounds like the monitor alarms in the NICU. Things that once seemed very important often become less so. So don't expect to be the same person you were before. Having a child, and especially a premature child, is a life-changing experience.

What Kinds of Reactions to Expect or Avoid

First, don't minimize the intensity of the experience you and your family are going through, especially if your preemie is sick and you don't know what the future holds. By acknowledging the wrenching emotions it brings, you're not being weak; just the opposite. Terror, grief, frustrating feelings of impotence, bitterness, and rage alternating with a sense of unreality and detachment, are frequent reactions to the trauma of a premature birth. The positive emotions that parents often feel can be overwhelming as well. Love can be frightening, too, when it's very strong.

Alienation is a common experience. It's not surprising: At the unexpected premature birth of their baby, parents are thrown into a situation in which they are extremely concerned about their offspring and yet feel excluded and unable to participate in her care. If a father was not present at delivery, sees his baby less than his wife does, or is ignored and not given much credence as a parent

by the medical staff, he may feel like even more of an outsider and have problems getting attached to his baby.

To top it off, parents can feel bad about their potent and sometimes contradictory emotions, which they may perceive as unnatural or unacceptable. Shame, guilt, and revulsion about your reactions can exacerbate the anxiety.

A common response to fear and anxiety is to avoid the situation that's generating the disturbing emotions. One typical escape for many fathers is work. Considering all the time you may have taken off during your baby's first, difficult days, your responsibilities may indeed be calling you back to the workplace. But it's important to ask yourself: Is there some leeway? Do you really need to stay there for such long hours now? Remember that this is one of the most critical periods of your life and your partner's. After it's over, you won't want to be left with regrets—or your partner to be left with resentments—that can linger and grow.

Another way that people protect themselves from too much hurt is through "anticipatory grief." They shield themselves from strong feelings of loss in the future by relinquishing attachment in the present. For parents of premature babies, this may take the form of avoidance: not visiting the hospital nursery, taking little interest in the details of your preemie's day, being overly pessimistic about his progress, not wanting to see photographs of him, even avoiding giving your baby a name. Anticipatory grieving is adaptive in that it helps lessen future pain. But it does so at the expense of emotional engagement with your child. Just remember: If you repress love in self-defense, you risk losing it altogether.

Another reason some fathers of preemies work excessively long hours or don't visit the nursery much is that they feel out of place there and are convinced that their presence isn't really needed. It may be because the mother is already spending so much time at the hospital, and the father believes his talents and expertise lie elsewhere. The hospital, with its sometimes opaque ways of doing things and rigid assertion of authority, can also be unsettling, especially to those fathers whose role in the family is to take charge and manage events. Most men in our society have been raised to think that the appropriate response to situations that are getting out of control is to take action.

This unfortunately flies in the face of the situation a father finds himself in with his preemie. Given how utterly unresponsive the situation is to any interventions you can come up with, it's easy to end up feeling incompetent and retreat, or to become aggressive and hostile just to assert some control. But if you have been feeling frustrated by your inability to make a difference in your preemie's well-being, just know that your assumption is probably wrong. Some research has found that a father's presence in the hospital nursery may improve his premature infant's growth, health, and long-term development (see *Fathering a Premature Baby* on page 343).

Finally, because this premature birth has completely disrupted your life, you should expect to have feelings you may be ashamed of, most commonly, jealousy and anger directed at your wife, your baby, or the doctors and nurses. You may even regret that your baby has survived.

It may help to know that many fathers and mothers have these thoughts. It's natural to feel angry and resentful when your world has been turned upside down. Acknowledging your negative feelings, at least to yourself, or better yet, talking about them with your partner, a close friend, or even a counselor, can be a relief and allow warmer feelings to surface. With time, your parental instinct and love for your preemie should overtake the rancor or bitterness you may feel, making them slowly, but surely, disappear.

How to Sustain Your Relationship, Your Partner, Your Kids

Avoiding a couples crisis

Studies have shown that a child's serious illness is one of the most disruptive experiences a couple can go through. Although most fathers and mothers are apt to feel the same strong emotions, they may feel them at different times and may rely on different coping mechanisms, which can create stress and put a couple off balance. For long months parents may not have much time for each other. Perhaps because of the stark contrast with pre-baby times, sometimes couples who were the closest can feel the most painfully distant.

When both partners are exhausted, physically and emotionally, resentments don't get talked out right away, as they ideally should. Small misunderstandings can lag on, and grow into big problems, increasing the risk of separation or divorce. Being aware of the danger can help prevent you from minimizing signals of distress so you can recognize and respond to them before they grow deep roots. If your partner accuses you of being emotionally distant from her or the baby, try to analyze whether there's some truth to it and the reasons for your behavior. If you can, confide your underlying worries to her. Tell her how much you care for her and the baby. You'll feel better—more of a team. Being sympathetic to each other and working as much as possible on communication with your partner, is the key to overcoming a crisis and maintaining unity and cohesion.

While for some couples a premature birth may destroy a relationship, for others it makes the relationship stronger. One study found that in the majority of cases, fathers and mothers of premature babies were each other's most vital source of support, sharing the special kind of love that parents have for their child.

Making your wife or partner feel supported and understood

To help make sense of your wife's or partner's reactions, you should realize that they too may be complicated by several factors. First of all, she may perceive the events surrounding the premature birth as a failure of her maternal abilities. She may blame herself for something specific that happened during the pregnancy or simply because she failed to carry the baby to term. Because a mother is hormonally and socially programmed to take complete charge of her newborn after birth, being separated from her infant can make her feel especially deprived and helpless. For that reason, mothers tend to feel more jealous of nurses than fathers do and have more problems working out their roles with them, while fathers tend to be more comfortable and confident about leaving their baby in the care of the medical staff.

Your partner may be physically debilitated after the delivery, particularly if it was an emergency or she was ill. Her weariness, sometimes worsened by postpartum depression, can last for weeks after the baby's birth. When a mother is sick or in a different hospital from the baby, it may be the father who sees the baby more frequently and is ahead of the mother in bonding with their newborn. If your wife or partner doesn't seem as interested in your preemie's medical details or progress, don't be taken aback. When she is able to spend more time with the baby, it won't take long for her to reach your greater level of involvement. If her emotional detachment lingers for more than a few weeks, though, it could mean that she's suffering from postpartum depression and should meet with a mental health professional to get help.

There are other reasons a preemie's father may feel his partner is simply on the wrong wavelength. He may be puzzled by her concerns with seemingly tiny details: a nurse's cold behavior or minor practical problems. If you feel that your wife is simply missing the point of what really counts right now, try to temper your disapproval with attempts to understand what might underlie her reactions. They could be her way of coping with unbearable fears. Or her guilt may lead her to interpret things as slights or personal attacks.

Most of all, try to reassure her that she's in no way responsible for the premature birth of your baby. "If I had stayed in bed . . ." "If I hadn't exercised . . ." "If I had told the doctor about those first contractions . . ." can haunt mothers of preemies for a long time. Let her express her guilt, fears, and regrets, and then patiently reassure her as many times as needed that it wasn't her fault. If you make an effort to empathize with your wife's feelings, she's more likely to be understanding of your own reactions, which can be as difficult to read for her, as hers are for you.

Helping your other kids

Take the time to focus on your older children. As you can imagine, they are going to miss their parents a lot during their premature sibling's hospitalization. A toddler may not understand why you're gone so much and may interpret your preoccupation with the new baby as abandonment or rejection of her, especially if she thinks her new little sister's or brother's difficulties magically resulted from her own misbehavior or feelings of jealousy. If your children are old enough to appreciate what happened, it's easy for them to feel deeply insecure about this unexpected turn of events, scared that something bad could happen to them or you, too. Putting your older children very high on your list of priorities can help redress some of their insecurities and need for attention. On page 215, you'll find some tips on how to help them cope.

Other things you can do

✳ **Get someone to help with chores, errands, and child care.** Since both you and your partner are vulnerable and distressed, dealing with mundane responsibilities may take more effort that you can muster. Calling on relatives and friends for practical help, even hiring someone temporarily, can preserve some of your precious energies and allow you to focus on top-priority items, like visiting your baby, dealing with medical issues, keeping up at work, and supporting your wife and older children.

✳ **Be your partner's eyes and ears.** Right after delivery, when your partner isn't able to move around much yet, you can be a bridge between her and the NICU, making sure she gets all the available information and telling her all about your baby. Take pictures, take notes, tell her where your baby is, who's taking care of him, and what he's going through. Deciding to spare her worrisome news may be a way for you to control your own fear, but is not a good idea, because it breaks down the lines of communication and understanding between you.

✳ **Spend time with your baby.** Whether your partner spends a lot of time at your preemie's bedside or not, the more you visit your baby, the more you'll feel that you're involved in and knowledgeable about his care. Learning how to hold, feed, and comfort your baby in the hospital can make you a better father and a more helpful husband or companion. Other fathers have said that learning how to care for their baby in the hospital helped them overcome feelings of powerlessness and bolstered their courage to carry on through this difficult time.

✳ **Keep contributing and keep your sense of humor when the baby comes home.** The pressures on you and your partner will change, but they won't diminish for some time. Premature children often require more patience and nurturing than full-term babies, even after they're discharged from the hospital. They may be more irritable and their daily rhythms more erratic. As even parents of full-term newborns learn, feeding, diapering and soothing are going to be your main preoccupations in the next weeks and months. So forget about regular family meals, uninterrupted sleep, and the rest of your daily routine, and be prepared to hone your survival skills. Contributing to family chores and joking about rather than criticizing your chronic lack of clean socks or that millionth pizza dinner will be greatly appreciated by your wife and kids.

✳ **Expect a temporary change in your love life.** The most likely victim of your frantic schedule is your intimate relationship with your partner. All parents go through a transition, a temporary change in their sex life, when a baby is born. But a premature birth may disrupt a couple's intimacy for much longer. According to psychologists, it's helpful to accept the idea that for a while you may not be the lovers you had been. When you feel romantic, your wife or partner may not be interested, and the other way around. Don't let this disharmony loom over you without acknowledging it, because it can lead to resentments. Take the pressure off having sexual intercourse, and try to express your love in other ways. If you don't force it, passion will come back.

Fathering a Premature Baby

All child psychologists believe in the utter importance of a father's involvement for his children's optimal development. Some interesting psychological research has focused on fathers of premature babies in particular. (If you are the male central figure in your preemie's life, even if you're not his biological father, everything here is relevant for you, too.)

The concrete power of a father's love

If your wife spends a lot of time in the hospital nursery, you may think your baby doesn't need you much right now. This is not true. One study found that premature babies who were visited more often by their fathers in the hospital recovered and grew faster—gaining more weight, leaving the hospital earlier, and showing better social development in their second year. Even when such things as the frequency of mothers' visits, how small or sick the babies were, and the socioeconomic conditions of the families were taken into consideration, the frequency of fathers' visits remained a significant factor in their preemie's recovery.

Visiting may bring some other benefits, too. The more frequently fathers went to see their preemies in the nursery, the more likely they were to be nurturing parents, involved in caregiving, talking to, and playing with their baby at the time of hospital discharge and at eight months of age. Fathers who visited more often were also less likely to view their preemies as difficult children at 18 months of age. One explanation for these findings, in addition to possible differences in attitudes or temperament that fathers and babies started out with, has to do with parental bonding: Having frequent contact with a newborn increases a parent's motivation and emotional involvement. So if you visit your baby as often as you can in the hospital, in the future you may take more joy in fathering him.

What fathers do in the NICU

Various studies have noted that fathers' behavior in the hospital nursery tends to be different from mothers'. For instance, fathers tend to touch their preemie less if he's younger than 28 weeks of gestation. They start doing kangaroo care later than mothers and seldom gaze at, speak to, or fondle their babies while they're holding them. This may have to do with deep-seated differences in parenting behavior between fathers and mothers, but it may also be from insecurity in handling a newborn, especially a fragile and seemingly vulnerable preemie.

Given the evidence that a father's presence can be comforting and healing, the challenge is to not be self-conscious about people around you. Remember that your preemie finds your arms and your voice especially soothing and beneficial.

Fathers and preemies, back home

Although patient and dedicated nurturing may not be considered a traditional male virtue, fathers of preemies beat that stereotype. Research has shown that fathers of preemies tend to be more involved than fathers of full-term infants, devoting a larger share of their time to the care of their offspring at one, 5, and 18 months.

Fathers show a distinctive style of interaction with their children, mainly dedicated to play—a more vigorous, arousing, and stimulating play than mothers tend to engage in. One study of nearly 1,000 preemies from ethnically diverse families found that a large majority of fathers played with their premature child every day, even when they didn't live in the same house. This held true at one, two, and three years of age, and the sicker a baby was at birth, the more highly involved in his care his father tended to be. There is evidence that both preterm and term children, especially from disadvantaged groups, thrive on this, having better social and cognitive outcomes than toddlers whose fathers are uninvolved.

Researchers can't pinpoint exactly what aspect

of paternal involvement is most beneficial to a baby. But based on a landmark experiment that showed that baby rats who were more frequently and vigorously touched grew up smarter, some have suggested that the high levels of physical stimulation provided by fathers during play might be the key to their children's improvements in cognitive development. So perhaps the things dads do, like tossing their kids high in the air or playing rough on the floor while moms cry "Not so high!" "Not so hard!" are not only typical family vignettes but also healthy educational experiences for the children!

It's also difficult to assess the influence that an involved father has indirectly, by giving love and support to his child's mother. But any experienced parent would say that this counts for a lot. In general, a father's impact is broad and deep—on all his children. But maybe, for a preemie, even more.

CHAPTER 6

IF YOUR BABY
NEEDS SURGERY

. . . .

Guiding parents through an event that is usually scarier than it needs to be.

. . . .

INTRODUCTION:
IF YOUR BABY NEEDS SURGERY

The idea of surgery is scary to everyone, especially to the parents of a small and frail preemie. Partly that comes from fear of the unknown—the mystery of the operating room, where a surgeon can look and reach inside the human body. In fact, most people feel relieved when they are told what a surgical procedure actually involves, because the reality is often more reassuring than what they imagined. You'll still worry until you see your infant fully recovered, but knowing more about his surgery may make you feel a little better.

There are some important things you need to know if your preemie needs surgery. You should ask the neonatologist or surgeon—or both if it will help you understand things better—to explain clearly what your baby's medical problem is, why surgery may help, and what its risks are. Ask how much experience the anesthesiologist and surgeon have doing this kind of surgery on a small premature infant. You may also want to ask whether your baby is likely to be in any pain and what will be done to soothe it. Some of the information in this chapter may help answer your questions. But because the complex technical aspects of surgery, anesthesia, and recovery can vary greatly depending on each baby's situation, you should rely on the doctors to explain exactly what's going on with your child.

QUESTIONS AND ANSWERS

Too Small for Surgery?

My baby is so small. How can he possibly withstand surgery?

Everyone's heart is touched by a premature baby who has to undergo surgery at a time when he would not even have been born. As if it weren't difficult enough to see him so tiny, struggling to make it outside the womb! If it's your premature baby who needs surgery, it can feel like the worst news you could possibly get. But in reality it isn't, as you'll soon realize.

True, it is challenging to operate on a human being who weighs only a few pounds and may also be sick. But pediatric surgeons and anesthesiologists have had years of special training, learning to care for newborns and preemies like yours. A pediatric anesthesiologist is familiar with the ways a preemie reacts to anesthetic drugs and the stress of surgery, and knows what doses and combination of therapies to use to see him safely through the operation. There are many surgical subspecialties in pediatrics, so if your premature baby is having a shunt placed for hydrocephalus, for example, he'll be operated on by a pediatric neurosurgeon, while if he's having surgery to close a PDA, a pediatric thoracic or general surgeon will do it. That precise specialization allows your baby's surgeon to develop very finely honed expertise and experience.

Today, surgery is commonly performed on tiny preemies, some weighing less than two pounds. Most of these operations are extremely safe and successful, with survival rates approaching 100 percent for many of them. Unless your surgeon tells you otherwise, you have every reason to be optimistic. The great news from recent studies is that even the most premature babies can tolerate the stress of surgery extremely well, without any increase in their rates of death or subsequent serious complications during their hospitalization compared with their equally tiny peers who didn't undergo surgery—something very comforting to know if you've been told that an operation is in your baby's best interest. Although it's stressful, you should try to look upon your preemie's surgery as a turning point in his life toward a better, healthier future.

For a premature baby's surgery to be as safe as possible, it is important for it to be done in a hospital with a neonatal intensive care unit and dedicated pediatric surgeons and anesthesiologists. Good teamwork among the NICU staff, anesthesiologists, and surgical team is essential to ensure that a baby gets the best care, particularly in the delicate time right after surgery as the anesthesia is wearing off, and over the next several hours or days as your baby's body adjusts to the stress of the operation. If your preemie has to be transferred to a different hospital for his surgery you may find it distressing, and the intensity and unfamiliarity of the environment may add to your anxiety for your child. But it probably won't be for long. Most babies who were relatively healthy before surgery bounce back soon, usually in a matter of a few days or weeks. Once his surgical problems are fixed, your baby may be able to return to his home hospital.

Most parents, understandably, would like to avoid surgery for their child if they can. Although the desire to protect your baby may make you feel defensive right now, you should try not to perceive the doctors as antagonists. If you tell them that you would like more time to think things over, and there's no immediate need to operate on your baby, they will almost certainly comply.

They know this is your child. No doctor or surgeon wants to take him to the operating room unless there's a clear benefit for him and until you, although worried, are also convinced of that.

Who Is in Charge?

My baby needs surgery. Who is in charge now, the neonatologist or the surgeon?

When a premature baby needs surgery, his already worried and bewildered parents may have to deal with another stressful change: the sudden appearance of new faces around his bed as the surgeon and maybe some surgical nurses and residents come to the nursery to meet their new little patient. Most of them will make sure to introduce themselves and talk to you. But since families are not always in the hospital, the surgical team may have seen your baby several times in your absence and then come back as old acquaintances, while you're still puzzled about who they are.

Most likely, after some initial unease with your baby's surgeon, you'll become more comfortable and develop a trusting relationship with him. But many parents have problems understanding who is in charge. Is it the neonatologist, the surgeon, or both? Who makes the decisions? Whom should you talk to? You'll be dealing with two sets of doctors, who will sometimes focus on different things and who may not always think alike.

Most of the time, your confusion can be solved by asking the neonatologist you know by now to explain your baby's situation and to tell you clearly who's in charge of what. In general, the surgeon is in charge of the surgical procedure, deciding exactly when it will be done, how to prepare your baby for it, and how to take care of the incision and any equipment he puts in (such as a VP shunt or a gastrostomy tube) afterward. Other than that, responsibilities may vary. In some hos-

pitals the neonatologist always remains in charge of a premature baby. In others the neonatologist and the surgeon share equal responsibility until a baby has recovered from the operation and the surgeon signs off. So for a while they'll collaborate on such medical decisions as when feedings will resume, when sedation can be lightened, and what lab studies to order. Finally, in other hospitals the surgeon temporarily takes over the care of a baby, with the neonatologist becoming his consultant for medical decisions.

Most likely, events will lead quickly and smoothly to your baby's surgery, and to your great relief as he recovers well. Sometimes, though, a baby's situation is more complex, and there is controversy about his need for surgery or how his medical problems should be handled during his convalescence. Parents may then hear somewhat different messages from the surgeon and the neonatologist. If that happens to you, try not to get upset and don't be afraid to lift your hand and question them. One solution is to ask to meet with both doctors together, the neonatologist and the surgeon, to figure out what's best. Everybody can benefit from that meeting, but most of all you will gain a better understanding of what's going on with your baby, and that's the most important thing.

Avoiding Pain and Discomfort

My baby has to have an operation. I can't bear to think what he'll be going through, and that he'll be in pain.

It should comfort you to know that shielding your baby from pain during and after a surgical procedure is a primary goal for the doctors and nurses taking care of him. Your baby's anesthesiologist, surgeon, neonatologist, and nurse will all be watching to make sure he's as comfortable as possible.

To keep a preemie stable and pain-free during surgery requires the special skills and experience of a pediatric anesthesiologist. You will probably meet your baby's anesthesiologist a day or two before his operation. She'll explain what will be done to keep your baby from feeling pain and tell you what to expect after the surgery. Both will depend to some degree on your baby's medical condition, the surgery that he's having, and the preferences and expertise of his doctors. Don't hesitate to ask about these or anything else regarding your baby if you have questions.

* **Before your preemie goes to the operating room,** the anesthesiologist will examine her new little patient and review his medical history. She'll want to be aware of anything that would influence the choice of anesthesia and be prepared for any problems that your baby might have during or after the operation. Apnea—an overly long pause in breathing—is a common complication in newborns, especially preemies, for a day or two following general anesthesia. In many cases, it can be prevented by giving a baby caffeine right before surgery (think of it as keeping the brain's breathing center awake). The anesthesiologist, working with your baby's surgeon and neonatologist, also will order any lab tests or other medications that have to be given right before surgery, such as antibiotics to reduce the risk of infection, and will give instructions on his feedings.

Fasting is required before having surgery to avoid the risk of aspirating food from the stomach into the lungs, but premature babies don't have to fast for quite as long as older children or adults. Preemies are allowed to have their last feeding of formula six hours before surgery or of breast milk (which is easier to digest than formula) four hours before.

Right before the procedure, the anesthesiologist or your baby's nurse will personally escort him in a movable isolette to the operating room, where he'll be delivered into the expert hands of the surgical team. Sometimes, the surgery is done right in the neonatal intensive care unit instead. Surgery in the nursery is common for laser treatment of ROP and some other relatively quick procedures, but can also be an option for longer and more demanding operations when the doctors want to spare a small, frail baby the additional stress of being moved to the operating room. If your baby will be having surgery performed in the NICU you shouldn't worry; the doctors and nurses will make sure they have all the equipment and personnel they need for a safe and smooth operation.

* **The operating room will be specifically prepared** to host a tiny preemie. To keep him warm during surgery, the room temperature will be raised—making it tropical for the team of adults working in there! He'll be kept covered as much as possible during the procedure with a cap, blankets, or even plastic wrap, which is great for keeping preemies warm. His intravenous fluids may be warmed, too, to avoid lowering his body temperature.

* **Most major surgical procedures in premature babies are performed under general anesthesia,** meaning that your baby will be "put to sleep." He won't be able to move or feel any pain during the operation, and he'll have no memory of it afterward. He also won't be able to breathe on his own until the anesthesia wears off, so he'll be on a ventilator during the surgery and possibly for a while afterward. He'll probably be given the anesthetic first as a gas that he breathes through a face mask (it takes only a few seconds to work), then as a liquid through an IV. After your baby is asleep, when it won't hurt him, the anesthesiologist

will put in any catheters and tubes that may be needed for the procedure.

While it's wonderful to know that your baby will be sleeping peacefully and feel no discomfort through the whole operation, general anesthesia always carries some risk of complications. The main ones are breathing, heart rate, and blood pressure abnormalities. Although small, that risk is higher for a young preemie than for a term newborn because of the immaturity of his organs.

For some short surgeries on body areas below the waist (such as hernia repair or circumcision), the anesthesiologist may use regional instead of general anesthesia. This involves inserting a catheter to deliver local anesthetics into the spinal canal (spinal anesthesia), or around the large nerves near the spine that transmit pain sensations from the areas where the surgeon is working (caudal or epidural anesthesia, similar to what many women receive during labor). The effect of both is to block pain sensations from traveling up to the brain.

Regional anesthesia can be difficult to administer to a preemie, but it may offer benefits. Since it numbs only a specific region of your baby's body, his respiratory muscles and the breathing center in his brain aren't affected, so he should still be able to breathe on his own and may avoid having to be put on a ventilator. His risk of postoperative apnea is also reduced.

Regional anesthesia is sometimes used together with general anesthesia to help lower the amount of general anesthesia that is needed, thereby reducing the risk of complications. The catheter to deliver regional anesthetics is inserted after a baby is put to sleep, so it doesn't hurt. As an added bonus, the regional anesthesia often lasts for several hours after the surgery; and in some cases, the catheter can be left in place and anesthetics administered through it to give a baby uninterrupted pain control over the next few days.

✳ **In the delicate postoperative time,** every preemie needs very attentive care. When the operation is finished, your baby will remain in the operating room or will be taken to a nearby recovery room, where he will be observed closely to make sure he remains stable as the anesthesia begins to wear off. Then your baby will be prepared for the trip back to the NICU. Some of the catheters, lines, and monitors that were used during the surgery will be detached or switched to portable medical equipment. When your baby is all set, the surgeon, anesthesiologist, and a nurse will accompany him back to the NICU. They won't leave until they've given the neonatologist and your baby's bedside nurse all the information needed to take care of him after his surgery: details about what went on in the operating room and any special instructions for your baby's postoperative care. While a baby is recovering from surgery, there will always be teamwork among the surgeon, the anesthesiologist, and your baby's neonatologist, but the exact assignment of responsibilities may differ from hospital to hospital.

After surgery, you should be prepared to see your baby in the newborn intensive care unit even if he was in a step-down unit before the operation. That doesn't mean the operation didn't go well. Preemies generally need to stay in a NICU after a surgical procedure to be monitored for postoperative apnea, pain, and any possible complications. Your baby may also be attached to a ventilator, not breathing on his own, for what seems like long hours or perhaps even days after surgery. That's because a preemie's immature liver and kidneys take some time to clear the anesthetics out of his body, so he may not wake up or breathe for a while, especially if he's given more pain medication in the NICU. Usually babies who didn't have previous breathing problems are off a ventilator within hours to a few days after their surgery. But babies who had respiratory problems before the surgery and whose lungs are not completely normal may have a harder time and take longer to come off the ventilator afterwards.

Postoperative pain in preemies can be treated very effectively, so you shouldn't worry about that. Be assured that the doctors and nurses will be watching for it carefully, since pain doesn't only hurt, but can also interfere with a baby's recovery. You can read about ways to assess how much pain a preemie is feeling and different methods of pain control on page 117; the same principles apply to your baby's care after his surgery. Your baby's doctors will probably use narcotics like morphine or fentanyl to keep him comfortable if he has severe pain. These drugs are excellent for easing pain but will make him sleepy, increase his risk of apnea, and possibly prolong his stay on the ventilator. Tylenol, which doesn't sedate a baby or suppress his breathing, is effective in treating moderate pain and is helpful once your baby's pain becomes milder.

After your baby's surgery, you can help to make sure that he receives any comfort and care that make him feel better. Sometimes parents are the best judges of how their baby is doing. Don't hesitate to ask what pain medication he's getting and what other relief measures have been taken. You should feel free to call a nurse or doctor if you notice that your baby is agitated; they may want to give him more pain medicine.

When you see that your baby is conscious enough to be aware of your presence, try to give him a gentle signal. Touch his hand and tell him softly that Mommy and Daddy are there, patiently waiting for him to get well. And when your baby is even more awake and a little better, ask the nurse if he can suck on a pacifier, be swaddled, or held in your arms.

Your Preemie Needs Surgery: Decisions and Precautions

When your premature baby needs surgery, in addition to being worried and upset you may find yourself under a lot of pressure. It would be helpful if you could stop the clock to discuss the matter more thoroughly with your family, talk again to your baby's doctors and to other physicians, and get more information before giving your consent to the operation. Even if your baby's surgery is not an emergency, you'll most likely feel that time is going too fast.

The questions below cover the essential information and support you should receive before your baby's surgery. If you are missing any of it, don't be shy about bringing your questions or needs to the attention of your baby's doctors. On the other hand, if you have all of this information and support, you can be assured that you and your doctors have done what you could to make the best decision for your baby.

1. **Do you know why your baby needs surgery, what the benefits and risks of the procedure are, how urgent it is, and what's involved in her recovery? In other words, do you feel you know enough to give informed consent for the operation?**

    All surgeries are invasive procedures, carrying benefits and risks. The doctors should explain clearly what your baby is going to gain from the operation, how soon it needs to be done, and what her convalescence will entail. Only your doctors can tell you exactly what you can expect for your baby, but most of the time the prospects for preemies who undergo surgery are very good.

    Sometimes surgery for a preemie is an emergency, needing to be done immediately to avert serious injury or death. But more commonly, you'll be told that even though your preemie's operation should be done soon, it doesn't necessarily have to happen right away. For instance, if your baby has hydrocephalus and her doctors say she needs a VP shunt, she may be sick and fragile, but she is probably not so unstable that you can't take a few days to think it over. Some surgeries, such as hernia repairs, are even less pressing. They need to be done eventually, but are often postponed for several weeks until a preemie is bigger, stronger, and better equipped to withstand the stress of surgery (usually, shortly before he's discharged home). Some procedures are elective, meaning that they are not absolutely necessary. For instance, a tracheostomy or a gastrostomy may be done to improve a baby's life and enhance her development or to make caring for him easier. They can sometimes be put off for a long time or even not done at all, so you can take as much time as you need to learn about the pros and cons.

2. **Do most doctors agree on the best treatment for your baby? If there are alternatives to surgery, do you know their risks and benefits and what will happen to your baby if surgery isn't done?**

    Don't be afraid to ask your baby's doctors whether all doctors would agree that surgery is the best way to treat your baby's condition. It is their duty to inform you about the risks and benefits of other possible treatments, and of not doing anything at all, even if they are convinced that surgery is the best way to go. Some families feel that if there is time they would like to consult another specialist or surgeon for a second opinion, but they may be afraid of offending their doctor. You shouldn't worry about that. Physicians don't tend to take a request for a second opinion personally. Indeed, if they're having to make a hard decision on how best to treat your baby, they may be relieved to share that responsibility with a colleague.

3. **Were you and your partner given enough time to reflect, have family discussions, and reach a considered decision about your baby's surgery? Are your values and feelings being taken into account by your baby's doctors? Has the medical staff been supportive?**

    You should not feel pressured to make quick decisions unless it's unavoidable because of your baby's medical situation. Even when there isn't time for much reflection, the doctors should give you as much time as possible, even if it is just a few minutes alone to talk things over. Before surgery, if your baby's medical condition allows, you should be able to spend time with her, take her picture, have your family visit her. After surgery, just being told that everything went well may not be enough to reassure a preemie's anguished parents. You should be told clearly and in detail what you need to know about the procedure and her expected recovery. Try to accept different personality traits and communication styles as part of the variety of human nature; some doctors and nurses will just be more patient and understanding, forthcoming, and supportive than others. Still, your needs should be accommodated by the nursery staff as much as possible, to sustain you psychologically and to make you a stronger, more informed advocate for your baby.

4. **Do the doctors and nurses know how to reach you shortly before, during, and after the surgery?**

    Sometimes the surgeon or neonatologist needs to talk to parents urgently about changes in their baby's medical condition or to get consent for additional procedures. For a day or so before and after your baby's surgery, when you're not in the hospital nursery, it will be important to let the medical staff know how to get in touch with you. Also, because the exact starting time and duration of most operations aren't known in advance, you should let the nursery staff know if you want to be notified when your baby goes to the operating room and when she returns, and if you want to accompany the team taking your baby to and from the nursery. This may not be done automatically.

It may be impossible for you to believe right now, but the memory of your baby's surgery will become less painful in the future. You'll always feel grateful, though, to the doctors and nurses who were most supportive and who gave you the information you needed to make the best decisions.

KINDS OF SURGERY A PREEMIE MAY NEED

On the following pages, you can find some basic information about the most common surgical procedures performed on premature babies along with their usual indications, outcomes, complications, and recovery. To get the full picture for your own baby, though, you need to talk to his surgeon and neonatologist. This brief overview is designed to help you know what to ask your baby's doctors and to understand what their answers mean.

Some preemies need surgery in their first weeks of life because of a congenital condition—a problem that was present before birth. If that's the case for your baby, his surgeon and neonatologist will discuss his specific medical problems and future prospects with you, as well as the risks and benefits of the operation. The operations that we discuss below are not for such congenital problems but are instead specifically for complications of prematurity.

Some risks are common to all surgeries: mainly infection, bleeding, damage to nearby tissues, and complications from general anesthesia. Today, thanks to the development of much smaller instruments, pediatric surgeons can sometimes safely perform minimally invasive surgery on their little patients. This technique involves making only tiny incisions in the skin and underlying tissues through which the surgeon inserts a thin fiberoptic cable with a viewing device and miniature surgical tools. Depending on where in the body it takes place, you'll hear this kind of surgery called by different names, such as laparoscopic (lapar refers to the abdomen and scopic to the scope, or tiny viewer, that the surgeon inserts and sees through as he operates), endoscopic (endo refers to the inside of a hollow organ, such as the bowel or bladder), and thorascopic (thora refers to the chest). Since the cuts are so small, the injury to surrounding tissues is limited, and recovery is sometimes quicker than after traditional surgery.

You should know that there's a chance with any operation that it won't be successful, because the surgeon can't accomplish what he set out to do, or the procedure doesn't end up benefiting the patient as hoped, or because the problem recurs and surgery needs to be redone. These risks vary from procedure to procedure and from patient to patient, so you should ask your baby's surgeon about them. He can tell you what he's planning to do to try to prevent complications and what could be done to treat your baby if they occur.

Most of the problems of prematurity that lead to surgery have been described in other chapters. It's a good idea to go back and read about your baby's underlying condition again, as some information in there might help you to better understand his surgical treatment.

It will be hard for you to feel at peace until your child comes out of the operating room and you hear the surgeon saying that everything went well. But in the meantime, try to be optimistic. Most of the time, preemies sail through their operations with flying colors.

Surgery to Close a PDA

Why it may be needed

If a premature baby has a large PDA (patent ductus arteriosus; see page 203) that cannot be closed with medication (either because the medication hasn't worked or because something about the baby's condition makes his doctors believe that using medication is not advisable), his doctors may consider surgery to close it. The operation is called a PDA ligation. Among the patients who have PDA surgery are some of the smallest and youngest babies in the NICU, because they often have breathing, blood pressure, or other problems that their doctors think might improve if the ductus were closed. Since there's uncertainty about the role a PDA plays in a preemie's medical problems and the benefits of closing it surgically, some doctors may prefer to wait and see whether the ductus closes by itself later. Other doctors may recommend going ahead with surgery right away.

How a PDA ligation is performed

A PDA ligation is performed under general anesthesia with your baby on a ventilator. (Some parents mistakenly think that a PDA ligation is heart surgery, but it's not; your baby's heart won't be touched at all.) To reach the PDA, the surgeon will make a small horizontal incision on the left side of your baby's back. He'll lift up your baby's lung to find the patent ductus, then close it tightly with a tiny metal clip or with stitches, neither of which needs to be removed. Within a few weeks after the ductus is closed, it will shrivel and go away, never to reopen again.

A PDA ligation also can be done thorascopically, a minimally invasive surgical technique that in experienced hands is as safe and effective as the traditional approach. In about one out of ten cases, the surgeon switches in the operating room from a thorascopic procedure to a traditional one, because he discovers that in a particular baby's case, the minimally invasive technique is too difficult or risky or that the baby isn't tolerating it well. There's no harm done to the little patient, who's safely sleeping under general anesthesia.

A few babies who are discharged from the hospital without having surgery may eventually need to have their PDA closed months or years later, if it is large and has not closed on its own. The older

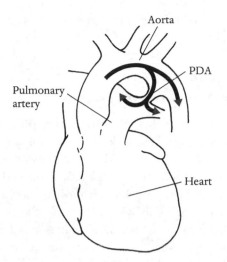

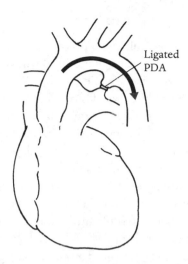

With a PDA, blood can flow back from the aorta into the pulmonary artery, overloading the heart and the lungs.

A PDA ligation closes the ductus, reestablishing normal circulation.

and bigger a child, the more likely his PDA can be closed using a less invasive procedure. As the child sleeps under general anesthesia or deep sedation, a tiny device to block blood flow through the PDA is inserted into an artery through a small incision in his groin and pushed into the PDA by means of a long catheter. Once there, the device blocks off the PDA, effectively closing it.

Outcome and possible complications

A PDA ligation, performed the traditional way or thoracoscopically, has a mortality rate close to zero and is nearly always successful in closing the ductus. Although complications are uncommon, they do sometimes occur. The risks are similar for traditional and thoracoscopic surgery. Very occasionally, the clip or stitches come loose shortly after the operation before the ductus shrivels up, and the PDA reopens. Rarely during the ligation, a major blood vessel—several lie close to the ductus—is nicked. If that happens, while the

surgeon immediately repairs the blood vessel, the anesthesiologist will give your baby a blood transfusion to replace the blood he's lost and will make sure that everything is done to keep his breathing, heart beat, and blood pressure stable. Another possible complication of a PDA ligation is a small tear in a lung, called a pneumothorax. This will heal naturally on its own in a few days. In a small number of cases, a PDA ligation may cause accidental damage to a nerve that passes near the ductus and controls the vocal cords and the movements of the diaphragm. An injury to this nerve could temporarily (for several weeks or months) or permanently give a baby a hoarse voice, increase his risk for accidentally aspirating food into his lungs (because his vocal cords may not close tightly when he swallows, allowing food to go down the wrong pipe), or make it more difficult for him to take deep breaths. Though it's natural to worry when you hear about a risk like this, you should keep in mind that it happens rarely, and that most such injuries are mild and end up healing on their own.

Recovery and healing

Due to the combination of general anesthesia and the pain medication your baby will get after surgery, it will take a while for him to wake up and breathe on his own. Usually a baby's condition improves gradually, beginning about 12 to 24 hours after the operation, with continued improvement over the next several days. Some babies, though, are sicker and more unstable for a couple of days after surgery as their lungs and heart recover from the added stress of the operation. Most babies resume breast milk or formula feedings in a few days.

How much better your baby ultimately gets—for example, whether closing his PDA allows him to come off the ventilator or not—will depend on how much the PDA was contributing to his medical problems. Often it's impossible to know this in advance: Doctors can be surprised by how completely a preemie's lungs recover once his PDA is closed. Unfortunately, they can be equally surprised by how little difference closing a baby's PDA can make.

If your baby had a traditional PDA ligation, the remaining scar on his back will eventually look like a thin, light line. If he had a thorascopic procedure, the tiny incisions made by the surgeon will become nearly invisible as he grows.

Surgery to Treat NEC

Why it may be needed

If a baby with NEC (necrotizing enterocolitis; see page 266), is not getting better within a couple of days of starting medical treatment, it can mean that parts of her intestine have torn or died. Once that happens, the damaged areas need to be removed and her abdomen drained of fluid and pus in order for the infection and inflammation to subside and the remainder of her bowel to rest and heal.

How surgical treatments for NEC are performed

Laparoscopy for diagnosis and planning: Sometimes it's hard to know if NEC is the right diagnosis, and if it is, whether a baby's bowel is damaged badly enough to need a major surgical procedure. To help with those questions and decisions, and only if your baby's doctors think it would be safe and beneficial in her case, the surgeon might perform a diagnostic procedure at her bedside in the NICU. Using local anesthesia, the surgeon will make a small incision in your baby's abdomen and insert a laparoscope (a fiberoptic instrument that allows him to look around inside the belly) and a little carbon dioxide gas to help him see better. With the scope the surgeon can directly see whether your baby has NEC, how extensive it is, and whether her bowel is torn and needs to be surgically repaired—valuable pieces of information for her care. Surgeons have only recently been doing this procedure on preemies with NEC, so there is little data yet on its risks and benefits, but some doctors feel it holds promise.

Peritoneal drainage: If a baby with NEC is extremely premature or very sick, doctors may believe that the stress of a major operation would be too much for her right away. Instead, her surgeon may do an initial, simpler procedure, called peritoneal drainage, which can be performed in her bed in the NICU under local anesthesia. The surgeon makes a small incision on the right side of the baby's belly and inserts a soft tube, called a drain, that goes into her abdomen and is secured to her skin with surgical stitches. The tube allows gas, infected fluid, and stool to drain out, lowering the pressure in her belly and helping to ease the inflammation.

More than one-third of babies treated with peritoneal drainage recover completely from NEC and need no further surgery. This encouraging outcome has led some surgeons to believe that peritoneal drainage should be the first choice of treatment for all babies with NEC. Other surgeons think that babies who are stable enough for surgery are better off having it done sooner rather than later because drainage doesn't correct NEC quite as rapidly, and a baby can thereby avoid the possible need for a second surgical procedure. Ongoing studies are comparing the two approaches. If your baby needs either peritoneal drainage or NEC surgery, her doctors will explain the pros and cons of both procedures and make a recommendation based on their experience and your baby's condition. Your opinion will also be taken into careful consideration when the treatment decision is made.

NEC Surgery: NEC surgery is performed under general anesthesia with your baby on a ventilator. The surgeon makes an incision, usually a few inches long, just above or below the belly button from one side of her abdomen to the other. He thoroughly cleans her abdomen and drains any abscesses, then carefully examines the whole length of her bowel from the stomach to the rectum, looking for holes and signs of damage. He removes any areas of intestine that are torn or irreparably damaged, while aiming to preserve as much bowel as possible so that your baby can absorb enough nutrients from her feedings later.

Sometimes it won't be obvious at the time of the operation whether an area of intestine can recover or not. In that case, the surgeon may leave it in, hoping it will heal. But if your baby's condition isn't steadily improving by about 48 hours later, he'll probably check on her bowel again with a second operation, called a reexploration or "second look."

If a baby has just an isolated hole in one part of her intestine or a few damaged areas that can be cleanly removed, and the rest of her bowel looks healthy, the surgeon may immediately reconnect her intestine. But other times, when the cut ends of her intestine are affected and need time to heal, it is safer and recovery is faster and more complete if they are not rejoined immediately. Instead, the surgeon brings the two open ends of the bowel out through a small incision in your baby's belly. That procedure is called an enterostomy, or "ostomy" for short (see illustration).

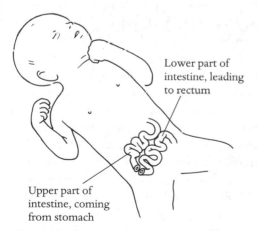

Lower part of intestine, leading to rectum

Upper part of intestine, coming from stomach

After the area of intestine damaged by NEC has been removed, the two open ends may not be rejoined immediately, to promote healing.

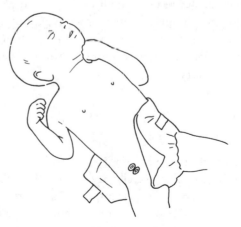

The two open ends of the intestine are brought out through the skin of the belly, forming an enterostomy.

To be told that your baby has been given an ostomy is shocking news. But be assured that it is only temporary. Usually in about six weeks your baby's intestine can be reconnected safely and tucked back inside where it belongs. In the meantime, having an ostomy allows the lower tract of her intestine to rest and heal, because food and stool won't be passing through it. Until her bowel is reconnected, your baby's stools will come out of the end of the higher intestinal tract, into a special bag taped to her belly. (The ostomy bag is usually completely covered by a baby's diaper, invisible to anyone who isn't changing her.)

Many babies will have their bowel reconnected and ostomy closed while they are still in the hospital nursery. In the meantime, parents can learn by watching the nurses how to clean and protect the delicate skin around the ostomy when they're changing the bag. If your baby is discharged home earlier, when she still has an ostomy, you can be sure that you'll be instructed carefully and thoroughly on how to take care of her.

The surgery to reconnect your baby's bowel (called an enterostomy closure, reanastomosis, or "take down") is usually a simple procedure from which babies recover rapidly, often within a few days—much quicker than from NEC surgery. Most of the time, the surgeon can go in through the previous incision, so your baby won't have additional scars.

Outcome and possible complications

Surgery to treat NEC is very effective in stopping the disease. The overall survival rate after NEC surgery is about 70 percent. (That figure reflects the average outcome of large numbers of babies, including those who are extremely premature and very ill. Bigger babies, especially those who weigh more than 1,000 grams or who aren't as sick, tend

to do even better.) Only one out of ten babies will ever have a recurrence of the illness.

How quickly your baby recovers after NEC surgery and how well she'll do in the long run will depend on how advanced her illness was before the operation and the amount of healthy bowel she has left. Right after surgery your baby's doctors will be able to make more precise predictions about her outcome. Babies who lose more than half of their intestine are at risk for a condition called short-bowel syndrome, and may need intravenous nutrition for a very long time. (If you are told that your preemie may have short-bowel syndrome, you can read a little more about it on page 269, and your doctors will explain what you can expect for your child.) Most babies will have an adequate amount of intestine left, and once they fully recover from their NEC will be able to eat and grow normally—usually in about three to six weeks. Preemies who have had severe NEC are at slightly higher risk of having developmental problems in the future.

The most common short-term complications of NEC surgery are infection, bleeding, and poor healing of the surgical incision, especially if some of your baby's fragile bowel develops new tears in it. Some babies with ostomies don't grow well temporarily and have metabolic disturbances because their upper intestinal tract is too short to absorb enough nutrients. These problems usually resolve when their bowel is reconnected. About 20 percent to 30 percent of babies will develop an intestinal stricture: a narrowing of the bowel due to scar tissue. A stricture usually shows up as feeding intolerance or a bowel obstruction several weeks after the episode of NEC has resolved and can be diagnosed by an X-ray study using a special dye. Intestinal strictures are easily removed surgically with a much simpler operation than your baby's original NEC surgery.

Recovery and healing

A preemie who has just had NEC surgery is usually very sick. You can expect that your baby will be on a ventilator for several days or more after the operation as she slowly recovers from her illness and the surgery. Your baby's doctors and nurses may notice the happy signs that she's getting better sooner than you do because her laboratory values will improve and she'll need less intensive medical support before she begins to look visibly better.

You should be prepared for your baby to have some swelling all over her body, which may get worse for a couple of days but then should gradually get better over a week or so. She will continue to receive antibiotics until any infection is adequately treated (usually about two weeks) and won't be given anything to eat except intravenous nutrition until her intestines are healing well. The doctors will be watching for the return of her bowel function, which will be heralded by her passing stool (the nurses will proudly display it to you in her ostomy bag or diaper!) and a clearing of the bile that is being drained from her stomach.

When the doctors think your baby is ready to eat again, they will reintroduce feedings very slowly and cautiously, using small amounts of breast milk or a predigested formula. Most infants after NEC surgery don't absorb nutrients well because it takes time for their intestine to fully recover, and those who have ostomies use only part of their intestine for a while. Your baby's feedings will be gradually advanced as she shows that she can tolerate them.

In general, you should be prepared for some fits and starts on the road to full feedings. But despite the terrifying experience of undergoing NEC surgery, it is likely that you and your baby will be feeling immeasurably better in a few weeks as she starts eating and growing well.

Surgery to Place a Broviac Catheter or Other Central Venous Line

Why it may be needed

Premature babies who need intravenous nutrition or medications for more than a couple of weeks may benefit from having a special intravenous catheter that is designed to be surgically inserted into a central (meaning major) blood vessel and used long-term. This kind of catheter—Broviac is the brand most commonly used, but there are many others—has a small cuff or rim around it that secures it in place under the skin. Compared to an uncuffed catheter (such as a PICC, described on page 161) or the small garden-variety IVs you're used to seeing, a cuffed central venous line is more stable and less likely to be dislodged. It is painless and convenient to use, and substances that could damage smaller and more fragile blood vessels, like high-calorie intravenous nutrition and some antibiotics, can be safely infused through it.

How surgery to place a central venous catheter is performed

Insertion of a central venous catheter is a minor surgical procedure. It can be performed under general anesthesia or deep sedation, either in the operating room or in the NICU. Either way, your baby will be sleeping peacefully throughout the procedure and won't feel any pain. The surgeon will locate a large vein, probably one in your baby's chest or leg. He'll make a small incision and put a soft plastic catheter into her vein, then carefully thread it forward so that its tip is in the correct position, in a very large blood vessel near her heart or in the upper chamber of the heart itself. The soft cuff around the catheter will be positioned right under your baby's skin where the tubing comes out, and stitched into place. The entry site on the skin will then be covered with a clear dressing and some tape, to keep bacteria out and prevent the line from being pulled out inadvertently.

Outcome and possible complications

Surgery to place a central venous catheter is usually very safe, even in small and sick preemies. A chest X-ray will be done immediately after the procedure to confirm that the tip of the catheter is in the right place and to make sure that no accidental tears were made in the lung nearby. The main possible complications from having a central venous line are infection (if the infection could not be cleared up with antibiotics, the line would have to be removed) and formation of blood clots in the catheter, which could block the line or possibly travel to other spots in the body.

Recovery and healing

Recovery is usually so rapid that often by the time a baby is back in the NICU or fully awake she's her old self—with only a new bandage and a different kind of IV line to show for her surgical experience. Most babies aren't bothered by the soft catheter, and after a while, most parents barely notice it's there. Best of all, your baby will be spared the pain of frequent needle sticks to put in new IVs. When she doesn't need a central line anymore, the catheter can be removed in just a few minutes at your baby's bedside. Eventually she'll have only a small scar.

Surgery to Treat Hydrocephalus

Why it may be needed

When a baby has hydrocephalus (see page 194), there's a danger that the buildup of fluid inside her skull could put too much pressure on her brain and eventually damage it. If your baby's doctors find that her hydrocephalus is getting worse instead of better over time, or if it is putting enough pressure on her brain to cause problems with her breathing or heart rate, they will want to drain off some of the excess fluid to relieve the pressure.

The most common and effective long-term treatment for hydrocephalus is a VP (short for ventriculo-peritoneal) shunt. A VP shunt is a small plastic tube that is inserted surgically and carries excess fluid from the ventricles in the brain, where it builds up, to the inside of the abdomen (or peritoneum), where it can be reabsorbed.

Most of the time in preemies, a VP shunt insertion is not an emergency. That's because their open skull bones can diffuse the increasing pressure by simply letting their heads expand, and there are other, temporary ways to drain off excess fluid. Surgery to place a VP shunt is often postponed for several weeks, until the doctors are certain that it's necessary and believe that a baby is big and strong enough for a shunt to be inserted safely and to continue working well over time.

For most preemies, the need for a VP stunt is lifelong.

How a VP shunt insertion is performed

A VP shunt insertion, in the hands of an experienced pediatric neurosurgeon, is a relatively simple and safe procedure. It affects only a very small area of the brain and carries almost no risk of damaging your baby's brain functions. It is always done under general anesthesia with your baby on a ventilator and usually takes an hour or two.

There are several types of shunts; your neurosurgeon will choose the one he thinks is best suited for your baby. The upper end of the shunt is first placed into one of your baby's ventricles by passing it through a small, crescent-shaped incision on the top or side of her scalp, then through a tiny hole in her skull. The surgeon then takes the other end of the shunt and tunnels the rest of the tubing just underneath her skin, passing behind one ear and down the side of her neck and chest to reach her belly. There the surgeon makes a very small incision below her ribs so he can insert the lower end of the shunt inside her abdomen. He'll coil some extra tubing in there, too,

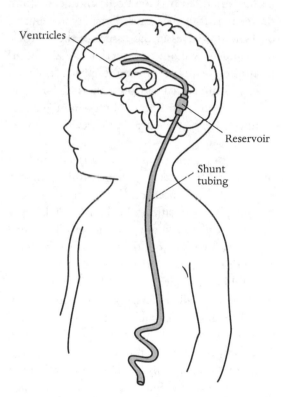

The upper end of a VP shunt, placed inside one of the ventricles, drains out the cerebrospinal fluid and carries it through long tubing into the abdomen where it is reabsorbed.

Adapted with permission of author Elizabeth Ahmann and illustrator Teresa Ahmann from *Home Care for the High Risk Infant: A Family-Centered Approach,* 2nd ed., Figure 18-2, p. 271; Aspen Publishers (1996, Gaithersburg, MD)

to make sure the lower tip of the VP shunt stays inside her abdomen (where it needs to be for the fluid coming from the ventricles to be absorbed) for as long as possible as she grows.

An important component of a VP shunt is the reservoir, or bubble. You'll notice it as a small bump underneath your baby's scalp near the incision. The reservoir contains a valve that controls the amount of cerebrospinal fluid flowing through the shunt and ensures that it doesn't drain too quickly or too slowly. The valve can also be used by the neurosurgeon to assess the functioning of the VP shunt.

An alternative procedure: endoscopic third ventriculostomy

Rarely, a preemie's hydrocephalus may be treated with an operation called a third ventriculostomy, which doesn't require the insertion of a shunt. Instead the neurosurgeon, using a fiberoptic endoscope so that he can see what he's doing, reaches inside one of the ventricles and makes a hole in it. This opening allows the cerebrospinal fluid to flow from the ventricle into the surrounding space to be reabsorbed. It sounds simple, but there's a risk of damaging part of the brain under the ventricle; and when hydrocephalus is caused by an intraventricular hemorrhage, as is often the case in preemies, the technique usually doesn't work well. At the present time, it's seldom performed on children under a year of age. If the pediatric neurosurgeon thinks your child is a good candidate for it, he'll thoroughly explain the benefits and risks to you.

Temporary surgical treatments for hydrocephalus

Hydrocephalus in preemies is usually a consequence of an intraventricular hemorrhage, due to blood clots or scarring that obstruct the flow or the reabsorption of cerebrospinal fluid. Often a preemie is too small or too sick when she develops hydrocephalus to have a VP shunt placed, or her doctors may want to wait for a few weeks until there's less blood and protein in the ventricles to see whether her hydrocephalus will resolve by itself.

When a preemie's hydrocephalus needs to be relieved before she's ready for a VP shunt, there are some simpler and quicker surgical procedures that allow for temporary drainage of the excess fluid. These techniques, called ventriculostomies, consist of placing a thin tube inside the baby's ventricles through which the cerebrospinal fluid can flow. The tube is then connected to either a plastic bag hanging on the baby's bed that collects the excess fluid or to a small plastic reservoir placed under the baby's skin from which the fluid can easily be withdrawn with a needle and syringe (called tapping, this is usually done by the baby's doctor once or twice a week). Alternatively, a pocket may be surgically created under the galea, the tough layer of tissue covering the bones of her skull, where the fluid can be naturally absorbed by her body (a subgaleal shunt). Each kind of ventriculostomy has its own pros and cons; your neurosurgeon will choose the kind he thinks will work best for your baby and explain what's involved. Insertion is usually a short procedure taking an hour or less and is performed in the operating room under general anesthesia.

Sometimes temporary drainage is all it takes and a preemie never needs a VP shunt. The doctors will know that they no longer need to remove excess fluid when any symptoms a baby has from her hydrocephalus have resolved, her fontanelle feels soft and flat instead of tense and bulging from the pressure of too much fluid, and the growth of her head slows to a normal rate. But if permanent treatment for your baby's hydrocephalus is needed, the neurosurgeon can easily convert the ventriculostomy to a VP shunt later, when she's bigger and stronger.

Outcome and possible complications

A VP shunt is nearly always successful in treating a preemie's hydrocephalus. Shunt malfunctions, leading to a recurrence of hydrocephalus, and shunt infections, are the most common complications after VP shunt insertion. A shunt malfunction can occur soon after surgery if the tubing becomes blocked by blood cells and debris from the hemorrhage that caused the hydrocephalus or if the tip lodges in the tissues of the ventricle or abdomen. A shunt malfunction can also occur months or years later if the tubing breaks or if a child gets so tall that the lower tip is no longer in her abdomen. A malfunctioning shunt requires another surgery (called a shunt revision) to replace or fix it.

Most shunt infections occur around the time of surgery, 70 percent of them within a month of the VP shunt insertion. Infections are serious because they can affect the brain and because they can lead to a shunt malfunction if bacteria and other inflammatory debris obstruct the tube. If a shunt infection can't be cleared in a few days by antibiotics alone, the shunt will have to be removed surgically (bacteria can hide in the tubing where antibiotics can't reach them). After the infection is successfully treated, your child will have another surgery to put in a new VP shunt.

Most neurosurgeons will not place a VP shunt in a preemie who weighs less than 1,500 to 2,000 grams. Complications are more common in the smallest babies because their delicate tissues don't stand up well to surgical manipulation, their skin is thin and easily irritated by the shunt tubing, their immune systems aren't strong in fighting off infections, and sometimes the smallest shunts don't drain well.

Your baby's long-term outcome will depend more on her condition overall than on factors related to surgery. The statistics are that 50 percent of preemies with VP shunts develop normally throughout early childhood. Some things that make a difference are the extent of the hemorrhage that caused the hydrocephalus, the presence of lasting, visible brain injuries on her head ultrasound (see page 325), the timing of the VP shunt insertion (waiting too long can be dangerous), episodes of shunt infection or malfunction (which sometimes, but not always, can worsen a child's neurological development), her size at surgery, whether she has additional medical problems, and how she has developed so far. You should keep in mind that many preemies who need a VP shunt have normal intellectual development. If they have a long-term developmental problem, it may be severe or mild and is more likely to involve their fine and gross motor skills.

Recovery and healing

Your baby will come back from the operating room to the NICU, probably still asleep and on a ventilator. She will be given antibiotics to prevent an infection and medications to keep her from feeling pain. Don't be scared if her head looks strange, with a patch of hair shaved off and sunken fontanels, because that's normal and just temporary. You'll probably see its shape change a lot in the next weeks and months until she looks just like any other preemie.

After a VP shunt insertion, you'll immediately notice the bump of the reservoir and the tubing under your baby's skin descending from the side of her neck to her abdomen. While it will look prominent to you initially, the shunt will become less visible as your baby puts on some weight and her hair grows. By the time she's a toddler, the shunt will be just a hard, very small bulge on

her head, invisible under her hair and completely unnoticeable unless you probe for it with your fingers. (In our experience, you'll have to warn anyone who gives her a haircut about it!)

For a few days after the operation, your baby may need to lie flat or in another position specified by the neurosurgeon so that the shunt drains at the best speed for her. Once you get the OK, though, you can handle or hold your baby as you would normally do. Remember that the valve doesn't have any contact with her brain and is so firmly secured that only the most extreme impact could jostle it around.

Most likely, your child will need her VP shunt for the rest of her life. (For more information on what having a VP shunt means for you and your child as she grows, see *Leading a normal infancy and childhood with a VP shunt* on page 463.) A few children eventually outgrow the need for a shunt as their ability to drain or reabsorb cerebrospinal fluid improves. But since removing a shunt requires an operation, which is more dangerous than leaving it in, doctors don't test for that and don't plan to remove it.

Most preemies recover quickly after a VP shunt insertion and in two or three days are more stable, alert, and active than before the surgery. Your baby will have some X-rays taken and maybe another head ultrasound to check that the shunt is intact and working, and in about ten days her stitches will be taken out. By that time many preemies are already fully recovered and doing great.

Surgery to Treat GE Reflux

Why it may be needed

Usually medical treatment and other measures are effective in keeping gastroesophageal reflux under control (see page 275). But for babies who have the most severe, persistent reflux, surgery could be the best route. Serious GE reflux can trigger potentially life-threatening episodes of apnea, bradycardia, and wheezing. A baby who spits up food into her airways may suffer from recurrent pneumonia, and the chronic inflammation in her lungs may make her breathing worsen over time. The acid from her stomach may also irritate the lining of her esophagus causing pain, bleeding, anemia, and feeding problems. And if a child vomits a lot, it cuts down on her food intake and may impair her growth.

How surgery for GE reflux is performed

The surgical procedure to treat GE reflux is called a fundoplication. There are different kinds; the most common is a Nissen fundoplication. It is usually performed under general anesthesia with your baby on a ventilator.

A fundoplication can be done using either a traditional or minimally invasive (laparoscopic) approach. The surgeon will make an incision in your baby's belly to get to her stomach, then wrap the round upper part of her stomach (the fundus) around her esophagus, securing it with sutures (see illustration). As a result, a valve is created. When your baby eats and her stomach is relaxed, food can go down her esophagus and into her stomach as usual. But after a meal, when the pressure inside her stomach increases as it grinds up food and propels it into the intestine, the part of the stomach wrapped around the esophagus pinches the esophagus shut and prevents food from backing up, keeping it in the stomach and intestines where it safely belongs.

Most babies who get a fundoplication will also have a gastrostomy tube (or g-tube) placed in their stomach as part of the procedure (see illustrations here and on the next two pages). The surgeon will secure one end of the g-tube inside your baby's stomach and tunnel the other end through the skin on the left side of your baby's belly. A g-tube is usually only a temporary measure to help a baby recover from surgery and make sure she is feeding and growing well afterward. It will help relieve gas pressure inside your baby's stomach and after a few days it can also be used for feeding, until your baby is ready to take in as much food or milk as she needs by mouth.

A simpler procedure: Placing a g-tube alone

Some older preemies who have feeding difficulties and can't eat enough by mouth to grow well may need a gastrostomy tube even without a

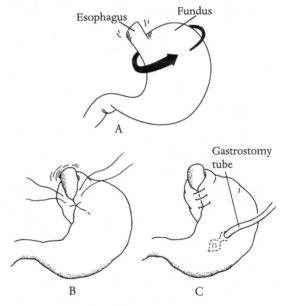

A: The fundus, the rounded upper part of the stomach, is wrapped around the esophagus.

B: A valve is created by securing the fundus with sutures.

C: A gastrostomy tube can be placed in the stomach, to help recovery and feeding.

Adapted with permission from Schatzlein MH: Gastroesophageal Reflux In Infants and Children, *Archives of Surgery* 114:505–510, © American Medical Association 1979

fundoplication. In that case, the procedure to insert a g-tube is much simpler, requiring only a very small incision in your baby's stomach. It is extremely safe and can sometimes even be done under local anesthesia in the NICU. (If an older preemie who has been discharged home needs to have a g-tube placed, he may be hospitalized for only a day or two after the procedure.) Most parents are initially upset by the idea of a g-tube, but once they see how their child's growth is boosted and mealtimes become more relaxed and pleasant, they feel better about it. Later, when it is no longer needed, the g-tube can be easily removed, and the opening will quickly heal.

Outcome and possible complications

GE reflux is successfully treated by a fundoplication in most babies (65 percent to 90 percent, with the best results in babies who don't have other abnormalities). How much your preemie's overall condition improves after surgery—for example, whether she stops wheezing or having bradycardia—depends on how much the GE reflux was contributing to her medical problems. Most of the time, you'll see some immediate improvement followed by more gradual progress over the next several weeks to months.

Like all surgical procedures, a fundoplication carries risks. The chance that your baby will die from the operation is very low, close to zero, but some other problems are more likely. Anyone who has had abdominal surgery can develop a bowel obstruction sometime in the future from scar tissue blocking the intestine. Complications specific to a fundoplication are gas bloat syndrome, an excessive accumulation of gas in the stomach that may last for several weeks after surgery but usually improves on its own; poor feeding for a while, possibly because a tightly wrapped stomach may make eating uncomfort-

able; and a loosening of the wrap over time, so that symptoms of GE reflux return. Children who have neurological impairments are more likely to have complications from the procedure, including a recurrence of GE reflux requiring a second operation later. Fortunately, the majority of babies won't have any of these complications.

Complications that are specific to the g-tube are leaking, irritation of the skin of the abdomen around the tube, and sometimes a buildup of granulation tissue (a bumpy kind of scarring that results from ongoing skin irritation and may be painful if touched). The best way to prevent these problems is by making sure that the g-tube doesn't move around too much. (Your baby's nurse will show you how to stabilize it. Usually tape and some gauze pads do the trick.)

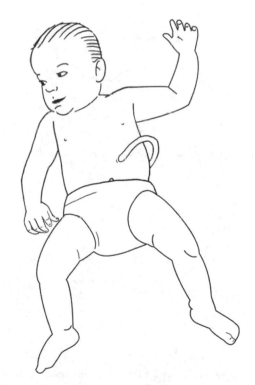

A baby with a g-tube, or gastrostomy tube.

Recovery and healing

Most preemies stay on a ventilator for a day or two after a fundoplication. To keep your baby comfortable, the nurses will be giving her pain relief medication, and will drain gas and fluid out of her stomach through the gastrostomy tube. After she's had some time to heal—usually from two days to two weeks—the doctors will try closing the g-tube to see if she can pass stomach secretions and gas through her bowel on her own. If she can, then they'll begin feeding her—by mouth if she seems ready and willing, or by putting some milk or formula in her stomach through the g-tube, gradually increasing the amount she gets at each feeding. Most babies who were eating well before surgery are back up to

their full feedings in one to three weeks. Others who weren't tolerating full feedings or nippling on their own before may take longer. Recent studies show that babies who had a minimally invasive fundoplication recover faster after surgery and can move more quickly on to oral feedings.

Your baby's gastrostomy tube will probably be left in for several months, until she is growing well with no signs of gas bloat or the need to supplement her nutrition with tube feedings. If your preemie is discharged home from the hospital with the tube still in place, don't worry: you'll be instructed on how to take care of it and what to do if it becomes dislodged. After a few weeks, and sometimes earlier, most g-tubes can be replaced with a gastrostomy button (Mic-Key is the most common brand), a small valve that sticks out of your baby's stomach just a little bit beyond her skin (see illustration). It's much more comfortable and convenient for her to wear and for you to care for than a long g-tube—and better looking, too. The procedure to change a gastrostomy tube to a Mic-Key button is usually quick and painless.

When the time comes to close your child's gastrostomy, the surgeons may just take out the button or tube and let it close on its own, or they may close it with a minor procedure from which she should recover rapidly. Your child will have one or two small scars on her belly—but she'll get great relief in return.

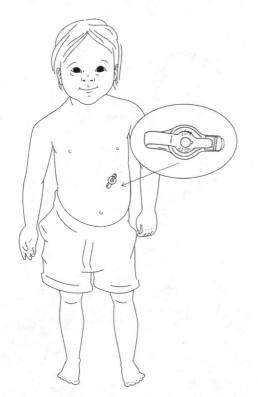

An active toddler with a button-type gastrostomy for his tube feedings.

Surgery to Treat ROP

Why it may be needed

The first line of treatment for ROP—laser therapy or cryotherapy (see page 304)—greatly reduces the risk that a baby's retina will pull away (or, detach) from the back wall of her eye and result in a severe loss of vision. But if despite treatment your baby's retina does detach, there are some surgical procedures that may help preserve or restore some of her sight. They are called vitrectomy and scleral buckling, and each is a way of repairing a retinal detachment. They are done by ophthalmologists who specialize in retinal surgery. Each procedure has advantages and disadvantages, and your baby's surgeon will tell you which one he recommends for her. Occasionally, both may be done at the same time.

How a vitrectomy is performed

While your baby is under general anesthesia, the surgeon makes several tiny incisions in her eye and removes the jelly-like substance that fills it (called the vitreous humor). He then cuts out the scar tissue that is pulling on the retina and causing its detachment so that the retina can lie flat against the back of the eye. Finally he injects a material into her eye to substitute for the vitreous humor that was taken out.

How a scleral buckle is performed

A scleral buckle is called that because the surgeon puts a band of silicone, like a belt, around the sclera (the white of the eye) to keep the retina from continuing to be pulled away from the back of the eye. It, too, is performed under general anesthesia. About six months later, after the retina has had ample time to reattach, most babies will have another surgery to cut or remove the buckle. This is usually a brief procedure with a shorter recovery time than the first one and is necessary for the eye to grow normally.

Outcome and possible complications

How effective a vitrectomy or scleral buckle is in reattaching your baby's retina depends on a number of factors, including how extensive the detachment is, where on her retina the detach-

ment is located, and how active her ROP is when she has the surgery. Reattachment rates from 30 percent to as high as 90 percent have been reported—you can ask the ophthalmologist what she predicts for your baby. The outlook is brightest if she has a small partial detachment away from the central part of her eye; approximately 75 percent of those babies end up with good vision. On the other hand, if the detachment is more central or more extensive, her vision is likely to be poorer. Still, restoring even a little vision, enough to distinguish stationary objects from objects in motion, for instance, or to perceive light, can be crucially important in helping a child become independent.

You'll have to be patient before you know the outcome (how many times do parents of preemies hear that?) because it can take several months or more to know whether your baby's retina has successfully reattached as hoped or not. Even then, reattachment is not the end of the story. To see well your baby needs not just an attached retina but a healthy eye in general, and the visual areas in her brain must be functioning well. A few weeks after the surgery, once your baby's eye is no longer swollen, a pediatric ophthalmologist can probably give you a sense of how good her vision is for ordinary daily activities (like reaching for an interesting toy, focusing on and tracking people's faces, or avoiding objects that are in her way). A formal assessment of this so-called functional vision will tell you a great deal about how well she can see. When she's older and can read a picture eye chart—around two or three years of age—a more precise measurement of her visual acuity can be made.

Overall, studies have found that of those babies whose retinas were completely reattached after surgery, about half had good vision, about half had poor vision, and a few were blind. Of those babies whose retinas were partially reattached after surgery, about half had poor vision and about half could perceive only light or were blind.

What's so important to keep in mind is that these outcomes, imperfect though they are, are still far better than if no surgery at all were done. Down the road, there may be another source of hope: experts say that technology to restore vision is on the horizon, with enough progress being made for them to believe it will be ready during the lifetime of infants being born now.

Although the thought of eye surgery is scary for parents, it is reassuring to know that complications from a vitrectomy or scleral buckle are rare. They include infection, bleeding, development of a cataract (clouding of the lens) or glaucoma (elevated pressure in the eye) after a vitrectomy and possible amblyopia (lazy eye) or nearsightedness after a scleral buckle. Nearsightedness is guaranteed if the buckle is not removed in a second operation later on.

Recovery and healing

After a vitrectomy or scleral buckle, your baby will get pain medicine, and for a day or two she may remain on a ventilator. To allow her retina to heal better, she may also need to lie in a particular position, often on her back or side, for about 48 hours following surgery. Her eye will be covered with a special ointment containing antibiotics and steroids to prevent infection and to limit inflammation, and will be patched briefly. When the patch is removed, you'll notice some swelling and redness, but within several days to a few weeks, these will disappear. Your baby's eye will continue to be treated with special drops for several weeks until the outside of her eye is fully healed. Because retinal reattachment and full healing of the inside of the eye can take several months, your child will get regular eye exams to check on the recovery of her eye and the success of the operation.

Tracheostomy

Why it may be needed

When it becomes clear that a premature baby will be on a ventilator or CPAP for many more months (usually because of severe BPD) or when there's an obstruction of her airway that needs to be bypassed (often because her upper airway is weak and collapses inward when she takes a deep breath), her doctors will consider giving her a tracheostomy. A "trach," as it is called for short, is an opening in the neck through which a tube is inserted directly into the baby's windpipe (trachea). The tube can then be connected to a ventilaor or CPAP device, or it can be left open for the baby to breathe through directly.

A tracheostomy will allow your baby to be free of the endotracheal tube that is now taped to her face and passing through her nose or mouth. Finally she will be able to practice all kinds of facial expressions (including smiling at you!), to eat through her mouth, to freely move her head around and discover the world, and eventually to sit up and move around despite needing a ventilator. All of these experiences, crucial for an infant's normal development, are severely limited by having an oral or nasal endotracheal tube. If your baby is getting a tracheostomy, you can look at it as a developmental step forward, truly in her best interest, despite the anxiety it may cause you. And it's reassuring to know that a trach doesn't have to be permanent. As soon as a child no longer needs it, her tracheostomy can be closed, leaving just a tiny scar on her neck where the opening used to be.

How a tracheostomy is performed

A tracheostomy is a delicate but quick procedure that usually takes about an hour and is performed under general anesthesia. The surgeon first makes a small horizontal incision near the base of your baby's neck. He sews two strings, called stay sutures or stay stitches, on each side of her windpipe, and makes an even smaller incision between them. Pulling on those stitches widens the incision in the trachea to form a small hole through which the surgeon inserts the tracheostomy tube. As you can see in the illustration, a tracheostomy tube is a short L-shaped plastic tube; one end goes down into the trachea, and the other end comes out your baby's neck. From the outside you can see the tip of the tube connected to two flat plastic wings to which strings, called trach ties, are attached. These strings go around your baby's neck and are tied together to secure the tracheostomy tube in place. The surgeon will select from different types and sizes of tubes so that your baby's is the most efficient and comfortable one for her. The long threads of the two stay stitches are brought out of the incision and temporarily taped to your baby's chest. They

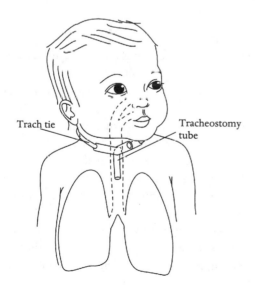

The L-shaped tracheostomy tube is inserted in the windpipe through a small incision in the neck.

Trach tie

Tracheostomy tube

are important only until her tracheostomy has completely healed: if her trach tube is accidentally dislodged before then, gently pulling on those sutures will reopen her windpipe enough to reinsert a new tube. (Once her tracheostomy has healed, this won't be a problem, as the trach tube will slide easily in and out of her windpipe.)

Outcome and possible complications

A tracheostomy is nearly always successful, and fortunately, surgical complications are very rare. They include an accidental tear in the nearby lung, which usually heals in a few days, and injury to the vocal cords or airway. If your baby's trach tube is accidentally dislodged in the first week after surgery before her neck and trachea have healed and her doctors are unable to reinsert it safely, they may have to temporarily reintubate her through her nose or mouth.

Infections of the trachea and lungs are more common in children who have tracheostomies. The most serious complications can occur if a baby's tube gets blocked with mucus and isn't promptly cleaned out. A child with a tracheostomy is dependent on the tube staying open so that air can flow through it in and out of her lungs. If the tube is blocked, she could suffocate. (To make sure that doesn't happen, the nurses will carefully suction your baby's trach tube at least every few hours and will replace it with a fresh one weekly. You'll be taught how to suction and replace your baby's tube, too.)

Although you've probably been aching to hear your baby's voice, at first you still won't hear her cry or talk. Eventually most children who keep their tracheostomies for more than a year or two do learn to talk around the tube, once they no longer need to be connected to a ventilator all the time. Your baby will likely have some delays in her speech, but don't worry—she will understand more than she can express. Once her tracheostomy is removed, her language skills should rapidly catch up.

Recovery and healing

Most babies are kept heavily sedated for several days after a tracheostomy so that they don't move their head or arms and accidentally dislodge the tube. For the same safety reason, you will also have to wait to hold her. At first the secretions being suctioned by the nurses from her tracheostomy may be a little bloody, but they'll soon clear. Usually a week after surgery, when the tracheostomy has healed and a smooth track has formed from your baby's windpipe to the opening in the skin of her neck, the surgeon will take out the trach tube, replace it with a clean new one, and remove the stay sutures. The sedation will be lifted, and your baby will be able to move around. From then on your baby's trach tube will be changed regularly, about once a week.

If your baby got a tracheostomy to bypass an obstruction in her airway and doesn't need to stay on a ventilator, once her tube is changed she'll have a device called a mist collar covering the trach tube in her neck. A mist collar moistens the air she breathes—taking over a job her nose and mouth would normally do—so that her airway doesn't get too dry. After a few months, when she's used to the trach, she may be able to go without extra humidification for a while.

If your preemie goes home with a tracheostomy, you'll be taught how to take care of it, what to do if her tube gets blocked or dislodged, and how to handle humidification. Many families will have some home nursing support for several hours a day or more initially, until they get used to taking care of their baby by themselves at home. Your baby's doctors will re-evaluate her lungs and airway regularly, to make sure the tube is the right size as she grows and to see whether she still needs a trach.

Remember that a tracheostomy, although demanding to live with, is almost always just a temporary measure to allow your child to grow and develop as normally as possible while her lungs and airways heal. Within a couple of years—and often earlier, before their first birthdays—most premature babies no longer need their tracheostomy. When that happy time comes for your child, her doctors will schedule an elective surgery at your convenience. The opening of her windpipe and the hole in the skin of her neck will be closed, and the small scar left behind will hardly be visible to those who don't know it's there.

Surgery to Repair a Hernia
Why it may be needed

An inguinal hernia (see page 310) occurs when loops of intestine—or sometimes, in girls, an ovary and fallopian tube—slip down from the abdomen where they belong through an open canal into the groin. Having a hernia doesn't usually cause a baby any discomfort, but it can be dangerous because the bowel could suddenly get stuck (incarcerated) down there, resulting in a bowel obstruction, which carries with it a high risk of infection and damage to the intestines, testicle, or ovary.

Surgical repair is the only available treatment for an inguinal hernia. If your preemie's hernia is not incarcerated, surgery will be scheduled when he's healthy and big enough for the operation to be done safely and successfully. If the hernia is incarcerated, the operation becomes urgent. Since repair of an incarcerated hernia carries different risks and is a more demanding procedure, you should rely on your baby's doctors for more specific information about it.

How a hernia repair is performed

An uncomplicated hernia repair in a preemie is usually performed under regional anesthesia, which blocks the pain in the area where the surgeon operates; the little patient is sedated and quietly asleep, but he can breathe on his own and avoid being put on a ventilator. If the hernia is incarcerated, however, general anesthesia, which requires a ventilator, is used. The surgeon makes an incision in the fold of skin at the base of your baby's belly, right above his groin on the affected side. He locates the open hernia sac, makes sure it's free of the bowel, testis, or ovary, and then cuts the sac and sews it closed. Sometimes the surgeon will explore the other side of your baby's groin as well to make sure there isn't a hernia there, too. (Preemies with a hernia on one side have about a 10 percent to 30 percent chance of having one on the other side as well.)

Alternatively, some surgeons use a minimally invasive—or laparoscopic—approach instead of the traditional open operation. To keep a baby still enough for this delicate technique, general anesthesia is usually needed. The surgeon makes a couple of tiny incisions in your baby's abdomen, then inserts a thin fiberoptic viewing scope to locate the hernia and some miniature surgical instruments to repair it. She'll also pump some carbon dioxide gas into your baby's belly to inflate it so that she has more room to see and work. One benefit of this technique is that the surgeon is able to look at both the right and left sides of the groin, so if your baby needs a hernia repair on the other side, too, it's possible to take care of both problems in one operation. If the hernia is incarcerated, the surgeon can inspect the bowel and repair any damage she finds. There are some cons, though, to the laparoscopic approach for repairing a preemie's hernia. One recent study found that it tends to take longer, cause more pain in the recovery period (partly because of the gas in the baby's abdomen, which goes away gradually), and results in more recurrences of the hernia than an open operation. If both techniques are performed at your hospital, your baby's surgeon will describe their advantages and disadvantages and tell you which approach she believes is better for your preemie.

If you want your preemie circumcised, it can usually be done conveniently and painlessly at the same time as a hernia repair. You can ask your baby's doctors about that possibility.

Outcome and possible complications

A hernia repair is a very safe and effective operation with zero mortality. Any early surgical complications that arise—bleeding, infection, or apnea from the anesthesia—are usually mild and treatable. Occasionally the hernia recurs, either because the canal could not be completely closed during the surgery or because the child has a medical condition (such as BPD or a VP shunt) that causes increased pressure in the abdomen and pushes the intestines down. Baby boys have a small risk of having a smaller than normal testicle after a hernia repair and of future infertility from an injury to the sperm duct. These complications are more likely after surgery for an incarcerated hernia than for an uncomplicated one.

Recovery and healing

After a hernia repair, a premature baby will be observed closely in the hospital for 48 hours for post-operative apnea. Older former preemies often have their hernias repaired as outpatients.

Recovery is usually very fast after this surgery, even if the hernia was incarcerated. Most preemies who were well before the operation are alert and eating several hours later. Pain is usually well controlled by regional anesthesia if your baby received it during surgery (the anesthesiologist can give a last dose at the end of the operation that will last for several hours) and after that, simply with Tylenol for a day or two. If your baby needs more, a dose or two of a stronger analgesic, such as fentanyl, may be given. By the second day after surgery, your baby's pain will quickly fade away. You'll notice some swelling and redness of his groin, which will resolve in a few days. There usually aren't any stitches to remove, just some tiny bandages which peel off when his wound is healed. Eventually the scars from a hernia repair turn into thin, barely visible lines.

Part III

A LIFE TOGETHER

CHAPTER 7

FINALLY TAKING YOUR BABY HOME

· · · · · · · · · · ·

Decisions and preparations for the moment you've been waiting for.

· · · · · · · · · · ·

PARENTS' STORIES: TAKING YOUR BABY HOME*

By the time of discharge, most families have adjusted to the unusual task of caring for their infant in the hospital. The huge effort and fatigue involved may feel to them like a fair price to pay to keep their baby safe. So when they are told that they can take their baby home, some parents react with incredulity. Happiness mixes with anxiety. They leave the hospital with their baby, delight and relief on their faces. But what they have lived through in the NICU can't easily be left behind.

I don't know these young parents' names, but I know their preemies: Eddie and Eve, who have been sharing my daughter's nursery room for many weeks. They are popular babies here in the hospital, beloved by some nurses. And I have become fond of them, too, of their shiny eyes, the color and shape of coffee beans. Their parents, who both work, usually come in the evening when I'm gone. But today they are both here, smiling, excited, and nervous, busily talking to doctors and nurses, trying to get everything in their heads. All parents on discharge day look like students who have to take the most important test of their lives. Today it's Eve's turn to go home, while Eddie still needs to stay. It's strange to see him feeding in his mother's arms, wearing his usual white hospital T-shirt—which makes all preemies look alike—while his sister, all dressed up in the cutest baby outfit, is napping in a car seat on the floor. Eve's already out of here. She might be taken for any other newborn leaving the hospital with her fam-

---

* *Parents' Stories* describes events and feelings that really happened or that could happen. Every situation is unique, of course, and you may relate to some parents' experiences and reactions more than others.

ily the day after delivery. But to more experienced observers, this mother and father look different. Not as newly un-pregnant, not as innocently exultant, weary but not as acutely exhausted. There's something about the way they hold that car seat that says there's so much already invested in this little baby lying here. After a last good-bye to Eddie in his isolette, his parents and sister are now leaving. A nurse tells them it won't be long before Eddie can go home, too. She also says the same about my daughter. But until that day arrives for your baby, you don't let yourself picture it, you don't feel entitled to believe it. You never know.

For parents, taking their preemie home from the hospital is not only psychologically demanding, it presents practical difficulties as well. Their schedules, their housing arrangement, their health, their jobs—all may pose problems. Sometimes guilt about the premature birth and its effects on the rest of the family can compound these obstacles.

"We're not ready!" This is what I should have told the doctor today. Instead, I said, "Oh, great!" on hearing the news that they will discharge my daughter Gillian tomorrow, six days before Christmas. She's been doing so well lately, every day putting a little weight on her still diminutive frame. As a result she's coming home much earlier than anybody would have predicted three months ago when she was born, an extremely premature baby. Now we're so relieved and proud of her, and we're looking forward to taking her home with us. But for this Christmas . . . well, my wife and I had other plans. We wanted to make up to Cooper for all that Gillian's birth has taken away from his life. Cooper is our older boy, six years old. He has spent weeks with relatives and friends, been picked up in the evenings by parents who have just come back from the hospital without any energy or cheerfulness left for play and bedtime stories. After all that, Cooper deserves the best Christmas ever. But how are we going to manage it now? How can we do the rest of the shopping, bake cookies, decorate the tree, pack all the presents, cook for the relatives and friends we wanted to be here for Santa's arrival (I haven't even rented the costume yet!) if Gillian comes home? Maybe we're ungrateful, I know. But this Christmas was meant to be only Cooper's.

All of the mixed emotions parents may feel at the time of discharge usually melt into a sea of joy, an immense sense of blessing, when they actually take their premature baby home into their life. The hardships of the recent past make every sensation clearer and stronger.

Now that for the first time, I'm stepping into our doorway holding you in my arms, my baby, I feel the intensity of this moment, I know its meaning. This is your home, where we have been missing you so badly, for long weeks after your rushed birth. Look, this is the phone we feared we might hear ring in the night, calling us back to the NICU. This is your parents' bed and your father's shoulder, where you can be consoled, cuddle, and nap. This is the hand of your grandmother, who has finally arrived from far away to touch you. Here there's no hurry, no sharp noises, no smell of alcohol. This is the sound of our voices, of our family life. This is your mother's breast, which you couldn't latch on to in the hospital. There was no privacy there, there were too many worries to deal with first, and we did. Now you can take your time getting acquainted with this breast: it belongs to you. This is how you breastfeed, my baby. I knew you would be able to do it here at home. This is how we all rejoice.

Leaving the hospital nursery to head into family life is another major change for already stressed parents, who may have little resilience left. Particularly in the first days and weeks at home, some parents find caring for their preemie a truly overwhelming responsibility. Anxiety about the baby's condition and demands can grow out of control without the safety net of the medical staff.

Ted has been home for one week now. The much-expected moment has come and gone, leaving me all alone with him—his father travels a lot. The weather is bad, I can't take him out, and it's best that friends don't come to see him yet, keeping their germs and colds away. I feel too tired to have visitors anyway! When I should sleep, I'm half-awake, ready to jump up at the first shrill of the apnea monitor. It rings two or three times a night, all false alarms so far. But sooner or later a real one will come. What if I pat Ted and he doesn't breathe? Will I be able to do CPR if he needs it? I read the instructions they gave me, trying to memorize the steps I performed on a doll. But I can't concentrate, I can't remember. Then, although he's feeding, I can't tell if Ted is growing. To me he looks as if he's getting smaller. But maybe that's because of his big clothes. I remember how good and reassuring it felt to hear the nurse announcing Ted's weight gain each day. Our pediatrician visit is next week. In the meantime, maybe I can go back to the hospital to weigh him again, as I already did once. The nurses were so happy to see us! They put a scale for us in the family room since you can't take babies from outside into the nursery. How weird that Ted could not go back to where he lived for so long! He was safe there. I felt safe, too. Is it possible that I'm missing the NICU?

Going home with a premature baby also means facing the world together for the first time. Your baby may not fit other people's expectations about how big an infant should be for her age. To avoid telling their stories to total strangers, for the sake of privacy as well as simplicity, many parents of preemies eventually try a shortcut. Nothing's wrong with that. But you should first test your new version with some predictable questions you may be asked.

—Hi! I haven't seen you in a looong time! How are you? Is this your baby in the carriage? A girl, I assume!
—Sure . . . this is our Melissa. . . .
—She's so cute, so little and perfect. . . . How many days?
—Mmmm . . . she's . . . over two weeks now. We came home from the hospital exactly two weeks ago.
—Oh! You know, I thought somebody in the building told me she was born some time ago. But I must be wrong, she's obviously a new baby! How much did she weigh?
—She was . . . very small. She's now about six pounds.
—Really? She doesn't look that tiny. . . . But she must be totally fine if they sent her home right away. Are you breastfeeding her?
—Yes. I breastfed her for six weeks, then I started supplementing her with formula. . . .
—Six weeks? . . .
—What did I say? Six weeks, six days—time's so jumbled now! Melissa doesn't let us sleep much. . . . I think I'm losing my mind here. . . .

After the trepidation, perplexity, and confusion of the initial time at home, parents begin to accept that things can now be normal, that their baby's well-being is under their control. Some of them even discover a new identity: the different person their baby's premature birth has made them.

I look at my baby sleeping in her bassinet, the phone rings and I don't answer, the clock ticks and I don't rush. Time had to be stretched before her birth, more had to be squeezed out of my life. For what, I think, had she not survived? All that mattered before is still appealing but with a paler tint, there in the background. How will I do without my eager grip on the world? How am I going to balance this unreserved love I never felt before? My friends find me well and seem surprised, knowing the peaks of anguish I climbed when my baby was born sick and small. I look at myself in the mirror and wonder why pain doesn't leave more visible traces. Inside I'm more aware now yet detached, as if nothing can ever hurt me anymore. I've reached the top already and returned. My baby's sleeping quietly. I'm at peace.

THE DOCTOR'S PERSPECTIVE: TAKING YOUR BABY HOME*

It's the question parents ask most often: "When will my baby come home?" And it makes me wish we had a crystal ball! Usually we tell parents to expect that their baby will come home around his due date. But it's not until certain things start—and stop—happening that we really know the momentous day is nigh. Here's what we're looking for before saying that joyful good-bye, and great good luck, to you and your baby.

Physical Exam and Laboratory Assessment

To discharge your baby home, we need to be certain she's outgrown the problems of prematurity that require skilled nursing care or a doctor's immediate intervention. That means, above all, that your baby's vital signs (her temperature, breathing, heart rate, and blood pressure) are consistently normal. We monitor babies to make sure of that, gradually tapering off the frequency and kinds of monitoring we do as a preemie becomes more stable.

The first thing to go, usually, is frequent blood pressure checks. Once healthy preemies without blood pressure problems are getting intermediate rather than intensive care, we may check their blood pressure only once or twice a day. We expect it to remain normal, and as your baby becomes more active, the readings are more likely to be falsely high. (If that happens, don't let it worry you; we'll simply repeat the reading when she's quiet or asleep.) A baby who's been off oxygen for more than a week usually no longer needs continuous monitoring of her oxygen saturation. (It will be checked if there's a problem.) When a preemie has been out of an isolette and warm and comfortable in an open bassinet for several days, we can stop monitoring her temperature so often and just check it a few times a day. Most preemies will remain on a cardiorespiratory monitor to detect changes in their breathing or heart rate patterns until they're close to discharge. But if your baby has stayed in the hospital for reasons other than prematurity (say she's convalescing but stable after surgery), even the cardiorespiratory monitor may be discontinued, and her vital signs checked intermittently just a few times a day.

We'll also want to see that your baby is eating well enough to grow and thrive. She should be gaining an average of 15 to 30 grams (one-half to one ounce) a day—and doing that without heroic measures on the part of whoever is feeding her! A preemie who's a very slow eater usually just needs a little more time in the hospital to develop the

---

* *The Doctor's Perspective describes how your doctor may be thinking about your preemie's condition and what she may be considering as she makes medical decisions. All of the medical terms and conditions mentioned here are described in more detail elsewhere in this book. Check the index.*

alertness and skill she needs to take in enough nourishment.

Some preemies will continue to have their blood drawn every couple of weeks or so until discharge to make sure they're not getting too anemic and that their bones are growing strong. And babies who are on medication may need to have their blood chemistry or medication levels checked periodically to make sure the doses remain appropriate as they grow. Toward the end of your preemie's stay, our daily notes in the medical record will get shorter, and there may not be much of import in her condition to talk about. There's only so much you can say about a baby who's just growing! That's what we're looking to see—not much excitement, just some nice, boring days.

Common Issues and Decisions

Outgrowing apnea and bradycardia: Because A's and B's are often the last remnants of instability to go away before a preemie is ready to be discharged, the last week or two in the hospital is often spent counting down the days without apnea. We want to see eight apnea-free days in a row to feel comfortable that her apnea of prematurity has truly resolved. Not infrequently, there will be occasional blips on the monitor, or changes in her heart rate or breathing while she's eating, that make one wonder if her breathing pattern has sufficiently matured. A question doctors often get asked is whether a particular episode that a preemie has had "counts" as significant apnea or bradycardia—meaning, will it hold up her discharge home? The answer isn't always straightforward, and will depend on the circumstances and the judgment of your baby's doctor. In general, we consider an episode significant if a baby requires stimulation to start breathing again or if her heart rate falls to fewer than 60 beats a minute. We don't usually count A's and B's that

occur with feeding, from spitting up or choking, unless they're severe and recurring. Babies tend to recover from these spontaneously and quickly, and if they happen at home, you or whoever is taking care of your baby will be able to handle it and help her out by stopping the feeding and giving her time to resume breathing normally again.

The days spent before discharge waiting for apnea to be outgrown can be a peaceful time for babies and their parents, but it can be nerve-wracking, too—waiting for an "episode" and hoping that it doesn't come. Occasionally parents don't trust that their baby's apnea is really gone for good, or get impatient about the eight-day countdown and ask if their preemie can go home early on an apnea monitor. Most of the time, we discourage that. Apnea of prematurity usually doesn't take much longer to go away after a preemie becomes able to eat on her own and maintain her body temperature—both of which have to occur before she's ready for discharge anyway. Monitors are clumsy and inconvenient, interfere with how you'd naturally interact with your baby (and natural interaction is probably the very best thing for her development), have not been proven to do any good, and may increase parents' anxiety if the alarm goes off a lot. We wouldn't want to send a baby home, apnea monitor or not, if it takes more than mild stimulation to raise her heart rate or get her to breathe again. (In the hospital nursery, she can get rapid and expert intervention if she needs it.) But if you feel very strongly that you just couldn't sleep without your baby being on a monitor, after all she's been through, then it may be worth it for your peace of mind.

BPD and home oxygen: Some preemies with BPD are actually quite well—growing nicely, their medical problems adequately treated, just needing some extra oxygen—and they can potentially be discharged home. But before that happens, there are several things we would need to make sure of. First, that your baby will be needing oxygen for at least a few more weeks; if not, it's not worth the effort and anxiety to set up oxygen at home. We'll try to judge that by looking at her breathing patterns when she's relaxed (calm or asleep) and when she's active (during her feedings or when she's fussing) together with how much oxygen she's getting and how rapidly she's been weaning from it. (Here's another time we wish we had that crystal ball!) Second, the amount of oxygen and medication she needs should be stable and predictable so that we can tell you what to give when. Adjusting therapies up and down to respond to frequent or erratic changes in your baby's condition is not something you can do reliably at home. Third, your family and home must be able to accommodate and handle home oxygen safely. There should be adequate room to store the oxygen equipment, so it's not inadvertently knocked or spilled and it's away from fire hazards. There should be no smoking in the house because the oxygen is flammable—and because breathing second-hand cigarette smoke can significantly worsen your baby's respiration. Parents and other caregivers (there should be at least two to cover times when one is sick or unavailable) must be willing and able to be trained to use the equipment, recognize and respond to signs of a problem, and provide CPR if necessary. There must be a telephone in your home, in case of an emergency, and assurance of good follow-up care with a local pediatrician and a clinic for babies on oxygen. Finally, you'll need to accept some help from a home health care agency, which will supply the equipment and periodically check on you and your baby to see how things are going.

You'd be amazed at how routine having your baby home on oxygen can seem once you're used to it. Some parents have said, for instance, that despite initially being taken aback by the appearance of the oxygen canister (some say it looks

like a missile!), after living with it for a while they were surprised when other people noticed anything odd. If we think that going home on oxygen is best for your baby, we'll certainly try to allay your fears. Still, you shouldn't hesitate to tell us if providing oxygen at home is too much of a burden for you and you don't think you can handle it. Discharging babies on medical equipment is not uncommon nowadays, but there's no reason to believe that all families should want or be able to do it. If home oxygen isn't for you, we can keep your preemie in the hospital nursery a while longer. (If you're still not ready to take her home after she's been stable for a long time, we may look at other places, such as rehabilitation hospitals, where she will be able to grow and recover in a more relaxed and enriching environment that's better suited for her development than an intensive care nursery.)

Feeding: If your preemie is getting fortified breast milk or special formula, we'll be deciding whether to change her feedings before she goes home. Most breastfed preemies who are nursing well can get all the extra nutrients they need in a couple of bottles a day of pumped, fortified breast milk. (We'll give you any extra breast milk you've stored with us to take home with you, along with a recipe for how to fortify it and instructions on how many bottles to give her.) Babies who are getting donor breast milk or preterm formula, once they're big and healthy enough to go home, are usually ready for transitional formula, which is more easily available and cheaper. It has higher concentrations of calories, salts, and minerals than regular term formula, but is less concentrated and less expensive than preterm formula. We'd usually make this switch a week or so before discharge to see that your baby keeps feeding and growing well. On the other hand, if your preemie has recently had feeding intolerance or problems with weight gain and has finally settled into a good growing routine on donor breast milk or special formula, we may not want to rock the boat right before discharge. In that case, we may send your baby home on special formula or donor milk with the intention of making the switch in several weeks, once she's more mature and doing well at home. The exact timing of that decision will be up to your baby's pediatrician, who will be weighing and measuring her and keeping close tabs on her progress. Mothers who will be exclusively breastfeeding at home but haven't nursed their preemie much in the nursery may be asked to room in for a night or two before discharge to make sure that mother and baby do fine with round the clock breastfeeding.

Medications: Preemies are commonly treated with medicine for apnea, BPD, or reflux. These problems gradually resolve; in fact, outgrowing them is one sign that a preemie is ready to go home. So as discharge day approaches, your baby's doctor will be deciding which medications to try to stop and which your baby should go home on.

We usually try to minimize medications (it's not like there isn't enough to do in a parent's day without having to remember and then give medicine to an often uncooperative child!), stopping them at least several days before discharge to make sure your baby continues to do well as the medication wears off. For intravenous medicines that she can't do without, we'll switch to oral dosing. You can't be expected to adjust medications frequently at home, so we'll want to see your baby stable on consistent doses for about a week or so before we'd feel comfortable discharging her. If your baby is sent home on medicine, her doctor may intend for her to gradually outgrow her current dose (which allows the medicine, in effect, to be tapered off) or may be planning to increase the dose as she grows. You can ask him to clarify what he's expecting to do. And don't worry—the nurses

will teach you how to give your baby the medications, and we won't write that "Discharge home" order until you've practiced and feel comfortable doing it yourself.

Follow-up: Before discharging your baby, we'll want to make sure that all of her urgent medical problems are corrected and that follow-up of nonurgent ones is arranged. For example, if your preemie has retinopathy of prematurity (ROP), we won't consider her ready for discharge until the ophthalmologist has assured us that she no longer needs very frequent eye exams and that therapy isn't imminent. Before sending your baby home, we'll make sure you know when her next eye exam should be and how important it is for you to make and keep that appointment. We'll also arrange for your baby to be seen or followed by any other specialist who diagnosed or treated an ongoing problem, to make sure the condition will be handled properly once she's home.

For preemies at risk for developmental delay, we'll arrange follow-up appointments in clinics that are specially designed to evaluate the growth and development of premature infants. Specific risk criteria will differ somewhat among hospitals and doctors but usually have to do with a baby's age and size at birth, whether she has had serious medical problems in the hospital, and whether there is a difficult situation of any kind at home. Our hope is to catch any problems early and put parents in touch with resources and services that can help. For the babies at highest risk (such as preemies with PVL or severe BPD), we may in addition set up home visits by a child service coordinator (a public health nurse or social worker employed by the state). Child service coordination programs are a tremendous benefit to families, and if you qualify for this service, we would strongly recommend that you accept it. Some parents feel insulted or nervous—thinking that we believe they can't adequately take care of their preemie themselves or fearing that their home or parenting skills will be evaluated and judged by outsiders. That isn't at all what we have in mind when we arrange for these services. We see them as opening your family and child up to opportunities and expertise that even the very best parents can't provide themselves.

We'll be asking you to choose a pediatrician and suggesting a time to take your baby for her first visit. For most preemies, this will be several days after discharge, for a weight check and to make sure you're both adjusting well to your new circumstances. Her pediatrician will want to see that she's eating and growing well and that any medical conditions she has are stable or improving. You may want to meet with your baby's new doctor even before she's discharged from the hospital, to get acquainted and to go over your concerns with the physician who in a short time will be responsible for most of her care.

Many parents wonder whom to call—the nursery or their baby's new doctor—when they have questions soon after discharge. We don't mind answering questions—and would enjoy hearing from you—but the answer, usually, is "her pediatrician." Please be assured that we're not trying to avoid you, just trying to manage your concerns appropriately and to assure continuity of care in the future. Unless your question is directly related to a problem that we followed in the nursery or you're calling to clarify instructions that we gave you, her new doctor should be able to handle it—and needs to hear about your concerns so he can get to know you and your baby. He may call us for more information or our opinion. But now is the time to pass the torch, as we hand over your baby's care to her own doctor at home.

Special requirements: Sometimes, caring for a former preemie takes some special skills and practice. If your baby is going home with medical equipment (oxygen, for example, or tube feedings) or will be getting other special treatments or medications, we may ask you to room in or at least spend a certain number of consecutive hours with your baby in the nursery before going home together. The idea is to give you a chance to care for your baby yourself, with lots of supervision and help readily available. We may also ask you to learn CPR so if any equipment your baby is dependent on doesn't work properly, you can support your baby until help arrives. Most parents welcome these opportunities for learning, but some are taken aback, interpreting our requests to mean that we don't trust them as parents. On the contrary, we're training you so carefully because we are willing to entrust a fragile newborn to your responsible and loving care. We wouldn't do that unless we thought she could be safe and thrive.

Family Issues

Parents occasionally think that they should continue the hygiene or isolation practices of the nursery to keep their preemie healthy at home. While it's true you shouldn't expose your nearly-newborn to people with obvious illnesses or take her into crowds of people during winter cold season, remember that she's going home just so that she can be exposed to lots of things that are missing in the hospital. We're discharging your preemie because that's what's good for her now—not just for your sake or because of hospital or insurance policies. Children develop better at home than almost anywhere else because that's where they're stimulated with all sorts of different sights and sounds and smells, get lots of loving and playful touch, and mingle with family and friends as part of a community. Your natural environment is a good environment for an infant. Use common sense to protect her—as any parent would—but don't think that your home is second best. If you make it too much like a hospital, you'll diminish how wonderful it is for your baby.

Some parents become extremely anxious about what they think is a too sudden switch from constant monitoring of their preemie in the hospital nursery to less than perfect vigilance at home. We promise you, we won't discharge your baby until we think she's strong and healthy enough to flourish away from the ever observant gaze and ministrations of nurses and doctors. To show you that the cardiorespiratory monitor is no longer needed, we may turn it off a day or two before she goes home—but sometimes it's needed for an up-to-the-last-minute apnea countdown, and to be honest, sometimes we forget! Try not to let this worry add to your tension and anxiety. Instead, you can view every extra day on the monitor as just another proof of how secure your baby is.

Oh, one last thing. Be sure to come back to visit us sometimes—and send pictures. We're more attached to her than you know. And who doesn't love to see their babies grow?

QUESTIONS AND ANSWERS

Preemie-Proofing

They say my baby's ready to go home. But what should we do to be ready for him? I feel like we should put him in a bubble to keep him safe!

Matching the bedding with the wallpaper, shopping for a cute mobile to hang over the crib, and having enough clothes and diapers in the drawers are the kind of things parents usually worry about in getting their household ready for a newborn. But taking a preemie home is a different story. Many families become concerned about the adequacy of their home environment and caregiving practices. After seeing their preemie tended to in a hygienic hospital nursery by specialized professionals, moving him from that safe haven to their house may cause them to fret.

Here is a first piece of advice: Don't worry too much. Your loving presence is the main thing your baby needs now that he's ready to begin home life with you. There are only a few arrangements and precautions, easy to remember and apply, for "preemie-proofing" your habits and house. Most are aimed at helping him avoid colds and other infections, to which he's still more vulnerable than other newborns in the first weeks or months after leaving the hospital.

In advance:

* Make sure you have a car seat appropriate for preemies (see page 388).
* If your baby is going home on a medication that needs to be compounded (mixed specially for him), ask your pharmacy whether they do compounding and, if not, to recommend a compounding pharmacy nearby.
* If your baby is going home during winter cold season and you've been told that he should be treated by his pediatrician with Synagis (a medication that helps prevent a common but especially dangerous respiratory virus called RSV), call the pediatrician and ask whether she needs to order it for your baby in advance. A pediatrician who takes care of lots of other preemies may have Synagis in stock, but others may need a couple of weeks to get it.

A few basic do's and don'ts at home:

* Do take your preemie outside, but don't expose him for long to strong drafts or direct

sunlight. When he's out and the sun is shining, protect him with a wide-brimmed hat or parasol. Don't apply sunscreen unless your pediatrician advises you differently; sunscreen isn't safe until a baby is around six months old when he'll have thicker skin.

* Avoid bringing him into crowded indoor places like churches, movie theaters, and shopping malls, where there's a higher risk of catching a cold or other infection.

* When you schedule visits with the pediatrician, ask for the earliest appointment of the day. If you're the first patient, you're less likely to be kept waiting in a crowded waiting room with sick kids.

* Ask relatives and friends who visit to make sure their small children keep some distance from your preemie, and not to visit if they have a cold, the flu, or any other contagious illness. If you or somebody else in the family has a respiratory infection, avoid face-to-face contact with your preemie or wear a disposable paper mask when you're spending time close to him, like during feedings. (You'll find inexpensive disposable face masks at any hardware store, or you can order them from one of the vendors of allergy products listed in *Resources,* page 590.) Older siblings should wash their hands when they arrive home from school, sports, or play dates. When sick, they should be kept away from the baby until they're no longer contagious.

* Wash your hands after blowing your nose, diapering siblings, or handling raw food. (Be careful about handwashing, but don't let it become an obsession. You don't have to replicate the hygiene practices of the NICU.)

* Post signs around the house if you need to, and be absolutely rigid with your family and friends: yours is a no-smoking household, for your baby's sake. All preemies, but especially those with BPD, shouldn't be exposed to smoke, aerosol sprays, or paint fumes. These irritants can cause wheezing, coughing, and difficulty breathing.

* The usual tips for cleaning and storing bottles, nipples, pacifiers, breast pump equipment, and milk or formula are perfectly apt for preemies as well as term babies.

* When you and your baby are away from home, a small package of baby wipes comes in handy for more than cleaning little backsides. Use them or a waterless gel cleanser to wipe off toys or pacifiers that drop on the floor, infant seats in supermarket carts, and so on. They're also great for keeping your own hands clean.

* If your baby is on an apnea monitor, be sure that you can hear the alarm from every room of your house (and read the In Depth section on monitors, page 434, for more safety tips).

Babies who have BPD are more susceptible to respiratory infections, which can be severe enough to cause them to be rehospitalized. For them, the precautions above should be continued through the first year or longer (ask your pediatrician). Here are some other special tips.

A few extra do's and don'ts for babies with BPD:

* Parents, siblings, and caregivers of preemies with BPD should get the flu vaccine every year, and a pertussis (whooping cough) booster shot if they were last immunized more than ten years ago.

* If your baby is on oxygen, carefully observe the cleaning requirements, particularly for the humidifier, and the safety recommendations (see page 396).

* Since it's important to avoid exposing your baby to strong fumes, make sure you follow the safety instructions when you use exterminating chemicals in your house and steer clear of very smelly floor waxes or cleaning products. If you

want to brighten up your preemie's nursery by painting it, do it well before she comes home.

* Here's a positive note: You do not need to find your beloved pets another home. Allergies aren't likely to cause problems, because babies under about a year of age can't mount a strong allergic response. If your baby has symptoms after that, her doctor will try to determine whether your pet or something else is to blame—and even if it's the pet, allergy medication rather than pet banishment may solve the problem.

Besides the guidelines above and any special instructions your doctor gives you, your preemie doesn't need anything different from what you'd normally do for a full-term baby. Most parenting books offer a review of what parents should do, at various ages, to try to prevent injuries. Your preemie simply requires that you follow the same baby-proofing schedule for his corrected age (the age he would be if he'd been born on his due date). Isn't it refreshing to be following the same advice as all new parents, after the special circumstances and consequences of your baby's premature birth?

Diapers and Clothing

Where am I going to find preemie diapers and clothes for my baby?

Finally, you're ready to shop for your beautiful baby. She deserves to be treated royally after all she's been through, and you deserve to indulge in the adorable outfits you've been admiring from afar for so long. But before you spend a lot of time and money shopping for special preemie-sized clothes and diapers, remind yourself of one thing: Preemies grow quickly. Your baby probably won't get much use out of them before she's ready for regular newborn sizes.

So try to resist the urge to invest in a complete preemie wardrobe. Consider buying just a few preemie outfits that your baby can don on special occasions. Remember that newborn-sized clothes can vary a lot in size from one brand to another and that the smallest of them may almost fit your baby. The rest of the time, just roll up the sleeves and ankles, and notice how within a few weeks your baby's arms and legs start to fill them out. All newborns, after all, spend most of their time dressed for casual comfort, in billowy nightgowns with drawstring bottoms, stretchy sleepers, and T-shirts, all often bought a size too big. The baggy look seems to suit them!

Many hospitals send parents home with a package of preemie diapers. (If nobody mentions this, be sure to ask.) Once those are used up, try moving on to the standard newborn size, rolling the diapers down at the waist to make them fit better. They may be roomy for a while, but chances are they'll work just fine.

The following are for parents who prefer preemie diapers and clothes with a more tailored look and for those whose babies are especially small at discharge:

Diapers: Two of the most popular brands of diapers, Huggies and Pampers, make preemie sizes. They are available at some large chains, including Walmart, Babies R Us, and Target, and from numerous web sites. Many varieties of cloth diapers in preemie sizes are sold online, also. Even more specialized are WeePee diapers, which were designed with thinner pads to try to minimize the tendency of some preemies' hips to turn slightly outward. They can be ordered from Philips Children's Medical Ventures at 888-766-8443 or www.childmed.com.

Clothing: As the number of premature babies born in the United States has increased, so has the interest of retailers in selling clothes for them.

For instance, some Walmart and Babies R Us stores have a large selection, Baby Gap sells some preemie clothes and so do a myriad of smaller online retailers. If you decide to make clothes for your preemie, be sure to use soft fabrics and avoid scratchy seams or accessories. And remember, no matter what your preemie wears, she'll always look pretty darn cute.

Choosing a Pediatrician

How do I choose the right pediatrician for my preemie?

When your baby has been cared for since birth by highly trained neonatologists and 'round-the-clock neonatal nurses, it can make any parent nervous to transfer her care to a plain old family physician or pediatrician who (a) isn't a specialist in preemies and (b) won't be living with you, standing next to your baby's crib 24 hours a day. Imagine!

What's hard to realize now is that your preemie is rapidly growing out of the phase in which she needs constant, specialized attention and into one in which she can safely be treated like other newborns of the same corrected age. If that weren't the case, her doctors wouldn't feel it's time to send her home from the hospital.

Nevertheless, some preemies will finish making that transition sooner than others. The challenge for parents of a preemie, then, is to select a doctor who will take excellent care of their baby both in the short run, while she still may face some special vulnerabilities or needs, and the long run, when you will want what everyone wants in a pediatrician: someone who will guide you through the long years of teething, sore throats, fevers, booster shots, sprained ankles, growth spurts, and teenage acne.

Before choosing a specific doctor, you should decide whether to look for a pediatrician or fam-ily physician. Pediatricians specialize in children, usually from babyhood into adolescence, while family physicians have a broader practice of entire families, children and adults alike. Family physicians don't consider themselves second best at taking care of children, but they do have less training in neonatology and pediatrics. (After medical school, family physicians divide their training between pediatrics and other specialties, so they spend less time in a neonatal intensive care nursery, usually less than a month compared to several months for pediatricians.)

Which kind of physician is right for you and your baby? That depends. If your baby is a big, healthy preemie with no special medical needs, then either should be fine. However, if you have a more vulnerable preemie who is receiving ongoing medical treatment (such as home oxygen or tube feedings), or who was sick in the hospital (for example, with BPD or hydrocephalus) and is therefore at higher risk for some future problems, then we would advise you to select a pediatrician, if possible. Being more specialized, pediatricians will generally have a better understanding of what your preemie (and you) have been through and what issues to look out for during the first few years when it's important to catch any possible problems early. Even if you have a family doctor you love, you may still want to find a pediatrician for the first year or two. Later your preemie can graduate to your family physician's practice.

Some parents become so attached to the doctors in the nursery, or so nervous about walking away from their expertise with premature babies, that they want to continue using the hospital staff as their pediatricians even after discharge. In many hospitals, it's possible to do this by taking your baby to the hospital's outpatient clinic. You might be able to see the doctors you already know, or others on the staff.

A word to the wise: While that can work well for families who live within a 30-minute drive of the hospital, it probably won't if you live farther away. A pediatrician is someone you should feel able to pop in on quickly whenever you're worried about a stuffy nose or high fever, someone you can pick up the phone and reach without thinking about long-distance charges, someone who can meet you in the emergency room or his office (or maybe even come to your house) in the middle of the night if your baby is crying inconsolably and you're scared, someone who is a knowledgeable guide to dentists, schools, and other resources in your community. Remember that more and more, your concerns are going to revolve around these basic matters that are part of the daily life of a pediatrician, not an intensive care nursery.

Having made these choices, it's time to gather names and to sort through the various doctors your insurance plan will cover until you find the best one for you. Some ways to do this:

* Ask your neonatologist for advice. She will be familiar with the doctors who are affiliated with your baby's hospital, and many others who know about preemies.
* If you live some distance from the hospital, it may be even better to ask around in your community, to find a physician who is locally respected and knows the other local doctors and social service providers you may eventually want to contact.
* Contact support groups for parents of preemies in your area or other parents of preemies you know. You'll probably tap into a useful reservoir of experience.
* Once you've focused in on one or two individuals, you may want to make an appointment to meet them in person. Most of the things to learn from the visit—whether your style and the physician's seem to be compatible, how night and weekend calls are handled, whether you feel more comfortable with a solo practitioner or group practice, and so on—are

no different than for a full-term baby. Many parenting books contain lists of questions and issues that may be helpful to consider.
* If your baby has special medical problems or needs, there's one issue you should not overlook: Some doctors welcome these patients and others, unfortunately, do not. It's best to find that out now rather than by being treated poorly later. When you talk to a prospective doctor, describe your baby's circumstances and ask straight out whether he's comfortable taking her on as a patient. Most likely he will answer your question directly, but if he doesn't, chances are you'll be able to read between the lines. If transportation problems will make it difficult for you to take your baby to his office, ask whether he will make house calls. Even today, some physicians in some circumstances do.

The doctor you choose will probably see your baby within a few days of discharge. Don't expect to feel as comfortable with him right off the bat as with the neonatologist who cared for your baby since birth. Give him a chance to show you that he knows a lot about babies, and will get to know and take good care of yours.

After a few visits, you should start to trust him and to feel that you've made a good choice. If not, go with your instinct and don't hesitate to make a change. A pediatrician is someone with whom you're going to have a long, intimate relationship, and it should be a good one.

End of Apnea

They say my baby can go home next week, but just last week she had some apnea. What makes her ready to go home now?

There are many factors that go into the careful decision of when to send a preemie home; you can read about them in *The Doctor's Perspective* on page 378. A common one is that a baby's apnea of prematurity must have resolved. That's determined by a baby's having gone for a set number of days—often eight, but practices at different nurseries vary—without any apnea or bradycardia.

Of course you wonder: How can a doctor ever be sure that an episode of apnea or bradycardia is the final one? What if there's another, unexpected one at home?

The first thing you have to understand (though many parents of preemies find it hard to believe) is that apnea of prematurity never goes on forever. Instead, it goes away gradually as a premature baby matures. You'll notice over time that the interval between episodes becomes longer and the apnea gets milder and milder, so that eventually no one even knows it's occurring, until it's completely gone. Research indicates that when a baby goes for eight days without apnea, it's safe to conclude that she won't have a significant episode again. (Remember that this applies to simple apnea of prematurity. If a baby's apnea is due to other health conditions, they may need to resolve before the apnea will stop.)

Therefore, many nurseries perform an apnea countdown, requiring a certain number of apnea-free days before discharging a baby. Don't be surprised if during the countdown period your baby sets off the apnea or bradycardia alarm but her doctors say the episode wasn't meaningful and doesn't affect the countdown. It may be that they realize her heart rate is just slowing as she matures (as it should) and therefore her monitor settings need to be lowered. Or perhaps she choked during a feeding and some fleeting apnea or bradycardia occurred—a normal reflex that has nothing to do with how regular and mature her breathing is and that isn't dangerous as long as the person feeding her pauses and lets her catch

her breath. On the other hand, if your baby has apnea that her doctors do consider significant, the countdown will have to be started all over again. It wouldn't be surprising for that to happen a couple of times, either.

At some hospitals, a preemie who is otherwise ready to go home but isn't quite making it through her apnea countdowns may be sent home with an apnea monitor. If that's the plan for your baby, you can read all about home monitors on page 434.

Car Seat

Why is a car seat test so important? Is a baby so much more likely to have breathing problems there than anywhere else?

It is well known that car accidents are the top cause of injury and death of children in the United States, and that car seats can prevent many of these tragedies. Occasionally, though, preemies riding in a car face a catch-22: Some may have trouble breathing in a car seat even though their breathing is perfectly fine when lying down or being held in an adult's arms.

The problem stems from the fact that many car seats are designed for bigger infants who weigh more than seven pounds. In these roomy seats, unless little preemies get extra support, they tend to slump down, their heads flopping forward or sideways—and as a result, quite a few have apnea, bradycardia, or oxygen desaturation.

That's why the American Academy of Pediatrics now recommends that all infants born before 37 weeks of gestation be monitored in their car seat for at least 90 minutes before leaving the hospital. If your baby passes with flying colors, you won't have to worry. If she shows signs of breathing problems, these are some things you should consider:

✳ **Make sure you have provided her with the optimal seat.** It could make all the difference to choose a different one since a small baby is least likely to slump in one that fits as it should. (The right fit will keep her safest in case of an accident, too.) A preemie needs a rear-facing car seat designed for small infants, not one that is made for children weighing over 20 pounds. On its web site, the American Academy of Pediatrics has a guide that lists most models sold and gives the lowest weight for which each is approved. You'll find it at http://www.aap.org/family/carseatguide .htm#. Many infant seats are approved for babies as small as five pounds, and a few are approved for babies as small as four pounds. To keep a preemie from slouching forward, a seat must have a distance of 5½ inches or less from the crotch strap between her legs to the bottom of the seat back and 10 inches or less from the lower harness strap to the seat bottom.

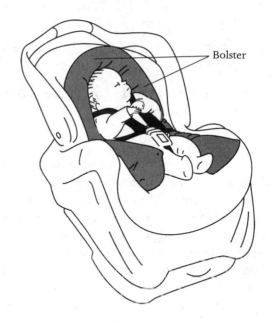

✳ **Use the bolster.** Many infant seats now come with bolsters that allow the tiniest babies to fit in them snugly. If your seat doesn't come with one, it's not safe to use a bolster that's sold separately; instead, you can pad around your baby with rolled-up blankets or cloth diapers to keep her snug and propped up.

✳ **Make sure to tilt the car seat halfway back** so that it reclines at a 45-degree angle.

✳ **If your baby still has breathing problems, she may do fine in an infant car bed** that allows her to lie down when she travels. Most nurseries have one available for testing preemies, and if it works well you can order one easily online.

✳ **Sometimes you just need to wait a few days or a week,** then try the car seat challenge again. A preemie's maturation proceeds in leaps and bounds, especially as she approaches term (her original due date).

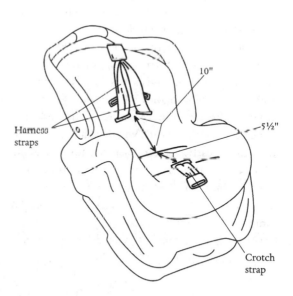

A special insert, which comes with some car seats, keeps a preemie propped in a safe position. In a car seat for a preemie, the harness strap should come out of the seat no more than 10 inches up from the bottom of the seat back. The crotch strap should come out no more than 5½ inches from the bottom of the seat back.

If You Want to Take Your Preemie on an Airplane

A word of caution: Some preemies may be well enough to go home, but not ready to ride in an airplane yet. This is because even airplanes with pressurized cabins (virtually all commercial passenger airplanes today) don't achieve an oxygen concentration as high as in typical room air at sea level. That means one needs to breathe more deeply or rapidly to take in the same amount of oxygen.

For a preemie whose oxygen saturation levels have been measuring close to 100 percent, a typical drop on the plane (between 1 percent and 10 percent) should be no problem. But for babies whose saturation levels in the hospital have been sufficient but lower—say, 90 percent to 95 percent—the further drop could be dangerous. Many neonatologists would advise parents not to take these babies on airplanes for several months after leaving the nursery. In addition, some very young infants, whether they were born at term or early, have occasional, unpredictable episodes of deeper oxygen desaturation after several hours of breathing oxygen at concentrations typically found in airplane cabins. So some experts extend that advice to even the best breathers among them. It would be equally un-wise to take your preemie to high-altitude places like Denver or the Alps, where air pressure is lower, also.

Another reason why planes are not preemie-friendly is that they increase the possibility of catching a cold or other respiratory infection. For economic reasons, some years ago commercial flights began recycling all or part of the air circulating in the cabin, and since then greater transmission of infections among passengers has been documented. All preemies are vulnerable to these illnesses, especially in the first winter of their lives.

If you are taking your baby on a plane ride, you'll face the decision of whether to buckle her into a car seat in the seat next to you, or just hold her in your arms. (On some international flights, she can lie in a special bassinet, provided by the airline, that attaches to the bulkhead wall opposite the front row of seats.) It's hard to know what's best; strapping her in is safest in the event of a severe jolt, but holding her saves you the cost of a seat and could possibly help her breathe more regularly. Your baby's doctor, who knows how strong her breathing is, can help you weigh the choices.

✳ **Until you're confident that your preemie has outgrown her breathing difficulties, minimize car trips,** and have an adult sit next to her in the back seat whenever possible, to keep an eye on her. (Remember that it is always safest for a child to ride in the back seat. Infants in rear-facing car seats should never be placed in the front seat of a car with a passenger-side airbag.)

A few additional tips are important for all preemies, reliable breathers or not. These may sound like small details, but they make a huge difference in your baby's safety:

* A preemie's car seat should have a three-point harness system (if it's an infant-only seat) or a five-point harness system (if it's a convertible baby/toddler seat)—not a shield or abdominal pad. In an impact, these could come into contact with a small infant's face and cause injury.
* Make sure the harness fits your baby snugly, and the retainer clip is positioned at the middle of her chest, not at her stomach or neck.
* You'll be happy to know that according to the American Academy of Pediatrics, a higher price does not mean a safer seat, and there's no best brand.
* Some local fire departments provide a wonderful free service for their community, and will fit the base of your baby's car seat into your car so that it's snug, secure, and positioned in the correct, safest way. Call your fire department to find out whether they offer this service and to make an appointment.
* Finally, don't become so worried about your baby's breathing that you make the mistake of thinking it would be safer for her to ride in the car held in someone's arms—it wouldn't!

CPR

I learned CPR, but will I really be able to do it? Or even recognize when my baby is having apnea?

Like Olympic divers demonstrating a perfect flip, experts in CPR always make it look so simple. But it's not simple when you're a parent learning it for the first time, trying to remember all of the precise moves. Breathing may come naturally,

but trying to make somebody else breathe doesn't come naturally at all.

Most parents who've just learned CPR feel like you: They aren't sure they could do it the right way in an emergency. Here's what we suggest.

* **Try to keep your memory of CPR fresh by practicing every couple of weeks.** Research has shown that parents who refresh their memory with hands-on practice using a doll (you should never use an actual baby) retain their CPR skills the best. You'll find free videos of infant CPR on the web (one example is at http://depts.washington.edu/learncpr/video demo/infant-cpr-video.html). You can remind yourself of what to do by watching every now and then.
* **Don't expect too much of your memory under pressure.** Even in NICUs, charts of emergency medications are sometimes posted near babies' beds so that doctors and nurses don't have to rely on their memories in the heat of an emergency. Since your memory may not function perfectly, you may feel more secure if you keep a copy of the CPR guidelines the hospital gave you (or a copy you make of the guidelines on page 589) in several places where you spend a lot of time with your baby—near her crib, in the kitchen, and also in your purse, diaper bag, or even glove compartment.
* **Be assured that although it's important to learn how to do CPR correctly, you probably will help your baby even if you don't do everything exactly right.** You'll most likely succeed in giving your baby some breaths (which will deliver oxygen into her lungs) and pressing on her chest (to pump the oxygen-rich blood to the rest of her body). Meanwhile, someone near you will be calling for help. If you are alone, start doing CPR before rushing

to the phone. Then after some breaths and chest pumping, you can take a brief pause and call 911.

How can you recognize whether your baby is really having apnea? First look for a change in her color. If she stops breathing or her heart pumps too slowly, her color will begin to change from pink to bluish gray. It's easiest to see a change in color by looking at her lips and tongue, since they're usually rosy. (Babies who are very fair can sometimes look a little blue around their mouths even when they're breathing normally because the veins show through their thin skin. As long as the inside of her mouth is pink, you don't have to worry—she's OK.) To check that she's breathing, you can glance at her chest to make sure it's moving and put your ear next to her nose and mouth to listen for breathing sounds. If your baby's pink and you can tell she's breathing, she's fine.

If you aren't sure, stimulate her a little with some gentle pats or rubs on her foot, belly, or back. You can also try changing her position since there are occasions when a baby may be breathing, but because her neck is kinked the air isn't getting into her windpipe. If she's eating at the time, take the nipple out of her mouth and give her a few seconds to recover and breathe. In case her airway is blocked, look to see whether any food or other object is in her mouth and, if so, remove it. (Don't just blindly sweep her mouth with your finger, since you could push an obstructing object farther down.) You can also suction out her mouth and nose with your bulb syringe or with a suction device, if you have one.

If these simple maneuvers don't work, try turning her over and patting or rubbing her back a little harder. The important thing is never to shake her so hard that her head moves back and forth like a rag doll. If more vigorous stimulation than you've already done is needed, that's the time to start CPR.

Home Nursing Care

The hospital wants to set up home nursing for my baby. What am I in for? I'm not sure I really need it.

If the doctors have told you that they want to organize professional home nursing for your baby, trust us: You should accept the offer. Your preemie is ready to leave the hospital, thankfully, but his care is still complex. Some temporary medical help from professional nurses can greatly ease the transition from hospital to home, assuring your baby's well-being until you're fully trained and comfortable enough to perform all of his care yourself. For many families that will be in a matter of a few weeks; for some, it may be longer.

Today increasing numbers of families are offered the option of home nursing care, which can shorten a hospitalization considerably. Your premature baby may need home nursing for respiratory care, such as mechanical ventilation or supplemental oxygen; for alternative feeding methods, such as parenteral nutrition or tube feedings; or because his medications or other special treatments are very complicated to administer.

Depending on your child's needs, his nurses will be in your home from just a few minutes once a week (for a weight or blood pressure check, for example) to most of the day and night. Most commonly, the nurses come more frequently in the first several weeks after discharge to make sure you are becoming familiar with the medical equipment and procedures. Then as you gradually take over your baby's health care, the nurses come less often; eventually, they'll come only for periodic supervision. In less common, more serious medical situations, the nurses may keep coming to your home every day for a much longer time, but at some point their hours will decrease, too, as your baby recovers.

Despite the great advantage of allowing your preemie to leave the hospital much sooner, it's best to be realistic about home care: It's not a stroll in the park. Here are some of the issues that may arise:

* **Pressure and demands on you.** At the beginning you will have to deal with many organizational issues, to make sure your home is ready for your baby and remains safe and hospitable. You'll be discussing everything with your home health care agency, from time schedules to the technical details of the medical equipment to the floor plan of your baby's room. The agency will expect you to learn enough about your baby's care to give the nurses the feedback they need, and then to take over the care little by little. As a result, there will be a lot of pressure and many demands on you. But always remember that the beginning is the hardest: Most parents describe an initial stressful, even chaotic, adjustment period lasting about four to six weeks. After that, most feel they've gotten their baby's care down to a comfortable, familiar routine.

* **Frustration and guilt.** Keeping up your self-esteem by reminding yourself of your unique and valuable parental role is very important right now. It will help you to control the frustration or guilt that home nursing can generate in some parents, who wrongly think they are not good enough to take care of their infant on their own. That's irrational, of course: The doctors' decision to set up a home nursing service is dictated by your baby's medical condition—not by any judgment about your ability as a parent. Despite the nurses' interventions and presence in your home, you are, as you always will be, your baby's primary and most important caregiver. The home nurses know that there are many people who are as qualified as they are to give professional care to

your baby, but only one mother or father. One of the things they want to do is to take over enough of the medical burdens to let parents be parents, not medical staff.

* **Loss of privacy.** For some parents, having a nurse in the house, sitting at their baby's bedside and observing their family life, is uncomfortable. You may become self-conscious about your personal habits, the appearance of your house, your lifestyle. One father told us that he was most bothered by something seemingly small: not being able to come downstairs in the morning in his pajamas. Others find that the loss of privacy disrupts more profound, intimate moments with their baby since not everyone is able to express love and tenderness in front of a stranger.

  Home health care nurses know this is difficult, and most try to be supportive, nonjudgmental, and respectful of your privacy. One thing that can help is to designate certain rooms of your house as private areas and to develop, together with your home care agency, a set of house rules regarding such things as where the nurse should store her food and what your policy is on television viewing. (There's a list of suggested topics for house rules on page 395.) Remember, though, that while rules are useful for communicating guidelines, a flexible and friendly attitude can help ease the initial discomfort of living alongside a stranger. To make your house a good work environment, remember to ask the nurses what they may need from you also. Over time, most parents succeed in developing a companionable and trusting relationship with their baby's nurses.

* **Psychological consequences for parents and siblings.** Negative feelings, such as anxiety and depression, can affect parents for a long time after a premature baby's birth and are especially common if a baby has a medical condition like

BPD that may take long months to get better. Not only are there practical problems in dealing with your preemie's special medical needs, but there's a nurse in your home as a constant reminder of your baby's ongoing health problems. It's natural to blame the nurse's presence for your stress, while in reality it's mostly due to worries about your baby.

If you have older children, they may resent the presence of the nurse, the disruption of family habits, or the tension they perceive in their parents. Their anxiety, jealousy, or anger may be expressed in temper tantrums or other aggressive behavior, health complaints, a regression in speech and behavior, or school problems. But they also may genuinely love their sibling and feel proud of themselves for helping out.

* **Parents who withdraw.** Occasionally, a parent will develop what has been called "parent dropout syndrome." This happens when mothers or fathers become so dependent on the nurses that they completely withdraw from their child's care, not even participating in routine acts like feeding or changing clothes and diapers. Less extreme and much more common is when parents simply resist learning the medical care techniques they should be able to perform on their own because they are too overwhelmed to focus and concentrate. If you notice that you're reacting this way, you should tell your nurses openly that you don't feel sure of your skills in caring for your baby. Home nurses are familiar with these parental reactions and generally handle them with patience and understanding. Since they know that you should be at the center of your baby's care, they will certainly help you to become more competent and overcome your insecurities. Another consideration is that sometimes nurses get sick or change jobs unexpectedly, and because it's not always possible for a replacement to be found right away, you may find yourself with the caregiving responsibility for a day, a week, or even longer. And when the new nurse comes, she'll look to you, as the one who knows your baby's needs the best, to help explain how best to care for him—how to read his signals, what caregiving methods he likes and doesn't like, and what schedule he's used to. Thus, a working partnership between you and the home nurses is essential for the sake of your baby.

* **Financial pressure.** Financial pressure on a family can obviously add to worries and resentment. Before your baby is discharged, you should talk to the social worker in your nursery to find out what costs you should anticipate for his home care and how you might meet them. Most of the direct costs, including nurses' and physicians' fees, medical equipment and supplies will be covered by your health insurance plan or Medicaid. But you should also plan for some indirect costs, such as higher electricity and other utility bills, perhaps some home remodeling, and loss of time and income for you, your partner, or another member of your family, since caring for a baby at home is demanding even with the help of a nurse. The social worker can help you find out what additional financial resources are available and which agencies in your community to contact for aid. Sometimes premature and sick babies are eligible for Medicaid even if their parents aren't, and for Supplemental Social Security income. Your home health nurse, who can see where you have extra expenses, can also be an advocate with your insurance company or government agencies.

* **Effect on your baby.** Having ongoing health problems and needing prolonged medical care can sometimes exacerbate a preemie's tendency to cry, fuss, and overreact or underreact to stimulation. Still, letting your baby complete

House Rules for Home Nurses*

Here are some points you may want to cover in a list of house rules for your baby's nurses. Let them know your preferences about:

1. **Entering the house:** Where to enter (with keys or not), where to store coats or personal belongings, where to park the car.
2. **Food:** Where the nurse should store her food, where she should eat in the house.
3. **Rooms:** Which bathroom the nurse should use, which rooms are private family areas, not to be entered.
4. **Phone calls:** Whether and how the nurse should answer your telephone, whether she may receive or make personal calls on your line, whether there is a limit on how much time she may spend on her cell phone.
5. **Visitors:** Which visitors you allow to visit the nurse or your baby in your absence.
6. **Television, computer, music:** How often, when, and where is watching TV, using a computer, and listening to an iPod or other music OK? May the nurse watch more TV or spend more time on the computer at night when she has no other distractions and needs to stay awake?
7. **Duties:** What you expect the nurse to take care of. Home nurses are generally responsible for keeping your baby's room tidy. Who will change your baby's clothes, change his diaper, feed him, bathe him, and put him to bed? When should these routines take place? Make clear what tasks you want to do yourself and how often.
8. **Discipline:** When and how the nurse may discipline your older children if they interfere with her work. Be specific! (Note that a caregiver other than the nurse must always be present to watch other children in your absence.)
9. **Information:** What kind of feedback and information about your baby do you expect from the nurse and how often?

*Adapted with permission from *Pediatric Nursing* 19(4): 375, copyright Jannetti Publications, Inc., Pitman, NJ, 1993

his recovery in his own home, where you can give him the attention, love, and stimulation he needs to develop well, is far preferable to spending many early months in the unnatural environment of a hospital nursery.

Although it may feel pretty daunting now, most families cope well with home nursing, appreciating that it is less disruptive than a long stay in the hospital. For many parents, it is also a great learning experience that enables them to become better caregivers. But those who benefit most, of course, are their babies, who get the opportunity to heal faster and develop normally in the warm, nurturing environment of their family home.

Getting Acquainted with: Home Oxygen

Some babies with BPD or other medical conditions still need supplemental oxygen when they're otherwise ready to be discharged from the hospital. The extra oxygen is usually a temporary measure, to be gradually eliminated as the baby's lungs heal and grow. If your preemie is in this situation, the good news is that while this process takes place, he can be at home with you, getting all the love, attention, and stimulation an infant needs to develop normally. And be assured you're not alone: Recent studies show that about 5 percent of all preemies—and around 30 percent of those born smaller than 1,000 grams—need to be sent home on oxygen.

Although this prospect might initially worry you, it doesn't mean that you have to turn your home into a hospital or become a professional nurse. You will be provided with all of the coaching and assistance you need. Most parents find they can lead a normal family life and quickly become familiar with the oxygen equipment, which is less intrusive than you may think. A baby on extra oxygen can go out for strolls (most home oxygen comes with its own carrying case or portable rolling rack) and even travel, with just a little organization first.

True, oxygen is one more thing you have to handle now. But most parents find that nothing is insurmountable. And sooner than you expect, your baby is likely to leave supplemental oxygen behind: Studies have shown that this therapy is seldom needed for longer than six months. If your child does need supplemental oxygen for a longer time, extra-long tubing will allow him to crawl or walk freely around a room, although he'll need supervision (like every other toddler!) to make sure he doesn't get tangled in the tubing and it doesn't get caught on furniture and dislodged.

How your baby's home oxygen therapy is organized

Starting before discharge and continuing at home, you'll be carefully instructed in:

* **the type of equipment** you're getting, including an oxygen source, a humidifier, a device to deliver the oxygen, and possibly a pulse oximeter or cardiorespiratory monitor;
* **how to use, adjust, clean, and check the equipment** for proper functioning and prevention of infections;
* **how much oxygen** to give your baby;
* **how much humidity** to provide with the oxygen;
* **when to give the oxygen:** continuously or just at certain times;
* **how to tell whether your baby is getting enough oxygen** and whether to give him more during more stressful activities, like eating or playing;
* **what to do in case of an emergency,** including how to handle technical failures of the equipment, and how to do CPR.

Although it sounds like a huge task now, you'll be getting lots of teaching, support, and practice. You'll have several hands-on training sessions before your baby is discharged from the hospital. And once you get home, you'll be able to count on the support of a home health service, routinely assigned to any baby discharged on oxygen. A nurse will be available to answer your calls 24 hours a day and to come to your home if problems arise. The home nursing team will also make routine visits to your home to ensure that you become progressively more con-

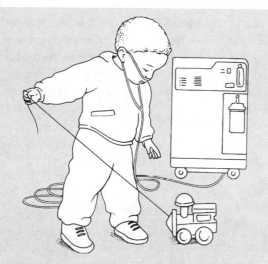

Thanks to long tubing, a supervised toddler on supplemental oxygen can move around freely.

Adapted with permission of Pediatric Services of America

fident in managing your baby's supplemental oxygen.

Because your training will be tailored to your baby's particular situation and equipment, you should rely on your hospital and home health nurses for specific information. But here's an overview of some of the most common, important issues faced by parents of preemies on home oxygen.

General safety issues

Thousands of families have used oxygen safely in their homes by observing some basic safety measures. Because oxygen is highly flammable, no smoking, fire, or sparks (including gas stoves) should ever be allowed in the same room with it, and radiators and heaters should be kept at least five feet from the oxygen source and your baby's bed. The room (or car, when your child is traveling) should always be well ventilated. Some parents like to put "Caution: No Smoking" signs on their portable oxygen tanks to warn passersby.

Oxygen equipment for indoors and outdoors

There are three possible sources of supplemental oxygen for use at home. Your baby's doctor will suggest the kinds that may work best for you. Most families end up using more than one, for different circumstances.

Oxygen cylinders. These are tanks filled with oxygen gas. If your baby needs oxygen only intermittently, up to twelve hours a day, they are your most cost-effective source. The tanks come in different sizes and can be stored for a long time. The largest are for use at home; the smallest, which are lightweight and easily portable, allow you to take your baby out for a walk, on a car trip, or on public transportation.

Once connected to a regulator (the device controlling the flow of oxygen from the cylinder), a portable oxygen tank should be kept upright whenever possible. The regulator and its connection to the tank should be protected from being accidentally knocked off because if gas at high pressure leaks out, the tank could propel itself forward dangerously.

When you travel by car, keep the oxygen tank vertical on a seat, well-secured with a belt or strap to protect it from any shock. Never put it in the trunk, where it may get knocked or overheated. When you take a walk with your baby, a backpack is a good way to carry a portable cylinder around. The tubing that runs from the cylinder to your baby should be safely taped in place (for instance, from the backpack to your shoulder, the handle of the stroller, and your baby's face) but not stretched tight. Some parents find it more comfortable to lay the cylinder down in a basket or rack under their baby's stroller. Just make sure that it's well-shielded from any jolts or shocks. If you want to avoid people's stares or questions, you can both protect and conceal the oxygen tank with a blanket.

You'll get information from your oxygen supplier stating how many hours of oxygen each size of tank will provide at a given flow rate. You'll learn to monitor and keep track of how much oxygen is left. Never leave the house without more oxygen than your baby needs in case of a car breakdown, traffic jam, or other unpredictable delay.

Liquid oxygen tanks. Oxygen at very cold temperatures (more than 300 degrees Fahrenheit below zero) is a liquid and can be maintained that way under pressure in special containers. Liquid oxygen is more convenient because it's more compact than the gas so more of it fits in a tank. If your baby needs continuous, low-flow oxygen therapy, it may be your best choice. Just keep in mind that because it will evaporate, it can't be stored for as long. Liquid oxygen tanks, like oxygen cylinders, come in different sizes. The smaller, portable ones can be refilled as needed at home. They require the same safety precautions as oxygen cylinders: they must be kept upright to avoid leakage, and protected from shocks. It's not necessary to store them in a cold place; the tanks themselves will keep the oxygen inside cold, but they should be kept where they won't overheat. You have to monitor their remaining oxygen supply so it doesn't unexpectedly run out. If some liquid oxygen spills, it should be kept away from the skin and eyes to avoid dangerous freeze burns. For the same reason, you should never touch the frost that may form on the tank.

Oxygen concentrator. This electrical device takes oxygen from room air and concentrates it. If your baby needs continuous oxygen at a high flow rate, you'll find it to be the most convenient source because the oxygen never runs out and you're spared the hassle of oxygen deliveries. The downside is that it will increase your electrical bills. A concentrator is a bulky machine that can be loud, but don't put it in a closet or closed storage place or use it with an extension cord or in outlets being used for other appliances, because of the risk of overheating and fire. If you get a concentrator, you'll also need to have a portable cylinder or liquid oxygen tank you can use when you take your baby out and as a backup in case of a power failure or machine malfunction.

Sources of humidification

Each oxygen delivery system is equipped with a humidity source. Adding water to the oxygen prevents drying and irritation of a baby's airways.

How your baby gets the oxygen

Nasal cannula. As you've probably seen in the nursery, a nasal cannula won't interfere with your baby's movements, feeding, speech, or interaction with the environment. It can be connected to long tubing, allowing you to carry your baby easily around the house, and later allowing him to move freely when he begins to roll over and crawl. (If you get extra-long tubing, be sure to tell

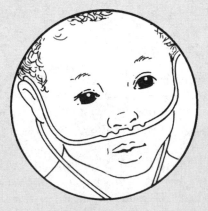

Clipping off the prongs and cutting extra holes in a nasal cannula can make it less irritating for a child's nostrils.

your nurse or doctor, because sometimes the oxygen flow rate will need to be increased.) The clear small tube can be held in place under a baby's nose with a headband, and if necessary, taped to his face with soft surgical tape. (You may want to do this, particularly at night.)

If your baby sometimes pulls at his cannula, it may help to run the tubing over and behind his ears, then slip it inside his clothes. (Don't restrain his hands, because being able to reach for and manipulate things is important for his development.) Nasal prongs that don't fit right—because they're too big or spaced too close together—can be irritating, and your child may need a bigger cannula as he grows. If he is between sizes, a little lubricating jelly around his nostrils may ease the discomfort. If that doesn't work and if your doctor gives you permission, you can clip off the prongs and cut additional holes in the cannula (see illustration on page 398), so it can still deliver oxygen without entering his nose.

Tracheostomy collar. Babies with BPD who have had a tracheostomy usually need extra oxygen for some time after they've been weaned from the ventilator. The oxygen is delivered through tubing connected to a collar positioned over the tracheostomy tube in the baby's neck. As with a nasal cannula, babies on "trach collar" oxygen can move about fairly freely, so their development is not impeded. At night, to prevent the oxygen tubing from being displaced when your baby turns, it can be anchored with a chest belt secured with Velcro.

Ventilator. A baby with a tracheostomy may be discharged home on mechanical ventilation, in which case he will get his oxygen through the ventilator. Home ventilators are electrical machines similar to those used in hospitals. If your baby goes home on a ventilator, you'll be extensively trained to use the equipment and troubleshoot problems. You'll also have a nurse assigned to assist you in your home for at least several hours a day, until you feel more comfortable.

Cleaning the oxygen equipment

To prevent infections, it's crucial to clean all of the oxygen equipment regularly, following the instructions provided by your home health agency. The filter of a concentrator, for instance, should be washed with hot water and mild soap at least once a week. It's particularly important to keep the humidification tubing clean since bacteria love to grow in its warm, moist environment.

Don't think that you need to maintain the same hygiene standards as the hospital, though! In the hospital, where the babies are more fragile and there are many more easily spread germs, the equipment is sterilized—while at home, your aim is mere cleanliness. That means you'll be washing and reusing many things that would be thrown away after one use in the hospital. You aren't hurting your baby; on the contrary, you are gradually exposing him to the real world and helping him develop a normal immune system.

In case of emergency

When a baby goes home on oxygen, the hospital or home health agency should inform the local electric and telephone companies to put his family on a special priority list in case of a blackout or rationing of service. Near your telephone for quick reference you should post a list of emergency telephone numbers: 911 or the local rescue squad; the fire department; the closest emergency room; your baby's doctor; the home health agency and oxygen equipment supplier; and the electric company's emergency service line.

Financial Considerations

Insurance plans and Medicaid usually pay for oxygen equipment, and most parents find that home oxygen alone poses little extra financial burden for them. What's not covered are the higher electrical bills generated by an oxygen concentrator, and any extra nasal cannulas or trach tubes and ties that parents have to buy beyond the limited number allowed by insurance or Medicaid each month. (Many families now buy some of the equipment they need inexpensively online, even on craigslist. Just be sure to check with your baby's doctor before you purchase anything. While it may be safe for certain kinds of equipment to be secondhand, other items should be unopened, and you may need to double check that you're getting the right size and brand for your child.) For babies with more complicated BPD, who need a lot of special care and medications, home nursing care is generally covered but only for a limited number of hours a day and for a short time after discharge from the hospital. And if your baby has lots of other medical needs and equipment, you may have other expenses that aren't covered—you may need to buy a van, for example, or even move to a different home. Be sure to check with the social worker in your hospital to find out exactly what your plan covers and whether you're eligible for any other government or private assistance programs that provide financial help or give you access to more services. Most of the time, some additional government funds are available.

Useful tips from parents to parents

There's nothing like direct experience to teach a parent how to deal with a baby on supplemental oxygen. Parent groups that you can find on the web may offer you invaluable practical or emotional support. In the meantime, to give you a head start, here are some key tips culled from families who have "been there":

* Choose a stroller with the biggest possible basket (to hold the oxygen tank) and with a canopy where you can store other things you have to carry.
* Some parents find they rest easier knowing their baby is on a pulse oximeter, so you may want to talk to your doctor about getting one. If your baby's oxygen tube gets squeezed or twisted during the night, and he doesn't get enough oxygen, this alarm will go off earlier than an apnea monitor.
* Once a baby on oxygen is able to roll over, it's possible for him to wrap the tube around his neck. An easy way to prevent this is to dress your baby in one-piece, long-legged outfits and run the tube down his back under his clothes, letting it out below the last button on the leg at his ankle.
* Most parents find that using extra-long tubing, about 50 feet, allows them to carry their baby freely around the house and is easier for them than switching back and forth between tanks in different rooms. Just make sure the path is kept clear and the tube doesn't get shut in a door.
* If your house has two floors, you may want to use two large tanks, one on each floor.
* Ask for a connecting piece between the nasal cannula and oxygen tube that can turn 360 degrees. That way, the tube is prevented from twisting too much when your baby moves.
* Some parents warn about the importance of having only metal pieces in the tank regulator. Plastic ones break more easily, creating an emergency. For the same reason, you may want to keep extra parts handy (nasal cannula, connectors, tubing), at home and in the car,

and bring some spares with you when you travel.

* Some babies on extra oxygen (usually those with other equipment as well, such as a portable ventilator or an apnea monitor) may qualify for a handicapped parking permit. You may not like the idea, but the convenience can be a boon when you have a lot to carry. Ask the NICU's discharge planner what papers you have to fill out to get one.

* Daycare centers don't usually accept babies on extra oxygen—and probably aren't the best childcare option for them, anyway, since babies in daycare are exposed to so many germs and tend to get sick more often, which can be a problem if parents need to work and don't have relatives or friends to help them. If you contact a parent support group, you may find someone who knows of a babysitting pool or will help you set one up. The organizational work you'll have to do at first may be worth it in the long-run, giving you extra time and your baby the opportunity to interact with other kids. Another option is to ask at your local hospital's special care nursery or pediatric nursing department whether any of the nurses would like to do some childcare. Often you can find a few nurses who enjoy the variety and fun, as well as the extra income, of taking care of a healthier baby at home.

* Some parents find it difficult to trust anybody to babysit for their baby. They end up very tired and stressed out, which isn't good for anyone in the family, baby included. If you have found somebody who is willing to be trained on your baby's oxygen equipment, you should try to accept the idea, and allow yourself to get some much-needed respite.

* If you qualify for more than a couple of hours a day of in-home nursing care, consider asking the nurses to come at night so you can sleep.

Assessing your baby's respiration

In time, you'll become a good judge of your baby's respiration and able to detect any evidence of distress. The most frequent signs are a change in color (a baby not getting enough oxygen becomes pale or blue), fast and hard breathing, pronounced flaring of the nostrils, and wheezing. Some parents may be taught to check their baby's oxygen saturation with a pulse oximeter. Your baby's doctor will tell you what to expect from your child and when you should be concerned.

Your baby will thrive on plenty of feeding, handling, and play, so you shouldn't restrict those activities unless you've been told to do so. Occasionally he may need to take a brief pause and rest, to give his breathing a chance to return to normal. (Be sure to tell the doctor if you notice that your child has any respiratory distress, because he might want to prescribe an increased amount of oxygen during certain activities.) It won't be surprising if your baby needs to have his oxygen increased when he gets a cold or other respiratory illness. But you shouldn't change your baby's oxygen settings on your own, either raising or lowering them for long, unless you've been instructed to do so by your doctor. Sometimes, parents might be tempted to turn off the oxygen because their baby looks fine to them. But even if a baby isn't blue, his oxygen saturation could be too low, potentially causing his growth to be slowed or injuring his lungs, heart, or brain.

Taking your baby off oxygen, therefore, must be your doctor's call. He will evaluate your baby's status, probably performing pulse oximetry during different activities and times of day. If he concludes that your baby is ready to be weaned, he'll reduce the extra oxygen slowly, usually over several months. Finally the time will come when you turn off your baby's oxygen once and for all, with thanks for its help but understandable relief.

Giving Medications

I'm supposed to give my baby medicine every eight hours. It's going to be such a hassle.

Yes, dealing with medications is going to be a hassle. But once you get used to it, within just a few days, it should be a little hassle, not a big one. It will become part of your regular routine, not much different than changing diapers, giving baths, mixing feedings, or giving daily vitamins.

These tips may help things go smoothly:

✳ **Before your baby leaves the hospital, make sure the nurses show you how to give your baby her medication, and that they watch you do it yourself to check that you're doing it right.** There are certain things you definitely will need to know, in addition to how much medicine to give and how often. If there's anything on this list that the nurses haven't mentioned, be sure to ask:

- How to position your baby when giving the medicine and where to place the syringe or dropper inside her mouth;
- Whether to give the medicine before, with, or after meals;
- Whether there's a little flexibility in the schedule;
- What to do if your baby vomits right after receiving a dose or you forget to give one;
- Whether to keep the medication in the refrigerator;
- Whether to expect side effects and what to do if they appear;
- What the plan is for stopping the medication.

✳ **Ask the nurses if you can take home a handful of syringes from the hospital.** They're perfect for measuring out infant doses. You can use each one many times if you wash them after each use.

✳ **Usually there's some flexibility in the medication schedule.** If you're told to give the medication to your baby "every eight hours," for example, it may be equally fine for her to get it three times a day—at roughly eight-hour intervals, but not exactly. That little fact will provide you with a lot of freedom. Instead of having to say, "Oh, no, it's noon. I have to wake my baby up," you'll be able to relax and finish what you're doing, or let her wake up on her own.

✳ **Look on the bright side. Many people believe schedules are good for babies, anyway.** If you're like some parents—especially those whose babies have to get their medicine with feedings—it's being tied to a clock-driven routine that feels most burdensome. But on the positive side, many parents and experts strongly believe that babies are happier and less cranky that way: They don't get overtired because they stick to a regular nap schedule or too hungry because they eat at regular times. Some people even think structure in infancy is the beginning of promoting self-discipline. Schedules aren't all negative for parents, either. You'll know you're free at specific times for other things rather than always being at your baby's beck and call. You may look forward to sitting down every morning with a mug of coffee at ten o'clock, or every evening to a precious dinner alone with your partner, relatively undisturbed.

✳ **Prepare your baby's medication for a day or two at a time, storing it in a safe place where it won't spill and labeling it if your baby gets more than one kind.** When it's time for a dose of medicine and you're rushing around with a crying baby or stumbling around half-asleep, you'll be glad you took a few quiet minutes in advance to get things ready.

✳ **Keep a running checklist of all the times you give your baby her medicine and hang it on the refrigerator or medicine cabinet (be sure to keep a pen nearby). Believe us, you'll be glad you did. Even the most organized parent occasionally forgets whether she just gave the medication a mere few minutes ago. If you aren't the only one giving the medication, keeping things straight with a careful record is especially crucial.

* **Don't give medicine in the dark.** It's too easy to make mistakes in measuring the dose and too hard to see whether your baby actually swallowed the medicine. In fact, if at all possible, try to schedule things so you don't have to give medicine in the middle of the night when you're groggy.

* **Don't panic if your baby throws up right after getting her medicine.** It happens to everyone. Here are some general guidelines to follow, but *only* after you've asked the nurse or doctor whether they apply to your baby's medication. If a baby throws up right after getting the medicine, give that dose again. (If it is colored, you'll be able to see that the medicine has come out.) If a baby throws up more than an hour after getting the medicine, don't give that dose again; she got it. In between, it depends. If you can see that some of the medicine has come out, the right thing to do could be to give another half-dose or to give no more and just wait until the next dose; it depends on how crucial the medication is and what the risks of overdose are (you should ask your doctor about them if he hasn't advised you yet).

* **If you miss a dose, never double or increase the next dose unless your doctor has specifically told you to do so.** This can harm your baby.

* **If you're very late with a dose of medicine, give it when you remember, then gradually modify the schedule back to the original times.** However, if the new schedule is con-venient for you—for instance, if it means you won't have to give the medicine in the middle of the night—you can stick with subsequent, eight-hour intervals at the new times.

* **Don't give medicine to your baby when she's lying down.** She could choke.

* **At your baby's checkups, ask the doctor whether it's time for the dose to be increased.** As your baby gains weight, she may need more of the medication for it to remain as effective—and her doctor may need a reminder.

* **Don't decide by yourself when to stop giving the medication.** If it's important enough for your baby to be sent home on, it's not something to fool around with. If your baby is having great difficulty taking the medication or you have the sense she doesn't need it anymore, you can certainly suggest to the doctor that you'd like to stop. He may consult with your baby's neonatologist or a specialist or may make the decision on his own, but ultimately this has to be a doctor's call.

Reflux

My baby has reflux. Any advice for dealing with this at home?

While reflux isn't usually a serious health problem, it can be an uncomfortable and messy one. Many parents of preemies with reflux say it can be draining to care for their babies.

Fortunately, most babies outgrow their reflux within the first year, and very few still have the problem beyond age two. In the meantime, here is some distilled advice from doctors and parents who've been down this road before:

* **Buy a whole stash of cloth diapers and always keep them handy.** You can use them to drape over your shoulder when you're holding your

baby to protect your clothes and to cover the upholstery of the chair you're sitting in. When your baby spits up, they're big and soft enough to clean her.

* **Don't move your baby around too much during or immediately after feedings.** This means no bouncy seats, baby swings, or physical exercise for an hour or so after meals.

* **When you put your baby down to sleep, lay her on her back as you would other babies—this is important for reducing the risk of SIDS (sudden infant death syndrome). But if her reflux is severe, ask your pediatrician whether an exception should be made for her.** Although it's true that reflux is reduced when a baby is in a tummy-down position, the evidence that tummy-down sleeping is associated with SIDS is so strong that the American Academy of Pediatrics recommends putting even babies with reflux to sleep on their backs. (Side-sleeping is not a solution, since many babies who are put to bed on their side roll over and end up on their stomach.) If your baby's reflux is unusually severe, though, don't hesitate to ask your pediatrician what he suggests. In an occasional baby, there may be an even greater risk on her back that refluxed food could get into her airway or lungs, causing her to choke or have breathing problems.

* **Some parents find it helps to raise the head of their baby's bed about 30 degrees.** Your local baby store may sell foam wedges to place under the head of the crib mattress. A cheaper alternative is to prop big books or towels under one end of the crib mattress or bassinet.

* **Hold your baby in as vertical a position as possible, rather than a reclining one, with a straight (not rounded or bent) back when you are feeding her and for a little while afterward.** Gravity will help keep the food

from coming back up. Many parents find this position less natural at first, but for babies with reflux, it's the most comfortable position there is.

* **Give your baby smaller, more frequent meals.** This often works wonders. But keep in mind that reflux is aggravated by long periods of crying, because the stomach fills up with air. So this tip can quickly backfire if your baby dissolves in tears every time you end a feeding before she's completely full.

* **During bottle feedings, burp your baby often.** Babies often swallow air from the bottle when they feed. A common guideline is to stop for a burp after every ounce or two.

* **If you are bottle feeding your baby and she gulps down her formula rapidly, she may do better with a different nipple that delivers the formula more slowly.** Choosing the best nipple for each baby—not so fast that she chokes or gags, not so slow that she becomes frustrated or tired—is usually a matter of trial and error. It's also worth trying a bottle with a liner designed so that babies will swallow less air.

* **If your baby's neonatologist or pediatrician approves, you can try thickening her feedings with rice cereal.** Eating thicker feeds improves reflux in some babies. Add one tablespoon of rice cereal per ounce of formula. You can also try a premixed formula with added rice, like Enfamil AR, but this won't work well if your baby is also on an antacid for her reflux because stomach acid is needed to activate the thickening agent in the formula. If you're feeding your baby breast milk, you can get a prescription for a special thickening product (such as Thick & Easy or Thick-It) to add to your pumped milk. (Rice cereal won't work because an enzyme in breast milk breaks down the cereal before it can thicken the milk.) If you notice that thickened feedings aren't helping your baby, it could be because

she is sucking more vigorously to get the thicker liquid through the nipple and taking more air into her stomach. Using a cross-cut nipple—one with an enlarged hole—can help with this, but don't cut it yourself; a hole that's too big will cause your baby to get too much milk at once and she could choke.

* **Some babies with reflux keep solid foods down better than liquids.** In some countries, it's traditional to introduce solid foods during the first month of life. (American physicians have worried that this may contribute to food allergies, but so far, evidence doesn't bear that out.) If you want to try it, be sure to talk to your pediatrician first about safe foods he recommends to get started and how to ensure that your baby continues to get the balanced nutrition she needs.

* **If you notice that your baby is turning dusky or blue during a feeding or if she is coughing or becoming congested, remove the nipple from her mouth and give her a chance to catch her breath.** Milk that backs up into her throat or nose can interfere with smooth breathing. If you find that a pause now and then isn't enough to keep her breathing well during meals, call your pediatrician right away. On the other hand, if your baby remains pink and her nostrils open and close slightly while she sucks, you can be sure that her breathing is just fine.

* **Ask your pediatrician whether he recommends medication.** There are several medications that your doctor may consider if your baby's reflux is severe. Most of them, like Baby Mylanta, Pepcid, and Prevacid, reduce stomach acid, so may help with any heartburn your baby may be feeling. It is not clear, however, how effective or safe they are in treating reflux that is less severe. Although some of these can be bought as pills over the counter, you should never give any medication to your baby without your doctor's permission and instructions.

* **If your baby is already taking medicine for reflux, check with the doctor to make sure that you're giving it at the best times of day and in the right amount.** If your baby's symptoms have gotten worse as he's grown, his dose may need to be increased. Or you may need to give the medication at a different time of day; most antacids work best if they're taken about 30 minutes before a meal.

* **Constipation can make reflux worse.** Babies who are fed thickened feeds often get constipated and that fullness in their intestines can exacerbate their reflux. If you notice that your baby strains to have a bowel movement and her stool is dry or hard, then a little daily prune juice might help. Be sure to ask your pediatrician first, of course. Giving your baby extra water to drink, encouraging her to move around more (or exercising her arms and legs for her), and massaging her tummy are other remedies for constipation that you and your baby's doctor might consider.

* **If an allergy is causing the reflux, switching to a predigested (elemental) formula might help.** You can ask your baby's doctor if he thinks this is the problem. It's unlikely if your baby is eating nothing but your breast milk. But some infants are allergic to the cow's milk proteins in infant formulas and breast milk fortifiers.

* **Keep in mind that reflux can be hard on a baby's teeth.** Over time, stomach acid that comes into contact with a baby's teeth can eat away at the enamel. Dentists suggest brushing your baby's teeth regularly, never putting her to bed with a bottle of milk or juice, and making sure she gets fluoride through your water or fluoride supplements once her teeth come in. All parents should follow these guidelines, but it's especially important for you.

If Reflux Is Severe

A few preemies have reflux that is unusually severe—more than an unpleasant but relatively minor and fleeting nuisance. It's a good idea to know the symptoms since severe reflux often goes hand-in-hand with feeding problems, which can linger even after the reflux disappears.

Your baby's reflux may be severe if:

* She refuses to eat, even when she's hungry;
* She often gags or chokes while she's eating (every baby does this occasionally);
* During meals or within an hour afterward, she arches her back or is irritable and appears uncomfortable;
* She has apnea or bradys during or shortly after eating;
* She vomits frequently (that is, after almost every meal);
* She wheezes or her nose gets congested while she's eating or shortly afterward;
* Even when she isn't feeding, she often swallows and grimaces;
* She suffers from chronic ear infections, drooling, or bad breath;
* She isn't gaining weight.

Feeding problems can arise because eating is often an unpleasant experience for babies with severe reflux, and—who can blame them?—they naturally adopt certain behaviors to avoid it. For example, a baby whose reflux makes eating painful may refuse to open her mouth to eat; may hold milk or food in her mouth or let it dribble out rather than swallowing; or may gag, retch, or vomit almost as soon as she begins to eat. If these behaviors persist over time and become habits, they can be hard to break, even after the reflux goes away.

So if you notice symptoms of severe reflux in your baby, talk to her pediatrician. He may want to start treatment, or to step it up if your baby is being treated for reflux already. He may even refer your baby to a feeding specialist who'll help nip any problematic behaviors in the bud.

* **Infant seats and car seats tend to worsen reflux because they cause a baby to slump down, putting pressure on her stomach.** If this seems to be a problem, you may want to look into getting an infant car bed. (You'll find a couple of options online; see the resources on page 591.) Or try tilting the car seat back partway, so it reclines at a 45-degree angle to keep your baby from slumping down.

* **When you're with your baby, don't wear clothes that must be dry-cleaned or that are irreplaceable.** You'll feel a lot less frustrated when your baby spits up if you can just toss your clothes into the washing machine or easily replace them if they're beyond washing.
* **Keep several changes of clothes handy for your baby.** If you want her to look and smell nice, you're going to be changing her outfits

more often than other parents do. White clothes are actually some of the most practical because stains can be bleached out. Don't splurge on gorgeous baby clothes that you'll be pained to see stained after just one wearing, but don't put away all of your favorite clothes, either. If your baby doesn't wear them now, she'll grow out of them before you have a chance to enjoy them. She may wear each piece of clothing for only a few hours at a time—but she'll look adorable while she does.

During moments of frustration, remember two things. First, all babies spit up, cry, and occasionally seem uncomfortable or irritable. While your baby may do more of these things, they're not as uncommon—and you're not as alone—as you may sometimes think. Second, your baby's body is maturing every day, gradually working to eliminate the problem. In just a few months, you'll probably notice that her reflux is better. And not long after that, it may well be gone.

Special Formula or Breast Milk

How long do preemies need to be on special formula or fortified breast milk?

Most preemies who are bottle fed today are sent home on a special kind of infant formula called transitional formula. The currently available brands are Enfacare and Neosure (by the companies that make Enfamil and Similac). They are designed to supplement premature babies' nutrition during the transition between preterm formula and regular formula,

Transitional formula provides 22 calories per ounce, less than the 24 calories per ounce found in preterm formula but more than the 20 calories per ounce in regular formula. It also has more protein, calcium, phosphorus, zinc, and other minerals and vitamins than regular formula and

a special kind of fat that's easier to digest and assimilate. Studies have shown that some preemies (mainly boys and those who weighed less than 1,250 grams at birth) grow better and have stronger bones when they are fed transitional formula for several months after discharge.

Whether to feed your baby transitional formula and for how long is a decision her neonatologist and pediatrician will make, taking into account your baby's age and size at birth, her medical history (such as whether she has BPD and needs extra calories, and how dense her bones have looked on X-rays and lab tests), and how well she's growing. It's common for preemies to stay on transitional formula for about 6 to 12 months. When your baby's doctor tells you that it's the right time for your baby to graduate to regular formula, it will be a milestone—another happy sign that your baby, after his special beginning, is settling into much-welcomed plain old infanthood.

Pediatricians differ on whether breast milk, too, needs to be supplemented for a while at home, because there hasn't been any good research on that question. Some doctors believe that after discharge preemies who are taking all their feedings from their mothers' breasts and are growing well don't need the extra minerals and calories from breast milk fortifier, so it's not worth interrupting or changing your nursing patterns to add it to your milk. Other physicians think that totally breastfed preemies do better if they get at least two bottles a day of transitional formula or fortified breast milk to supplement the milk from their mothers' breasts.

It's easy enough to do if you're sometimes pumping your milk and giving it to your baby in a bottle; you simply add a fortifier (which may be a special product or just some powdered transitional formula) to your pumped breast milk. This usually isn't advised for longer than a couple of months—until a preemie is big and strong enough to respond to his own body's signals to increase the amount of milk he takes when he's nursing if he needs additional nutrients. As long as your baby is being exclusively breastfed, he'll be prescribed vitamin D (alone or in a multivitamin), iron, and maybe fluoride drops to supplement the few nutritional elements that are relatively lacking in breast milk. These can be discontinued when he's eating adequate amounts of solid food; ask your pediatrician when that will be.

Some babies, such as those with BPD or heart problems, need lots of energy to grow but do poorly if they get too much fluid. If that's true for your preemie, your pediatrician may tell you to prepare regular formula with less water to increase its caloric content. This is also a convenient alternative for some healthy preemies who aren't eating quite well enough just yet and whose parents might otherwise find themselves spending hours on feedings when they go home. (Don't do this unless your doctor instructs you to, however. A baby can get sick if he doesn't get the right amount of water and nutrients, and for most babies, the standard formulation is best.)

Here's what you may be told to do by your baby's doctor.

With powdered formula:

* to make regular 20-calorie-per-ounce formula, mix one scoop of powder with two ounces of water
* to make 22-calorie-per-ounce formula, mix three scoops of powder with five-and-a-half ounces of water
* to make 24-calorie-per-ounce formula, mix three scoops of powder with five ounces of water

With concentrated liquid formula:

* to make 20-calorie-per-ounce formula, mix one ounce of concentrate with one ounce of water (or mix the usual 13-ounce can of

concentrated liquid formula with 13 ounces of water)
* to make 22-calorie-per-ounce formula, mix a 13-ounce can with 10½ ounces of water
* to make 24-calorie-per-ounce formula, mix a 13-ounce can with 8½ ounces of water

If your baby needs even more calories or special nutrients, the pediatrician can give you a recipe to further enrich his formula. Whatever instructions you receive from your doctor about your baby's nutrition you should follow carefully, never taking the initiative and changing the concentration or doses on your own. Overconcentrated formula is difficult to digest and can cause dehydration and other serious problems. Supplements can be very dangerous if not given according to your doctor's prescription.

Obsessed with Your Baby's Weight

My husband thinks I'm obsessed with feeding my baby. But I've got to make sure she keeps gaining weight.

To her parents, a preemie's small size often comes to represent everything that is scary or dangerous about her condition. With the daily weighings in the hospital, the jubilation or consternation over ounces gained or lost—well, no wonder you're obsessed with feeding her! Even a small spit-up may upset you, as if those few lost calories could be the precious ones that make a difference. But now, even your husband, who has gone through all of this with you, is telling you to relax. What might help you do that?

First of all, you may need to acknowledge and accept that you're going to have special feelings about your daughter's nutrition for a long time. In fact, when the time comes to make the transition from breast milk or formula to baby foods, you may feel more anxious, since it means leaving a reassuring, known feeding schedule for an uncertain new one. Many parents of preemies continue paying special attention to how their child eats for a long time—and nobody should blame you for that. Being vigilant is something practical you can do to ease your fears and ensure that she's getting good nutrition.

But you also need to realize that it's perfectly normal for your baby to eat more at one meal and less at another. It's one way her body regulates itself, matching her fuel intake to her energy demands. If you consistently overlook her signals saying she's hungry or feeling full, you can short circuit this important regulatory function. So try hard not to ignore your baby's cues, even if she's saying (heaven forbid!) she's not hungry. Remember that following her cues was the guiding tenet when she was fed in the hospital nursery, and it should continue to guide you at home. Rather than thinking that you have to get your baby to eat a certain amount at each feeding, try to see her food intake as averaged over one- to two-day cycles. Chances are that the varying amounts she eats at each meal will balance out over time. Your baby's doctor can tell you the minimum amount of food she should eat each day, on average, to grow and develop well. As long as she takes in that much, you don't have to press for more. Feeding experts say that your overriding goal should be to make mealtime a pleasant experience—one she'll want to repeat again and again. (Force-feeding can actually be counterproductive, leading to more feeding refusals in the future.)

Another reason not to push a preemie to eat more than she wants is research showing that overly fast growth in early infancy is associated with the development of insulin resistance and type 2 diabetes later in life. Babies who are formula fed are more likely to grow excessively than breastfed babies, who tend to be leaner. (But if your premature baby is experiencing fast catch-up growth—meaning she's getting closer to the weight and height of term babies her age—on her own, without your pushing her to eat more at every meal, you shouldn't interfere in that natural, often desirable process. The key is not to force it.)

If you need more reassurance, ask your baby's pediatrician to go over her growth chart with you. She's doing fine if she's growing at a steady rate along a standard growth curve or gradually catching up to her full-term peers. It might also help to ask the doctor how important it is for you to continue doing your utmost to feed her or whether you can relax your vigilance. Some preemies, such as those with severe BPD, often have trouble eating and need all the calories they can get, while others do just fine on their own. Tell your doctor if there's something about the way your baby feeds that is worrying you (such as how she sucks or reacts to eating from a spoon). But if he tries to reassure you by saying that a bottle or baby food jar occasionally left unfinished is not the end of the world, believe him.

If you can, look at this attitude of yours with a sense of humor. A self-deprecating joke here and there about your constant attempts to stuff the poor baby like a Thanksgiving turkey can lighten your spirits and give your relatives and friends insight into your reaction to one of the most stressful issues for parents of premature babies.

Whom to Call with Questions

I've already called the NICU twice because I was worried about my son, and it turned out to be nothing. Now I'm nervous again, and I don't know if I should call.

If you're often tempted to call the NICU or already have, you're certainly not alone. Studies have found that a great number of parents make telephone calls to their baby's hospital for several weeks after discharge. The NICU staff understands this need. Some nurseries even have a specially assigned nurse to deal with families of discharged babies.

But acknowledging a common behavior doesn't mean that it's the best thing to do. Your baby's pediatrician, with whom you should schedule a visit a few days after discharge, is the one who should field most of your questions and concerns. Don't hesitate to call him with any worries about your baby's behavior, daily activities, breathing, feeding and sleeping patterns, digestion, or possible illnesses. Actually, your baby's doctor needs this information to get to know his new little patient, and you need to begin to interact with him to develop a comfortable, trusting relationship. Don't forget that pediatricians are trained in caring for young babies, including preemies just home from the hospital. If he needs any specific information about your baby, he will call the doctors in the NICU. They've probably already spoken to him or sent him information about your baby, and will be happy to confer with him as needed.

One time when it is appropriate for you to call the NICU is when you have questions about instructions you received at the time of discharge—regarding your baby's medications, for instance—but only until your pediatrician has had an opportunity to review your baby's caregiving schedule and to take over the responsibility of managing it.

Of course, you should definitely not hesitate to call a doctor, whether it's your pediatrician or the NICU, if a problem you know your baby has is getting worse or if she has a fever, is unusually lethargic, exceedingly irritable, isn't eating, or is having difficulty breathing. Often you'll find that these are false alarms and your worries are unfounded. (One of us called the NICU terrified about her son's high temperature, only to have it pointed out that the cause was at least two layers of excess clothing!) But sometimes parental

instinct can detect the first signs of a real problem. It's better to get your concerns addressed and suffer a little embarrassment if it's nothing than to let a potentially important problem pass.

Missing the NICU

I thought I couldn't wait to take my baby home. But now that we're here, I think I actually miss the NICU.

It may seem strange to you to miss a place you wanted so much to leave. But think of it this way: You couldn't wait for your preemie to be discharged from the hospital mostly because that meant he was finally safe, a normal infant going home with his family. What you couldn't picture in advance was the tremendous weight of responsibility you would feel taking care of a fragile and demanding baby at home. Looking back, the NICU doesn't seem so scary anymore, more like a safe haven where they knew what to do to make your baby well and, as a result, to make you feel good, too.

It's true that the dozens of daily questions you have about your baby's breathing, crying, feeding, spitting up, and sleeping can no longer be answered right away by a reassuring nurse or doctor. You have to screen through your concerns and choose only those that really need to be addressed. There are no monitors to tell you with their silence that everything is fine with your baby here at home. You have to rely on your judgment. Or if your baby is on a home monitor, the sense of security you get from it may be confounded by the stress of false alarms and the hassle of managing it on top of everything else.

Loneliness can add to your frustration. Most premature babies are discharged around their due date or before, so they're still not very responsive, or respond with mostly negative signals like crying, fussing, or refusing to sleep. Here at home there are no other mothers or fathers to interact with, tell your story to, distract yourself with their problems, make you feel you're not alone in dealing with a preemie. Although the social interactions you had in the NICU may not have seemed very important to you at the time, now you may realize that they added a brightness to your day. And since it's safer not to take your preemie to crowded places and to curb visitors for a while, you may not have many chances for distraction.

Not least, there's the sheer fatigue of caring for a young baby. There are no quiet nights and few quiet moments anymore. Who wouldn't miss that?

The important thing to realize is that your reaction is completely normal. You need some time to develop confidence (and competence) now that your baby is home with you. Give yourself a chance to adapt and settle down, and you'll see your insecurities slowly disappear. Although giving birth to a preemie leaves indelible marks on a parent's soul, these initial difficulties caused by his homecoming are, we promise you, quick to pass. They will, sooner than you may expect.

Older Siblings

I've read that it's good for an older child to be a helper with a new sister or brother. But I'm so afraid that my daughter will hurt my preemie.

After all that your baby has been through, you probably have a tendency to think of him as more fragile than he really is. Unless your baby has special needs or equipment, such as home oxygen or a tracheostomy tube, you can treat him pretty much the same as a full-term newborn except for being a little more vigilant in protecting him from colds and infections.

Because of your baby's premature birth, your older daughter may get even more out of helping with him than most older siblings do. Some researchers have suggested that siblings of preemies, having felt powerless during the family crisis, want to help take care of the baby (and even their parents) as a way of sharing the burden. Also, given your entirely natural feelings of protectiveness toward your baby and desire to make up for his separation from you, you're probably spending even more time with him than most mothers do with their second child. It's easy to keep postponing your older child's needs. But it isn't easy on your daughter, who may have felt left out or less loved during all of the weeks or months of hospitalization, and may have expected the homecoming to finally put things right. By involving her as much as possible in the new baby's care, you can put her back at the center of your attention and make her feel special again.

Still, it's true: Unless your older child is nearly a grown-up herself, she probably isn't capable of handling any baby on her own. Toddlers and young children simply don't have the coordination or power of concentration to keep an infant's neck supported at all times, to watch him every second while he's on a high changing table or bed, or to hold both bottle and baby comfortably and safely during a feeding filled with countless squirms and distractions. No matter how eager your older child is to help or how much you want her to feel included, your most important job is to keep your children safe, and right now that means drawing the line at anything your older child could do that might be harmful to your newborn. You can be sure that your daughter counts on you to set these limits, which she has no way of knowing on her own.

But there are plenty of more limited, safe, and fulfilling ways that older siblings can help. Here are some, and you'll think of many others:

* You can ask her to help get the baby's room ready for his homecoming, and to give her brother a tour of his new home when he arrives.
* During diapering, she can bring you the diaper, coo and talk to the baby while he's on the changing table, and help attach the diaper's tabs once you have them in place.
* When the baby is unhappy, you can suggest that she try making funny faces, singing songs, or caressing him. If he stops crying, be sure to point out how successful she was.
* You can ask her to choose the baby's clothes or bibs.
* She can hold the bottle for a few seconds during feedings (or longer, if it's going well).
* She can hold the baby in her lap when she's sitting down and you're supervising.
* She can help you push the baby's stroller when you go out for walks. Remember, though, to supervise her closely, because out of enthusiasm she could pull down the handle and tip the stroller backward.
* You can ask for her opinion when you're trying to interpret the baby's gibberish or cries.

It's a small thing but will count for so much: if you give your daughter positive feedback by pretending to talk for the baby and thanking her for being a great big sister, you'll probably see her face light up with pride. If she does something wrong, try not to criticize her. Instead, gently show her the right way to do it or find some other role for her to play.

Also, stop and check yourself every few days: Are you spending as much time as you can with your older child? Have you spent some time alone with her today? Are you helping her to feel how much she's loved and valued? Are you viewing your baby as overly vulnerable and fragile, as many parents of premature babies have a tendency to do?

No matter what you do, of course, you aren't going to be able to make your family exempt from some inevitable sibling rivalry and acting out. Just consider that part of your welcome to normal life with two children!

Questions about Your Baby's Age

People keep asking me how old my baby is. I don't know what to say!

Most kids would find it awesome to have two birthdays, as preemies sort of do: the date they were born, which is their legal birthday, and their due date, which you could call their developmental birthday. To preemies' parents, though, the situation is just confusing. The simplest questions, like "How old is your baby?" or "At what age did your son start crawling?" are, well, not so simple.

From the standpoint of developmental milestones—when your baby should be rolling over, reaching for objects, sitting up, babbling, walking, and so on—what counts is his due date, not his birth date. Nobody notified Mother Nature to reprogram his innate developmental schedule when he came out a little early. So for the first couple of years when assessing whether a preemie's behavior and size are appropriate for his age, experts use his adjusted or corrected age. To calculate this, figure out how old he'd be if he'd been born on his due date. Or, if you find it easier, take his actual age and subtract however many weeks or months he was early. Thus, if your baby is four months old but was born two months early, his corrected age would be four minus two, or two months.

Nothing is simple, though. Some characteristics and abilities of a baby do develop partly from experience, such as his ability to eat (food in the digestive tract speeds up its maturation), his immune system (exposure to germs gears his body up to fight off certain infections), the maturity of his skin (its tough outer layer develops more quickly on exposure to air), and his familiarity with language and objects. These and any other traits that respond to stimulation and postnatal experience may be more advanced in your baby than in a two-month-old term baby.

OK. How to answer those questions? That depends on what if anything the inquirer is really getting at (is it just passing small talk by an admiring stranger in a supermarket or someone trying to figure out whether your baby should be crawling by now?) and how long an answer you're in the mood to give. The appropriate answer to any question concerning your baby's development is: "His adjusted age is two months." Of course that may lead to further questions and explanations. If you want to avoid them, don't feel dishonest about simply saying: "He's two months." It's the truth, if not the whole truth—and there's no reason that parents should be expected to tell their baby's entire private life story to everyone they meet!

But when you're in the mood to open up and reminisce about your baby's monumental experiences, the most accurate—and intriguing—answer you can give is: "He's two months going on four." Like people who are said to be 16 going on 30 because they are biologically young but emotionally and experientially older, your baby is a rich, fascinating interweaving of two ages.

Daycare

I'm thinking of going back to work. Is daycare safe for my baby?

From a medical standpoint, it's best to avoid daycare if your premature baby has been home for just a short time. Anyone who has watched the way children transfer toys from one mouth to another and hover intimately within a few inches of each other's little faces, runny noses

and all, can see why. Every child picks up more germs and therefore comes down with more mild infections—from colds to ear infections, conjunctivitis (pink eye), diarrhea, and rashes—once she enters daycare or school. That's unavoidable no matter how carefully the program is run.

How risky daycare will be for your premature baby depends on how fragile she is. If she's a big, healthy preemie, you can figure that her immune system is about on par with or a little more advanced than her adjusted age. So if on an adjusted basis she's at term now, it would be like sending a newborn to daycare. However, if she was born before 34 weeks of gestation, she lacks some or all of the infection-fighting antibodies that normally pass through the placenta from the mother in the last trimester of pregnancy. Most of these maternal antibodies pass to the fetus between 28 and 34 weeks of gestation and give older-born preemies and term babies some extra protection. They're gradually cleared from a baby's system within the first year or so of life, after which the baby's immune system is on its own.

One particular problem for preemies is a common respiratory virus called RSV (short for respiratory syncytial virus). Most children and adults who catch RSV simply have the symptoms of a cold. But infants, and especially preemies, are particularly susceptible to getting seriously ill from it. In some cases, RSV worsens into pneumonia or bronchiolitis, and can cause breathing difficulties severe enough to require hospitalization. So if you have to send your preemie to daycare, or even to a babysitter who takes care of other children, be sure to ask her pediatrician whether she should get treated with preventive immune therapy for RSV (see page 487). This is given as a monthly shot during the season when RSV is especially common: late fall, winter, and early spring. After your baby is more than six months old or gets through her first cold season, her special vulnerability to RSV will be much less. Also, now may be the time for her pediatrician to schedule the first of the three shots she needs against rotavirus, a common childhood virus that can cause severe diarrhea and vomiting, especially in premature babies.

If your baby has BPD, she is more fragile and the risks of sending her to a daycare center are much greater. At least for the first year or so, you should try to find another option. Remember: even when it looks to you like your baby's BPD has gone away—she is no longer on oxygen and is not acting sick—she has less reserve in her lungs than other babies, and when she catches something, she'll have a tendency to get sicker. For a baby with BPD, many common childhood diseases may require rehospitalization and even become life-threatening. This won't be true forever; most children outgrow their BPD, and your pediatrician can help you decide when daycare is safe.

What should you do if you decide that a large daycare center isn't safe and you have to return to work? If it isn't possible to arrange one-on-one care for your baby, the next best option is to find someone who cares for a small number of children in her own home. For referrals, check pediatricians' bulletin boards, ask your friends and neighbors, and look in the Yellow Pages or online for childcare referral services. Just as you would do with a large daycare center, make sure to visit and see the small center in action (arriving at a time when you aren't expected, if possible), and check several references before sending your child.

Every extra month you give your preemie in the relative protection of her home will allow her immune system to become more mature and better at fighting off infection. You can help by keeping up to date with her immunizations, getting a booster shot yourself for pertussis if it's been longer than ten years since you were immunized (your baby is not immune to pertussis until she

has had her second or third set of vaccinations, after she's four to six months old, and if you get it you could pass it on to her), getting a flu shot in flu season for yourself and for your baby, once she's older than six months, and asking all of her babysitters to get one, too.

Though you probably can't wait for your life to get back to normal after the upheaval of your baby's early birth, be patient if you can. Even if your choice of baby care is limited right now, you'll have a lot more flexibility soon. Be proud that you're taking every precaution to help your baby get through her important first weeks and months at home in good health.

The Right Stimulation

I want my baby to have the best chance to thrive. How can I stimulate her in just the right ways?

No developmental expert or pediatric neurologist can tell you exactly what to do with your baby and when, because a simple prescription isn't available. But don't let that worry you: You won't need one. To quote Dr. Spock, the child-rearing guru of our parents and grandparents, "You know more than you think you do," and your own parental sensitivity and intuition are your greatest, most effective tools.

Just keep in mind the following, general guidelines:

* **Your goal should be to stimulate all of your preemie's senses without overloading them.** A baby's brain and body develops as it's used. Stimulation provides fuel for her development by giving her the kinds of everyday experiences she needs to sense, move, learn, and think— and to practice her evolving skills.
* **The best time to interact with your baby is when she has her eyes open and looks calm and attentive.** This quiet alert state, as it's

called, is more likely to occur when she's well-fed and burped but before she becomes drowsy again or starts crying because she's too tired. This is when she is most receptive to stimulation.

* **At first, your preemie may have only two or three periods a day when she's in a quiet alert state, open to stimulation.** If your baby is often irritable and overloaded, you may be able to increase her quiet alert time by keeping her swaddled more. If she tends to be a sleepy baby, you may find that she's more receptive after an activity that is gently arousing, like a bath. But don't press too hard or get concerned if she isn't ready for much interaction just yet. Every infant has a different threshold for stimulation. Being sensitive to your preemie's responses when you interact with her is one of the keys to helping her flourish.

* **When you notice that your baby is quiet and alert, try approaching her slowly,** placing your face about eight inches away from hers where she can focus best. You might lie down on a bed or the floor with her, on your side, so she can see your face well. (Your baby's brain is programmed to prefer human faces to any other interesting objects.) Smile and change your expression often. You can also stimulate her vision by showing her bold black and white toys or pictures.

* **By the time she gets home, your preemie should be mature enough to handle having more than one sense stimulated at a time.** So while lying face to face, you can also talk to her softly in a high-pitched voice (infants can hear high-pitched sounds better and seem to prefer them), sing a calm song, play some music, or read her a simple nursery rhyme (babies like rhythmic sounds). At other times you can add touch by giving her your finger to hold or stroking her body while she's looking at you.

* **By moving her neck, arms, and legs gently, exercising and stretching** her shoulders, hips, elbows, wrists, knees, and ankles, you can help her overcome any stiffness that may have occurred from lying in only a few positions in the hospital nursery. Now may even be the time to try some infant massage (see page 329), if you haven't done it already. Remember that babies find light touch arousing and deeper, slower strokes calming.

* **One of the best kinds of stimulation is also one of the most natural: holding your baby as you walk around the house.** She will enjoy the movement and close contact with your body, and will begin to get acquainted with the different people, lights, sounds, views, and smells around her. If you are thinking of using a fabric sling or Snugli-type baby carrier, be sure to talk to your pediatrician first, since there are concerns about their safety for preemies. You may need to wait until your baby is older and a more mature breather.

* **When you are holding her in your arms, try when you can to keep her shoulders flexed by placing her arms together in front of her chest.** A flexed position is good for calming her and also for relaxing the splayed-out shoulders and hips that many preemies develop after prolonged lying on their backs in the hospital. Similarly, instead of laying your baby down flat on her bed or on the floor, make a little nest of rolled blankets around her to keep her shoulders and hips from turning outward. This will make it easier for her to bring her hands forward later on when she wants to reach for things, and will help her get into the position she needs to learn to crawl and walk. (You'll need to do this only until she's able to assume a flexed position by herself, usually when a preemie is three to four months adjusted age.)

✳ **Tummy time is really important for your preemie when she is awake and supervised since she spends so much time on her back when she's asleep.** Tummy time can help her develop a stronger neck and shoulders, loosen neck muscles that may have gotten tight from lying turned to one side in the hospital, and build the abdominal and other muscles she needs to roll over, sit, and crawl. Her crib or, even better, a blanket on the floor will provide a good flat surface for this kind of exercise. Place her on her stomach with her arms forward, elbows not wider than her shoulders, an interesting toy six to eight inches in front of her to get her attention. In the beginning, she may last only a minute or less before getting tired, but that's OK; you can do it many times a day, even after each nap and diaper change. You can slowly increase how long you spend on the exercise. Occasionally you can also place her on her tummy when she's in your lap.

✳ **The single most important guideline we can give you about stimulating your baby is to proceed slowly and carefully** with each new kind of interaction, always paying attention to how she reacts to see if she appreciates what you're doing. Your preemie will give you clearer clues than she used to as to what she likes and what she finds too stressful. If she goes on looking at you without averting her gaze, continues to breathe smoothly, doesn't grimace, strain, arch her neck or back, or begin crying, you'll know that she likes what you're doing. At around six to eight weeks corrected age, your baby's smile and cooing will show up to light up your days and tell you that you're doing the right things.

From her due date on, your preemie's needs are not much different from a term infant's. You can consult a regular parenting book to find strategies that foster infant development. There are many things to do to help her reach and explore the world with her hands, grasp objects, and discover new textures, sounds, shapes, and forms. More complex body movements and postures, like rolling and sitting, which may seem to you so incredibly advanced right now, will be within your baby's reach before you know it. Just remember to always correct her age when you consult developmental charts, in order to avoid unrealistic expectations. Also remember: by showing her how pleased and proud of her you are, you'll foster her autonomy and self-esteem and support her efforts to master new tasks.

Fussiness

Is it true that preemies are a lot fussier than other babies?

Yes, several studies have found that preemies are more likely than term babies to behave in ways their parents find difficult to deal with. Premature infants have been described as less adaptive to new people and situations, less regular in their feeding and sleeping patterns, more likely to cry for reasons their parents can't fathom, more difficult to soothe, and more withdrawn. In other words, fussy babies! But generalizations are always of limited value. While fussiness may be more common among premature babies, that doesn't make it true for all of them.

Even a preemie who had serious complications and a difficult hospital course can turn out to be a no-fuss, self-calming baby and an excellent feeder and sleeper. So try not to be influenced by warnings about preemie fussiness, and to understand your baby's behavior and temperament without preconceived ideas. Some of his demeanor will depend on how you react to his cues and behave toward him.

(*Continued on page 420*)

If You Are Adopting a Preemie

If you're adopting a preemie, most of this book applies just as much to you as to a biological parent. But you'll have other issues and emotions as well, arising from the special nature of your parenting experience. Although no one can predict exactly what these will be for you, below are some of the most common, along with some ideas to help you deal with them. Some apply only to parents who arranged the adoption before the baby was born, while others apply to all adoptive parents of preemies.

Feelings of guilt

A sense of guilt is something that goes with the territory when you have a premature baby. Birth mothers berate themselves for things they did or didn't do during their pregnancy that they imagine contributed to the premature birth. Although people may assume that adoptive parents are free of that burden, not all are. You may find lots of reasons to blame yourself: for choosing the wrong birth mother, for example, for not checking carefully enough on her health, diet, and behavior during the pregnancy, or for doing something that led to your having to adopt in the first place. Some adoptive parents identify so strongly with the birth mother throughout the pregnancy that they simply have a general sense of failure, like most biological mothers of preemies do.

But these feelings of guilt surrounding a premature birth, although natural, are often overly self-critical and unfair. More than one out of ten births in the U.S. is premature, many occurring in instances when parents took all precautions. If you are blaming yourself, try to remember that your response is normal but not necessarily rational, and as soon as you can, shift your energies toward taking the best possible care of your wonderful child. Your baby's doctor can help put in perspective any specific doubts that you have.

Feeling trapped

Legally, adoptive parents have the freedom of an option that biological parents lack: to back out of the adoption before the waiting period ends, deciding that they are not ready or able to take into their family a baby who was born prematurely and could have future problems. Emotionally, however, you may feel differently. Some adoptive parents have been through years of trying to conceive and then adopt a child. They may feel trapped in the situation because of their long, difficult struggle and intense desire to have a child or because they feel responsible for the commitment they've made.

Few would deny that it's best to go into parenting willingly, with one's eyes open. One great resource for you is the social worker in the NICU, who is very concerned with getting the baby placed in the right home. Talk to her directly or, if that's not possible, ask your adoption agency to be your intermediary. Ask questions about your baby's medical and developmental outlook, and be honest about your own needs and what you think you can handle. Remember, most premature babies grow up healthy and normal. But don't feel callous or irresponsible if you decide that this adoption is not the best thing for you or your family; if it isn't, it wouldn't be the best thing for the baby, either. If the baby faces significant risks, it may help you to know that there are many families willing to adopt babies who may have special needs. Your baby will find a home.

On the other hand, if you feel "stuck" mainly for the same reason that biological parents do—you already feel that this baby, a bundle of uncertainties and hopes, is all yours—then your preemie is one lucky baby. In that case, your strong commitment and love is going to get you through these early, anxious days to happier family times ahead.

Bonding with a difficult preemie

If their premature infant is irritable and fussy, as preemies frequently are in early infancy, some adoptive parents wonder whether they are having more trouble bonding than a biological parent would. Many assume that biological parents feel immediately loving and attached to their babies, starting with a magical moment in the delivery room. Maybe they do in fairy tales! In real life, it sometimes takes longer for love to grow. Some birth parents feel guilty about this and worry that something is wrong with them, when in fact what they—and you—are going through is entirely normal.

A popular, simplistic concept of bonding—that it is supposed to occur instantly the first time you hold your baby in your arms—is now considered an inaccurate representation of the parent-child relationship. The deep, lasting attachment that binds parent and child takes time and nurturing to grow. It develops over weeks, months, and even years, as each responds to and returns the other's caring and love. Just as falling in love at first sight (or, for that matter, how the first few dates go) is a poor predictor of the depth of a couple's love later on, the same is true of babies and their parents, biological or adoptive.

Interestingly, some social workers who work with premature babies and their parents observe that adoptive parents often feel more positive about their babies than birth parents do, perhaps because they've had to work so hard to have a baby. But that doesn't mean you won't have negative feelings—everyone does. Anger, anxiety, disappointment, and detachment are all typical feelings of parents of premature babies. Many of these feelings arise from grief, as parents of preemies, adoptive or biological, mourn the loss of the roly-poly infant they imagined, the joys they would have had in the early days or months, their fantasy of perfect radiant health, now and in the future. It's also normal to feel anger toward your baby for putting you through all this, although parents find it hard to admit because it seems so unacceptable. But don't assume that you're feeling negative emotions any more strongly than biological parents. You probably aren't.

It's of greater concern if your feelings remain predominantly negative for several months or you have thoughts about harming your baby or yourself. In that case you should talk to a mental health professional or to your baby's pediatrician right away. Some experts believe that adoptive parents can suffer from postadoption depression that's very similar to postpartum depression. Professional help could make all the difference in how you feel about your baby and how your relationship develops.

An immediate maternal or paternal response

Other adoptive parents are amazed at the opposite reaction: how immediately they feel a profound protectiveness toward their infant. Even on early visits to the NICU, they may feel an instinctive urge to cry out, "Don't hurt my baby!" whenever a doctor or nurse goes near him with a needle. The intensity of love for a child is an incredible feeling, and adoptive parents aren't immune to that neon emotional light flashing, "This is *my* child." If you're wondering whether you're strange to have such a forceful attachment—well, welcome to parenthood.

Needing to be "perfect" parents

Some adoptive parents say they feel pressure to prove that they're "perfect" parents. That's really impossible to do and you certainly shouldn't feel you have to in order to justify your place in this baby's life. Unfortunately, no one can criticize themselves like new parents, especially ones with high standards for themselves. Most new birth mothers and fathers are riddled with self-doubts, too.

The thing is that all parents make mistakes—lots of them. First children are especially stressful, because no new father or mother comes to them with any parenting experience, and everybody learns through trial and error. Make that child a preemie, and you have even more opportunity to torture yourself as you deal with a variety of medical, behavioral, and parenting challenges that parents of term babies don't have to face. If you're a caring enough parent to be worried about this, the chances are that you're an excellent one. Time will bear that out.

Not treated equally in the NICU

Some adoptive parents find that they're prevented from visiting their newborn preemie in the hospital, or not given much medical information by the NICU staff. If you're lucky, you won't encounter these obstacles. But as you know, every adoption takes place under different circumstances. While there are many agencies, lawyers, birth mothers, and hospitals that encourage adoptive parents to get involved with their babies as soon as possible, others insist that they keep some distance until the waiting period has passed.

One reason for this reserve toward the adoptive parents is to avoid pressuring the birth mother, who can still change her mind about giving up the baby. Another is to protect the adoptive parents from becoming too attached, and possibly suffering severe loss and disappointment if the birth mother revokes her decision. Also, some birth parents have an agreement that their confidentiality will be maintained, and that's hard to do in a hospital where babies wear name tags. (The adoption agency or lawyer will tell the hospital when the baby's name may be changed to yours.) And there's an important legal issue involved: Until guardianship of the baby has been officially transferred, the birth parents are the only ones who can be given confidential medical information or consent to medical and surgical procedures. Once you become your baby's guardians, of course, you can neither be kept away from your baby nor denied information about him, and you'll participate in decisions about his care. If anyone on the hospital staff is confused about this, talk to the social worker or your agency or lawyer and ask them to help clear things up.

It can be incredibly frustrating if you're kept away from your baby at a time when you think he needs you. If you're encountering limits that you think are unreasonable, approach the nursery's social worker (the staff member who is best able to intervene), either directly or using your agency or lawyer as an intermediary. Even if you're told that you have no rights to see your baby until he is discharged from the hospital, the social worker may be able to arrange an exception for one or two visits. Ask her for a photograph to keep close to you until you can be with your baby. Also ask whether the hospital has a program of volunteers who are assigned to hold and cuddle babies, and if so, whether your baby can be included until you're allowed to be with her often yourself. Remember that the waiting period is usually over in a few weeks, and that your baby will benefit from your presence even more as he gets a little older.

Breastfeeding an adopted baby

It's not easy to induce lactation if you haven't recently been pregnant; it takes hard work and perseverance, and even then many mothers are not able to do it. But others do manage to produce enough milk to at least partially breastfeed their infants, and feel a tremendous sense of satisfaction in giving the advantages of breast milk to their babies. (You can read about how these advantages apply to preemies on page 138.) If you're interested, ask La Leche League (telephone 1-800-LA-LECHE) for literature and a referral to a specialist in lactation induction so you can learn what's involved. But keep in mind that breastfeeding is by no means mandatory—either as a source of good nutrition for your preemie or as a way to show her you love her—and only a small fraction of adoptive mothers try to do it. It's impossible to tell in advance how much milk you will be able to produce, because that varies widely for mothers who induce lactation, as does the amount of time it takes to get there. You should carefully consider the tremendous physical and emotional effort involved before you go down that road. The important thing is to get enough information so that you can make the choice that's right for you.

There are other ways of getting many of the advantages of breastfeeding. One is to arrange for your preemie to get breast milk from a milk bank, as explained on page 170. For the physical intimacy of the experience you may crave and that your baby will thrive on, you can try using a supplemental nursing system (see page 257) or holding your baby skin-to-skin (see kangaroo care, page 249), which will provide much of the same closeness.

Living day by day with your premature baby, you'll find plenty of other useful things you can do to enhance his development, growth, and happiness. Many are covered in the rest of this book, which is for all parents, no matter how their baby comes to them.

A simple reason that explains a lot about preemies' behavior is their immaturity. It's no wonder, since most preemies leave the hospital a few weeks before their due date. As a result, their sleeping and waking times are often unpredictable, their feeding patterns irregular, their responses limited or disorganized, and their energy levels low. It's not surprising then that preemies as a group are reported to be less adaptable and sociable and to get upset more readily than term infants. Just give them a little time!

Environment plays a role, too. A difficult temperament is more common among those preemies who were smaller and younger at birth. These infants have gone through long hospitalizations and are more likely to have suffered severe illnesses and complications. When stimulation is excessive or painful, as it can be in the NICU, some preemies become easily startled and prone to extreme agitation, or become absent and withdrawn to block out the stimulation. These behavioral patterns can linger for a long time, even after a baby goes home and is no longer subjected to disturbing medical procedures, only to his parents' loving attention.

Thus, try to be patient: What you notice in the first weeks or months is often just a passing stage while your baby matures and develops before showing you his true nature. While you may have heard your friends say that their newborns' personalities and temperaments were immediately obvious from their very first days, research has shown that a premature baby's behavior is less stable during his first years of life than a term baby's. It's not until they pass their first birthday, or sometimes their second, that preemies are rated by their parents to be as stable in temperament as children who were born full term. (According to parents, by the time they enter preschool, the vast majority of preemies have not only achieved a stable temperament but have gone from being difficult infants to easy children.)

The so-called "goodness of fit" between a baby and his family is also important. Some parents adjust more quickly to the needs of a more demanding premature baby and get more satisfaction from parenting. They are likely to rate their babies as less difficult, and to find them more responsive and less irritable. (Studies show these tend to be parents who have good family and social support, a steady income, and are more religious.) How much is a baby's behavior shaped by his family's positive or negative attitude rather than the other way around? That's hard to assess. But a parent-child relationship is a circle of mutual influence, leading to change and development by the baby and his parents. What counts is finding a common behavioral rhythm through understanding and communication.

It may help you adapt more quickly and may ease your stress if you know what's normal in a premature baby. Be prepared to encounter some difficulties in these daily activities:

* **Sleeping.** Healthy premature babies are expected to wake up and fuss about every two hours until they're three to four months corrected age (a long time, if you ask us!) By about six to eight months corrected age, they will have settled into longer periods of sleep, to everybody's understandable relief.
* **Feeding.** Nearly half of all parents of preemies complain about some feeding problems during their baby's first year, ranging from the infant's getting tired too easily while feeding, to difficulty reading his hunger signals, to persistent reflux. These problems can be especially frustrating to parents of preemies, who are

concerned about their baby's need for catch-up growth.
* **Crying.** Premature babies' crying reaches a peak of frequency and intensity at three to four months corrected age, later than term babies. Although the first months at home with a baby who fusses a lot and is difficult to console can be really vexing, over time you will learn how to interpret all the different meanings of your baby's cries—including when he's crying for no reason at all that you can find, just an inability to be easily soothed that's typical of prematurity. The good news is that most parents of preemies report that inconsolable crying tends to disappear all of a sudden after a few months—an extremely welcome surprise!

In the meantime, parents who find their preemies fussier most commonly complain that they don't know when to do what. They find their baby's cues unclear, so they don't know when to play or quietly cuddle, feed or put him to sleep, soothe or leave him alone. It may appear to be a constant series of misunderstandings: Their baby crying inconsolably (when his parents expect him to sleep) then suddenly falling asleep at the wrong times (for instance, during feedings) or turning away (when his parents try to comfort or play with him). Feeling that you don't know how to care for your baby can be extremely frustrating, and you may come to feel incompetent and rejected.

What can you do about it? First, recognize that preemies are less predictable and harder to read than term infants. It's not just you, or your child. Then, try to learn to decipher your preemie's behavioral signals (see page 234). Not all parents learn this in the hospital, overwhelmed as they are by other worries. Finally, follow your baby's cues and allow him to call the shots when you can. Don't worry that you're spoiling him now; it's way too early for that to happen. To feel comfortable and secure, he needs to know that his needs will be recognized and met, and that his family can be trusted to be available, gentle, and empathetic (quite a difference from his experience in the hospital, unfortunately, where busy nurses and doctors often had no choice but to handle him in ways he wished they wouldn't, and on their schedules, not his).

To soothe your baby and help him to sleep, try the following techniques. You'll gradually discover what works best for him:

* Offer him a pacifier or the tip of one of your fingers to suck on, or help him bring his own hands to his mouth.
* Calm him with your touch by holding him quietly, providing him with physical boundaries, or swaddling him snugly in a blanket to make him feel secure. (See page 233 for more details of calming techniques.)
* Studies show that infant massage (see page 329) can often calm fussy preemies and helps to develop a strong bond between parent and baby. In particular, try tummy massage, designing an imaginary "U" on your baby's abdomen, to help relieve gas and soothe abdominal pain.
* Try to relax your baby with your voice, talking or singing softly to him. Experts on bonding say that babies who are attached to their parents come to know and love the sound of their voices.
* Don't assume that a quiet room with dim light is what your baby needs to fall asleep. After the constant noise of the NICU, he might be better soothed by background music, the soft sounds of a TV, running water in the sink or tub, or the monotonous humming of a hairdryer, vacuum cleaner, or white noise machine.
* A ride in the car (always in a car seat) or a walk in the stroller may provide your baby with just the right level of sound and movement he needs to console himself and fall asleep.
* Hold your baby close to your body to combine the soothing effects of touch and motion. Some parents end up carrying their preemie everywhere during the first months. If you feel like it, you can gently jiggle your baby around or dance with him, making sure you're always supporting his head. (Don't, however, use a sling carrier without asking your pediatrician first, since slings may not be safe for preemies until they are older and more stable breathers.)
* To calm and soothe fussy older preemies, some hospital nurseries use hammock-style motion beds that can softly bounce and swing a baby both up and down and side to side, re-creating motions a baby might experience in the womb or in your arms. You can try one and see whether it works for your baby; if it doesn't, after a few days you can return it (see *Resources* on page 591). You can also try firmly rocking your baby in a low baby seat, swing, or car seat placed on the floor, but beware that while some preemies like this, others become more nervous rather than calmer. If your preemie is one who doesn't like it, you may want to try again in a few weeks—his preferences may have changed.
* Vigorous rhythmic touch, which arouses some babies, pacifies others. Some parents confess they feel weird when they give hard pats on the back or forceful tummy rubs in public, but these work marvels to calm down some preemies.
* When your baby is asleep, let him slumber undisturbed as long as possible. Play with him or try to engage him actively only when he seems to be completely awake.
* Try to control your frustration and anger at your baby's crying by using deep breathing or other relaxation techniques. Instead of

getting agitated and nervous along with your baby, which may just prolong the outburst, try to slow down your movements, lower your voice, and talk in a sweet, loving tone. (Psychologists believe that showing that you understand his distress and are there for your baby will also help with his future emotional development.) Above all, if you ever get so upset that you feel you want to shake your crying baby, lay him down immediately on his back in his crib, leave the room, and calm yourself down, calling on a family member or a neighbor for help if you are alone. Remember that shaking an infant may do irreparable damage.

* To prevent burnout, take turns with your partner and get any help you can from relatives, friends, and other caregivers. Plan to regularly take some time off for yourself: Visit a friend; go to the gym or a yoga class; exercise at home in another room while someone else is taking care of your baby (all the better if you can't hear him crying—some background music can help with that!); or simply take a long bath or shower. Don't feel guilty about this because it's for your baby's good, too. By relaxing and replenishing your emotional energies, you'll be ready to go back to your baby with renewed parental love and a positive attitude.

* Make sure to choose a babysitter who can deal with your baby's fussiness or excessive crying. You'll need someone who has lots of patience, ample maturity and experience with very young babies. No matter how highly babysitters are recommended or how well you know them beforehand as family members or friends, you should observe them interacting with your baby a few times before leaving them alone with him.

Every time you find yourself thinking how difficult and exhausting it is to care for this infant,

just stop for a second, rewind your mental tape, and say instead: "My baby needs more help from me than I expected." Does being aware of the special behavioral characteristics of preemies change your perspective? It probably will. And remember that although this especially fussy time feels very long, it will pass and you'll gradually come to enjoy your baby more and more.

Is Your Baby Remembering Pain?

Every time my baby smells an alcohol wipe, he starts to cry. Is he remembering pain from the NICU?

Some parents of preemies notice that their babies have unusual reactions to pain. They say their babies seem oversensitive to pain, or they seem undersensitive. Just as you wonder whether your child is associating the smell of alcohol with the pain he felt during medical procedures in the nursery, when disinfectants were used, other parents say their preemies are scared by the sound of tape being torn, as it would have been before an IV or endotracheal tube was put in, or by the sight of doctors in scrubs or white coats.

There's no sure way to tell whether your child is simply disturbed by the irritating smell of alcohol or is actually associating it with the pain he felt in the hospital nursery. There's little research so far on whether preemies remember pain or whether early painful experiences have any long-term effects.

A few things have been discovered, though, that make parents' concerns plausible. We already know that newborns can recall some sensations from the past. Studies of full-term newborns have shown that they can recognize the sound of their mother's voice and music they heard while in the womb. Since the sense of touch develops even earlier than hearing, it's quite possible that pain could be remembered by preemies, too.

In fact, one study of 32-week preemies who had already spent four weeks in the NICU found they were more apt to have racing pulses in response to painful heel pricks than newly born 32-weekers (as if the earlier-born ones were already traumatized by medical procedures performed during their hospital stay). It's hard to know if this was a conscious reaction or just a physical reflex. Interestingly, they grimaced less than the newborns, as if the repetitive painful experiences muted their behavioral responses to pain.

A recent study of newborn rat pups—whose neurological maturity is similar to 24-week human preemies—found that early pain altered their developing nerve fibers in ways that left a lifelong legacy of greater sensitivity to pain. It isn't clear whether the same permanent change occurs in humans, but in one small study of full-term newborns, boys who were circumcised without a topical anesthetic were found to react more strongly to the pain of immunizations when they were four to six months old. Another small study of full-term babies found that infants who had their heels pricked repeatedly during their first few days of life not only appeared to feel more pain from heel pricks later, but learned to expect the pain, grimacing much more than other babies when their skin was cleaned beforehand.

So while it's too early to draw any definite conclusions, there are some clues that preemies may remember the pain from the NICU—not necessarily in terms of conscious recall but through changes in their bodies that affect their perception of pain and reactions to it. If your baby seems to cry in response to a certain sound, smell, or event, try cuddling and comforting him while he's experiencing it or afterward; perhaps you'll gradually change his association to a more positive one—and if not, at least you'll show that you are a source of support and love when times are hard.

Some parents worry that early pain could result in long-term emotional problems for their child. Clinical studies haven't specifically addressed that link. Yet one psychologist who specializes in research on pain in preemies and follows preemies as they grow up points out that what amazes her most is not how burdened they seem by their early experiences but how refreshingly, normally happy and well-adjusted most of them turn out to be. It's hard to be pessimistic if you see these children later and witness their incredible resilience and ability to recover.

To be sure, there could be rare, severe situations when long months of pain, especially in preemies who lack the persistent presence of a loving caregiver, might leave permanent scars on a child's personality. But if your baby went through the common experiences of a preemie in the NICU—if he was on a vent for a while, got his share of needle sticks and suctioning, even had some complications that needed one or more surgeries but have since resolved—you needn't be afraid of these severe emotional consequences. More likely you'll be taken aback by the gleeful and indomitable child your preemie turns out to be.

Your Baby's Appearance

Will my preemie ever look like other babies?

Most of us have a baby image in our head that's based on the picture-perfect cherubs in ads and on newborn diaper packages. While exceedingly cute, they're about as similar to most real-life infants as gorgeously turned-out fashion models are to your next-door neighbor: not very! Most real babies have some of the following common imperfections: a conehead, birthmarks, infant acne, protruding ears, receding chins, and too much or too little hair, to name just a few. And yet they're undeniably beautiful—just not perfect.

Do Preemies Have Scars?

Yes, many preemies are left with some physical reminders of their days in the NICU, but in most cases the scars are so small that only their parents notice them. And although it may seem amazing to you now, many parents and children come to treasure those scars, hoping they won't disappear completely; like battle scars, they're souvenirs of an experience that was central to their lives and took great strength to get through.

For example, tiny pinpoint scars are common where intravenous needles were placed, usually on the back of the hands or elsewhere on the arms or legs. There can be pinpoint scars on the heels, also, where blood was drawn with heel sticks. These tiny scars fade even more with time. Occasionally, a spot will harden into a firm bump, but that doesn't do any harm.

Very young preemies whose skin was particularly immature and sensitive at birth may have light-colored scars where removal of tape or the monitor leads abraded their skin. These become less noticeable over time. If your child is prone to getting raised scars, these and other scars may be raised and bigger.

If your baby had any tubes inserted—for example, a tracheostomy or gastrostomy tube or a chest tube—there may be small scars that follow the typical course of any surgical scar: They start out reddish and raised, then fade to white, and finally become flat or slightly sunken lines or dimples. If your child had several chest tubes, and some had to be placed close to her breast tissue, her adult breast could be somewhat abnormally shaped. If the problem is severe, cosmetic surgery could be done to correct it. The same is true for a large surgical scar that is unattractive—there are plastic surgery techniques that can improve its looks a lot.

If fluid or medication infiltrated deeply from an IV line, your baby may have a scar where it occurred. Since scars tend to pull the skin tighter, if one is directly over her ankle, wrist, or elbow joint, it could hamper her movement somewhat. Most of the time, exercising the joint gently and regularly will alleviate the problem.

These are the most common scars—that is, until your preemie starts climbing jungle gyms, riding bicycles, and running down sidewalks!

Some preemies who are on their way home, though by no means all, have a few of their own characteristic traits. One is a more oval-shaped than round head that's flatter at the temples, so their faces are long and narrow. (This may come from lying on their sides in the hospital when they would have been floating freely in the womb.) They may also have wide-set eyes

(their narrower faces and less mature, flatter noses make their eyes look wider apart) and a pale complexion (because of anemia—normal in all infants, but deeper and longer-lasting in preemies). And the heads of some preemies are flatter in back, with bald spots, from lying on their backs.

To be sure, all of these traits can be pretty

subtle, so most people would see just typically cute kids, no different from anyone else, although a neonatologist might be able to point out an occasional former preemie in a crowd. Some of these preemie characteristics go away quickly (in several weeks for the paleness, for example), and some go away gradually over months to years as a child matures, possibly lasting through childhood.

Other differences? A premature baby who was on a ventilator for a long time may have a higher than usual arch or groove to his palate, probably from the pressure the endotracheal tube exerted. This lessens as a child matures, too, and is usually nothing to worry about. It shouldn't affect his speech (though it may make for difficulty eating foods like peanut butter, which will stick to the roof of his mouth—but who's never had that problem?), and nobody but his dentist would notice. Avoiding pacifiers and sippy cups in children older than a year will help this resolve. (To avoid spills, you can give your child a cup with a flip straw instead.) Later, usually when a child is seven or eight years old and has permanent teeth and a well-developed jaw, if a palate groove disrupts his bite or causes teeth overcrowding, it can be treated by an orthodontist. (Former preemies apparently need braces only somewhat more frequently than term children. In a recent study, about a third of term-born children had braces while about half of prematurely born children did.)

Premature babies—especially smaller ones who spent time on a ventilator or those with high bilirubin levels—may have some minor imperfections in the enamel of their baby teeth, making them look discolored or imperfectly shaped. Most of the time only the baby teeth are affected. If you want to read more about teeth, see page 482.

As for size, some preemies always remain small, but the vast majority attains normal height and weight sooner or later. You'll find more about growth on page 456.

Your baby may well have none of these traits.

In that case, people will just have to take your word for it and marvel that he was a preemie.

Shouldn't I Feel Happier?

Everyone assumes I'm ecstatic now that my baby is home. The truth is I feel relieved, but I can't say I feel happiness.

Some parents of premature babies, during their first weeks and months at home, find themselves wondering: How come I'm feeling sad when I should be rejoicing? Why isn't my baby's presence and well-being enough to make me happy?

You may feel uneasy or just numb, a legacy of fear about what the future might bring. If you can't answer a resounding "yes" when friends ask if you're overjoyed or blissful about being a new mother or father, you may wonder whether something is wrong with you or with your feelings about your baby. There isn't. Some parents, when their child has just escaped danger, are simply too wounded and carrying too much baggage for that. Of course, there are plenty of joyful and tender moments, when you hold your baby in your arms or watch him peacefully sleeping. You may feel relieved, yes. Grateful, yes. Even that you have grown wiser with a new perspective on what's truly important in life. But you don't feel that elation, that lighthearted pleasure so many parents of term babies experience when they bring their infant home. You've been through too much and still feel too vulnerable for innocent, shiny-eyed happiness.

In order to understand and accept your unexpected reaction, you should realize that you have been through a multifaceted experience of loss, although your premature baby is alive and well at home. Parents of preemies need to grieve the loss of the healthy full-term newborn they pictured they'd take home, as well as the normal pregnancy, delivery, and birth they were expecting. Don't forget that your parenthood, too, was premature, and you probably missed out on some important and meaningful social rituals that would have helped prepare you to take your baby home. You may not have completed your parenting class, had a baby shower, exulted in a celebration after delivery with your family and friends. Your deprivations were many and deep, and you should acknowledge them without feeling guilty, to allow yourself to heal and move on.

If you've just come back from the hospital, it's also natural for you to feel burdened or even overwhelmed by the responsibility of taking care of your baby at home. Parents of preemies tend to feel nervous and uncertain for a while about their baby's condition and future well-being no matter how healthy he is now. A long and painful NICU experience sometimes interferes with the timing of the normal deepening of attachment between parent and child, and anxiety and fears may further weigh you down. All of this doesn't mean that you don't love your baby! But acknowledging what you've lost can help explain some of the ambivalence and confusion you feel surrounding your preemie's discharge.

The good news is that in general these negative reactions gradually subside. Researchers have found that most parents of preemies have regained their emotional balance by their baby's first birthday; a minority of them need longer but generally feel that their anxiety has finally subsided by the time their baby turns two. This time frame for emotional recovery is totally normal. In the meantime, just be wary of a deep state of bereavement that interferes with your normal functioning and lasts longer than a few weeks. It could be a postpartum depression (see page 285) that should get treated before it becomes a threat to you or your family relationships.

Of course, you also shouldn't forget that you don't need to be a parent of a preemie to feel less than elated after your baby comes home. Some parents of term babies, even though they may have had far easier experiences than yours, find that they don't experience storybook bliss, either. They face sudden new sources of stress in their lives, from caring for a needy baby to physical exhaustion and steeper financial responsibilities. All of these adjustments may lessen the joy of new parenthood, postpone their falling in love with their new child, or simply exacerbate the normal baby blues. But almost always, the great joy of parenthood eventually prevails, as it most likely will soon for you, too, with the added pride of having achieved it after walking a much harder path.

Feeling Protective

Now that my baby is home, I want to envelop her constantly in my arms, just the two of us, perfectly safe.

After putting your desire to take care of your baby on hold so often during her hospital stay, now you can finally let your maternal instinct pour over her. If you don't feel like doing anything but staring at your baby, if you just want to be alone with her to protect her from any possible danger or disturbance, if you resent your family's demands because you don't want to be distracted, that's understandable. You're making up for lost time.

Some parents of preemies get worried by what they perceive as disturbing feelings in themselves, such as resentfulness toward their family, irrational fears, excessive protectiveness toward their baby, and a desire for isolation. If you respond like that, you're not unusual. And you're going to regain your balance soon. What you're going through now is normal and temporary. Studies have shown that levels of anxiety and depression among parents of preemies are highest one week after discharge and already begin to diminish by the second week at home.

(Continued on page 429)

Parental Responses that Are of More Concern

A few parents remain unable to adapt to their preemies, developing worrisome long-lasting responses that can be disruptive to their child's development and well-being. These extreme parental responses are not common. But many mothers and fathers of preemies will recognize some hints of what they feel, although in milder forms.

* **Vulnerable child syndrome.** There's no doubt that preemies are vulnerable at the beginning of their lives, and their parents rightfully worry a lot about them. But when a premature infant goes home and is growing and developing well, his parents should gradually relax. If over the first months or years of a child's life, his mother or father continues to worry excessively about his health, taking him to the doctor at the slightest sign, discouraging his desire to actively discover the world, denying him contact with other people to avoid illness, and limiting his participation in activities to avert possible dangers, this overprotectiveness can impede his normal development. Kids growing up in such an atmosphere can become insecure, shy, dependent, and lacking in self-esteem. Later, in school, they may have poor social skills, a childish demeanor, and frequent academic and health complaints. Vulnerable child syndrome is not a direct consequence of an infant's prematurity. Rather, it is an abnormal parental reaction that is probably due to personality traits in the parent, who becomes convinced that the premature birth justifies her or his own attitudes and behavior.

* **Post-traumatic stress disorder.** People who have gone through a traumatic experience involving the possibility of imminent death or serious injury to themselves or a loved one are at risk of developing post-traumatic stress disorder, or PTSD. You may think that this occurs only in war veterans or victims of earthquakes, but don't underestimate the stress and threat that parents of preemies face (see page 339 for what one army officer said about his experience as a father in the NICU). Experts believe that a premature baby's birth and hospitalization can be stressful enough to cause this reaction, too.

One symptom of PTSD is the reliving of pieces of the traumatic experience through flashbacks. A flashback can be triggered by an experience—such as a beep that sounds like the alarm of the monitor in the NICU, a phone ringing in the middle of the night, or a baby's new illness—or it can occur for no apparent reason. More than just a haunting but distant memory of the NICU, a flashback feels like you're back in the experience, reliving it intensely all over again. Another symptom of PTSD is avoidance; for example, you might avoid driving anywhere near the hospital where your baby was in the NICU or never look at his early baby pictures. At its extreme, avoidance could lead to skipping follow-up doctor appointments or denying real problems or symptoms your baby has, putting his health in danger. A third symptom of PTSD is heightened arousal, a kind of high alert or constant fear. It may be specific—a fear that your child might die or get sick again, leading you to be overly protective—or more of a generalized sense of hypervigilance and anxiety pervading your daily life.

Now a word of caution. Almost all parents of premature babies experience one or more of these reactions, and it doesn't mean they're suffering from post-traumatic stress disorder. Only when these symptoms become persistent, interfering with normal functioning during the day and sleep at night, or when they are accompanied by other psychological problems like depression or substance abuse, would a person be diagnosed with full-fledged PTSD. There are particular kinds of psychotherapy and medication that are effective in treating it, so be sure to seek professional help.

✳ **Parental burnout.** Preemies, who are often more withdrawn and irritable than term babies, can be less rewarding for parents to care for. Sometimes a mother or father who has tried hard to interact with a preemie without positive results just burns out and stops trying. In some families, the initial normal period of low stimulation (appropriate for a very young premature baby who's easily overwhelmed) never evolves into the more interactive relationship that the baby becomes ready for as he matures. In others, a preemie's inscrutable dislikes or frequent discomforts make his parents feel incompetent and rebuffed so they give up trying to meet their baby's needs and refrain from almost any stimulation. Burned-out parents act cold or absent toward their babies and hold, touch, talk to, look at, and smile at them much less than other mothers and fathers. It may be hard to tell what comes first, the baby's lack of positive responsiveness or the parents' bias. But either way, it's a dangerous situation. Developmental psychologists warn that an absent and withdrawn parental attitude can impair a child's development if it continues as the preemie grows older.

✳ **Risk for child abuse.** Preemies are more apt to be abused than other children, mainly due to a combination of parental risk factors (such as a lack of social and family support and a history of violent experiences and reactions to stress) and the common behavioral characteristics of premature babies (who can be fussier, more difficult to console, and more withdrawn). Put these types of parents and children together, and the situation can sometimes degenerate into a serious crisis.

If you think that you or your partner fits one of these descriptions, it's important to talk about it with your pediatrician or a mental health professional.

Most heightened negative emotions that you have should subside within nine to twelve months after discharge, though higher than normal levels of anxiety about your baby's health can sometimes last for up to two years. Most likely, over the next few months you will become gradually less distressed and more attentive and responsive to the rest of the world. You'll get back to your old emotional self, although painful memories of the NICU and negative feelings may periodically resurface—just temporarily—for many months or years to come.

Even though you feel you want to focus all of your energies on your baby now, beware of trying so hard to get his attention that you overstimulate him. It is a normal parental reaction, since premature babies can be less responsive and more withdrawn than term babies in their first weeks at home. But because preemies don't handle excessive stimulation well, this can do more harm than good. To defend himself, your preemie may become even more withdrawn, leaving you frustrated and disappointed. The antidote is to try to adapt your reactions to your baby's cues, being sensitive to signals that she's either ready to interact or overloaded with stimulation. (Some descriptions of preemies' signals that may help you are on page 234.)

In the meantime, talk to your partner about how you feel so he can understand what you're going through and be patient. Try to avoid cutting him completely out of your private nest with your baby. If you have older children, make sure your partner or their grandparents give them extra love and attention while you adjust, and start spending more time with them as soon as you can. Soon you'll be ready to face the world again—and all the relatives and friends you'd now like to keep out.

After this initial period of adaptation, you'll be able to look at your baby more objectively, too. Preconceived ideas can be damaging: If you expect your premature baby to be frailer, less responsive, or more demanding than a term baby, it may influence the way you interact with her, inhibiting her now and affecting her future behavior.

Right now your feelings are probably normal and healthy. But if you ever become uncomfortable with them, thinking they're excessive or not subsiding appropriately, you may want to consider the intervention of a mental health professional. Behavioral therapy (a kind of short-term, focused psychotherapy) has been beneficial for other parents in such circumstances. Joining a parent support group or arranging for one of your baby's nurses to babysit (you can ask in your nursery whether any of the nurses would like to do this) can also help. You may get precious clues about your premature baby's needs, behavior patterns, and habits as well as valuable insight into your own feelings. Being alone with your baby and doing everything by yourself might be most appealing to you right now, but later on, isolation is exactly what you should try to avoid to be the excellent parent you want to be.

MULTIPLES

One Twin Home Earlier

One of our twins came home two weeks before the other. Will he always be more advanced?

Being discharged from the hospital is not a race in which the premature twin who's first out of the starting gate is also the one who'll likely pull further ahead in the long run. In stable premature babies, the physical requirements for discharge—being free from apnea for a certain number of days, eating well, gaining weight steadily, and maintaining their body temperature in an open crib—are usually achieved somewhere between 34 and 40 weeks of gestation. There's no known connection between the age that a preemie develops these maturational abilities and the time when he reaches his later cognitive or motor developmental milestones, such as smiling or sitting up. Over the next few years, you'll get used to seeing your twins' differences: One may talk earlier while the other may be a more adventurous and active toddler. Still, you won't be able to predict whether the first one will be more eloquent in sixth grade or the second one more drawn to sports. So long as both twins, according to the doctors, are doing well, it's misleading to interpret a slightly shorter or longer hospital stay as indicating that one is generally more advanced or physically gifted than the other.

It's a different situation when an unevenness in growth or development in premature twins is due to a serious medical condition in one of them. If one twin has to stay longer in the hospital because he has more severe BPD or had to undergo surgery for NEC or hydrocephalus, for example, then he may be at higher risk than his sibling for later health problems or a developmental delay. But since babies have amazing resilience and an extraordinary capacity to recover, you shouldn't label one baby as weaker or more vulnerable at such an early age. Time will tell you whether there is a developmental difference between your twins or not.

In the meantime, it can be a real hassle for parents to take care of one twin in the hospital and the other at home. Often, parents don't trust anybody else to take care of their newly discharged preemie, yet bringing him back to the nursery with you for visits may feel overwhelming—and may not even be allowed. The hospital staff expects—and you should accept without guilt—that you won't be able to visit as often as before. If you can find a relative, friend, or volunteer who'll regularly spend time with your preemie in the hospital, it may help reassure you that you're not abandoning your little one in the nursery. Some parents find that their babies' staggered discharges, if they're only separated by a week or two, can even be beneficial, allowing them to adapt to the home routine with just one preemie at first. If you look at your experience from this point of view, you may be grateful to the baby who took his time for the extra breathing space he gave you before making your hands really full.

By the way, since one of your twins was discharged earlier than the other, they may have gotten their first vaccinations on different days. But now that they are both home, you'll be spared some visits to the pediatrician if they get future shots at the same time. Since the timing of vaccinations is somewhat flexible, don't hesitate to ask your pediatrician whether she can work out a way to put your babies on the same schedule. With a little advance planning, she'll probably be able to do it.

Daily Schedule for Multiples

Any suggestions for a daily schedule to take care of triplets?

What could sound better to parents like you, whose life is a never-ending waltz around feedings and diaper changes, than the mere possibility of a daily schedule? You already know that taking care of three babies at the same time requires commitment and strength. But organization and experience can help a lot, too, to conserve your precious energy and spare you some worry.

During the first weeks at home, when your triplets are still waking up for at least one feeding in the middle of the night—and maybe at different times—you need as much help as you can get from your family and friends. Don't be proud: Ask if it's not offered. You can return the favor later when your life is more in control.

To know what's going on with each of their babies, some parents of triplets find it useful to keep track of each baby's daily events. One way to do this is to make copies of the feeding and changing form in Appendix 4, on page 588, and use one for each day. Or you can take inspiration from it and draw up your own version, adding in other activities, such as bath time or one-on-one time with Mom and Dad. Parents say it can be a lifesaver when you feel so tired that you're afraid you'll lose your mind and forget essential information.

Getting your three babies to follow a regular and possibly uniform routine and to sleep through the night is going to be a slow work-in-progress. Some lucky parents of triplets say that it's possible to have them on a feeding, playing, and sleeping schedule by the time they're about 12 weeks corrected age, and not long after that to see them sleeping six to eight hours a night. But some other families don't get to the blissful point when parents can finally enjoy a good night's sleep until their babies are ten months old or more. A great place to give and get advice, to and from other parents like you, are web sites and forums organized by nonprofit organizations like MOST (Mothers of Supertwins), which you can find at www.mostonline.org, or Triplet Connection, at www.tripletconnection.org.

Here's what some families of triplets, quads, and quints have to say about the crucial issue of scheduling:

* If you're trying to get your triplets into a uniform routine, slowly try to encourage them to follow the same timing by letting one cry longer before a feeding or putting one down earlier. If one baby has woken you up at night for a feeding, wake the others up to feed them, too. (You'll be reluctant to do this at first, but believe us, it will save you sleep in the long run.)

* The assembly line method will help you get organized and perhaps free up some spare time while training your triplets to adapt to a regular routine. You can apply it to everything from daily tasks like diaper changing to bathing, nail-clipping, and more fun activities like one-on-one time, reading, or playing with each of your babies, as long as it doesn't become too rigid or obsessive. (Speaking of bathing your babies, you need not do it every day. In fact, many parents of triplets and even some parents of twins or singletons give their baby a bath only once or twice a week, which as long

as you're cleaning his diaper area when you change his diaper is perfectly adequate to keep a young infant clean.)

* Accept the fact that when a child is sick, his schedule will probably change. Try to be patient, and return to the schedule as soon as possible after he's better.

* If one baby seems to want to play, feed, or sleep at a different time, put the little maverick in another room if you can to avoid disrupting his siblings' more uniform schedule.

* If you're nursing and supplementing with formula, always feed your babies formula for their last meal before bed. Formula takes longer to digest than breast milk, so your babies' stomachs will be full longer. (This also works out well for mothers who have plenty of milk in the morning, but then see their supply dwindle as the day goes by.) When your babies begin eating solids, they'll sleep even longer between feedings.

* To further encourage a longer night's sleep, you can try keeping them awake with lots of lights on for several hours before the last evening feeding at 10 or 11 p.m. For some other babies, instead of keeping them awake in the evening, it works better to put them to bed about thirty minutes earlier than usual after a relaxing bath. (There's no harm in trying both ways.)

* Use only disposable, top of the line, premium diapers at night. Some babies wake up just because they feel wet.

* Once they're about three months corrected age, try keeping them awake for a longer time after each feeding to wear down their energy a bit more and encourage longer intervals of waking and sleeping. (This works for some babies; others just get crankier and sleep less. You can try it and see.)

* Remember that babies' schedules tend to change a lot with seasons and growth spurts,

so even if you think they're finally settled, don't declare victory until they're nine or ten months old.

* You're asking too much of yourself if you also try to fit in such extra things as making a home-cooked dinner every night, keeping your house spotless, or grooming and dressing your kids (or yourself) to look ravishing. Give yourself a break: For now, safe and loving childcare is enough.

Even if you do all the right things, sometimes babies just aren't ready to follow a consistent schedule yet. So don't blame yourself if your little ones don't cooperate. At a certain age, due to a combination of development and growth, something will click, and they'll magically become more consistent and easier to care for. According to many parents of triplets, despite the fatigue, it all happens too fast.

IN DEPTH

The Cardiorespiratory Monitor: A Noisy Companion

Is it an intrusive nuisance or a gift that will keep your child safe? Will it add to your stress or to your peace of mind?

A lot will depend on your mind-set going in. Some parents resent their home monitor because they had been eagerly looking forward to walking away from the hospital and leaving all aspects of having a sick or fragile baby behind. They wanted to move on to a normal family life, which didn't include a high-tech machine next to their baby's crib. Other parents cherish their monitor because they feel so nervous, after all they've been through, that normalcy isn't their top priority anymore: security is. The monitor allows them to relax during the day and sleep at night without being plagued by worries about whether their baby is breathing and fine.

In truth, for most parents, it's a mixed, love-hate relationship. If the doctor has recommended that you take a monitor home with your baby, read on to understand more about what's in store.

Why the Doctors are Recommending a Monitor

One of the most common reasons for a preemie to go home with a monitor is that she's otherwise ready to leave the hospital, but is still having episodes of apnea or bradycardia. Although apnea of prematurity usually disappears by the time preemies are 36 to 38 weeks of gestational age, occasionally it persists even after their due date, especially in preemies born extremely early. Doctors know that it will go away eventually and that an otherwise healthy baby is better off at home with her parents, where she can get the physical contact, positive stimulation, and love that they are best at providing.

Some other reasons a home monitor may be recommended are that a baby has apnea from other causes, such as reflux or seizures; she had an apparently life-threatening event, or ALTE, as doctors call it (an incident when her breathing unexpectedly faltered, for reasons that may or may not have been identified); she has BPD and needs home oxygen; she has a tracheostomy tube; there is a family history of SIDS (sudden infant death syndrome). Often, parents' needs are taken into consideration, too. If you have been through a lot since the birth of your baby and are afraid that something might happen if you take your eyes off her, the doctor may weigh strongly the sense of security a monitor can provide.

While a home monitor cannot prevent a problem from arising, it does alert you if there is one. An alarm will sound if there's too long a pause in your baby's breathing or her heart rate slows down or speeds up too much, telling you to intervene and help.

Will a Monitor Protect Your Baby from SIDS?

Home monitoring has not been shown to prevent SIDS even though it alerts you that your baby has stopped breathing. Researchers still don't fully understand SIDS; indeed, it is defined as an infant's sudden death that remains unexplained even after all possible causes have been investigated. Respiratory problems may be one cause of SIDS, but we know it's not the only one.

Simply having apnea of prematurity does not in itself put a baby at increased risk for SIDS. While SIDS does occur more often in prematurely born infants, researchers have never found a causal relationship between apnea of prematurity and SIDS, which usually occurs at an age when apnea has passed. Bronchopulmonary dysplasia doesn't put a baby at increased risk, either. A baby's risk *is* higher if she has had an ALTE, was exposed in the womb or in her home to cigarette smoke or drugs like opiates or cocaine, is put to sleep on her stomach, in an overheated room or on very soft bedding, and, possibly, if she's from a family with a history of SIDS. A baby's risk is lower if she is breastfed, shares a bedroom with an adult (sharing a bed, though, is controversial; some studies show that cosleeping increases the risk of SIDS, others show that it reduces it), and if she's given a pacifier at bedtime, for reasons that aren't yet known.

Researchers understand so little about SIDS that even though they can't demonstrate that home monitoring reduces its risk, they also can't say for sure that monitoring hasn't helped some infants. Since home monitors may give anxious parents some peace of mind, many doctors recommend them for babies at risk.

Why Home Monitoring May Be a Hassle

So, you want the real scoop on the disadvantages of home monitoring? Here are the main complaints that come up:

✴ You're going to get occasional false alarms. They're inevitable, but scary—and incredibly frustrating when they wake you in the middle of the night. What's important to realize is that while some families get annoying false alarms several times a day (tempting them to smash their monitor against the wall), others get them only once a week or less. So read about how to cut down on false alarms below, to give yourself a much better chance of being among the lucky ones.

✴ You can't sleep with your baby when she's on an apnea monitor because your movements could make the monitor think she's breathing when she isn't.

✴ Trips to the store are harder. But you'll do it: A home monitor, which is about the size of a textbook, can run on a battery pack while you're away from home and comes with a carrying case that can go right into the car or the basket under a stroller.

✴ If your baby is on a monitor all the time, you won't be able to carry her casually in one arm while you make coffee, set the table, or meander around the house. (Of course, you will be able to carry her around with you any time she doesn't need to be hooked up to it.)

✴ You may have to postpone daily tasks that are too noisy to allow you to hear the monitor if it goes off and get to your baby quickly. Vacuuming and showering, for example, may have to wait until your partner or someone else is home.

✴ Finding and trusting a babysitter is harder. You'll need to find a steady babysitter who isn't scared off by the monitor, can learn to use it reliably, and could handle an emergency if one occurred.

✴ Having a home monitor can be expensive: generally from $200 to $300 a month, but almost all health insurance plans and Medicaid cover the charges. It's important to find out whether your plan covers only certain, specified equipment providers so you can tell the hospital's discharge planner.

* A home monitor promotes the image of your baby as a fragile, vulnerable child. This can affect how you perceive her and interact with her, and how your friends, relatives, and strangers do. All new mothers have to put up with their share of intrusive looks and questions, but the monitor may make your share a little bigger than most. Just remember that most infants on apnea monitors are healthy, with a very manageable temporary problem. Your baby just has a high-tech companion to keep her company, along with her stuffed animals.

Why Home Monitoring May Be Worth It, Anyway

Simply put, a home monitor can offer you peace of mind. Even parents of full-term newborns sometimes find it hard not to rush out of bed during the night to check that their babies are still breathing. Parents of preemies, with their lingering anxiety, often find it even harder to sleep well or to relax and enjoy their babies. With the extra feeling of security provided by an apnea monitor, some of their fears may fade more quickly. In fact, one study found that far more parents continued to use the monitor beyond the time recommended by the doctor than stopped early.

You'll be especially grateful to have the monitor when your child gets her first cold and, like all congested babies, is struggling noisily to breathe. As you leave her in her crib at night, the sight of those little flashing lights that blink with her breaths and heartbeats will do your own heart good.

Getting Organized

Don't worry if you're inexperienced with machines or simply have so much to do before your baby comes home that the thought of organizing one more thing seems impossible. You'll find that almost everything concerning your baby's apnea monitor will be well organized for you.

The machine. Home monitors are usually not supplied by the hospital but by an outside provider of home health care. Your discharge planner will arrange for a representative of the provider to meet you at the hospital, train you in how to use the machine, and leave it with you a few days before your baby is discharged. You'll be given a telephone number where you can reach someone 24 hours a day in case you have questions or problems once you get home. (Although you'll be encouraged to call during office hours, don't hesitate to call at any time if you have a question that seems urgent.) Some hospitals encourage parents to spend one night rooming in with their babies to make sure they're able to use the monitor properly.

The machine may seem complicated and daunting when it is first introduced to you. But even the most technologically challenged parents (we know from personal experience!) become familiar with their apnea monitor quickly. You'll master it, too.

Home monitors sound an alarm if your baby stops breathing for more than a certain number of seconds; her heart rate is too fast or too slow (your baby's neonatologist will determine the settings for your baby's machine); or there's an equipment problem. One kind of apnea, called obstructive apnea, won't set off the apnea alarm but will set off the slow heart rate (bradycardia) alarm. This kind of apnea happens when a baby's airway is obstructed. The baby moves his chest to breathe, but little air gets through, and his heart slows down as a result.

You'll be asked to keep a record of all alarms. This, along with any data that stays in your monitor's memory, will be a valuable tool when you and your baby's doctor are deciding when to discontinue the monitor or whether to adjust medications. (Most machines can download the data they've recorded over a phone line, transmitting it straight to the doctor for her to review.)

Instructions from the doctor. Your baby's neonatologist will tell you exactly when to keep your baby hooked up to the monitor. For some babies, it's recommended that they be on an apnea monitor almost all the time. Others need it only while sleeping. Also ask the doctor how long she thinks your baby should stay on the monitor and what the criteria are for discontinuing it.

CPR training. Most hospitals give CPR training to all parents and caregivers of babies being sent home on a monitor. Make sure to ask about this if no one has mentioned it. If you have a regular babysitter, arrange for her to attend a training session, too.

Getting set up at home. There isn't much you have to do. You must have a telephone, in case of questions or an emergency. You'll have to choose a good place for the machine. It should go on a hard surface near your baby's bed, close to an electrical outlet and where your older children or pets are unlikely to touch it. (In case they do, home monitors have a sibling alarm that lets you know when there's been tampering by curious fingers or paws.)

After you set up the machine, test to make sure you can hear its alarm (which sounds something like a smoke detector) in all the rooms in the house. If it isn't loud enough, call the provider and ask for a remote alarm, which runs on a long wire to the monitor, or pick up an infant intercom from your local baby store.

Important safety precautions. Home apnea monitors are extremely safe as long as you follow the safety precautions you're given. Most important: never bathe your baby when she has the monitor on because of the risk of electrical shock. And keep the wires from getting wrapped dangerously around your baby's neck by running them inside her clothing to emerge between two snaps or buttons near her ankles or, if it's a short outfit, near her crotch. If her outfit has no snaps or buttons there, just poke a tiny hole in the fabric yourself, to bring the wires through.

Planning for emergency. The vendor will give you letters to mail to your local electric and telephone companies asking them to put your family on a special priority list in case of a blackout or rationing of service. Post a list of emergency numbers near all of your telephones: 911 or the local rescue squad, the closest emergency room, your baby's doctor, the equipment provider, and the electric company's emergency service line. And post a copy of CPR guidelines (the ones you get from the hospital or on page 589) in several places around the house: next to your baby's crib and changing table, in the kitchen, and anywhere else she spends a lot of time.

Those Pesky False Alarms

Like most machines, apnea monitors are not perfect. No matter how hard you try, false alarms can't be completely avoided. When babies squirm (which they do more and more as they get older), leads can slip out of place. Activities like stretching or a bowel movement can cause natural, trivial bouts of bradycardia. Sometimes the sound of the alarms themselves (or the baby's own somewhat delayed natural regulatory systems) stimulate a

(Continued on page 439)

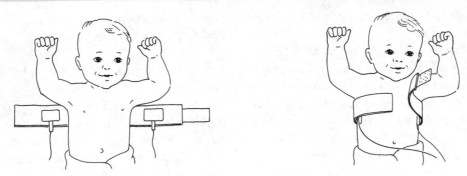

Place the leads on the belt according to the instructions you received and fasten it snugly, but not too tightly, around your baby's chest.

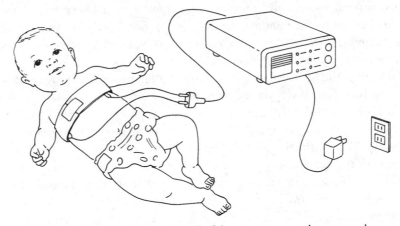

Before turning the monitor on, always check to make sure that all of the wires are properly connected.

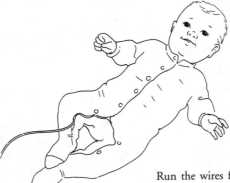

Run the wires from your baby's chest down to her crotch or leg, under her clothes, and bring them out between two snaps or buttons.

Adapted with permission of Mallinckrodt Inc., Pleasanton, CA

baby who's having apnea to breathe again, so by the time parents reach their baby's crib, it seems like the alarms were false.

Here are some ways to keep false alarms to a minimum:

* False alarms often arise when leads are in the wrong place, either because they weren't placed properly or because the belt was too loose to keep them from sliding around. (You can tell that a belt fits right if you can fit a finger snugly but comfortably between it and your baby's chest. If a belt is too tight, it might restrict your baby's chest movements.) So if you're not positive you put them on right, don't be lazy: start over and do it again.
* Every time you turn the monitor on, take a few seconds to check that all wires are firmly connected.
* If you have any doubts about whether a lead or wire is still in good shape, don't hesitate to throw it away and use one of your spares. That's what they're there for. Call the home health care provider right away to ask for a replacement, since you should always have spares on hand.
* When you're in the house, plug the monitor into a wall socket rather than using the battery. Low-battery alarms are almost completely avoidable.
* Don't apply oil, lotion, or powder to the areas of your baby's chest where the leads go. The leads could slide around or not function properly.
* As babies get older, their heart rates naturally slow down, which may set off more bradycardia alarms. If you notice that you're getting more false alarms, ask your doctor whether the alarm settings on the monitor should be lowered.
* If you get a lot of false alarms, ask your provider or your baby's doctor to help you

figure out why. If your baby is an abdominal breather—she moves her stomach more than her chest—the leads may not be picking up her chest movements so it may help to place them a little lower. (If leads are too high, they can also get stuck under a baby's armpits, where they won't detect chest movement as well. As a baby gets older, the leads may have a tendency to rise under the armpits.) Also, if your baby tends to breathe shallowly the leads may miss some of her chest movements. Your home health care provider or doctor will be able to tell if she's a shallow breather by looking at a download of your monitor's memory.

Remember: never, ever ignore an alarm and assume it's false without checking on your baby. If you get a lot of false alarms, that can be tempting—but there have been sad cases proving it's dangerous.

How to Respond to an Alarm

If you have any questions about how to recognize whether your baby is breathing or what to do about it, turn to page 391 for a quick summary. Although it's important for you to know and practice CPR, it's also reassuring to realize that most babies on monitors never need it.

If you respond to an apnea alarm, but you see or feel your baby breathing and she looks fine, it's probably just because of one of the problems described above. Aside from thinking about how to minimize these false alarms, you don't need to do anything.

Useful Tips from Parents to Parents

Here are some additional tips from parents who have been in the trenches with a home monitor:

* After your baby falls asleep in your arms, you won't want to wake her up again by putting on the monitor. So, place the leads and wires on your baby before it's her bedtime, ready to plug in quietly after she falls asleep.
* Although some parents try keeping the leads and wires on almost all the time, there are disadvantages. For one thing, as your baby is picked up and moved around, the leads may slip out of place, subjecting you to more false alarms. For another, many babies have sensitive skin. They may need a rest from the leads and belt, which can be irritating. Most babies can take a monitor break when you're watching them closely, like during playtime. If you're uncertain about whether this is safe, ask your doctor.
* Some babies' skin is especially irritated by stick-on leads. If you notice this, ask your provider about switching to nonadhesive leads that are held on by a belt. If you stay with adhesive leads, try varying the locations slightly on your baby's chest. Since stick-on leads can pull, or even tear at the skin when you remove them, try this gentle way to do it: Place your baby in the bath with the leads on (but, of course, *never* with the wires attached!) to let them soak and loosen, and remove them while she's in the tub. If any bad sores develop, talk to your pediatrician.
* Some parents say they get more false alarms with stick-on leads; others that they get more with the ones that are held on with a belt. If false alarms are a problem for you, it's worth trying the other method.
* When your baby has a cold or a fever, expect her to set off a few more apnea and bradycardia alarms simply because she's weaker and breathes more shallowly than normal or has a stuffy nose. You only need to worry if the alarms are frequent or significantly increasing, and then you should call your pediatrician immediately.
* Always keep the monitor plugged in at night. That way it will be fully charged whenever you want to use it in the daytime, away from home.
* Choose a stroller with a basket underneath, and make sure it's big enough to hold the monitor.
* If you're flying with your baby, call the airline ahead of time to say you'll have a monitor with you. Take a doctor's prescription for the monitor with you to the airport and allow extra time since security may want to inspect it. On the airplane, ask a flight attendant whether you can use it at all times or if it must be turned off during takeoff and landing.
* If you're having trouble finding a babysitter you trust, contact a local preemie support group. Members may know of a babysitter you can try, or you may be able to take turns babysitting for each other's babies. If you don't have a local preemie support group, your monitor's provider may be able to put you in touch with other parents.

When to Stop Using a Monitor

Unfortunately, although parents would find it reassuring, there's no precise formula for determining when a baby no longer needs to be monitored. Many doctors recommend monitoring until a baby is six months old, after which the risk of SIDS and serious apnea are usually very small. Some doctors wait until babies have been off all medications for apnea and have gone at least two months without any serious episodes of apnea or bradycardia. Others also wait until the baby has shown that she can tolerate stress, by smoothly enduring immunizations or an illness.

Based on his clinical judgment, your baby's

doctor will at some point decide that it's time either to stop the monitor completely or to wean your baby from it gradually, perhaps by using it only at night. Actually, it's often more a matter of weaning the parents, who've come to rely on the monitor for their sense of security. The first few nights without the monitor may be hard for you. But after that, it will become clearer and clearer that your baby is safe not because of the monitor, but for one simple reason: because she is healthy. The machine served its purpose well but is now, thankfully, superfluous.

CHAPTER 8

FROM PREEMIE TO PRESCHOOL (AND BEYOND)

. . . .

A time to watch your baby's health and development—
and gradually begin to relax and enjoy!

. . . .

PARENTS' STORIES:
FROM PREEMIE TO PRESCHOOL*

People say that babyhood goes by so fast. "Enjoy her now, soon she'll be six months old and you won't know how she got there," new parents are told. But if you have a preemie, common truths may not apply. When a baby comes home from the hospital she may be only a few days older than her due date—but she already has a history that weighs like years on her little shoulders, and on her parents'. Once they bring their baby home, mothers and fathers must squeeze out the little energy they have left after weeks or months in the NICU to take care of a baby who's often more demanding than they ever imagined. First months flying by? Forget it. A mother posted this note on the Internet, where some parents seek companionship and advice from other parents of preemies who understand what they're going through:

Date: Tue, 08 Nov 2010 09:22:42–0700
From: WXXXX <WXXXI@KXXXX.com>
Subject: Ticia update

Hi everyone, winter's come so early in our area that Ticia and I had to go under cover sooner than expected. I'd al-
ready planned to keep Ticia home until the chill is gone, but I was really convinced when our pediatrician warned

---

* *Parents' Stories* describes events and feelings that really happened or that could happen. Every situation is unique, of course, and you may relate to some parents' experiences and reactions more than others'.

us about the risk of RSV and bad respiratory problems. Here's my list of rules: no trips to the mall, no eating out, no visitors allowed at home, strict handwashing and safe distance from Ticia for everyone who dares to come over (basically, only my mother-in-law and my sister. But not her kids!). DH says I'm crazy. [DH stands for "dear husband."] I'm not crazy yet, although I may go insane by the end of the season. I'm so lonely! My only pastime is reading your messages. I'm so thankful to all of you for sharing your thoughts and experiences with your babies.

Here's an update on Ticia: She's 5 months corrected age now and weighs almost 10 pounds. She's smiling and reaching for things. It's so cute! The problem is with her weight. Her doctor doesn't seem very concerned as long as she's growing regularly, which she does, just very slowly. We're feeding her solids and adding in oil for calories, but she's not taking much, like she never has. Let's keep our fingers crossed and hope she puts on a bit more weight. Sleeping through the night also, we're not there yet. She fusses and fusses, four hours is the longest time she can go without a bottle. Any suggestions about that? I wish I could take her out for a walk. But it's snowing. Love to you all :-)

Wendy (mother to Ticia, 28-weeker, now 5 months old CA), Minnesota

Just when they thought they'd escaped the stethoscopes and uniforms, a few parents have to face what they fear most: a rehospitalization. It's scariest when an unexpected illness or emergency surgery brings a former preemie back to that dreaded place. But even if the trip back to the hospital has been planned in advance and the stay is short, the shock it creates is still enormous. The hospital hits deep, to the core of a parent's heart, where the bruise is still tender.

It's 2 am, and I'm walking in the corridors of "our" hospital, like a ghost with too much caffeine in his veins. I've spent a few hard hours. Sitting by my son's bed, I've been staring at the pulsing lines of his heartbeat on the monitor until my eyes hurt. After 11 months, a bad dream from the NICU has come true. But there's nothing to worry about now, everything went well, the surgeon said. Shaun woke up three hours after surgery and cried only a little bit, still drowsy from the anesthesia. A nurse helped me change him and lift him off the bed without disconnecting his IV. He's so big and heavy, nobody could tell he was only 3 pounds when he was born. He took his bottle in my arms then went peacefully back to sleep. A small bandage on his head is all you can see from the surgery. They shaved a patch of hair but left the rest of his locks intact. He's doing fine. So I came out to stretch my legs under the glaring fluorescent lights that can turn days and nights into the same suspended time. That's the entrance to the NICU we went through so many times. Somebody's washing his hands. Is he a father? If he had to come back in the middle of the night, maybe there's bad news about his baby. I follow him. I don't see any nurses or doctors I know well, and that's best, since I would probably break down if someone asked me why I'm here. I look through the glass doors into the large rooms at the rows of isolettes, at the babies and the nurses handling them. There's where Shaun spent most of his six weeks in the NICU. And here's the father I just saw coming in. He's holding an infant not much bigger than his fist close to his chest. He's smiling. Maybe he's just catching up with his preemie, taking a night turn. I feel relieved for him. I feel relieved for myself, too. Tomorrow morning Shaun will go home, you know?

When a preemie's first birthday arrives, his family may be taken by surprise. "Aren't you going to have a party, a family gathering?" relatives and friends ask. But parents often have mixed feelings. Yes, it should be an occasion for rejoicing, but they may not feel like celebrating. Why is that?

New York, June 9, 2009

Dear L., today is your first birthday, but it doesn't look like a special day at our house. There are no balloons, no children with their parents coming in for a party. You don't know that they should be here, busy as you are crawling around, tasting the new thrill of independence, and that's fine for now. I'm writing you this birthday card for when you're grown, and you'll ask to see a picture of your first birthday. You know, in the last few days summer has come. Exactly a year ago, I was ready to stop working, to go to the beach to enjoy my growing belly. I was dreaming of swimming like a seal, with you swimming inside me. How perfect. I needed a maternity swimsuit but didn't have time to find one. When I walked into the hospital with your dad, feeling contractions, they made me lie down on a bed without even letting me take off my shoes. That evening, you were born. This morning, a year later, I took you for a stroll in the park. People were looking at us, smiling. But if they knew that today was your first birthday, they would ask me: Why aren't you home making a party? Did you get him presents? A birthday cake? I'm afraid I don't have the strength to light that candle. Maybe next year, or the following one. But it will always be the beginning of summer.

Happy Birthday. I love you. Mommy

Many couples say that after the births of their children they had to give up some things they enjoyed doing before. Some parents of preemies, though, take that normal process too far. Parenthood, if achieved with a lot of struggle, may grow absorbing and exclusive, shutting out the rest of the world, including even one's partner or closest friends. For a while, that can help keep emotions under control.

After the premature birth of our twin girls two years ago, my wife, Sarah, changed so much. Before, she had a great business and social life. "Boy, what a woman you found," my old friends would say. Not to mention my parents, who seem to like her more than they like me. When Sarah got pregnant with twins, she decided that when they were born, she would leave her partner in charge of the store for a year. More than two years have gone by now, and she's still home. All she wants to do, she says, is be with the girls. Her friends call me to find out why she's disappeared. She's become detached from everything—sometimes, I'm afraid, even from me. And tonight on the phone with my sister Judy, she freaked out. Judy called to tell her something about her baby, who's just three weeks old. I heard Sarah saying: "How dare you complain about him? You're so ungrateful." Then she hung up. "Nobody understands how incredibly lucky they are," she cried angrily, fighting the tears. "I feel the same way you do about Judy's baby," I said. "What do you mean?" Sarah inquired. "Seeing them handling that chunky baby so casually annoys me. We couldn't enjoy our girls when they were little," I explained. "But we're enjoying them now, aren't we?" she whispered. There was so much love in her voice that I felt I could be a part of it. Wouldn't it be nice if I could always count on a soft, emotional side of myself to reach out to Sarah? Tonight I did great.

At some point, a child's premature birth fades into the background. A time comes when parents become self-conscious about mentioning that event unless specifically asked. Despite the fact that their memories are still vivid, mothers and fathers begin to live a life in which their child's prematurity has apparently disappeared.

I'm here in the playground, watching Ricky play with Dave and Martin. Ricky is my son. He's two and a half now. (Although I don't say it anymore, I really consider him a little younger than that, because he was a preemie born nine weeks before term.) Dave and Martin are Ricky's pals. Dave is the oldest of the trio; he's tall and strong, just turned three. I tried to lift him the other day, but he was almost too heavy for me, much heavier than Ricky. Ricky is at the 15th percentile for weight and height, so he's on the small side for his age, but I don't worry about it as much as I used to. He loves to jump in the sandbox with Dave; they can't stop giggling while they bounce. I'm still terrified that Ricky might hurt himself, but I know he needs his share of bumps and bruises, so I let him do the things he likes. Martin, who's just two months younger than Dave, is a quieter little guy. He always brings a fire truck to the playground, to trade with the other kids' toys. He speaks very well and now is saying something to Ricky, who's sitting in the sand pushing his truck. Ricky knows it's a red truck: all of a sudden, he's learned all the colors, putting to rest my anxiety that he might be color blind. He's not different from the other kids, we know that. But to us, there's always something that we never felt with his sister, who was born at term. It has to do with our secretly comparing him to the other children, checking on his speech, his movements, his achievements. To us, Ricky walks around with a big sign on his shoulders that says: "I was a preemie. Everything that seems predictable and uneventful to you is not. I'm an extraordinary child." What strikes me most is that people can't see it.

Many adults who were preemies are oblivious of their difficult starts, blissfully unaware of the obstacles they had to overcome. But memories of that tiny baby remain alive within their parents, usually hidden and muffled by time and life events, occasionally to reemerge when nobody expects it.

In December 1998, astronaut Robert Cabana successfully led a historic space shuttle mission, the first to carry material into space to build the international space station. Bob Cabana's parents were so proud of their son, a brilliant Navy pilot flying his fourth shuttle mission, ". . . especially," as his mother tearfully told a local television news station, "since we didn't know if he'd make it past his first year." Mrs. Cabana spoke of her son's premature birth fifty years before. Great men can be born premature too, you see? And parents of preemies may not know if they're crying from remembered pain or present joy.

THE DOCTOR'S PERSPECTIVE: FROM PREEMIE TO PRESCHOOL *

Although we'll gladly give you the doctor's perspective once again, you'll probably find that it carries a lot less weight now as your preemie is growing up. Just before her birth or when she was in the hospital nursery, her doctor's assessments were so revealing—and necessary—for you to understand how your child was faring. But now that months, or maybe even years, have gone by, doctors don't loom as large in her world. You, her community of family and friends, and a few other professionals, such as teachers or child-development specialists, have taken over much of that role. Of course, some health risks may be higher for her, and she may still have some conditions that relate to her prematurity, but most of the medical problems that older, former preemies have are those we can see in any child.

* *The Doctor's Perspective* describes how your doctor may be thinking about your preemie's condition and what she may be considering as she makes medical decisions. All of the medical terms and conditions mentioned here are described in more detail elsewhere in this book. Check the index.

Physical Exam and Laboratory Assessment

How often your preemie is seen as she grows older and by what kind of doctors will depend on the problems she's had. Most preemies who were born at 30 weeks of gestation or more and who sailed through their hospital stays without unexpected problems will be treated almost like term babies. We'll ask you to schedule regular "well baby" checkups and immunizations with her pediatrician, and you'll be instructed to call the pediatrician for the same illnesses and questions that any new parents would. At first her doctor visits will occur a little sooner and more frequently than a term baby's (especially during her first winter, when she may get monthly shots of a preventive treatment to help her fight off RSV, a common respiratory virus that can affect preemies more severely than term babies), but those will soon taper off. Except for social calls (many NICUs have reunions, and we're always hoping for a visit from our graduates!), your baby's neonatologist probably won't be seeing her again.

Preemies who were born very early and who are at higher risk for developmental problems will, in addition to regular pediatrician visits, be followed in a clinic for NICU graduates. There neonatologists and other specialists in child development will pay special attention to areas that former preemies may have problems with. Because preemies often have growth delays, we'll be asking you about her eating behavior and diet, and we'll carefully plot her length, weight, and head circumference on her growth chart. Since most preemies are still anemic when they leave the hospital and severe anemia can impede growth, we'll look at her color to see if she's pale and may check her blood count. Because preemies can have difficulty with respiratory infections in their first year or two, we'll be evaluating her breathing and ask how she handled any colds. We'll also remind you that the whole family should get a flu shot every year and make sure her immunizations are up to date. We'll check her blood pressure to make sure it's not too high. And we'll evaluate how her teeth are coming in, because a preemie who had a tube in her mouth for a long time or who had less than optimal nutrition for a while may have dental problems that it helps to catch and treat early. If your preemie went home with specific problems—an oxygen requirement or reflux, for example—we'll be assessing whether to step up or back down on any treatments for them.

In particular we'll be evaluating your child's development, sometimes with formal examinations, other times by simply observing her behavior. (Is she interested in her environment? Does she recognize her name? Does she focus on objects, smile and babble socially, react to loud noises? Are her movements fluid and easy? Does she use both hands or favor one, maybe because it's stronger or more flexible than the other? If she's playing with a truck, is she simply spinning its wheels, or is she pretending it's going somewhere?)

We'll ask whether there are any behaviors you've been concerned about or thought were odd. Any concerns that you bring up we'll consider carefully, even if you try to dismiss them yourself. For instance, if you say that your toddler doesn't hear what you tell him to do half the time, but it's probably just because he's stubborn, we'll still want to check his hearing. Parents, we've found over and over, are usually right about their child, and doctors who listen to parents are much better at picking up problems early.

Some preemies will also be followed by other medical specialists or professionals in their first years of life. Preemies who had ROP or were born extremely early will be checked regularly by an ophthalmologist. Infants who didn't pass their hearing screens in the nursery will be reexamined, and a few will end up needing therapy for hearing loss. Infants who had surgery may be seen by their surgeons a few more times to make sure all is going well. Those with other problems, such as seizures or BPD, may be seeing neurologists or pulmonologists.

Keeping up with many medical appointments can be hard, especially if you have trouble with transportation or finances. Be sure to let your preemie's follow-up clinic know if this is a problem for you: They may have resources to help or be able to put you in touch with county or other services that could make a big difference.

As your baby recovers and grows, he'll gradually shed therapies and physicians, and those that remain will become familiar and habitual. So what may seem like an overwhelming schedule of appointments now will soon become more manageable.

Common Issues and Decisions

Stopping medications and therapies: When we know that recovery is going to be a gradual or long process (in children with BPD or severe reflux, for example), we'll taper therapies slowly, and decrease medications little by little. (Usually we'll wait a few weeks after stopping one medicine before discontinuing another.) Your observations about your child's need for continued therapy are important in this process, so be prepared to be a partner in making treatment decisions. Of course, you'll be asked to report back if there's any worsening in your baby's condition after a therapy is reduced or discontinued. For conditions with a risky period that will pass (such as an infection), we'll usually stop therapies more abruptly. Your doctor will decide to do that when she thinks your baby is out of the danger zone.

There is always some trial and error to this, so don't be surprised or consider it a failure if a treatment that was stopped is restarted. Your

baby may show us that he's not tolerating the weaning from a medication or that he hasn't yet reached the critical time when he no longer needs a therapy. If that happens, we will probably just wait a while and try again later. How much later? You and your doctor will work that out, but often there's little science to it; it's what some call the art of medicine.

If your baby doesn't come off his therapies in the broad time frame we expect, we'll wonder if some other problem could be complicating things. For instance, a baby with BPD who's anemic or who has difficulty eating may have trouble weaning off oxygen. So we might do some tests and perhaps add a new medicine, hoping that it will speed up his recovery. If you find a particular medication or therapy especially onerous, let us know. Sometimes—although not always—there will be a substitute or a different way of doing things that's easier for you to live with.

You shouldn't be surprised if there are times when it seems your baby backslides, when you're adding therapies rather than taking them away. Preemies with a chronic condition, even while it's continuing to slowly resolve, tend to have some ups and downs along the way, including episodes when they may need additional treatment or even a hospital stay. Try not to get discouraged about this, and try to focus on the big picture. Once you find a doctor you trust, never hesitate to ask her to help you put things in perspective.

Growth: It's OK if your preemie remains smaller than his full-term peers as long as his weight, length, and head circumference are growing proportionally and his rate of growth is normal. A normal rate of growth corresponds to good nutrition, which is necessary to build strong, healthy muscles, bones, lung and brain tissue, and all the other organs he needs to develop well. Catch-up growth, which is faster than normal, may seem like it would be more desirable, especially if your preemie lost some ground during his hospitalization. But these days, doctors are not so sure. Some long-term studies show that preemies with overly rapid growth in infancy are more likely to develop diabetes and heart disease later (as adults do who gain too much weight, even if the preemies never became fat). So we won't encourage you to push your child to eat more than he wants, simply to catch up to his full-term peers. On the other hand, we wouldn't want you to slow down your baby's growth on purpose by withholding food (until he's old enough to ask for potato chips and candy, that is!). In most cases, following your baby's lead is likely to yield what's right for him. As long as your preemie continues growing along his own growth curve, we'll be able to reassure you that he's doing fine.

If your preemie's size is falling further and further behind, though, we'll worry that he's not getting all of the nutrition he needs. Doctors call this "failure to thrive" (an awkward medical term that describes only his physical growth; it doesn't mean he's not thriving emotionally from your love and attention). Growth problems are not uncommon in children who are chronically ill. In preemies, we see them most often in those with severe BPD or cerebral palsy because they often have symptoms that interfere with eating and tend to burn up a lot of calories with their illness. The treatment, usually, is more nutrition. We'll have your baby evaluated by specialists in feeding and nutrition, who may recommend feeding therapy, changes in his diet (such as a special high-calorie formula or the addition of certain nutrients), or possibly even tube feedings.

Sometimes, more food isn't the only answer. A preemie with BPD won't grow well if he needs more oxygen. Children who are anemic may grow faster if their blood count is raised. If your baby's poor growth isn't simply a matter of his taking in too few calories or having a medical problem we already know about, then we'll do further evaluations (possibly including a brief hospitalization, where his activity, diet, elimination, and lab tests can be closely monitored) to try to get to the bottom of the problem.

Development: An important part of a pediatrician's job is recognizing which children are developing normally and which are not. But actually determining whether your preemie has a significant, permanent disability can take months, or even a couple of years. As you'll read later in this chapter, many preemies in their first year of life have abnormal muscle tone that gradually goes completely away. It's common for kids who have been ill to have some mild delays in both growth and achievement of skills that often resolve. Sometimes a problem in attaining a developmental milestone is actually a behavioral problem in disguise: A child may be extremely passive or hyperactive, or an overprotective caretaker may be interfering with his learning.

Be sure to keep in mind that the developmental tools available for evaluating infants are not nearly as accurate in predicting their future abilities as those for older children. If your baby scores just a little low on them, especially if he's evaluated before 18 to 24 months of adjusted age, you should take heart—he still has a good chance of falling squarely into the normal range later on. We become fairly certain that a baby's developmental delay will persist or be severe only when his score is extremely low or his abilities are very obviously impaired.

Even if your child has a delay that is mild and probably temporary, we may still refer him for special services so that he can improve his skills right now. Early intervention and stimulation can lead his brain to create new neural connections that will help him reach his developmental milestones, even if he does so a little later or in a somewhat different way. It's important for him to catch up as soon as possible so that he can continue to move forward. If you can, you should try to see a referral for special services as a positive opportunity for growth, not a disheartening comment on your child's future. In fact, most children's future abilities, achievements, and opportunity for a wonderful, fulfilling life will still be wide open, whether they have ongoing disabilities or not.

Starting school: If your preemie was born at less than about 28 weeks of gestation, even if he's been discharged from preemie follow-up clinic as normal, you might still want to have his hearing and vision checked and have him evaluated by a developmental psychologist before he enters kindergarten at around age four or five. Some people think this is unnecessary. But it's something to consider because quite a few of these youngest preemies have subtle disabilities or attention problems. It can take a while for teachers to realize that a child's poor performance, lack of confidence, or disruptive behavior doesn't reflect his intellect or personality but that he's having trouble at school. If you catch the problem early, you can assist your child before he begins feeling like a failure or a bad kid. There are lots of techniques to deal with learning disabilities and attention problems, and most kids can do very well in school with a little help. You can ask your pediatrician or the public health department where and how to make an appointment. You may also want to use your child's adjusted age rather than his chronological age to determine when he's ready to start school.

Family Issues

Making time for discussion: If you have a lot to talk to your baby's doctor about, you should consider scheduling a special longer appointment just to discuss things. It's very frustrating if you're hoping to get your concerns addressed in detail and the doctor is trying to rush out of the room, seeming to brush you off with superficial answers and reassurances. (Hopefully, that's only because of the time constraints in every pediatrician's schedule. Think about how you would feel if you had one of the subsequent appointments and were kept waiting a long time because the doctor was running late.) You may even want to leave your child at home if the doctor doesn't have to observe her directly. You'll both appreciate the more relaxed atmosphere, in which you can concentrate without feeling guilty for taking up too much of his time and he doesn't feel pulled in multiple directions.

Getting all the therapists and doctors you need together to have fruitful discussions can be extremely frustrating if your child is seeing several professionals and there isn't someone to coordinate his care. The preemie follow-up clinic will help with this, but after your child graduates there may be a vacuum, especially because currently, insurance doesn't pay for this valuable service. If you have an activist pediatrician, she may do it, or it may be that you as a parent—difficult as it is—will need to become the advocate for and manager of your child's comprehensive care. It's a hard job to take on, not only because it can take a lot of time, effort, and research but also because it means pressing—even sometimes arguing or disagreeing with—experts and being a stubborn "squeaky wheel." If you find yourself in this situation, don't hesitate to turn to family support groups for help. They're there so that you can lean on and learn from parents who have "been there, done that."

Waiting to find out if there's a problem: The long drawn-out process of waiting to know whether your child has a permanent developmental disability or not can be extremely nerve-racking, and many parents will wonder whether their doctor is holding back important information along the way. We can assure you that most doctors do not. Most of us believe that would be unfair to parents, who want desperately, and deserve, to know their own child. But a doctor may not share every bit of uncertainty with parents, either. That, too, would be unfair, putting you through emotional agony over often trivial or nonexistent issues. If we don't say everything we're thinking or wondering about, it's usually not to hide anything; when our judgments are really indefinite and can go either way, we sometimes don't even know whether we should be worried or not! That profound uncertainty can be very hard to express without generating unnecessary fear in a parent. On the other hand, if you're worried about something, such as mental retardation or cerebral palsy, and we don't address your concerns, please ask. We're perfectly willing to discuss our observations and conclusions, even without being clear or definite, if talking about those things can help you organize your thoughts or put your fears in perspective.

Your doctor shouldn't be offended if you ever want to get a second opinion. Judgments about something as weighty as your child's future deserve exploration and confirmation. Hearing from different doctors may help you understand or accept a diagnosis or recommendation for treatment, and if opinions differ, you'll have an idea of the range of uncertainty you're dealing with.

Vulnerable child syndrome: The tremendous caution that may once have saved your preemie's life has probably now lost its value and become counterproductive. So take a deep breath: Now's the time. You've got to stop thinking of your child as a preemie!

It's hard, of course, because your perception of your child as extremely vulnerable doesn't necessarily go away, especially if he has lingering medical needs. You may feel an overwhelming desire to keep him away from anything risky or to give him everything he wants so he doesn't suffer any more than he already has. Although this is a natural parental impulse, it can get out of hand. We'll be asking you where your child sleeps, how you manage discipline, who besides you takes care of him. Not that there's a right or wrong answer to any of those questions. But if, for example, you don't want your child in your bed yet he stays there because "he refuses" to sleep by himself, there's a problem. If you can't place limits on your child's behavior because, as some parents fear, "If he cries too hard he'll get sick," then you've abandoned an important aspect of your parental role, and he's become a far too powerful child. By treating your child as though he's fragile and vulnerable, you close off some very important opportunities, both physical and psychological, for him to grow and develop at his best.

It's every parent's burden that the future of their children is uncertain. You worry about the possible consequences of prematurity; we all worry about car accidents, cancer, and bad teenage choices. But like every parent, you should try hard to keep your fears in perspective. If your child doesn't have a chronic illness (and even if he does, in every way you can) you should start treating him normally. Because that's what you want him to be and what he probably already is—a normal, or better than that, an extraordinary, wonderful, unusual, and precious child, one who will gradually make his own way out into the world.

QUESTIONS AND ANSWERS

Turning Out "Normal"

How could we be so lucky? Our daughter, who was born so early, seems to be totally normal.

Actually, as amazing as it may seem, you aren't unusually lucky. The vast majority of today's preemies turn out to be healthy, normal children, no different from their friends or schoolmates—except, of course, that not many kids had the same kind of start they did.

So unless their baby is at especially high risk because of an early health problem, a good outcome is exactly what most parents of premature babies should expect.

To you, though, your child will never cease to be a walking and talking miracle. Like other parents of former preemies, you may find that you stare at her in awe as she does perfectly normal things that other parents would hardly notice. You may know every little inch of her face and body by heart, every hair and joint and scar. It's not that you love your preemie more than other parents love their children but that you never take her or her good health for granted. So maybe you are especially lucky, after all.

Adjusting Age

When should I stop adjusting my preemie's age?

The general rule of thumb used by many pediatricians and preemie follow-up specialists is to stop correcting a preemie's age when she is two to three years old. The rationale is that a difference of a few weeks or months (depending on how early your baby was born) is very significant in infancy. Put a three-month-old and a six-month-old next to each other, and it's easy to see that they

have little in common. But by the time a baby grows into a toddler, the difference becomes less and less meaningful. It's hard to tell a 26-month-old from a 29-month-old—and whatever differences in behavior or appearance there may be at that point are just as likely to be due to the wide range of individual characteristics as to a few months difference in age.

But a rule of thumb shouldn't be taken too literally, and this is no exception. There's no magic or scientific reason for preemies to catch up at precisely age two, or age three, or at any other point in time. Some of your child's attributes that develop as a result of experience rather than an innate developmental timetable will catch up with term babies sooner. (See page 412 for some examples.) Others may do so later. For example, some researchers who have studied the long-term growth patterns of preemies have suggested that in evaluating a preemie's height and weight, it's misleading to stop correcting so soon. Catch-up growth can take much longer. So professionals may decide how long to correct your child's age depending partly on what aspect of her development they're looking at.

And remember: the two-year mark applies to an average preemie. If your child was one of the youngest-born preemies, born at 24 weeks or less, her big age gap may remain significant for longer. If she was a 34-weeker, her smaller age gap may become unnoticeable way before her second birthday arrives.

Actually, you are probably the best judge of when to stop correcting your child's age because you're the one who sees where she falls in relation to her full-term peers. If your child's development is progressing normally, but she's still generally lagging by a few months, you probably still need to correct.

Of course, you may have doubts whether some lags are due to developmental delays rather than simple prematurity. Just remember that there's a wide range of normal when it comes to the timing of childhood achievements. Every parent harbors worries, openly or secretly, about something their child is doing a little later than other children her age. It would be nice if all preemies could reach every one of their milestones sooner rather than later, to save their parents some worry. But since no children do that, talk to your pediatrician or the experts at your preemie follow-up clinic. If they tell you that your child is developing normally, believe them!

The truth is that your child is *always* going to be several weeks or months younger than her full-term peers. So, it's not that you'll ever really stop adjusting. There may be times, even later on, when it may make a difference—for example, when it comes time for kindergarten. If your child is just on the edge of age eligibility for a given school year, some developmental experts suggest that you use her adjusted age to determine when to enroll her. (Since some preemies have minor learning disabilities or problems that show up only when they get to school, this is one circumstance in which it may be best for them not to be the very youngest in a group.) But most of the time, after a while it just won't make much difference anymore.

Rehospitalization

My baby is back in the hospital. I feel like I failed to take care of her.

It's natural for you to feel that way, but you're probably being unfair to yourself. Unfortunately, it isn't rare for premature babies to be rehospitalized. Researchers have found that about half of all preemies who weighed less than 1,000 grams at birth have to go back into the hospital at some point during their first two years of life, most

often because of respiratory illness. Even excluding those with chronic lung disease, who are most fragile, the number is still steep: about 40 percent. (As with so much else relating to prematurity, preemies who were older and bigger at birth are much less likely to get that sick.)

So rehospitalization is just one more hill that many preemies and their parents have to climb. Parents sometimes suffer almost as much as their babies, with the following, common emotions:

* **Guilt.** Nothing can cause more self-doubt than having something happen to your baby on your watch. But you can only do what's possible. It's not possible to shield your baby from germs that are everywhere or to will her health problems away. You also can't be expected to do everything right all the time (no parent does!). So don't blame yourself for some real or imagined mistake that you can identify now with 20–20 hindsight. And don't assume that other people—your spouse, relatives, or even the doctors and nurses—are wondering whether you took poor care of your baby. Most people realize that preemies are more fragile and that the usual pat advice and judgments don't apply to them. Indeed, it's very likely that what you deserve is praise—for recognizing when your baby needed medical help and getting her to the doctor or hospital, the right place for her to be. That is exactly what a good parent should have done.

* **Anger at your baby's doctors and nurses.** Anger is a natural reaction when you're feeling frustration and pain, but try to be fair, too. You may be angry that the hospital staff, in your opinion, discharged your baby before she was ready, didn't tell you how vulnerable she was, or didn't do more for her in the first place. There may be some truth in any of these, but most likely the staff made the best decisions possible under the circumstances.

(Continued on page 455)

Through the Doors of a Preemie Follow-up Clinic

For some parents whose preemies have been home for a few months, taking them back to the hospital's follow-up clinic can be like a nostalgic trip back to an old home with old friends. For other parents, having to go back to that hospital, if only for a follow-up visit, can be a source of anxiety and painful memories. If you're not at ease, be assured that the doctors and nurses can understand that and will try to make you feel more comfortable. Your baby will probably be greeted warmly by a clinic staff that is proud to see one of their growing graduates and genuinely concerned about her progress.

While every preemie follow-up clinic is a little different, and they go by different names, the basic idea is always the same: for a team of doctors and specialists across a broad range of disciplines, all of whom have experience with preemies and understand your baby's start in life, to look closely at her to make sure she's healthy and developing well.

Around the time your baby is discharged from the hospital, you'll be told about preemie follow-up clinic and scheduled for a first appointment. If you aren't, that's because, happily, your baby is not considered at risk for developmental problems. On the other hand, it shouldn't make you nervous if your baby is asked to come. It simply means that she meets one of the standard criteria set by the clinic, possibly relating to her weight or gestational age at birth or a medical problem she had, designating which babies are at a somewhat higher than normal risk for a persistent complication of prematurity. Most follow-up clinics include many more babies than necessary so that they don't risk missing any.

Some hospitals don't have their own preemie follow-up clinics but instead rely on a web of state- and county-provided developmental services. If that's the case, your baby will be referred for an assessment by an expert in child development (this will usually be done in your own home), who will arrange for any evaluations or therapies from other specialists she thinks are needed. Alternatively, you may be advised to rely on your baby's pediatrician to refer her for an evaluation if any problems arise.

What can you expect at your first visit to a preemie follow-up clinic? It will take place a few months after your baby's discharge, usually when she's two to six months of adjusted age. Don't count on being there briefly, as if for a quick half-hour doctor's appointment. Block off your whole morning or afternoon, plan to feed your baby there, bring a snack and a book for yourself and also a couple of toys to pass the time in waiting or exam rooms that may not be well-stocked with amusements.

Your baby will be seen by several professionals. A doctor (usually a neonatologist or developmental pediatrician) will do a medical exam. An expert in child development, who may be the same doctor or another specialist, will evaluate your child's cognitive development (thinking and learning), motor skills (movement, balance, and coordination), and behavior. The most widely used standardized tool for assessing a baby's development between birth and two years of age is called the Bayley Scales of Infant Development. It involves giving your baby a variety of tasks to do, to assess her performance relative to other babies her age. (Don't feel bad if she can't do some of the things she's asked to do. She'll purposely be given some tasks above her age level that she won't be expected to perform.) Other professionals, possibly including a physical therapist, occupational therapist, psychologist, audiologist, or speech therapist (see pages 495–496 for a brief explanation of these specialties), may also examine your child. In addition, your clinic may provide a nutritionist to assess your child's diet and counsel you about her nutritional needs, and a lactation consultant who can help you with breastfeeding.

Based on these evaluations, the experts will assess whether your child is growing and developing normally or whether there are areas in which she needs extra help. If you are receiving any early intervention services already, they will talk to you to evaluate how they're going. A social worker or case manager will help to coordinate whatever services your child needs with the organizations that supply them. He can also help you to get government or other funding for which you are eligible. (Keep in mind that you may qualify for additional funding if there's a new diagnosis or a change in your family situation.) Not least of all, he'll ask how your family is doing and whether you need any other assistance.

Finally, you'll be told about specific next steps you should take including any other medical evaluations your baby may need and when to return for her next appointment. Every clinic has a standard schedule for visits, although extra appointments can always be inserted to meet a child's needs.

At some point your preemie will graduate from the preemie follow-up clinic. Some clinics prefer that all preemies keep coming until they reach a certain age, while others dismiss babies earlier if they are developing normally, to be followed by their pediatrician. Even if a child continues to need special services, she will outgrow the preemie follow-up clinic at about two or three years of age, depending on the clinic's policies. At that point, she may start going to a developmental clinic for older children, which might be part of the same hospital or a state-run center with similar resources. Or if a child has one particular overriding medical problem, she will be dismissed to be followed at a specialty clinic (for example, a neurology clinic for a child with seizures or a pulmonary clinic for a child with bronchopulmonary dysplasia). The specialists there will be expected to pick up any developmental problems that might arise in the future.

Many parents wonder whether their baby needs to go to a regular pediatrician in addition to the follow-up clinic. The answer is yes. Your baby still needs her immunizations and regular pediatric checkups, when her doctor will do some things that are outside the scope of the follow-up clinic—from checking for ear infections to getting routine blood or urine tests. She still needs a doctor who will treat her normal childhood illnesses. The staff of the clinic will be concentrating on any medical problems that are specifically related to prematurity and on assessing your baby's development. So while she will get double the weighings and measurings and there will be some other overlap, much of what's done in the two kinds of checkups will be different.

If you live far from your follow-up clinic, either because you've moved or had to travel a long way to the hospital in the first place, your neonatologist can tell you whether there is another preemie clinic closer to you. But it may still make sense to go back to your original hospital's clinic at least for the first appointment to tie up any loose ends—and, as an added benefit, to get the chance to show off your growing baby to her fans on the staff.

Discharging babies home helps their development by placing them in a loving, enriching environment with their parents, removes them from the infection risks that are present in all hospitals, and makes beds in intensive care nurseries available for critically ill infants. If you're feeling bad about blowing up at one of the doctors or nurses, be assured that you aren't the first parent in this situation to do so, and the staff probably understands what you're going through.

* **Physical and emotional exhaustion.** Some parents find the second hospitalization harder in some ways than the first one, feeling like they have no strength left to handle another round of anxiety and stress. Make sure to pace yourself: Take breaks from the hospital, even if you just go to a coffee shop for a few hours, or go home and sleep for the afternoon. Tell your partner, who may not realize how much you need his help, how you're feeling. You might ask him to fill in for you at the hospital for a while, or just go there with you and hold your hand. If you feel that you need additional support, contact a parent support group whose members understand what you're going through or talk to the hospital social worker.

* **Worry that this additional hospitalization is too much for your baby to take.** One thing parents of preemies come to realize over time is how strong and resilient babies are—sometimes more so than their parents! Although it's painful for us to see our babies having to struggle, you can be sure that premature babies are tough little fighters. Once your baby is home again, you'll give her plenty of time to rest and get the comfort she deserves in your arms.

* **Feeling less confident and more worried after your baby gets home.** It may take time for you to relax again. Your baby is probably stronger than ever—she's older and more physically mature, after all—but it's normal for you to have more of a sense of vulnerability. Parents who have gone through this say it can take weeks or months before they regain the sense that everything is going to be OK. As time passes, you will, too.

One thing that can be extremely productive, after this crisis is over, is to ask yourself whether you handled your baby's illness or emergency as best you could. Do you feel you need any additional information on how to care for your baby or to detect a problem? Would you do anything differently next time, if there's ever an emergency again? Asking these questions constructively is a great approach, since parenting of any baby is a life-long process of learning.

Understanding Developmental Delays

When they say preemies sometimes have developmental delays, do they mean temporary or permanent ones?

The term developmental delay (which means that a child isn't reaching certain developmental milestones as quickly as most of his peers) can mean either one, and preemies get both. Permanent developmental delays, or disabilities, are often not diagnosed for sure until a preemie is a year old or more. That's because in preemies, a delay is often truly transient, causing their parents some temporary hand-wringing, then fading into memory with no lasting consequences.

For example, it's common for preemies to have developmental delays resulting from temporary abnormalities of muscle tone—and then to grow out of them. Some preemies are a little weak early on, and may be slower to roll over or sit without support. Others develop stiff joints or tight muscles, causing them perhaps to be stiff when they stand up or to be unable to bring their hands together to hold their own bottle. Preemies who aren't grasping their bottles at 6 months are often doing it perfectly normally at 12 months. And preemies who don't begin walking quite as early as other children, if they don't have a permanent motor disability, will walk perfectly well when they do.

Nobody knows exactly why these transient muscle tone abnormalities occur so often in premature babies. They may be related to different patterns of brain maturation in preemies. Or they may be related to a preemie's experience: For example, a long stay in a hospital bed may make certain muscles weak and joints tight from lack of movement.

Experience may also play a role in delays in acquiring other skills, such as eating with a spoon or making speech sounds. Preemies who are on ventilators for several months or who have tracheostomies, for example, may not have gotten any early practice in eating or speaking. Any illness, even a relatively mild one, that makes a preemie less active in working her muscles and exploring the world, can cause a temporary developmental delay.

In general, temporary problems usually cause only mild delays. Permanent disabilities often cause more significant lags, of many months or years. A child with a motor disability, such as cerebral palsy, for example, with practice and training might walk at the age of 30 months. Some milestones may never be attained. (Keep in mind that a child who has an impairment in one area will often reach milestones in other areas a little late but perfectly well, with or without the help of special therapy. For example, a baby who doesn't see well may learn to walk later than other children, but may eventually walk just as smoothly and quickly. A child with a mild or moderate hearing loss may be delayed in her speech, but learn to talk well with appropriate intervention.)

If you are concerned about a delay in your child's development, don't keep it to yourself! In some instances, a pediatrician or physical therapist will be able to reassure you that the quality of your child's movements or play is normal so the delay is most likely temporary. (You can read about getting a developmental evaluation through your state's early intervention program or local school district on page 494.) If they suspect that there could be a more serious problem, or can't draw any conclusions until they observe your child's progress over time, you may still feel better getting support and help for your child from experts rather than stewing about the problem alone.

Growth Predictions

I'm average in height, but my two-year-old preemie is only at the fifth percentile. Will she always be small?

Everybody is enchanted by toddlers who come in adorably small packages, calling them "peanut" or "pipsqueak" in the most affectionate way. But your daughter won't necessarily be keeping those nicknames forever. The only thing anybody can say for sure about her eventual height is that it's still too early to predict. Preemies start out small but most of them then catch up, or come close later on.

Medical researchers are still studying the long-term growth of preemies, so we're bound to learn more over time, but here's a snapshot of what's known to date. At the time their due dates arrive, preemies are smaller on average than full-term newborns. More than half of them are below the normal range in height and weight (meaning below the third percentile on the regular growth charts used for term newborns). Some preemies are born small for their gestational age so they have further to go to catch up, but even the others find it hard to take in enough calories to grow as fast in the outside world as they would have in the womb. That's especially true if they're sick, because sick infants need even more calories to grow but take in fewer.

This picture gradually changes. Some preemies, especially those with chronic lung disease or feeding disorders, continue to lag in growth even after their due dates, but most begin to grow just as fast as their full-term peers. Then, at some point during the next months or years many preemies begin growing even faster than other babies, making up for their slow start. Because of this catch-up growth, by eight months of corrected age only about one-third of the preemies in a large study were still below normal in weight and about one-quarter were below normal in height. By eight years of age, although most preemies were still somewhat smaller than their full-term peers, only 8 percent of them were below the normal range in weight or height.

Premature babies who are born small for their gestational age, have shorter parents, or have neurologic abnormalities are more likely to remain small. Standard growth charts for preemies, which reflect their different growth patterns through age three, can be found in the appendix on pages 584–587. (To see how your baby measures up, be sure to use the right chart: there are separate ones for boys and for girls, as well as for preemies who were born weighing more, or less, than 1,500 grams.)

The good news is that catch-up growth doesn't always stop during a preemie's childhood, but often continues on through adolescence. One series of studies followed preemies with a birth weight of 1,500 grams or more, comparing them over the years with a similar group of children who were born full-term. From age 8 to age 20, the preemie girls almost entirely caught up in size, ending up on average around five feet three inches tall and 143 pounds—only about half an inch shorter and four pounds lighter than the girls born full term. The preemie boys didn't get quite as close to the full-termers; at the age of 20, they were on average a little more than an inch shorter and 24 pounds lighter than their full-term peers. But even the boys were no slouches! At an average of five feet eight inches tall and 152 pounds, these young men were well within the normal range.

Another series of studies focused on the growth of the very smallest preemies, those with a birth weight of less than 1,000 grams. These children also experienced remarkable catch-up growth from age 8 to age 20, although they did remain on average lighter and shorter than preemies who were born bigger and at a later gestational age. In young adulthood, these smallest preemies were about two inches shorter and 15 pounds lighter than their full-term peers. But 90 percent of them were still within the normal range of weight and height, and measurements showed that their bodies were well-proportioned.

For many people, body image plays an important role in self-esteem and social identity. How do former preemies feel about their physical growth? According to interviews with the boys and girls in these studies, their body image is just as good as that of their counterparts who were born at term. And other studies looking at the adjustment of shorter-than-normal children and adolescents found that although they may occasionally be teased about their height, being short doesn't interfere with their social opportunities, achievement, or emotional well-being.

So don't worry too much about your baby's earliest measurements, and be assured that she has a lot of catch-up growth ahead of her. In the meantime, enjoy her, and don't assume that if she is small, it will ever stop her. Maybe she'll be a gymnast instead of a basketball player.

The Option of Growth Hormone Treatment

If your child was born small-for-gestational-age, or SGA, and by the age of two years is still under the third percentile in height without showing signs of catch-up growth, she may be a good candidate for human growth hormone treatment, especially if the heights of others in your family indicate that she should be taller. Many studies have found this therapy to be safe and effective in boosting the heights of SGA children (in addition to children with growth hormone deficiency) into the normal range.

If your child is treated with growth hormone, she'll be followed by a pediatric endocrinologist. You'll be trained to give her an injection with a tiny needle (kids say they can barely feel it), which you'll do daily for several years, usually until she has gone through puberty and reached her adult height. The earlier the treatment begins—ideally before the age of five—the more effective it is, but even children who start later can often grow a lot. Children who have a genetic predisposition to be taller tend to grow the most. Because growth hormone therapy has been approved by the Food and Drug Administration for treatment of SGA children it is probably covered by your health insurance plan, but it's still a good idea to make sure beforehand.

Maybe she'll be the smallest of her friends but have the biggest personality. One of our preemies was a tiny toddler, and we used to quote a line from a song about Madeline, the famous gutsy little French girl of the children's books. "Though she's very small," the song goes, "inside, she's tall."

Picky Eater

My tiny toddler has never been a good eater, and now he's getting worse: All he wants is Cheerios. Is there something I can do to make his diet more nutritious?

As long as your pediatrician assures you that your child is consistently growing at a pace that's adequate, even if he's still smaller than other kids his age, you shouldn't worry much about his diet. A rich, varied diet would be nice, but children have an amazing ability to grow on what seems to their parents to be far too little food.

To be sure, some preemies develop serious feeding problems that prevent them from growing adequately. Most of the time, severe feeding problems are related to other medical conditions, such as reflux or cerebral palsy. If this is true for your child, he should be evaluated by experts who can diagnose his specific problems and give you advice on how to deal with them (see page 511). More likely, though, your preemie is afflicted with the same pickiness that's common in full-term toddlers and children. Of course, some have worse cases than others. When you talk to your pediatrician about it, ask her whether your child's nutrition might be too limited, and if she reassures you, try to relax. (Cereals and pastas—perennial toddler favorites—have a lot more nutrients in them than many parents realize.) If not, you can try the practical advice below to make your child's diet more varied.

When children tend to eat only one kind of food, it may just be that they have gotten into a comfortable, pleasurable habit that's hard to break. Or it might be something else: Another explanation for pickiness could be a lack of coordination. Cheerios are so simple to pick up that they are one of the first finger foods a baby can eat by himself. In addition to being delicious, they also melt in the mouth and are easy to swallow, so a predilection for them can come from a lack of coordination in a child's fingers, chewing, tongue motion, or swallowing. This is perfectly normal at a young age—it's why bibs were invented! But if you're worried that your child is more uncoordinated than most other children his adjusted age, an occupational therapist can determine whether he has mild finger or mouth coordination problems, and if he does, can help him overcome them.

Sometimes a toddler won't eat certain foods because he doesn't like the sensations he gets from them. For instance, he may reject ripe bananas because he is repulsed by touching slimy foods or by feeling sliminess in his mouth. Fingertip and lip sensations are wired to areas of the brain that are very close to one another, so if a child doesn't like to touch food with a particular texture, he often won't want to eat it, either. The same child might reject a new food just because of its shiny look, which he may associate with sliminess.

It's very common for children and adults to be unable to tolerate certain sensations of touch, taste, sight, sound, smell, or motion (fingernails on a blackboard, anybody?). In most cases, a longer list just reflects an especially sensitive personality. At the extreme, you may hear this trait called sensory processing disorder (see page 507). Former preemies seem to be more prone to sensory processing issues than children born at term. Occupational therapists who are trained in sensory processing and feeding-related problems can help children become more comfortable with the sensations they find difficult.

Whether your preemie has a case of extreme fussiness at the table or the garden-variety level of pickiness that's so common in children, there's a lot you can do to help without making eating into a battle. Using common parental sense and some creativity in the kitchen, you can help him grow perhaps not into a foodie, but a pleasant enough dinner companion.

Here are some practical suggestions:

* **Establish a schedule.** Toddlers and young children usually do well with three meals and two to three snacks a day. Try not to give your son juice and sweets as snacks, to prevent him from taking in relatively empty calories that can ruin his appetite for more nutritious food. Save sweets for after a good meal.

* **Make experimentation possible.** At meals, present him with two or three different options, and let him experiment with new foods. Also, sneak healthy food like vegetables onto your child's plate. Try mixing pureed butternut squash into macaroni and cheese or hiding little pieces of cauliflower in mashed potatoes. Play with similar colors and textures, sprinkling shredded carrots into tacos along with cheese, or being really bold and hiding spinach in brownies. Even some picky toddlers love those old favorites, pumpkin and zucchini bread. In recent years, some successful cookbooks have come out with creative ideas on this topic. You'll find them in *Resources* on page 592. Take inspiration from them and feel good about these innocent deceptions, which arise only from good intentions!

* **Entice your child with fun and interesting foods.** Here is where you can let your imagination go wild: Try cutting sandwiches with cookie cutters; make faces of animals out of fruits and vegetables; sprinkle designs using crumbly foods; use decorative toothpicks, corncob holders, or funny straws; or transform a pretzel, carrot stick or apple slice into a spoon.

* **Give choices and create games.** Harness your inner child and think back to when a seed-spitting contest made eating watermelon more fun; when it felt exciting and powerful to choose which color popsicle you got. So let loose and have a "How loud can you crunch?" contest. Ask your child whether he wants to eat the nose or the eyes first (of a vegetable face); which spoon (apple slice, pretzel) or toothpick he wants to use. Make food towers (by stacking cheese, tomatoes, or crackers) and challenge your child to eat them down.

* **Be persistent (but cool).** If your son seems to hate some foods (green vegetables, perhaps?), keep putting that kind of food on his plate meal after meal but don't insist that he taste it, and don't be discouraged if he doesn't. Some children need to get used to the sight and smell of certain foods before actually trying them. Patience and coolness in the face of rejection, some parents say, is the key to success.

* **Don't serve too much.** A good rule of the thumb is to serve a child one tablespoon of each food for each year of his age and then give a little more if he likes it. At 18 to 24 months, typical serving sizes for some common foods are:
  - four to six ounces of whole milk;
  - one-fourth to one-half cup of hot or dry cereal;
  - a half-slice of cheese;
  - one-half cup of yogurt or cottage cheese;

  - a half-slice of bread or two to four crackers;
  - three or four tablespoons of pasta, rice, beans, eggs, fruits, or vegetables;
  - two to four tablespoons of chopped meat or fish.

* **Add calories to the foods your child likes.** To increase the calories your child takes in, you can try such tricks as:
  - Adding a little butter, cream, oil, or grated Parmesan cheese to foods;
  - Putting cheese sauce on vegetables;
  - Adding finely chopped hard-boiled eggs to pasta or rice;
  - Adding condensed milk or powdered whole milk to yogurt, cream cheese, or hot cereals;
  - Spreading crackers or bread with peanut butter.

* **Limit the length of meals.** Some parents have found that limiting mealtime to 30 minutes helps make a child's eating pattern more regular and structured. Let him play around a little with his food and feed himself as he pleases without getting upset about messiness, but after 30 minutes, even if he didn't eat enough, take his plate away and let him leave the table. Don't worry that he might get too hungry before the next snack or meal: he needs that experience to help him establish a schedule.

* **If he doesn't eat his dinner, don't give him something better later.** If you're afraid your child hasn't eaten enough, it's tempting to give him something he's sure to enjoy as a substitute, just to get some food into him. But a child will quickly learn to hold out at meals if it means he'll be given more "good stuff" later. Instead, put his uneaten dinner in the refrigerator and present it to him again when he's hungrier.

* **Avoid nagging or conflict.** Try not to let your anxiety turn each meal into a conflict. Don't talk too much about food, don't punish or scold your son for not eating, and don't bribe

him to eat. (A sweet treat to reward him after a healthy meal, though, is fine.) Otherwise, you're giving him the message that when he wants to assert his control, food is a good arena in which to do it.

* **Never force-feed your child.** This can bring on immediate negative consequences, such as crying, gagging, or vomiting, and lead to long-term feeding refusals. A wise maxim to follow is that the parent decides what to put on the plate; the child decides what to eat and when he's full.

Flu Vaccine

Should my preemie get a flu vaccine?

When it comes to flu vaccines, the same guidelines apply to all babies, whether they were preemies or not. Yearly flu vaccines are now recommended for all children through 18 years of age. A baby can get her first flu vaccine once she's six months old, when her immune system is mature enough to react to it. If a baby is younger than that when she enters her first flu season, then pediatricians advise that all of her family members and anyone else who cares for her get the vaccine to protect them from catching the flu and giving it to her. (Doctors look at a preemie's actual age, not her corrected age, for purposes of vaccines.) Since newborns—and especially preemies—may not handle a respiratory infection as easily as older children, it really is important to follow these precautions.

Keep in mind that even though many people say they have the flu whenever they're suffering from a bad cold, influenza is actually a specific virus. A flu vaccine will protect your baby against certain strains of influenza, but not against every winter cold.

Ready for Daycare?

I purposely kept my daughter out of daycare because I was afraid of her getting infections. Now that she's two years old, is daycare safe for her?

It's an unavoidable fact that any group of little ones is a perfect setup for the quick spread of germs, and children in daycare or preschool come down with more colds and minor infections than children at home with their parents. So if you mean will your daughter be safe from getting sick often, the answer is no. But will she handle the colds and illnesses as well as any other child? If she is otherwise healthy, there's no reason she shouldn't. Once a preemie is a year old and has gotten through her first winter, you no longer have to worry about her being especially vulnerable. She has roughly the same amount of infection-fighting antibodies as full-term children of her corrected age, with an immune system that is as mature.

Of course, some full-term toddlers get sick more often than others or suffer from wheezing or painful ear infections every time they come down with a common cold. So whether to send a child to daycare is always an individual decision.

The one thing it's important to realize is that preemies who are still on oxygen or medications for BPD are definitely more fragile. They have less reserve in their lungs and are more prone to wheezing, so if they get a cold or respiratory infection, they will get sicker than other children. They also need more calories to grow, so diarrhea (one of the other common maladies that kids in daycare come down with) may cause them more problems. If your daughter has BPD, you'll have to make a trade-off between the advantages of daycare (the social and developmental stimulation she'll get from being around other children and adults, and the time it frees up for you) and the more frequent sicknesses she'll undoubtedly get. Make sure to talk this decision over with her doctor, who can help you understand the benefits and risks.

Also talk to the doctor if your child has a history of BPD but is no longer being treated for it. She may still tend to get a little sicker than other children when she catches something because her lungs may not have fully recovered, but in most cases, she won't be so fragile that she can't lead a perfectly normal life, including going to daycare.

The latest, reassuring research has found that high-quality daycare programs can actually be beneficial in promoting a child's learning abilities until she's old enough for kindergarten. (Researchers have also found that a child's behavior is likely to be more advanced but only up to the age of three; after that, children in daycare tend to have more behavior problems.) Especially if your child is getting early intervention services because of some developmental risks or delays, you may want to look for special developmental daycare programs, which offer more organized skill-developing activities. If you don't know of any, ask at your child's preemie follow-up clinic or look online for childcare referral services.

No matter what kind of program you choose, be sure to observe it in action and check its references, licensing (having a state or local license generally provides some safeguards, at least in terms of safety, sanitation, and caregiver-child ratio), policies on medical checkups and immunizations for the staff and kids, and enforcement of health rules (for example, whether toys are regularly disinfected, caregivers wash hands after diaper changes and before serving food, and pacifiers and bottles are labeled and kept separate). Since some of the good programs have waiting lists, it's never too early to start looking at them and to apply for a spot.

Possible VP Shunt Problems

I worry so much about my child's VP shunt. What can go wrong with it?

Parents of a child with a VP shunt have wrenching doubts every time their child gets sick, as all kids do. Is it just a virus, an innocent upset stomach, or is it the shunt, they wonder in anguish. You may find it reassuring to review some things your baby's neurosurgeon and pediatrician have already told you about how to recognize a shunt problem (see page 465), and to hear from some parents like you, who know how hard it is to live with the knowledge that their child's well-being depends on that essential, but still foreign, object implanted in his body yet have still found it possible to describe their everyday lives as normal (see page 463).

Despite its reliability and resistance to damage, a shunt system may occasionally fail and need to be changed. When a malfunction is only partial, meaning some cerebrospinal fluid is still being drained by the shunt or absorbed by the body, the pressure inside the brain from hydrocephalus rises slowly. A toddler may not show any symptoms other than his head enlarging more quickly than normal over a few weeks or months. In other instances, the shunt malfunction is total, and the rapidly increasing pressure on the brain can make a child feel very sick with a headache and vomiting. In the most serious cases, a doctor may find that a child's blood pressure is high, his heartbeat slow, and his breathing irregular. If that happens, it is a medical emergency.

The most common reasons for shunt failures are breaks in the tubing, blockages (by blood clots, scarring, or nearby tissue in the ventricles or abdomen) that plug up the shunt and keep it from draining, or movement of the shunt tubing so that it's no longer in the proper position in the abdomen, usually because a child has grown so tall.

(Continued on page 464)

Leading a Normal Infancy and Childhood with a VP Shunt

All parents have mixed feelings about their child's VP shunt, but some have an especially hard time accepting it. Although they understand that there's no other good option, they may become overly concerned about its presence and its effects on their child's life. But keep in mind that the shunt is not an impairment in itself; on the contrary, it's a very effective way to prevent the consequences of hydrocephalus on the brain, and even to reverse some of them, greatly improving the chances that your child will grow and develop normally.

From personal experience, we can reassure you that you're going to feel a lot better when your premature baby becomes a toddler. By then, many of your initial uncertainties about your child's development will be resolved. Even if he has some problems or delays, you'll have become familiar with early intervention, established relationships with follow-up specialists, and know what to expect. You do have to be prepared for the possibility of a shunt revision in the future—most preemies outgrow their shunt within a few years—but the bigger and stronger your baby is, the less anxious you need to be about his having to go back to the operating room.

Emotionally, you'll be especially vulnerable during your child's first year, still feeling the aftershocks of stress and sorrow caused by his premature birth and illness. The shunt inside his body, which initially you may not even want to acknowledge with your touch, will become little by little more familiar and acceptable to you, just as it disappears from the sight of anyone who doesn't know it is there. The time will actually come, sooner than you expect, when you realize that the shunt is no longer a threatening presence in your thoughts. It's important for you to let that

natural adaptation happen. If someone close to you has a tendency to revive your anxiety about your child's shunt, be firm and tell that person that you don't need such aggravation. You need, instead, to stay calm and optimistic, to allow your child to live his life to his maximum potential. There is nothing he cannot do simply because of his VP shunt.

Here's a brief overview and some parent-to-parent advice about some other issues that come up when you're raising a child with a VP shunt:

* During their baby's first couple of years, some parents decide that it's easier to avoid daycare than to go through frequent shunt infection scares. Daycare won't increase your baby's chance of developing an actual shunt infection, but it certainly will increase his chance of having symptoms—irritability, fever, vomiting—that *look* like a shunt infection but are really due to other common illnesses. Those scares can be really hard on parents! If you can't arrange for babysitting in your home, consider sharing a sitter with a few other parents or choosing a small family daycare setting so that your baby is exposed to only a few other children.

* To avoid infections, some doctors and dentists recommend that a child with a VP shunt take antibiotics before dental procedures and surgeries although research supporting that practice is lacking.

* Your child should get periodic vision and hearing screens, as well as developmental evaluations (these are done routinely in many preemie follow-up clinics) to catch and correct any problems early.

* If you have to move to another city or state

and you're worried about leaving behind your trusted neurosurgeon, ask him for advice before you go. He can suggest how to organize your son's follow-up and refer you to a colleague or medical center close to your new address. After the move, if a shunt revision is necessary and your child has only mild symptoms, he might be able to travel back to his original neurosurgeon for the surgery if you wish. But be sure to ask your insurer about this and about any limitations on your choice of doctor or hospital. Your concerns are not uncommon: Some families even consider moving to be near a particular doctor or hospital.

* Don't treat your son differently because of his shunt. It won't be dislodged or damaged in the course of daily activities, so he can play, run, participate in team sports, swim, and dive just like any other child—even become a competitive athlete if he has a passion and gift for it. Some doctors discourage contact sports like football, but if he wears a helmet, you can even allow him to do that. A helmet is necessary when he bicycles, skis, or rides a skateboard. (What wise parent would allow a child to go without one?)

* Your child needs to know about his VP shunt. As soon as he is able to understand a simple explanation, you should tell him. Have him touch the little bump of the valve on his head and the tube tunneled under his skin down to his belly. At the same time, you should reassure him that everything is OK. Don't scare him by talking about the possibility of surgery for a shunt revision, but if it happens, tell him that it's normal and he's going to recover fast.

* As long as you understand your son's condition and are confident about the VP shunt's effectiveness and safety, you'll be able to explain it reassuringly to his siblings, friends, and teachers. Don't fear that he may be treated differently because of it: Since the shunt isn't visible, most of them will quickly forget about it. You'll find that their attitude toward your child will depend almost entirely on yours.

VP shunts for tiny preemies are necessarily short, and even though neurosurgeons use extra-long tubing and coil it inside a baby's abdomen to allow for future growth, the catheter usually needs to be replaced with a bigger one at some point. Although it's possible to check on a VP shunt with X-rays or an MRI, this isn't done routinely unless a child has symptoms. If your child's doctor suspects a shunt malfunction, he may order a shunt series—a series of X-rays of the tubing going from the head to the abdomen—to make sure there are no breaks in it and that everything is still in the right place, or a brain MRI, to see whether fluid is building up excessively in the ventricles.

Another possible cause of malfunction is a shunt infection. Most infections occur in the first six months following shunt surgery, but they can happen at any time. Even if a shunt infection doesn't interfere with how well the shunt is working, it may not resolve until the shunt is removed (usually temporarily) because bacteria can hide in the plastic tubing and evade efforts to eradicate them. Such a big step—temporarily taking out a child's shunt—is worth it if an infection isn't clearing up rapidly, because an unchecked infection could cause neurological damage or even death. An infection can be diagnosed with a spinal tap, usually done by a pediatrician, or with a ventricular tap, done by a neurosurgeon. The doctor inserts a tiny needle into a baby's back or ventricle and withdraws some cerebrospinal fluid, which is sent to a lab to be analyzed and checked for bacteria. The doctor can also measure the pressure when he does a tap to see if it's become too high.

Sometimes, doctors can't definitely prove or disprove that there is a shunt malfunction or infection. In that case, they may observe your child closely and wait to see if he improves or worsens. Or, if their suspicion of a shunt malfunction is high, even if they're not certain, the doctors may recommend surgery to prevent complications, which are more likely the longer an infection or hydrocephalus goes on.

If your child does have a shunt infection, he will be treated with intravenous antibiotics for several weeks in the hospital, under the watchful eyes of nurses and his neurosurgeon. Either a partial or a total shunt malfunction would be corrected with a shunt revision. On average, a child will need two or three shunt revisions during infancy and childhood. Although it's scary and upsetting to go through, a revision gives your child a new functioning shunt and almost always returns him to his previous wellness.

When to Call the Doctor about the VP Shunt

When I see something I fear might be caused by a problem with my child's VP shunt, I never know when it's time to call the doctor.

It's terribly worrying when you're not sure whether your child is in trouble or not. If it helps, know that you're not the only one who finds this baffling. Even doctors can have a hard time telling whether a child with a VP shunt has just a run-of-the-mill illness or the shunt is to blame. If your child doesn't look very sick, a wise approach is to wait until your first impression is confirmed, rather than calling the pediatrician right away. For your peace of mind, though, remember that you're justified in making as many phone calls

and visits to your baby's doctor as you need, even if they result in false alarms, to avoid missing a real emergency. Over time, as you make such decisions again and again, and learn from their outcomes, you'll become more sure of yourself.

In the meantime, here are some general guidelines on which symptoms should concern you and which should not:

Fever. Always call the pediatrician if your child has a fever higher than 101 degrees Fahrenheit. Most of the time, the doctor will end up diagnosing a viral infection or another common illness rather than a shunt infection. Remember, though, that in an infant, particularly a preemie, it's possible to detect a fever caused by nothing but a hot room and too many clothes. Undress your baby, leave him undisturbed for fifteen minutes, and then check his temperature again.

Full fontanel. A puffy, bulging fontanel (the soft spot on a baby's head) when the baby is held upright and not crying or straining is a typical sign of hydrocephalus in infants who still have open skull bones (a natural protection against pressure on the brain). If you notice tension in the fontanel when your infant is lying down, but it disappears when you put him in a vertical position, it's a false alarm. So don't panic, wait until your baby is calm and pick him up and check again. Very large and visible scalp veins and wide-open spaces where the skull bones should come together can also be signs of increased pressure. But keep in mind that the shape of your infant's head will change a lot in the first months after surgery, even if his shunt is functioning perfectly.

Enlarging head. Even after the fontanels close, a toddler's skull bones are not tightly fused together, so his head can still enlarge quickly if the shunt malfunctions. (As a child grows older, this leeway gradually disappears.) Neurosurgeons and pediatricians don't advise parents to check their children's head circumference, since the common spurts and sputters of growth may unnecessarily worry parents, and the measurements performed at the pediatrician's office and plotted on your child's growth chart are sufficient. If you feel compelled to measure more often, though, you should use a flexible tape measure divided into centimeters. Place it across your child's forehead over his eyebrows, then wind it around his head at the widest point. Take three measurements, one after the other, to be sure of your result.

The normal rate of head growth will vary depending on the age of your child: faster (about one centimeter a week) for infant preemies and slower (about one centimeter a month) for toddlers. To know whether your son's head is growing at a normal rate for his age and sex, you'll need to plot your measurements over several days or weeks on the appropriate head circumference chart (see pages 584–587). A single measurement made at only one point in time is not an accurate guide, since a child who had hydrocephalus may have had a bigger head to start with but now has one that is growing normally over time.

Headache. Many parents are greatly relieved when their child begins to speak. While an infant can only cry if he hurts, or become fussier, a toddler is able to point to where he has pain and an older child describe what he is feeling. A headache caused by a shunt malfunction can be severe or mild, intermittent or persistent. Be especially wary of a headache or a sense of heaviness that wakes your child from sleep, is worse when he's lying down or in the morning, or is accompanied by vomiting or nausea. In those cases, you should call the doctor.

Vomiting. Babies spit up for a million reasons that have nothing to do with shunt malfunctions. Over time you'll get to know your baby well and usually will be able to tell if he vomited because he ate too fast or too much or because you bounced him or for some other reason. In an older child, vomiting is more unusual and therefore more worrisome for a possible shunt malfunction. A single episode of vomiting or nausea, though, should concern you only if it's accompanied by some other sign of shunt malfunction or infection. In cases of repeated vomiting, you should always call the doctor. Most of the time, the doctor will be able to reassure you that your child's vomiting is likely caused by a flu or common virus.

Abdominal pain, diarrhea, constipation. A bloated or painful abdomen, sometimes with fever or diarrhea, may signal a shunt infection and should immediately be reported to the doctor. A VP shunt can cause bowel blockage, but this is a very rare complication, and you needn't be concerned about mild constipation without pain or vomiting. But you should help your child try to maintain regular bowel movements with a diet rich in fiber and fruit and vegetables, because persistent constipation can interfere with the VP shunt tubing in the abdomen.

Lethargy. Lethargy can be a hard symptom to ascertain in an infant, particularly in a sleepy preemie who tires easily, falls asleep in the middle of feedings, and needs to get all the rest he can. But if your baby doesn't wake up at his regular times or doesn't seem hungry, then you should watch him more carefully to see whether that pattern continues. In an older child, difficulty waking up or excessive sleepiness is more telling. Don't get anxious, though, about an occasional longer nap or night's sleep; your son probably is simply tired and replenishing his energies. Do worry about a consistent trend, especially if it's accompanied by headache and vomiting, and call the doctor.

Poor feeding. This is another confusing sign for parents of premature babies, who may not be the most vigorous eaters. Often, if a baby eats less at one meal, he'll balance it out by eating more at the next one. But if your baby seems much slower in his sucking than usual and doesn't seem hungrier over the course of several feedings, call the doctor.

Abnormal gaze and eye movements. A shunt malfunction can give a baby sunset eyes, so called because the gaze is cast downward. (The iris, positioned at the bottom of the eye with the white visible above it, looks like a setting sun.) If you notice this, you should call the pediatrician. Children with hydrocephalus can also have mild visual problems even with a properly functioning shunt. They include nystagmus (rapid involuntary eye movements) and difficulty following or focusing on objects. After an evaluation by an eye doctor, which your baby should have at about six months of age, you'll know whether he has any of these problems, and you can look out for any change from what's normal for him.

Seizures. Children with VP shunts are more likely to have seizures, which are usually treated with medications. But seizures can also be a symptom of a shunt malfunction or infection. Therefore, if your child has more seizures—or different kinds of seizures—than usual, you should call the doctor.

Irritability and changes in behavior. A baby or child with a mild, persistent headache or nausea from a shunt problem may become fussier or more difficult. Sometimes a change in temperament or behavior, like increased irritability or problems at school, are caused by pressure from hydrocephalus. But what toddler doesn't have a temper tantrum every now and then? What kid doesn't occasionally fail to pay attention at

---

Symptoms of Shunt Malfunction

Up to one year of age:
* full fontanel
* enlarging head

Sometimes also:
* vomiting
* poor feeding
* irritability
* lethargy or excessive sleepiness
* abnormal gaze and eye movements
* seizures

Toddler or older child:
* enlarging head
* headache
* vomiting
* lethargy
* abdominal pain
* sunset eyes
* irritability
* behavior changes
* loss of previous motor or cognitive abilities
* seizures

Symptoms of Shunt Infection

Alone or together with any other symptoms of shunt malfunction:
* fever over 101 degrees Fahrenheit

Sometimes also:
* redness and tenderness around the valve and along the catheter
* abdominal distension
* diarrhea

school? Overreacting to subtle common swings in behavior is unfair to yourself and your child. A significant change in your son, one that could indicate a shunt problem, will become evident to you even if you take a more relaxed and optimistic attitude.

Loss of previous motor or cognitive abilities. Sometimes a shunt malfunction can impair a child's normal development without other acute symptoms. If you notice that your child is no longer able to do something he used to do well, like sitting up, pulling himself to a standing position, walking steadily, or naming a familiar object, you should watch him carefully. But also remember that ups and downs are a normal pattern of development. A child doesn't learn to do something and immediately master it, rather, he needs to practice a new skill a lot, before he can perform it consistently. So you should inform his doctor only if you continue to see a change. If your son does develop an impairment caused by a shunt malfunction, you'll be understandably anxious, but he has a good chance of overcoming it when the shunt is revised and the hydrocephalus is again under control.

Keeping these guidelines in mind, it's a good bet that you will still find yourself calling the doctor plenty of times. When you do, be sure to say that your child has a VP shunt before describing his symptoms; doctors and nurses will give your call immediate priority. Your pediatrician will refer you to the neurosurgeon if that's what's needed. There's also nothing wrong with calling your neurosurgeon directly if you have a particular concern or question. A pediatric neurosurgeon who cares for children with VP shunts has made a long-term commitment to his little patients and is well aware of their families' practical and emotional needs. Knowing that he's always there,

ready to revise your child's shunt if necessary, can make you feel much safer.

Seizures

My daughter had a seizure in the NICU, and recently she had another seizure with a high fever. Does this mean that she'll have more?

In most parenting books, you'll find a section on febrile seizures (as the convulsions that children can get with high fevers are called), for the simple reason that they're fairly common. About one out of every 25 toddlers gets one, and preemies are even more susceptible than term-born children. Although they're terrifying to parents, doctors don't worry about febrile seizures much at all. Not only are they harmless, but children who get them have only a tiny risk of developing epilepsy, a disorder in which seizures recur without fevers. Up to 98 percent of these children will never have to worry about seizures again after outgrowing their febrile ones, usually well before their fifth birthday. (The peak period for febrile seizures is from 18 months to 24 months of age.)

But of course, if your preemie also had a seizure in the hospital nursery, it's natural for you to wonder whether the outlook for her is different. The answer is: It depends, but there's a good chance you're worrying unnecessarily.

There are only three factors that make a young child who has a seizure with fever more likely to develop epilepsy. One is if she has a cognitive or motor impairment, since this would indicate that there is some underlying injury in her brain. If your child has no cognitive or motor impairment, the great news is that neither her neonatal seizure (which could have occurred for all kinds of long-gone reasons) nor her febrile seizure, nor even the fact that she had both make her any more likely to have epilepsy. In fact, even if she had more than one neonatal seizure or she has recurring febrile seizures (about one-third of toddlers who have one seizure with a fever go on to have at least one recurrence), it won't make any difference. On the other hand, if your daughter does have cerebral palsy or a developmental delay, then it could be that both her seizure in the NICU and her seizure with a fever at home were triggered by the same underlying brain injury—and the likelihood of future seizures does rise.

The second factor that would increase your child's risk is if her febrile seizure was atypical. Typical, or so-called simple, febrile seizures last for less than 15 minutes (most commonly, they last for just a minute or two, and some can be as brief as a few seconds) and affect a child's whole body. The child would stiffen up and arch her back, her arms and legs would jerk repeatedly, and she would briefly lose consciousness. A seizure is atypical if it lasts longer, affects only portions of the body, such as just an arm or a leg, or just the right side, or recurs within twenty-four hours.

The third factor that would increase your child's risk is if you have a family history of epilepsy.

Now, if your child has one or more of these risk factors, please be warned against excessive pessimism! The chances that she'll have epilepsy are still small. For example, of all children who have atypical febrile seizures, only an estimated 10 percent to 20 percent develop epilepsy later on. Your child's doctor can give you an idea of her risk, based on her particular circumstances.

In any event, you should read up on febrile seizures to make sure you know what to do if she has another one. It's important to prevent any accidental injury or choking. And you should talk to your daughter's doctor, who to be safe may want to do some tests to make sure that the seizure wasn't caused by any problem other than the fever itself.

Worrying about Cerebral Palsy

Everyone tells me I don't have to worry, but I still keep dreading that my child has cerebral palsy.

Like many other parents of preemies, you may not even have known what cerebral palsy was before your baby was born. Once you learn that it is one of the most feared consequences of prematurity, though, it can be hard to get out of your mind. If your baby isn't sitting up by herself on the very day she turns six months of age, you ask yourself: Will she sit up tomorrow? When you see her clench her hands into little fists, you worry: Is this simply an adorable gesture or a bad sign of things to come?

In cerebral palsy, or CP, a person's muscles don't move in a naturally strong coordinated way. It's due to a permanent injury to the brain—which may have occurred before, during, or after a baby's birth—that prevents it from sending the signals the muscles need for well-coordinated movement. CP ranges from very mild (sometimes almost imperceptible) to severe, from affecting only one limb to affecting the whole body. Temporary movement problems, which infants eventually outgrow, are not cerebral palsy.

As a rule, cerebral palsy can neither be diagnosed nor definitively ruled out until a baby is 18 months to two years of age. If your baby is already one and a half to two years old and the way she moves is normal for her age (according to you and her doctors), you can put your fears aside for good. She does not have cerebral palsy. It should reassure you to know that if your baby is younger and doesn't have visible signs of brain damage or other risk factors for cerebral palsy, such as hydrocephalus or birth asphyxia, the chances that she will have cerebral palsy are tiny. And even if she has a known risk factor, she still has a chance—possibly a good one, depending on her situation—of being normal.

It's important to realize that abnormalities of muscle tone and reflexes are extremely common in preemies during their first year. At least two-thirds of babies born at less than 1,500 grams have them—while only 5 percent to 10 percent will actually have cerebral palsy. It's not known whether these problems are due to long hospital stays that weaken muscles and joints from lack of activity, early brain injuries that are healing, or different patterns of brain maturation in babies who are born early. But in most cases, these abnormalities are just temporary, gradually resolving by the time a baby is 12 to 18 months old. On the other hand, it's also possible for an infant to have normal muscle tone very early on and then develop abnormalities later in the first year.

Because a preemie's abnormalities are so often fleeting, a diagnosis of cerebral palsy is generally made before 12 months only if a premature baby had a known brain injury, such as a severe intraventricular hemorrhage or periventricular leukomalacia, and she moves some parts of her body very differently from others. From 12 months to 18 months, a diagnosis of CP is usually made if a child has a combination of a few of the following: different or asymmetric movement patterns in different extremities, delayed motor skills, movements that are abnormal in quality (for instance, unusual, awkward, or stiff), and reflexes that persist beyond the expected age. (You can learn about these characteristics and what they look like on page 471.) In general, premature babies with cerebral palsy have increasingly obvious abnormalities of muscle tone, movement, and reflexes and increasingly long delays in reaching motor milestones, especially from 6 months to 18 months of adjusted age. It's not that their CP is worsening; it's that as a child grows, more complex movements are expected of her and abnormal tone interferes more.

Even the most sophisticated brain imaging, such as ultrasound or MRI scans, are of limited help in forecasting which preemies will get CP. Because the part of the brain controlling movement lies right next to the ventricles, cerebral palsy is frequently associated with a Grade 3 or Grade 4 intraventricular hemorrhage or periventricular leukomalacia. But a brain scan can't accurately predict the future for an individual baby. Early head ultrasounds or MRIs that show no brain lesions don't definitely rule out a later disability. (There could be an injury that isn't visible on the scans.) And early ultrasounds or MRIs that do show abnormalities don't rule out normal development. (An infant's brain has an amazing capacity to recover from injury. Until the healing process is complete—and the timing of that is not very predictable—you can't tell whether there will be a permanent problem.)

So don't assume, as many parents do, that the doctors are hiding something when they say that they need to observe your baby's progress for a while before giving a diagnosis or a thumbs-up. And don't think that it's ominous if physical or occupational therapy is recommended to help with your baby's muscle tone problems. Although many muscular abnormalities will resolve on their own, it still can be good to work on them early so that they don't interfere with your baby's reaching other developmental milestones. For example, a mild amount of toe-walking might eventually go away on its own, but could delay a child's starting to walk independently. Stiff shoulder muscles can prevent a child from reaching for objects well. Not only is this frustrating for a baby, but motor delays can even impede cognitive development if they go on for too long, by restricting the range of a child's experiences.

We urge you to try not to look at every behavior of your baby as a possible diagnosis: You will risk missing out on the joys of this wonderful period of parenting and possibly even transmit your anxiety to your baby.

(Continued on page 474)

Typical Characteristics of Cerebral Palsy: What's Worrisome and What's Not

Typical characteristics of cerebral palsy are abnormal muscle tone in some or all parts of the body; infant reflexes that last beyond the time when they should disappear; delays in reaching motor milestones; and abnormal quality of movements (meaning they're not as fluid and varied as they should be). If your baby has one or two of the characteristics described below, join the club and don't worry—most preemies do, and it rarely indicates a long-term problem. When a baby has many of them, however, the possibility of CP increases. It may reassure you to have your baby's doctor discuss with you what kinds of delays or symptoms are more significant than others.

Muscle tone abnormalities

When muscle tone is abnormal—either too rigid and stiff or too limp and floppy—some movements can become difficult.

One problem that may occur in some preemies after a long hospital stay is a stiff neck, or as you may hear the doctor call it, "torticollis" (Latin for twisted neck). Although some babies with cerebral palsy have torticollis, in most young preemies it's a temporary problem with a simple cause: Lying on their back for a long time in the nursery, babies who are old enough to turn their heads often prefer to look in one direction— because that's where the action in the room is or where a fascinating picture is hanging—and end up with a stiff, shortened muscle on that side of their neck. This kind of torticollis almost always goes away within about four to six months if you do daily gentle stretching exercises with your baby. The physical therapist will teach you what to do and will warn you that your baby probably won't like the exercises much but that it's important to be persistent for the problem to resolve. You can also help by attracting her attention with mobiles, toys, and pictures strategically placed so that she turns her head to the other side.

Another abnormality often seen in preemies is high muscle tone in their legs, causing them to keep their knees stiff, toes pointed, and hips rigid when they're lying or standing. Typically this is evident by three months of adjusted age and begins to resolve by 12 months. A little bit of toe-walking may last until 18 months, and if it does, your child may start to walk late but isn't likely to have a long-term impairment. If the high tone is extreme or lasts beyond 18 months to 24 months, though, particularly in a child who has other neurologic problems, cerebral palsy becomes more likely.

Many preemies have temporarily stiff shoulders, especially those who spent a long time lying on their backs in the hospital, on a ventilator, without moving much. Called retracted shoulders, they're held back, like an exaggeration of good posture. If a baby's stiff shoulders go along with stiffness of her whole upper body, she's likely to have some developmental delays (when doing things that involve bringing her arms and hands forward, for example) but not cerebral palsy. If stiff shoulders are accompanied by a limp upper body, though (the stiff shoulders may be a baby's way of compensating for her limpness, to improve her head control), she does face a significantly higher risk of having cerebral palsy. In either case, physical therapy to relax her shoulder muscles may help a baby bring her hands together to hold a bottle, reach for objects in front of her, sit, and crawl.

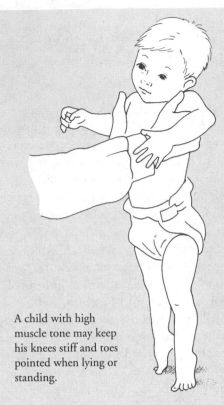

A child with high muscle tone may keep his knees stiff and toes pointed when lying or standing.

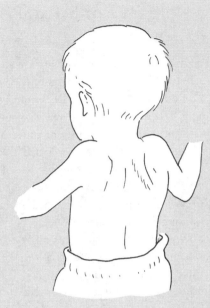

A child with retracted shoulders, held out and back.

Adapted with permission of Judy Bernbaum, M.D., from *Primary Care of the Preterm Infant* by Judy C. Bernbaum and Marsha Hoffman-Williamson, Mosby 1991

Abnormally low muscle tone (most often, limp trunk muscles) is less common than abnormally high tone but more concerning. If your baby has it, you would notice her head flopping back when you pull her by the arms into a sitting position; even after two to three months of age, her head would bob when she was sitting up; and even after six months of age, she would slump when sitting supported. You may see your baby compensate for this floppiness with retracted shoulders or by locking her knees and hips when she is held in a standing position. Low muscle tone can make reaching many milestones—from rolling over, to sitting, crawling, and standing—more difficult. Some babies with low muscle tone will be just fine, but others will end up having cerebral palsy or, even if the muscle tone problems later resolve, cognitive problems, such as learning disabilities or mental retardation.

Delays in reflexes and balance responses

There are numerous reflexes that are programmed to appear then disappear in a specific normal time sequence in infants. (One example is the palmar grasp: place your index finger across the inside of a newborn's palm and she will automatically flex her fingers around your finger. Another is called the Moro, or startle, reflex: when a newborn feels like she is falling, she throws out her arms and then brings them back to her chest a few seconds later. Both reflexes are programmed to disappear by about four months of adjusted age.) In babies with CP, infant reflexes may last many months longer than normal. So-called balance responses, which help infants keep their position when their balance is threatened, also normally appear on a pre-programmed schedule. For example, most infants develop head righting, the ability to keep their head upright when their position changes, at about four months. Balance responses may be lacking in some babies, such as those with CP, who don't have appropriate muscle tone.

Many perfectly normal babies have delays in the disappearance of some reflexes or the appearance of balance responses. Only if this goes along with other symptoms is it considered worrisome.

Delays in reaching developmental milestones

Because there is a wide range of normal timing, even if your preemie isn't rolling over, reaching out for objects, sitting up, walking, or otherwise attaining some motor milestones as early as other babies you know, she may still be within the normal range. To pediatricians, the following delays in motor development would typically be of concern:

* **At 3 months:** poor head control
* **At 6 months:** cannot sit, even with support; keeps hands clenched in fists; does not bring objects to her mouth; only grasps an object momentarily
* **At 8 months:** cannot sit without support
* **At 12 months:** is sitting, but can't move from sitting position onto hands and knees or to standing without falling
* **At 18 months:** does not walk; tries to walk on toes

Just remember that in full-term babies, long delays are often more worrisome than in preemies, whose temporary abnormalities of muscle tone can make certain kinds of movement more difficult. Also remember that for a preemie, adjusted age is what counts.

Quality of movement

A child who has stiff muscle tone or developmental delays may still be perfectly fine. Often a skilled pediatrician or physical therapist can tell parents that, despite the stiffness or delay, the quality of their child's movements is normal: fluid, varied, and coordinated.

Although all children deviate from normal movements when they're learning new skills, once they master them, they should use their muscles and move in standard ways. Some examples of movements that are abnormal in quality:

* Rolling over in only one direction or stiffly extending the trunk and neck to start and complete a roll; sitting only in a W position (see illustration) when on the floor; or sitting only back on tailbone, with legs stiff and straight in front of them;
* Lying, sitting, or standing only in a frog-legged position with legs splayed wide apart;
* Crawling with hands fisted or in an asymmetrical pattern (using one side of the body differently from the other);
* Pulling stiffly to stand or using arm strength only, without coming up one foot at a time;
* Capable of reaching for things well with only the right hand or the left (a preference for using one hand is OK, though);
* Standing on toes most of the time or overly stiff at the knees;
* Cruising (walking while holding on to furniture) with legs stiff at the knees.

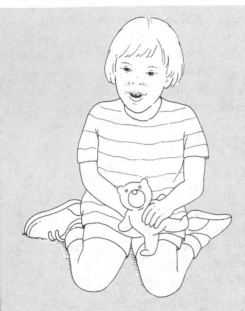

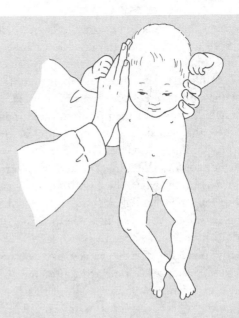

W-sitting may indicate abnormal muscle tone, although all children occasionally sit in the W position.

A child whose legs are splayed apart, frog-like, may have abnormally low muscle tone.

Adapted with permission of Judy Bernbaum, M.D., from *Primary Care of the Preterm Infant* by Judy C. Bernbaum and Marsha Hoffman-Williamson, Mosby 1991

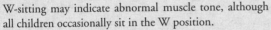

There are certain motor skills that children may achieve early *because* of movements that are abnormal in quality. Babies with stiff muscle tone may be able to roll over as early as two months of age or to stand holding on to something as early as four months. To be safe, mention to her doctor any motor milestones that your baby reaches long before you'd expect. And even though it's easy to feel proud of your baby's accomplishments, you shouldn't encourage them if they rely on atypical movements. They could interfere with her developing the right muscle and movement patterns for other motor skills.

On the other hand, if you are really worried that your baby fits into the categories on page 471, by all means talk to your pediatrician about your concerns. You know your baby better than anybody, and your concerns should always be taken seriously.

The doctor may put your fears to rest, telling you that your child's movements are a lot more normal than you think. If he tells you that he needs to keep an eye on your baby's motor development over time or suggests that she get a thorough developmental evaluation, remember that these are not necessarily bad signs or reason for pessimism. Even if your preemie's movement problems are only temporary, as they often are, she'll benefit from being watched carefully to see if she needs a boost from physical therapy. If you do learn that your baby has a lasting problem, you'll get the benefit of expert advice and she will get the benefit of early intervention, giving her the best chance of reaching her full potential. (You can read about living with cerebral palsy on page 520.)

Eyesight After ROP

My three-year-old had ROP and wears glasses. What can we expect for her vision?

That depends on your daughter's unique medical history, including how mild or severe her ROP (short for retinopathy of prematurity; see page 301) was and why she needs glasses now. The best person to ask, therefore, is your daughter's eye doctor. He will be able to make some predictions about her future vision and describe any increased risks she faces because she had ROP.

Because eye problems in preemies can be complex and diagnosing problems in very young children—who aren't articulate about their eyesight (or anything else!) yet—can be tricky, your child's eye exams should be done by a specialized pediatric ophthalmologist, or at least one who is very experienced with young children. During the first few years of a child's life, when the visual pathways between the eyes and the brain are being established, eye problems that go uncorrected for too long are more likely to cause some permanent loss of vision. So making sure that your daughter gets follow-up eye exams at the recommended times will be very important.

In the meantime, you can get a sense of where your daughter might fit within the general possibilities outlined below.

* **Mild ROP** (Stage 1 or 2) heals itself without treatment. If your child had mild ROP, you can feel relieved that the outlook for her future vision is excellent. If she's wearing glasses now because she's nearsighted, you do have to keep in mind that many people's nearsightedness worsens as they get older, but genetic factors

(whether thick glasses run in your family) are likely to play a larger role than her past ROP when it comes to the course your daughter's nearsightedness will take. In any case, she'll have lots of company: nearly one-third of all high school graduates are nearsighted, and the usual options of glasses and contact lenses will most likely be available to your daughter for correcting it.

Nevertheless, it's very important for parents not to get complacent during their child's early years, because any preemie, and even more so a preemie who had ROP, faces a higher risk of developing two of the most common childhood eye problems: strabismus (crossed eyes) and amblyopia (a lazy eye). These problems can almost always be treated successfully when they're caught early; with glasses and simple surgery for strabismus or glasses and eye patches for amblyopia. (Treatment may be more difficult if factors other than ROP are contributing to your child's vision problems, as they could be if she has a brain injury.)

So any child who had ROP should have her eyes reexamined no later than her first birthday and again when she turns three—and even sooner if her parents notice anything unusual. The doctor will pay particular attention to whether she is developing better vision in one eye than the other, since this is how amblyopia can arise.

By the time your child is about four years old, if there's no sign of strabismus or amblyopia, it's unlikely that she'll ever get them. Of course, she should continue to wear her glasses and, like any child who had ROP, she should get yearly eye exams to find and treat any problems early. But chances are you're home free and there will be no further complications from her ROP.

* **Moderately severe ROP** (Stage 3) is likely to leave a child's retina with some scarring or

distortion. Even if it is microscopic and does not affect her vision, it does mean there's a higher risk of future eye problems to look out for. Many children with moderate or severe ROP have more complicated vision problems, because they're more likely to have been sick and had a brain injury in the nursery (from an intraventricular hemorrhage, for example) that contributes to their difficulty seeing.

If the doctor tells you that your daughter's retinopathy of prematurity went away without causing noticeable injury to her eye, follow the guidelines for mild ROP mentioned above: eye exams when she turns one year old, three years old, and annually thereafter. If the doctor can see some leftover scars or changes in your daughter's retina, either from laser treatment or the ROP itself, he'll give you guidance on her additional follow-up care.

Feel assured that if you are careful about checkups, the chances of any further complications are small. Still, although the vast majority of children with moderate ROP won't get them, you should be aware of two serious conditions that can arise in the future: glaucoma and late-onset retinal detachment. Glaucoma occurs because changes in the structure of the eye from severe ROP can interfere with the drainage of fluid from the eye, causing pressure to build up. There are various treatments for glaucoma, ranging from eye drops to special surgical procedures. A late retinal detachment occurs if, despite the best medical treatment, there is pulling on the retina as the eye grows because scar tissue or some leftover retinal abnormalities keep some part of the retina more firmly attached than the rest to the wall of the eye. Thankfully, if retinal detachment occurs in a teenager or adult, the prognosis is far better than when it occurs in infancy, especially if it is repaired quickly. Thus, to be safe, it's important for your daughter to continue going

for her annual retinal exams throughout her adolescence and early adulthood.

* **Severe ROP** (Stage 4 or 5) affects the structure of the back of the eye differently in every individual. Most children who had severe ROP will have serious visual impairments, even with glasses, although some will have enough vision to help in walking around and daily activities. In some children, eyesight will be stable over time, while others will have progressive changes or even need further surgery. If your daughter had severe ROP, she should be followed by an ophthalmologist who specializes in children with retinopathy of prematurity. The ophthalmologist will tell you how often she should come for checkups. Also, make sure to read about how to give your child the best opportunity to develop normally and happily with her visual impairment on page 503.

Risk of Future Developmental Problems

My toddler is perfectly healthy. Is he still at risk for the developmental problems that premature babies get?

A premature baby who by 18 to 24 months of corrected age is healthy and doesn't show any signs of major disabilities (cerebral palsy, intellectual impairment, vision or hearing loss) is no longer at risk for the most severe developmental problems caused by an early birth. So you can relax about that.

There are some milder developmental delays—or minor disabilities, as doctors classify them—that may show up only later: subtle difficulties with balance and coordination; slightly lower than normal intelligence; learning disabilities; or problems with attention or behavior. Frequently, these minor impairments aren't discovered until a child is in school, when he's faced with different kinds of pressures and demands from those at home. For example, learning disabilities may not show up until a child is required to do complicated mental tasks, such as reading, spelling, or arithmetic; hyperactivity or attention problems may become obvious only when a child is asked to sit still in school for many hours; and the lack of motor precision needed to write legibly or play team sports well can highlight problems with agility and coordination.

According to recent studies, up to 50 percent of premature babies with a birth weight less than 1,500 grams will develop one or more minor disabilities. Not all preemies are at equal risk; as usual, the smallest and youngest and those who had the most medical complications are most susceptible. But before you start worrying too much about your son's future, keep in mind that minor learning disabilities and behavior problems are also common in children born at term (about 12 percent have them) and can be found even in children who are highly intelligent and gifted. Doctors call these impairments minor for a reason. It's not because they're not important but because children who have them, with appropriate strategies and interventions, can adapt very well. Although these problems may transiently disturb a child's academic progress or social interactions, they need not significantly affect his eventual accomplishments or quality of life. In a study by Canadian researchers of adult former preemies, even the smallest, those born at less than 1,000 grams, were almost as likely as full-term babies to attain the traditional measures of a successful, fulfilling adult life: pursuing a college education, living independently, being employed, being married or living with a partner, and having children. These reassuring findings should make all families truly hopeful that their tiny babies will grow into accomplished and happy young adults.

If you have any concerns about your toddler's development or behavior, don't hesitate to talk to his pediatrician. If she says your child is functioning at his peers' level, you should let your anxiety go, allowing him to develop skills and his unique character traits at his own pace, as any full-term child does.

No matter how well your preemie is doing, if you need more reassurance, you can ask your doctor to schedule him for a full multidisciplinary developmental evaluation. This is often done at age three, before a child enters preschool, or at age five, before he enters kindergarten. A multidisciplinary evaluation is usually performed by a developmental psychologist, a speech-language pathologist, a special educator (who will evaluate a child's learning skills), an occupational therapist, and a physical therapist. It is an extensive, and therefore expensive, kind of testing that may or may not be covered by your health insurance plan or by the government, depending on your child's circumstances. So you may want to inquire about that first.

If you decide not to have your child evaluated, don't kick yourself about it later if a learning disability shows up when your child is in school. There will still be plenty of time for effective intervention. And try not to blame yourself or anyone else for not having detected the problem earlier. First of all, a baby or toddler can't be tested for the kinds of sophisticated information processing he'll be required to do in school. Also, many children compensate for minor impairments so well that they're not readily apparent. If they're noticed at all, they may be considered just a variation within the normal range.

Some support from a specialist—an occupational, physical, or visual therapist, speech pathologist or psychologist—may be all your child needs to catch up if he has a problem that is slowing him down in school. In our personal experience, weekly occupational therapy sessions for a year in fifth grade was what one of our preemies needed to make up for some delays in fine motor skills and to develop better penmanship. Our other preemie, who was shy and anxious, made tremendous strides in self-confidence when she was given the responsibility of raising a puppy to become a seeing-eye dog. Of course, some minor disabilities are lasting. But the capacity of a child's brain to adapt and create new circuits continues through late childhood and into adulthood, as people who make dramatic recoveries from head injuries or strokes can testify.

Most of all, your parental attention is what's going to give your child the best chance. Many studies confirm that the environment in which a preemie is raised has a huge effect on the development of his brain. Enriching stimulation from a nurturing, attentive family or from a good-quality daycare program can balance out some biological risk factors, enhancing a premature child's intelligence and making behavioral problems less likely. In the meantime, try not to transmit to your child a sense of anxiety or to let apprehension about the future deprive you of the daily surprises, hopes, and pleasures that make parenting such a wonderful experience.

Troublesome Behavior

My toddler can be really impossible. Does that come from his being born prematurely?

Possibly, but more likely it comes from his being a normal toddler. Toddlers specialize in being impossible, no matter how much time they spent in the womb. If you have any doubt about that, just open the nearest parenting book and notice how much advice it contains for parents who are worrying that their toddlers are hyperactive or overly moody or negative or rigid or aggressive. Or, alternatively, for parents who are concerned that their toddlers are the opposite of everyone else's: fearful, hypersensitive, passive, and shy.

No matter how much you know about the common behavior patterns of young children, they can still surprise you when you encounter them close-up in your own child. Toddlers flip-flop from sweetness to violent tantrums at the flick of an invisible switch. They go through periods of extreme negativism and can lash out when they're frustrated, sometimes biting, scratching, and hitting like wild little animals. Some seem like bundles of frenetic energy with an irresistible need to run until they're exhausted. Many resist any changes in their cherished daily routines, making parents yearn for the good old days when they could vary their lunch and dinner menus or go to more than one playground. Remember that even from a very young age, personalities differ, so your child may exhibit some of these characteristics more than his playmates or siblings, while still behaving like a normal toddler.

However, if your child's behavior is so extreme or long-lasting that it worries you or interferes with your relationship and feelings for him, then you should talk to your pediatrician about it. Even though the behavioral development of the majority of preemies is entirely normal, studies have documented more behavior problems in the smallest, youngest-born preemies than in children born at term.

In the first year of life, preemies are reported to be more irritable, less responsive, and less predictable than other infants. (You can read about this and how you might deal with it on page 416.) Fortunately, many of these fussy babies grow into perfectly normal toddlers. Parents of premature toddlers who do have behavior problems typically describe their children as excessively fearful (separation from parents, in particular, may cause great insecurity), or overly active, having difficulty staying still for quiet play or meals. Some parents mention poor self-control coupled with a stubborn willfulness, making the "terrible twos" battles extreme. Of course, it is hard to draw a line between normal temper tantrums and overly aggressive outbursts, so you shouldn't automatically assume that your child's behavior is a reaction to his early birth.

In the majority of children, these difficult behaviors in early childhood soften or vanish spontaneously without any lasting effect. On the other hand, parents and teachers reported in one study of six-year-old children that nearly 20 percent of former preemies had behavior and emotional problems compared with about 3 percent of full-termers. Preemies are more likely to have shorter than normal attention spans, feelings of anxiety, depression, or shyness, and difficulties in their peer relationships. (Preemie boys have more attention and peer problems; preemie girls are more prone to feeling anxious, depressed, or withdrawn.) In preemies with an intellectual disability, hyperactivity and behavior problems are also more common.

Recently, suspicions have been raised that the rate of autism might be somewhat higher in preemies: In a recent study, about 10 percent of two-year-old former preemies scored positive on an autism screening test compared with 6 percent of two-year-olds who were born at term. (This number doesn't count preemies known to have impairments that could be confused with autism.) For a parent with a difficult toddler, this news can be scary, but don't be misled into worrying unnecessarily. A screening test isn't conclusive: many who screen positive won't actually be found to have the disorder as time goes by. Still, it's a good idea to start treatment as soon as possible, even before the diagnosis is confirmed, because autism experts are convinced that early treatment is important for a child to develop to his full potential. In the meantime, you may be able to allay your fears by asking your son's pediatrician or an expert at his preemie follow-up clinic whether any aspects of his behavior are worrisome—or whether they are frustrating, yes, and difficult, yes, but entirely normal.

As preemies reach adolescence and young adulthood, just as in their elementary school years, most are found to have no or only mild behavioral or emotional problems. They continue to be at greater risk than their peers for attention problems and more prone to anxiety, unhappiness, and social withdrawal. On the other hand, preemies are less likely to engage in risky behaviors (such as smoking, drug use, and early sexual activity)—so you can finally sit back and relax while other parents get a turn to do the worrying! But experts debate the reasons why. The glass half-full view is that this is reassuring news, indicating that former preemies are resilient, sensible, and strong; the glass half-empty view is that it's more a matter of overprotective parenting or reflects the anxieties and social isolation of the preemies themselves.

Happily, teenage preemies rate their self-esteem—one of the most important measures of well-being at this age—as high as teenagers who were born at term. Even though parents and teachers continue to report higher rates of inattention in preemie boys and depression in preemie girls, the teens themselves participate as fully in school and social activities as their full-term peers and see themselves as no different. Research hasn't yet established whether prematurity is associated with any severe psychiatric illnesses later in life.

A variety of biological and environmental factors have been blamed for preemies' greater risk of mild behavior and emotional problems. Brain injuries in the newborn period, both obvious ones that result in cognitive difficulties and more subtle disruptions in brain development, may play a role. Some complications of prematurity, such as bronchopulmonary dysplasia or feeding problems, make difficult temperamental traits more likely. Parents may also contribute, by overprotecting their preemies because they view them as fragile or vulnerable. Some parents may be less willing to discipline their children, not wanting to deny them anything after their suffering in the NICU. Some may allow their preemies to rule the roost, because they've labeled them as stubborn, strong, or fighters because of their early will to survive. If you think you fit these descriptions, just being aware of it, and perhaps talking to a friend or counselor, may help you control your anxiety and change your behavior.

What's most important now is feeling good about your child. Thankfully, the world is vibrant because it is full of many different personality types, and while you might be drawn to some more than others, it would be hard to get any two adults to agree on what type is best. Children with attention problems often go on to become successful, high-achieving adults. People who are less social and more introverted can make excellent friends, form wonderful, intimate relationships, be highly creative, and excel in many professions. Included in history's greatest figures are many former preemies—some who were extroverted and combative, others who were introverted and contemplative, some who behaved well by society's standards, and others who pushed the limits. If you would find it reassuring—or, like us, simply find the history fascinating—you can read about a few of them in *I Was a Preemie, Too* on page 569.

It is a good idea, though, to keep your eyes open for any lasting behavior or emotional problems as your child gets older since you will probably be able to help him by getting guidance early. For example, if he is withdrawn and resistant to change, experts suggest that you should try to expose him to different experiences and people in secure environments. Find the right balance: experiences that are difficult enough to stretch him but that make him only mildly, not excruciatingly, anxious. Get excited when he tries something new that is difficult for him, and tell him how proud you are.

You can probably help a lot, but you shouldn't expect to change his personality or feel frustrated if he doesn't become the captain of his sports team. If your toddler is especially aggressive, impulsive, and impetuous, your goal now should be to channel his growing autonomy in the right direction. Experts suggest using firm but noncoercive methods to manage his behavior, such as giving time-outs or withdrawing rewards when he becomes disruptive and giving token rewards, such as points toward a special desired activity, to reinforce good behavior.

If social problems at school go along with a learning disability or if you feel that your child's behavior significantly frustrates his need to interact with other children and his teachers, then it may be worth having him evaluated by a pediatric psychologist, who will judge what kind of therapy may be beneficial to him. You can ask your pediatrician for advice or a referral. Together, you and the experts may be able to lessen his behavioral difficulties and help him put his personal qualities to best use.

Clumsiness

My three-year-old is constantly bumping into things and falling over his feet. Are former preemies clumsier than term children?

Some are, but by no means all. Chances are your child is like every other three-year-old—so busy exploring the world that he doesn't pay enough attention to obstacles in his path, like furniture and walls. That's often true of toddlers, who are very energetic, not aware of their still imperfect control of walking, running, or other movements, and most of all, unafraid of the painful consequences of their falls!

If by age two your preemie has not been diagnosed with a motor problem, such as cerebral palsy, affecting his strength, muscle tone, or agility, and if he's been reaching his developmental milestones at the normal times, then you shouldn't worry that he'll have some serious chronic problem with coordination. Toddlers tend to refine their gross motor skills, like running, skipping, jumping, and climbing, at their own pace, so young children of the same age can differ markedly in how fast, agile, strong and balanced they are. In preschoolers there's also a wide range of coordination in fine motor skills, involving the muscles of the face and hands. Fine motor skills determine visual-motor control (needed, for instance, to catch a ball or eat without making a mess), and hand and finger dexterity (affecting writing and drawing abilities). Only in later childhood do kids' motor skills tend to level out.

Still, there are several reasons—ranging from temporary delays that a child can naturally outgrow to slight abnormalities that can be diagnosed and treated by a specialist—why some preemies might be clumsier than children born at term during their early childhood years:

* Some preemies have slightly turned-in or turned-out legs and feet, making them a little pigeon-toed or duck-toed. This usually goes away by school age. In the meantime, those whose feet turn in tend to be clumsier, and those whose feet turn out tend to be slower. (Being pigeon-toed, by the way, runs in families.)
* Clumsiness can result from the temporary abnormalities of muscle tone that are so common in premature infants. Even if a preemie's tone is now normal, if his muscles were tight when he was learning to roll over, stand up, or walk, he may have gotten used to shifting his weight differently and developed ways of moving that are less fluid or graceful. Because these awkward movements aren't due to an ongoing disorder, former preemies will naturally imitate and practice more graceful movements as they grow older, gradually becoming indistinguishable from their peers. If a child's high or low muscle tone persists, physical therapy is very effective in improving motor control, balance, and body strength.
* Since motor skills and vision are closely related, there might be a subtle eye problem that hasn't yet been diagnosed. For instance, problems with depth perception or double vision can contribute to or cause poor coordination. An ophthalmologist can diagnose these conditions and prescribe corrective lenses, vision therapy (a kind of physical therapy for the eye), or recommend other treatments.
* Ear infections can disrupt the vestibular system and impair a child's sense of balance so that he trips or falls more often than usual. If your child has a history of ear infections, talk to your pediatrician about his clumsiness and ask whether he should be seen by a pediatric ear-nose-and-throat specialist.
* The natural exuberance of toddlers can be heightened in preemies, who may have even shorter attention spans and be more impulsive. As a result, they may just run into things more! This can be perfectly normal, but if you think your child is much more active and easily distracted than other toddlers, talk to your pediatrician about your concerns. Preemies are more prone to hyperactivity and attention deficit disorder, which are difficult to diagnose before school age. He might keep a closer eye on your son, and recommend an evaluation by a child psychologist when the right time comes.
* Minor lasting impairments in gross and fine motor skills are found in about a quarter of former preemies by the time they are eight years old. These children don't have significant disabilities but are more apt to be described by their parents as clumsy, to have worse penmanship, and to be less coordinated and athletic than their term-born peers. Mild motor disabilities often show up later than more severe ones, which are usually evident by the time a child is two years old.

If, when your child is five, you notice that he's still not keeping up with the other children in games, sports, writing or drawing, or if his movements looked normal when he was a toddler but appeared clumsier when he started school, you should mention it to your pediatrician and consider getting a referral for a developmental evaluation. (This can be done free through your local health department or public school district.) If your child's developmental evaluation shows some delays in gross or fine motor skills, your local public education agency will arrange for him to receive any special therapy or equipment he may need. Or you can ask your pediatrician to refer you to a private therapist, whose fees might be covered by your health plan.

Physical and occupational therapy can greatly help a child's coordination, and it's never too late for successful treatment. Physical therapy is aimed at gross motor skills, improving balance, muscle tone, strength, and endurance. Occupational therapy focuses on fine motor skills, enhancing a child's eye-hand coordination and his ability to use a pen, spoon and fork, or any other tools. Even if physical activity will never be your child's strong suit, it's important that he get help so that he can keep up in gym and not worry about being teased. And penmanship, as well as other good manual skills, are essential for your child to be successful and feel good about himself at school.

Your child also needs support from you, his family and friends. Try to accept his awkwardness and deal with it gently, never emphasizing it, and reassuring him if he has any concerns about it. So he's a little less dexterous than some other kids. Focus on his strengths; he surely has many, even if athletic strength isn't one of them. To enhance his coordination and self-confidence, encourage him to do noncompetitive sports, and enroll him in a relaxed extracurricular physical education program, if you can. Besides sports, playing a musical instrument, dancing, doing karate, or any activity with rhythm and body movement may do marvels for your son's well-being and self-esteem while enhancing his motor skills. Who knows? Maybe one of these pursuits will even become your child's forte!

Teeth

Our baby's teeth are coming in late, and a few of them look funny. Does being premature affect a baby's teeth?

If you correct your baby's age, you'll probably find that her teeth aren't coming in especially late but at just about the right time. Most preemies get their first teeth around six to ten months of age, just like term babies do, but counting from their due date rather than their birthday. If you're still worried, a pediatric dentist can reassure you that she's not missing any teeth. Then be prepared to sit back and relax for quite a while. When it comes to teeth, you'll have to correct your daughter's age for many years, longer than for other developmental milestones: According to studies, most former preemies don't catch up to term-born children in tooth eruption until they are nine years old. Only later will you be able to count on the tooth fairy's usual calendar.

The enamel (the hard white coating) of preemies' baby teeth is often slightly underdeveloped or irregular, causing some teeth to be shaped a little unusually, or to have opaque white spots. The upper front teeth are most often affected. This happens mainly because a premature baby's teeth are becoming mineralized right around the time of her birth. The supply of calcium and phosphorus—the principal minerals in tooth enamel—may be disrupted not only by an early delivery (a fetus gets huge amounts of calcium and phosphorus from her mother through the placenta) but also by low oxygen and high bilirubin levels, some medications, and a less-than-perfect diet. Thus the younger and sicker a baby was at birth, the more likely she is to have some abnormalities in her enamel. Early trauma to the gums can also cause problems. Some researchers think that when a baby is put on a ventilator, the instrument used to insert the breathing tube presses against her gums and may damage the developing teeth inside, or that the presence of the breathing tube itself may cause damage.

Since a tooth with an imperfect coat of enamel is in theory more prone to cavities, you should be especially careful about brushing your daughter's teeth twice a day and never put her to bed with a bottle unless it contains plain water. Ask your pediatrician to refer you to a pediatric dentist, if he hasn't done so already; preemies need to have their first dental visit scheduled early, around their first birthday. The dentist will be able to reassure you about the effectiveness of good oral hygiene: studies have found that former preemies, despite their common enamel defects, don't have a higher incidence of tooth decay than children born at term. Frequent dental checkups will help you pick up any problems soon and get the maximum possible protection (such as fluoride treatments and sealants) for your daughter's teeth.

Preemies' permanent teeth have enamel irregularities less often than their baby teeth do, although still about twice as often as those of term-born children. But most of these imperfections are so small that they are practically unnoticeable to anyone but a child's parents or dentist. If your daughter finds her teeth really bothersome when she grows up, she can get porcelain veneers or another cosmetic treatment to give her a perfect smile. Just remember that several beauties with irregular teeth, such as Madonna and Kate Moss, refused to fix theirs, preferring their own special smiles and original beauty.

Emotional Aftershocks

My daughter is two years old now, happier and healthier than ever, but I'm still feeling the aftershocks of her premature birth and hospitalization. Will I ever be able to recover my old self and put my life back together?

You're certainly not alone in suffering the lingering effects of a premature birth. Plenty of parents of former preemies have said that although much of the distress caused by their baby's birth receded after a few months, it never vanished completely. Having seen their newborns so frail and struggling to live without being able to help them can leave many parents with an enduring sense of insecurity. The effect of having gone through such a painful, life-changing experience can stay with families for many years, and often forever.

The aftershocks of a child's premature birth can take many forms. Some parents report recurring dreams; intense reactions to certain sounds, images, or smells that remind them of the NICU; or a reappearance of pain and fear when their children are sick, even with trivial illnesses like colds. Just hearing that their child is ill may bring uncontrollable tears. Some parents admit that they've given up friends, hobbies, or jobs so they can spend all of their time with their precious children, who have become the sole focus of their lives. Others can't deal with the idea of becoming pregnant again because of the painful memories it stirs up or the fear of having another preemie. More than half of the parents in a series of follow-up studies of extremely premature babies in Canada said that they hadn't had more children and that their decision was influenced by having experienced the premature birth.

Another ripple effect can be marital problems, especially if partners have different ways of coping with emotional distress. If one parent was unable to talk about her grief or fear, the other may have felt isolated and abandoned. One partner may have resented the other's anger, or guilt, or obsession with medical details, or retreat into work. Turning the page, forgiving and reconciling, may be harder than usual because the painful episodes occurred when both parents were particularly vulnerable and needy. A couple may not even be completely aware of the role that their premature baby's birth played in their eroding relationship. But fortunately, after having gone through such a difficult experience together, many more couples end up finding each other again and feeling closer than end up separating.

Suffering that lingers underneath the surface and is periodically refueled by events that rekindle feelings of sadness and loss has been called chronic sorrow. The expression was first applied to parents of children with special needs. Those parents struggle, often for their whole lives, to gradually let go of various plans and dreams and come up with others that are meaningful. Even for parents of relatively healthy premature infants, chronic sorrow may last through infancy and for several years afterward while preemies are still perceived as fragile and at risk for health and developmental problems. During this period, a rehospitalization, a developmental evaluation, a baby shower or birthday party, even a banal situation like watching toddlers play in a sandbox, may revive old anxieties and sorrow.

Some psychologists have compared the reactions of parents of preemies to post-traumatic stress disorder (PTSD). That comparison makes sense to the many parents who have been haunted by nightmares or terrifying flashbacks brought on by seemingly innocent things like an unexpected nighttime telephone call, seeing a striped baby hat, or even just walking out the door. Like soldiers returning from war, they too may find themselves constantly on the lookout—perhaps waking up to check on their baby several times a night or scouring every surface their baby may come

in contact with to free it of germs. Some parents of former premature babies report that they have difficulty falling or staying asleep, are jumpy and irritable, and have problems concentrating: reactions that are typical of both post-traumatic stress disorder and depression.

Chances are, you recognize yourself in some of these descriptions—nearly all parents of preemies do. You would not be diagnosed with PTSD or clinical depression, however, unless you suffered from a sizable cluster of severe, frequently recurrent or persistent symptoms. You can read more about PTSD on page 428 and if it does sound like you, know that psychotherapy and medications have been found to be very effective treatments. And even if you're having a milder reaction to your premature baby's birth, that doesn't mean you aren't suffering or that you wouldn't benefit from some kind of professional counseling.

Although the psychological aftershocks of a premature birth may last through your child's toddler years, you should expect them to become progressively milder. Psychologists studying the reactions of parents of preemies have found that by two years after a baby's premature birth, their mothers, on average, are no more anxious or depressed than mothers of term babies. Mothers of preemies who have more health problems tend to have longer-lasting psychological distress. (Just remember that you're experiencing some things that all parents go through with a new baby and raising a child. Adding a new member to a family is stressful, even when it's mainly full of delights. And ripples in a child's health or happiness can make any mother or father emotionally vulnerable.)

To make your recovery easier, it's important to communicate with relatives, friends, and trusted counselors who can understand your feelings and help you make sense of them. Spending all of your time with your child may soothe some of your anxieties, but it will give rise to others. Remember that to be a good parent you need to be able to enjoy yourself and show your child how partners, friends, and meaningful pastimes can enrich one's life. It's a good bet that if you reach out, you'll be rewarded; in the Canadian follow-up study, more than half of the parents of preemies said that they felt more understood by their friends and relatives after the premature birth.

If you don't feel that you're making emotional progress or if your recovery is too slow for comfort, counseling can often help to resolve some lingering issues. Definitely seek counseling if you find that your fears are getting out of hand, if you can't function at home or work, or if you find yourself in a deep state of bereavement that doesn't abate. You can get treatment for what could be a bout of depression. If your partner is the one who's suffering, don't hesitate to ask your family doctor to refer him to a therapist.

Couples counseling can be beneficial if you're experiencing marital problems. Don't be skeptical—it really can work. Sometimes just by committing to work on their union, a couple realizes how much their relationship still means to them and takes the first crucial steps toward each other. Counseling can help point out how elements in both partners' histories and emotional makeup influenced their reactions to their child's premature birth. Don't lose hope: Many couples, with or without the help of therapy, succeed in working their way out of this crisis and reconcile. Parents who cling to each other during the hardest times or who are able to get back together after a crisis often build the strongest families.

Most parents say that giving birth to a premature baby has deeply changed them and their attitudes toward other events and life choices. Everyone's path is different, but you'll probably also realize that your suffering has not been useless and that you've grown in awareness, maturity, ability to assign things their proper value, and basic human understanding. Although it may not feel soon enough—time will heal you, too.

Thinking about Another Pregnancy

We've always wanted to have another child, but we're scared of having another preemie.

Of course you're scared—anyone who had been through this wrenching experience would be afraid, for themselves and their future baby, to think of it happening all over again. But that's exactly why you should know that the outlook isn't all bleak.

You might have heard that after one premature delivery, a woman has a 20 percent to 50 percent chance (studies vary) of having another preemie. But depending on the circumstances of your first delivery, your chances of bringing your next pregnancy to term could be much better. If there's a known preventable or treatable reason that you gave birth early, you may be able to do something about it. Be sure to discuss this with your obstetrician—the sooner the better, because there are changes you might want to make before you conceive for them to be most effective. If you don't know why you went into preterm labor, you still may be able to reduce your chances of having another preemie by getting progesterone shots, a treatment that is the greatest recent breakthrough in the quest to prevent prematurity.

In *Previous Premature Delivery* on page 17, you'll find more details about how to minimize your risk after having had a preemie already. Also take a look at Appendix 1 on page 575 for a list and brief explanation of what doctors currently think are the main risk factors for delivering prematurely. With this information in hand and your obstetrician's guidance, you may identify things to do differently before or after you become pregnant again—and you may feel reassured.

If you and your obstetrician conclude that a second premature delivery is likely, you'll know much better than you did before what you're up against and what kind of hurdles you, your family, and your new baby may have to face. Take some time to ponder, alone and with your partner and other trusted friends and counselors, what it might be like to add a second preemie to your family—and what it might be like not to. Armed with greater knowledge and understanding, you can make a careful, considered decision.

IN DEPTH

What You Need to Know about RSV

You've probably had RSV many times in your life. Short for respiratory syncytial virus, RSV is a very contagious virus that gives most people a plain old common cold. (Any cold you catch may be from RSV or from one of a few dozen other cold viruses.) Most children get RSV at least once before they're two years old.

While RSV isn't discriminating in whom it infects, it does affect some people differently from others. In older children or adults it usually triggers nothing more than a cold, but in infants it can be more serious. The virus may cause not just an upper respiratory infection, with symptoms like sniffles, sneezes, and fever, but also a lower respiratory infection, such as pneumonia or bronchiolitis (an infection of the small airways in the lung), with breathing problems that can be serious enough to require hospitalization. Some babies even need to go on a ventilator while they fight off the virus. In a few cases (less than 5 percent), it can be fatal.

Although the chance of the average preemie having such a serious problem is very small, it's worth knowing about RSV and the preventive therapies that are available, in case your child is at high risk.

Which Babies Are at Risk

RSV is a seasonal virus that you don't need to worry about much in the warmer months. It's mainly around during the cold season, making an appearance typically in October and departing in April.

The two groups that are most likely to be hospitalized with RSV are preemies and full-term infants with chronic respiratory conditions. Both are prone to breathing problems, and preemies have two additional disadvantages. Their airways are very small, so any swelling or mucus there is more apt to cause problems with breathing. Also, their immune systems are immature, and they lack some or all of the protective antibodies against RSV that they would have received from their mothers in the last trimester of pregnancy.

Not all preemies are at equal risk, though. Most vulnerable are those who are under two years old and have bronchopulmonary dysplasia (BPD) or congenital heart disease. Next come other preemies who don't have BPD or heart conditions but are less than six months old when the cold season starts. As these preemies get older and bigger, their vulnerability declines. Once they are past their first winter, if they are healthy, the chance that they'll get seriously ill from RSV is remote.

These numbers may help put things in perspective. In a study that followed premature babies for one cold season, about 8 percent of preemies who were healthy and younger than six months old and about 13 percent of those who had BPD and were younger than two years old were hospitalized with RSV.

Other risk factors that come into play are:

* Preemies who were born earlier, especially at less than 28 weeks of gestation, are more vulnerable than those who were born later;

* Boys are more at risk than girls;
* Formula-fed preemies are more at risk than those who are breastfed;
* Preemies who are in group child care or have school-age siblings are more likely to be exposed to the virus;
* Preemies who have a smoker in their household may be at greater risk of being hospitalized if they catch RSV.

How to Recognize Whether Your Baby Has RSV

The first symptoms of RSV are usually those of a cold, such as a runny or stuffed nose, sneezing, coughing, or fever, along with general symptoms of sickness like irritability, lethargy, or poor feeding. If your preemie has BPD or is less than six months old, or if you're just feeling worried, don't hesitate to take her to the doctor at this point. He'll make sure she's handling the cold OK and can do a simple test to find out whether she has RSV by swabbing her nose with a tiny Q-tip. If he has the necessary laboratory equipment, he may even be able to give you the results on the spot. Some parents find it's worth going to the doctor to find out that their baby doesn't have RSV just so they can relax. But even if your baby does have RSV, it probably won't progress beyond a slight cold. Most likely, you and your doctor will just watch your baby more closely.

If her RSV does get worse and becomes a lower respiratory infection, you'll notice that your baby will have more trouble breathing: She may wheeze, suck in her chest deeply, her nostrils may flare widely with each breath, and she may breathe rapidly or have spells of apnea. If you notice any of these symptoms, call the doctor right away. He's the best judge of whether your baby needs help with her breathing or other medical support and whether it would be safer for

her to be in the hospital while she fights off the virus.

Treatment of RSV

Just as there's no cure for the common cold, there's no cure for RSV. When a baby gets the virus, the important things are to keep her nourished and breathing adequately while her body's immune system does its job of fighting the infection off.

If your child has cold symptoms, you can help her breathe more easily by keeping her room humid with a humidifier or vaporizer (be sure to clean them every day according to the instructions because their humid surfaces are a great breeding ground for bacteria and fungi that could make your baby's breathing problems even worse) and by elevating the head of her bed a little (you can place some towels or a stack of books under one end of her mattress). Saline nose drops can also be a big help (why humidify just her room, and not her nose itself?) by thinning the mucus and rinsing out her nose. You'll find them in drugstores sold in squeeze bottles. Try to keep your baby well hydrated, which at her age doesn't have to mean large quantities of fluids. Even a few teaspoons of liquid every hour, whether milk, formula, water, or Pedialyte (a liquid that contains salts and sugar and is sold in many drugstores and baby stores), is usually enough.

If your child is wheezing, it probably indicates that she has bronchiolitis. The doctor may try treating her with an inhaled steroid or bronchodilator (the same medications that might be used for asthma) to help open up her airways so she can breathe more easily. Studies are mixed on whether this helps with RSV, so if your child develops more than very mild respiratory distress or her oxygen levels are low, the doctor will probably recommend that she go to the hospital where her breathing can be monitored carefully. She may not need much more than monitoring and plenty of fluids through an IV. If she's having a lot of trouble breathing, she'll also get supplemental oxygen or, in rare cases, will be put on a ventilator.

Having your preemie rehospitalized, when you've had her home so briefly, can be heartbreaking. For parents whose baby had a rough hospital course the first time, it can also be terrifying. But if you can, try to see the hospital as the safest, most comfortable place for her to be, where she'll be supported, enabling her to do the best possible job of battling the virus. You can read more about rehospitalization of preemies on page 452.

Keep in mind, so you won't worry excessively, that it's normal for babies with RSV to get sicker before they get better. Within a week or so, most babies recover enough to go right back home with their parents.

Should You Isolate Your Child?

All of this makes it tempting to want to build a protective wall around your child, isolating her from the sneezes, coughs, hands, and kisses of well-meaning but germ-ridden people. That's understandable. If your child is still at a point where she's at risk of getting very sick from RSV, taking a certain amount of precaution, especially in the late fall, winter, and early spring, is wise—such as keeping her out of daycare, forbidding visits by friends or relatives who have colds, and washing your hands frequently. But also remember that there's a limit to how much isolation is good for you or your preemie. You'll find some suggestions on page 383.

Prevention of RSV

Vaccines can prevent illnesses like measles, mumps, and whooping cough, but unfortunately, there is not yet a vaccine for RSV. The way a vaccine works is to stimulate the body's immune system to produce its own infection-fighting antibodies against an illness. A second-best but still valuable measure is to get the antibodies from somewhere else. That's what a preventive treatment, called Synagis, provides for RSV: special RSV-fighting antibodies. Research has shown that this treatment doesn't stop babies from getting the virus altogether, but does cut by about half the number of babies who get so ill that they need to be hospitalized.

Synagis is given to a baby as a shot, in a doctor's office. Babies go for three to five monthly shots during RSV season, usually getting their first dose in November and their last in March.

The American Academy of Pediatrics recommends Synagis for your baby at the start of RSV season if:

* She has BPD, is less than two years old, and has received medical treatment for respiratory problems within the past six months;
* She was born at 28 weeks of gestation or less and is younger than 12 months old;
* She was born between 29 and 32 weeks of gestation and is younger than six months old;
* She was born between 32 weeks and 35 weeks of gestation is younger than three months old, and also attends group childcare or has siblings at home who are younger than five years;
* She has heart disease, moderate to severe pulmonary hypertension, a congenital abnormality of her airway, or a neuromuscular disease that affects her breathing.

True, the protection Synagis offers is far from perfect: Some babies will still need to be hospitalized; and of those who are, there is little evidence that they will have a less serious illness than they would have otherwise. But there is only a minor risk of adverse reactions, such as fever or pain at the site of the shot, and the overridingly valuable chance that this treatment could help avoid a serious illness and hospitalization.

A few pointers to plan your baby's Synagis treatment may be helpful. Since you'll have to make monthly trips to the doctor, where it's possible your baby could pick up some germs that she would have avoided if she'd stayed home, try to make the first appointment of your pediatrician's day when there will be fewer kids in the waiting room and you're least likely to be kept waiting. The cost of the treatment is steep, over $1,000 a month, so be sure to find out whether your insurance will cover it, as most do. Finally, many parents hate exposing their baby to even a little extra pain from a shot each month. If your baby is going to be getting monthly anti-RSV injections, you may want to give her a pacifier dipped in sugar water right before and during the shot. This simple homespun remedy has been shown to be an effective pain reliever for preemies. A few other nonmedical ways to relieve pain in preemies are explained on page 118. And if they seem to help your child, you can also use them for any other shots or blood drawing she might need as well.

CHAPTER 9

WHEN PARENTS HAVE SOMETHING SPECIAL TO WORRY ABOUT

. . . .

Learning more about some possible consequences of prematurity.

. . . .

INTRODUCTION: WHEN PARENTS HAVE SOMETHING SPECIAL TO WORRY ABOUT

If your child has special needs, you are going to need more detailed information and support than this chapter can give you, but it is a good place to start. You may need to learn to deal with a radical change in perspective, practical problems you've never thought about, and new, powerful, and contrasting feelings—possibly without role models to follow. You and your baby will need time to adjust, to find your own path, advisers, special sources of information, and support. Learning more about a disability may frighten you initially but may also make you feel better, because reality can often be more reassuring than what you fear. Most of all, you will discover that there's a lot you can do to help your child live well with his condition and develop to his full potential.

Much as it might comfort you, you shouldn't think of early intervention and other special services as a cure. What they do is help a child work with and around his disability so that the disability doesn't unnecessarily impede his development in other areas. For example, a child with very poor sight will be given special lenses to improve his vision as much as possible. But providing him with nonvisual ways of taking in information will probably make a greater difference. A child with a motor disability that affects his face and mouth will be given exercises to build up his strength and flexibility. Some children may never be able to speak clearly, but they may be taught to communicate extremely well by typing on a computerized communication board, even with a single finger. By giving a child alternative ways to develop knowledge and skills, special services can be the impetus that gets a child's development back on track, helping him do his best.

You are likely to find that doctors (except those who specialize in child development) are not the best source for finding and negotiating the maze of possible resources for your child. The school system, the public health department, your child's service coordinator, your hospital's social worker, and other parents with children in similar situations will often be a lot more helpful and informed. A word of warning, though: Be sure to be careful about things you hear from nonprofessional sources. Claims of miracle cures—or the opposite, major problems that pop up suddenly and unexpectedly—are often not based entirely on fact. There are innumerable web sites on special needs and many of them are useful for opening up possibilities and pointing you in interesting directions. But always be wary of possible inaccuracies and of marketing and promotional web pages—for a therapy, a device, or professional services—that at a first glance may appear like objective sources of information but are really designed to sell you something. When you come across a promising lead, by all means follow it up and be aggressive and innovative in looking for resources for your child, but don't leave your critical faculties behind.

You are probably going to find that accepting your child's limitations is a process that gets easier over time and comes more naturally than you might think. Just consider examples from your own life. You may never speak a foreign language, or climb a mountain, or paint a portrait—and by now that's probably OK with you. It's just not part of who you are. What you do often and well, though, probably means a lot to you and to the friends and loved ones who know you well. You'll find a similar thing happens with your child—you'll help him hone some skills, come to value the things he can do, and dismiss the things he can't. Every child, with or without special needs, has weak areas and strong ones. Your responsibility will be to provide your child with opportunities for growth by helping him improve his weaknesses, for sure, but mainly by focusing on his strengths. That is what most parents naturally do anyway.

Your attitude will rub off on your child. It may surprise you to know that in a survey asking people with disabilities what one thing they would change about themselves if they could, most chose something other than their disability. It just shows how one can celebrate the person one is and be fulfilled in the life one has.

QUESTIONS AND ANSWERS

Why Do We Need Early Intervention?

I'm energetic, I read a lot, I'm going to be home with my child. What can an early intervention program possibly do that I can't?

If your child has been referred to an early intervention program, you shouldn't think that your parental skills or dynamism have been underestimated or disregarded. On the contrary, your personal qualities are going to be put to good use because a main tenet of early childhood intervention is that nobody has a more powerful effect on a baby than his parents.

According to government regulations, early intervention services are family-centered, meaning they are there to assist a baby and his family, providing them with information, skills, and support. A referral for early childhood intervention can be made by you—the parent—or by your baby's doctor, nurse, social worker, caregiver, or any other specialist. But from this point on, you alone are going to be in the driver's seat because your participation is needed for each of the steps that follow, and nothing can happen without your consent.

After the initial referral, an early intervention service coordinator will contact you and begin to work at your side. She will listen to your concerns, help you schedule a screening evaluation for your child, and inform you about the care he can get through the early childhood intervention program. Later you will meet with your service coordinator and some members of the team who did the evaluation to organize your individualized family service plan—an early intervention plan that's especially designed for your child, you, and your family. You will choose a time and place to meet that's convenient for you; if you like, you will lead the discussion about your child's needs, what you and the specialists think would work best for him, and what your expectations are; and you'll also be able to invite your extended family, friends, or anyone else whose opinion you trust to the meeting.

Convincing data on the efficacy of early intervention services in premature babies come from a nationwide study called the Infant Health and Development Program, involving nearly 1,000 preemies who were randomly assigned to get either routine medical care or intensive early intervention services until they were three years old. The early intervention services consisted of parent support group meetings, home visits several times a month (to help families better understand child development, provide appropriate toys and activities for their infant or toddler, and deal with behavioral or other problems), and attendance at a developmental daycare center for at least four hours a day, five days a week, beginning when the child was 12 months old. Compared with preemies who got just regular pediatric follow-up, at

three years of age those who also got early intervention had on average higher IQs and were rated by their parents to have fewer behavior problems. The improvement in intelligence was greatest for preemies who weighed more than 2,000 grams at birth, although smaller preemies benefited, too. The improvement in behavior was significant only for preemies whose mothers did not have a college education.

Long-term follow-up research on the same group of children showed that the benefits of early intervention lasted through childhood and young adulthood in the bigger former preemies but not in the ones who weighed less than 2,000 grams at birth. Don't let this discourage you if you have a smaller preemie; it may simply be that some interventions need to be carried on longer for the youngest preemies to get lifelong benefits, and your child could benefit more than the average child in the nationwide study.

Early intervention services are usually provided by an infant-toddler development specialist (a specially trained psychologist, social worker or graduate of a school of education). The infant-toddler development specialist will work with you and your child to help him develop at his best, and may also get help from professionals from other disciplines (see pages 495–496 for a summary of what each one does) who will bring additional valuable experience and expertise as well as knowledge about useful resources.

You'll be counted on to practice exercises at home, as that's the best way for your child to learn new skills. You can also make up creative games that build on the exercises or make them more fun, so you'll have ample opportunities to help your child take his developmental steps forward. And since you'll be the main source of information on your child's situation and progress and be involved in all decisions concerning your child, you should always feel in charge.

(Continued on page 498)

Getting Acquainted with:
Early Childhood Intervention Services

The idea behind early intervention is that when it comes to children's development, preventing is better than correcting. Whether a child has a diagnosed developmental delay or is simply considered at risk for one, the earlier an intervention program is begun, the better the results.

The reason is that every individual skill or ability can influence a child's overall developmental progress. For instance, a baby who has trouble moving may not be able to explore his environment freely. As a result, his learning will be more limited, so he may understand fewer things. Even his language skills can suffer because his lack of exposure provides him with fewer concepts and words for objects and activities, and he may have additional trouble communicating because with a movement disorder his body language may be less expressive. As he grows older, his independence and sense of self-worth could be affected, too. Fortunately, many developmental delays can be prevented, corrected, or at least lessened if the right stimulation and exposure occur.

Who is entitled to early intervention

Early childhood intervention services for babies and toddlers are mandated and funded by the federal government under the Individuals with Disabilities Education Act (IDEA). Although IDEA guides how states and public agencies provide early intervention and special education services, the particulars of each program differ somewhat from state to state. In every state, infants and toddlers between birth and three years of age are entitled to early intervention services if they have a diagnosed developmental delay (meaning they lag behind other children their age) in either:

* Physical development (growth, and fine and gross motor skills);
* Cognitive development (thinking, learning, and problem-solving skills);
* Communication (understanding language and using it);
* Social-emotional development (ability to socialize);
* Adaptive development (self-help skills, such as feeding).

Children are also eligible for early intervention if they have a condition that carries a high probability of a future developmental delay, such as periventricular leukomalacia (PVL), severe chronic lung disease (BPD), or hearing loss. Each state has its own interpretation of developmental delay and its own list of high probability conditions. For example, in some states, all premature babies with birth weights of 1,500 grams or less are included, as are bigger preemies with complicated medical histories and difficult family situations. In other states, only much smaller or sicker babies are considered at risk.

To find out more about your state's early intervention program, you can call the state agency in charge of the program. In your state, it may be part of the Department of Education or of Health and Human Resources, or it may be a distinct department of its own. Your county health department, public school guidance counselor, and preemie follow-up clinic can also give you information and tell you where to call. Other excellent sources of information for you are national organizations dedicated to supporting children with special needs, such as NECTAC (National Early Childhood Technical Assistance Center: on the web at www.nectac.org or by phone at 919–962–2001) and NICHCY (the National Dissemination Center for Children with Disabilities: on the web at www.nichcy .org or by phone at 800–695–0285). Both organizations' web sites have useful links for each state.

Referral

Premature infants are usually referred for early intervention services by their hospital at discharge, a preemie follow-up clinic, or another medical professional. Parents, relatives, or anyone who's in close contact with a child can request a referral from his pediatrician or even initiate one themselves. (For information, check with NECTAC or NICHCY, above.) Don't be intimidated by the paperwork that may be required, and don't let anybody or anything discourage you if you think your child needs to be evaluated: Developmental experts are convinced that a parent's concern is the most powerful indicator of a developmental delay. On the other hand, parental consent is required at each stage, so you have the right to refuse evaluations and services or even to leave the program at any time.

Once your child has been referred, he'll be assigned a child-service coordinator, who will contact you. The child-service coordinator's job is to listen to you, give you information about your child's rights and the services available through the early intervention program, and assist you in scheduling a free evaluation to determine whether your child is eligible.

This first evaluation may be a simple screening by the child-service coordinator or another specialist, or a more extensive evaluation by several specialists. Premature babies are usually evaluated soon after their discharge from the hospital, after a referral is made by their neonatologist. If your baby is doing well and doesn't have a condition that is known to cause developmental delays, the child service coordinator may decide simply to reevaluate him periodically, or conclude that further follow-up is unnecessary. (A second referral can always be made in the future if you or your baby's doctor see a need for it.)

After an evaluation, if your child does qualify for early intervention services, the child-service coordinator will invite you and your family to a meeting to work out an individual family service plan. This written document will include:

* your child's medical history;
* the results of his latest developmental evaluation;
* information about your resources, concerns, and developmental goals for your child;
* an overview of the early intervention services your child needs;
* a list of the public or private professionals who will provide them, how often, and where;
* any applicable financial arrangements.

Eligible children and their families are entitled to a child-service coordinator at no cost. Other early intervention services beyond that are usually free for children on Medicaid, but most private insurers don't cover them fully, or at all. Many early intervention providers will help out by charging for their services on a sliding scale based on the family's income.

Meet the early intervention team

Your child's early intervention team may include, along with an infant-toddler development specialist, professionals from such diverse fields as:

* **physical therapy,** to help with his gross motor development—strength, balance, coordination, and the ability to control his movements and get around;

* **occupational therapy,** to improve his fine motor and self-help skills—the ability to manipulate things with his hands and to feed, dress, clean, and otherwise care for himself. Occupational therapy can also help if your child has sensory processing problems; see page 507;

* **audiology,** to assess his hearing and provide hearing aids;

* **speech and language therapy,** to help him understand and develop speech or to address feeding problems;

* **vision services,** to assess his vision and provide glasses or special lenses;

* **special education,** including sign language classes for hearing-impaired children, early education for blind children, and stimulation-enriched environments for infants at risk for cognitive delays;

* **psychology,** to facilitate cognitive and behavioral development, given a child's particular temperament and activity level;

* **nursing,** to provide home health care and specialized medical services;

* **social work,** to assess the impact of a fragile child on a family and to help locate and arrange for special resources, such as financial aid, transportation, specialized schooling, and respite care.

Several professionals may work with your child, individually or together. Alternatively, one therapist (usually an infant-toddler development specialist) will be assigned to your child and will provide a wide range of interventions with periodic input from her colleagues. The child-service coordinator is responsible for encouraging communication and sharing of expertise among team members and for flexibly addressing the family's needs and preferences.

The best setting for early intervention services is an environment that is natural for the child, for example, his home or a childcare center. Since the main occupation of a child is playing, which is crucial for his overall development, age-appropriate and skill-appropriate play is an intervention tool, as well as one of the primary goals of therapy. Some children may benefit from the presence of other children, while others may respond better to therapy if they are alone. The choice of setting is worked out by the service coordinator and the family, with the family having the right to modify the location and to choose from public or private specialists.

At any time, parents, the child-service coordinator, or another medical professional may request a complete formal evaluation of a child's development. If for some reason you're not happy with the specialists assigned to your child, you may also request changes there, although some options may be limited, depending on the resources in your county and region.

When does early intervention end?

The opportunity to assess whether the goals for your child are being met comes every six months when you and your coordinator meet to review his individual family service plan, and also when your child gets a complete developmental evaluation. Most early intervention programs schedule a complete developmental evaluation at around 18 months of age (some states do it earlier, some later). It can be done at your preemie's follow-up clinic or at your county's public health department or child developmental evaluation center. (Public developmental evaluations are usually excellent, so you shouldn't feel that private is better.

Plus, they're free.) When these evaluations take place, most parents feel that early intervention is a success story because the benefits, whether small or large, all can improve a child's quality of life. Once a baby or toddler is consistently reaching the developmental milestones appropriate for his corrected age, he'll be discharged from early intervention.

Sometime after your child's second birthday, it will be time to start thinking about preschool. If at that point he's still receiving early intervention services, you and your coordinator will plan together to have him evaluated by the local Commission on Preschool Special Education (CPSE). This step is very important to make sure that there's no interruption in the developmental support he's receiving and to ensure a smooth transition to the school system.

Like early childhood intervention services, public special education services are mandated and funded by federal law. The public preschool education system in your state may be called childcare, Head Start, Universal Pre-Kindergarten, nursery school, or something else. (If you are considering sending your child to a private preschool, be sure to discuss this with your child service coordinator so that you can hear the pros and cons of being outside the public system.)

The preschool special education evaluation will include an interview with you and a physical and psychological assessment of your child. If he is found eligible to receive special education support, the local CPSE will devise an individual education plan for him that lists both short-term and long-term goals and recommends any services, adaptive equipment, or special transportation that he needs. The school system will then provide these to him for free. (If you disagree with the decision about your child's eligibility,

If Your Child Didn't Qualify for Early Intervention

Sometimes a child won't qualify for early intervention services but his parents or doctor are still convinced that he needs extra help. That's not surprising: Unless the evaluator said that your child is normal, not qualifying doesn't necessarily mean there's nothing wrong. What it means is that your child's developmental delays, if he has any, are not severe enough to meet the program's criteria. The same is true for public special education services.

Even if your child isn't eligible for early intervention, if you think that he could benefit from professional help, don't hesitate to try to get it. What you can do is ask your child-service coordinator or local early intervention office for its list of providers (your pediatrician can help you locate therapists, too) and call them directly to arrange for private therapy for your child. Fortunately, Medicaid will often pay for these private services even when a child's delays are too mild to qualify for early intervention. Private insurance is less apt to cover them, unfortunately.

you may request a second evaluation free of charge.)

By law, the priority of preschool special education is to offer a child the extra help he needs to be included in a mainstream preschool classroom. The idea is to make sure that he gets not only expert attention but also the daily interactions with other kids that he needs to blossom.

According to many parents with experience, you should beware of one pitfall: It can be hard to tell people about shortcomings you perceive in your own child. So not surprisingly, some parents find themselves exaggerating to the therapists what their child can do or practicing things they know he'll be evaluated on so he'll perform better. Although this is a natural reaction, you should try hard to combat it. It may briefly make you feel more comfortable to present your child as more polished than he actually is, but it won't do him any good if he doesn't get the help he needs.

On the whole, you should feel glad that you're not your preemie's therapist and that the early intervention team is there to fall back on. If you were the sole provider, it would be easy to let a home therapy program completely take over your daily routine. But constant pressure and excessive attention aren't beneficial to your child in the long run, and they can drain you of energy, causing frustration and making the rest of your family feel neglected. Free play, activities, and interactions with family and friends are just as important as planned intervention for your child's development. With professional support, when the time for exercises and therapies is over, you can forget them—letting your child be just a child, with you, just his loving, committed parent, by his side.

Hearing Loss

How well can a hearing aid restore my child's hearing?

A hearing aid amplifies sounds, making them louder, but can't restore hearing as thoroughly and immediately as glasses can restore vision. Since making sounds louder doesn't always make them clearer, hearing and speech therapy is also needed to help a child understand what he hears.

As soon as your preemie is fitted with a hearing aid, he should begin working with a speech and language therapist, who will follow him throughout childhood. The therapist will help him learn how to listen to sounds and make the most of the hearing he has (95 percent of hearing-impaired children have some) and to develop his language skills, using spoken language only or a combination of speech and sign language.

Although hearing loss is usually a life-long condition, with patience and training an infant can benefit greatly from a hearing aid. If you've never met people with hearing loss before and seen what successful, enjoyable, normal lives they lead, you may not be imagining your child's future to be as open and bright as it is. Very few endeavors will be closed to him.

On the other hand, you shouldn't underestimate your child's needs. The sooner a baby is fitted with a hearing aid and begins hearing and speech therapy, the better he will be able to talk and to understand spoken language. If a hearing loss is not discovered and compensated for by about six months of corrected age, a toddler can develop significant speech and language delays, and over time his cognitive abilities may be affected. In some cases, the isolation caused by an unrecognized hearing impairment may lead to behavior problems, such as lack of attention, hyperactivity, aggressiveness, or poor social skills.

Thus, if your preemie didn't pass his hearing screens in the nursery, you should have him evaluated as soon as possible by a pediatric audiologist (a professional trained to diagnose and treat hearing impairments), who can get a complete picture of his type and degree of hearing loss and determine what kind of amplification or other special intervention he needs. If the audiologist thinks your baby might have a condition that could be improved with medicine or surgery, she'll also refer him to a doctor specializing in the ear (usually an ear, nose, and throat doctor).

If your child has a mild hearing loss (difficulty hearing soft or distant speech), he may not need a hearing aid while he's still an infant since adults will talk to him mainly from close by while they're holding him. When he grows into a roaming toddler, however, he'll probably need a hearing aid or FM system (see page 501) to hear well from a distance. Children with moderate hearing loss, who can understand face-to-face conversation but have trouble in groups, or those with severe hearing loss, who can hear only very loud, close voices and sounds, are the ones who benefit most from amplification and hearing and speech therapy. Children with profound hearing loss, who can perceive only very loud sounds or vibrations, may not get as much from amplification as children with a less marked hearing impairment. But if a cochlear implant is a possibility for your child (see page 502), he should be fitted with a hearing aid or FM system or both as soon as possible, and followed with therapy now to get the best results in the future.

It's important to keep in mind that time matters. Most children with hearing loss can learn to talk well provided they get amplification and therapy early. Young children develop speech by imitation and practice, so they have to be exposed to language to learn it. By eight weeks of age, normal infants can distinguish the sounds of their own language from other languages, and by six months, all of the basic sounds have been learned. Up to six years of age, children can ac-

quire complete linguistic fluency, but after that, their ability quickly fades. (If you've ever studied a foreign language as an older child or adult, you know that struggle!) This period for language development should not be missed if your child is to master either speech or sign language (sign language is a complete language of its own, not just a translation of spoken words). People with hearing loss who are not exposed to sign language early enough can still learn it but don't totally master it.

Studies have found that children diagnosed with hearing loss and treated before six months of age achieve much better speech than children who are diagnosed later, from the seventh month on. When tested at one to five years, the children who were identified earlier showed language skills in the normal range, even when their hearing loss was severe. So if your preemie is home by about three to four months of corrected age, you can wait until after he's discharged from the hospital to address his hearing problem. But if a baby with hearing loss is going through a very long hospitalization, his family and doctors should consider getting him hearing aids and speech and language therapy while he's still in the hospital nursery, so the crucial window for intervention is not missed.

Language Education for Children with Hearing Loss

Is it true that children who are hearing impaired should learn sign language before speech?

If your baby has hearing loss, it is important to make up your mind soon about the educational program you want for her. There are two main options:

* The total communication approach, in which a baby is taught to use a combination of sign language and speech at the same time. Chil-

dren wear hearing aids, but more importance is given to sign language than to speech;

✳ The auditory-oral approach, in which a child is taught to use only oral speech with the help of lip-reading or other cues. A variation is the auditory-verbal approach, which discourages lip-reading and stresses the importance of learning to understand words by listening to their sounds.

Total communication allows a child with hearing loss to learn sign language very quickly and easily and to fit in well in the deaf community. Because a young child's skill in using his hands develops earlier than his ability to manipulate his mouth, learning to sign usually means earlier use of language. (An added bonus: Being able to express his wants can really reduce a toddler's frustration and make for a more harmonious household. In fact, many experts advise parents to try this with their children who aren't hearing impaired, but are still too young to speak.)

A child using total communication will attend a school for the deaf or special classes where the teacher and other students use American Sign Language (ASL, the official language of the Deaf community). His parents and the people who interact with him often, such as siblings, grandparents, and regular babysitters, should also learn sign language. But while he will become perfectly fluent in ASL, which is as rich and expressive as any other language, his understanding of spoken language will often lag far behind. Why? Because without clearly hearing the sounds of speech, it's difficult to imitate and learn them. Since sign language has no written form, he'll eventually need to be taught to read and write English as a second language so that he can advance academically and the world of books will not be closed to him.

Auditory-oral education requires more from a child. It can take great patience, time, and effort for a hearing impaired child to learn to

understand and speak fluently. "Bathe your child in sounds," the Center for Hearing and Communication recommends to parents who have chosen auditory-oral education for their children. If later in life he wants to become part of the deaf community, he will have to learn sign language as a second language, and it will never come as naturally to him as it would have if he had learned it as a baby: a regrettable thing, according to the deaf. Experts from the auditory-oral field, though, argue that only with this kind of education is a child with hearing loss really free to choose between the mainstream culture and deaf culture or to participate in both, because if sign language is taught first, most hearing impaired children will lose the motivation to struggle to learn to hear and talk. With the auditory-oral approach, children can attend special classes with other hearing impaired childen or can attend mainstream schools with or without the help of a special educator for extra tutoring.

Not all children will do equally well with both approaches, and each option has advantages and disadvantages. You should carefully weigh them with your child's audiologist, speech and language therapist, and experts from organizations for the deaf (see *Resources* in the Appendices, page 593). Your decision on your child's education will be influenced by the degree of his hearing loss and by the programs that are available in your area. Be assured that either choice can be excellent, provided that your child is given a chance to develop at least one kind of language very well and that the significant people around him are able to talk to him using the same kind of communication.

When your child has been diagnosed with a hearing loss, he may also have been referred to the Early Childhood Intervention Program in your state. If not, you can contact it directly (see page 494). He'll be assigned a child service coordinator who will help him get the appropriate evaluations to assess his developmental needs.

(Continued on page 503)

About Hearing Aids

Modern hearing aids, thanks to microchips, digital technology, and sound processors, have some very sophisticated features. For example, they can be programmed to amplify only certain sounds—the softest ones or those of a certain pitch; to automatically adjust very loud and disturbing noises, to protect the wearer from discomfort; or to diminish background noise, making human speech coming from in front and close by easier to hear and understand. Still, a regular hearing aid doesn't help much when it comes to understanding somebody speaking from more than three feet away because other background voices and noise will be amplified as well.

An FM system can help solve those problems. It consists of a wireless microphone worn by a person who's speaking and a receiver worn by the hearing impaired listener. With an FM system, a child with hearing loss can listen to his parent's or teacher's amplified voice, avoiding most of the background disturbance. Most children with hearing loss do best with an FM system when they're in school because classes can be very noisy. But many infants and children will also benefit from wearing an FM system at home—when the family is having dinner, watching TV, or even all the time.

The audiologist will choose the most appropriate kind of hearing aid for your baby. The smallest and most invisible ones, which fit inside the ear, are not used for young children for practical and safety reasons: they would need to be changed too often to properly fit a rapidly growing baby's ear, and their hard plastic cases break too easily from falls and knocks.

Young children can be fitted with a BTE (behind the ear) hearing aid. A BTE consists of a plastic hook holding a small case that goes behind the ear and a tiny tube that conveys the amplified sounds into a soft mold that fits in the ear canal. Earmolds are custom-made after taking impressions of your child's ear, a simple process that only takes about 15 minutes. They will need to be periodically readjusted throughout childhood, and especially frequently during infancy—every six to eight weeks when your baby is growing rapidly and his ear canal is changing a lot in size and shape. Some BTE hearing aids also contain FM systems (the FM receiver is barely half an inch long and connects to the bottom of the hearing aid). A child can use either the hearing aid function or the FM function, or the two together (for instance in a classroom, when he's listening to the teacher wearing the FM microphone and also wants to hear other sounds or voices).

To help your child with his hearing aid:

* Make sure the earmold fits snugly in his ear to avoid feedback noise (an unpleasant whistling sound).
* Ideally, hearing aids should be in the ears and working during all waking hours (except in the bath, where they can get wet) to help a child develop his listening and language skills and, if he is to get a cochlear implant later, to prime his brain to hear really well. So keep an eye on your baby's hearing aid to make sure it hasn't been dislodged during movement or play, or that little fingers haven't been tampering with it.
* Young toddlers in particular have a tendency to pull out their hearing aids. It's fine to give your child five minutes of rest occasionally, but otherwise be sure to keep placing the hearing aid back in his ear, even if it's driving you crazy to do it again and again for what can feel like

What Is a Cochlear Implant?

If, after being equipped with a hearing aid, your child still isn't able to understand speech without lip-reading, he may be a candidate for a cochlear implant. A cochlear implant is a device implanted surgically in the inner ear that picks up sounds from the environment, electronically codes them, and directly stimulates the auditory nerve—the nerve that sends sound signals to the brain where they are heard. Incoming sounds are transmitted to the cochlear implant by a microphone system that fits in a small case and may be worn either behind the ear like a hearing aid or carried in a chest pocket or backpack. Sometimes a child will get two cochlear implants, one in each ear. The Food and Drug Administration regulates cochlear implants to make sure they are safe and effective.

Cochlear implantation is now considered standard treatment for severe to profound deafness. When surgery is performed early and a child receives intensive hearing and speech therapy and has a committed family who supports and stimulates him, he is likely to develop an understanding of speech and to learn to talk, even on the telephone. Before being able to speak intelligibly, though, a child may need a long course of therapy. Many children continue to show improvement even three years after surgery.

Experts point to some beneficial effects of cochlear implantation even when speech doesn't fully develop. Many children's first reaction, stimulated by this new taste of verbal communication, is an increased interest in learning sign language. And a greater awareness of voices and sounds coming from the environment may greatly improve a child's cognitive development and social responsiveness.

Despite its positive effects, cochlear implantation remains controversial in the deaf community, especially when it is performed on children who can't choose for themselves whether they want it or not. Some deaf adults, who argue that they know better than any hearing person what it's like to be deaf, criticize cochlear implantation as an invasive procedure that doesn't cure deafness and prevents a child from leading a normal life among either the hearing or the deaf. They also believe that deafness is not a disability but an alternate way of life, and that a deaf child can grow up without feeling or being in any way handicapped if he is nurtured in American Sign Language and allowed to participate fully in deaf culture. (If your child is severely to profoundly hearing impaired, it is worth learning about and understanding these arguments so that you can make the best choice for your child. See page 593 for some references to organizations for the hard of hearing.)

If cochlear implantation is a possibility for your child, his ear doctor will give you the information you need, discuss the pros and cons of the procedure with you, and refer you to a cochlear implant center. A child becomes eligible for a cochlear implant only after he's 12 months old and has tried hearing aids together with hearing and speech therapy for at least three to six months. So, you will have enough time to make an informed decision.

a thousand times a day! Some parents say that it helped a lot to take a few days off from work in the beginning to pay close attention to the hearing aids and by constantly putting them back to help their child get used to them more quickly. Remember that all children need to adjust to the new amplified noises and to sounds they may not have heard before, which can make them feel nervous or anxious. But eventually they do adapt well to their new hearing experiences.

* A BTE can create feedback when a child is lying down if the microphone is covered. It's OK for you to take it out at night and nap time so that he can sleep undisturbed. This also helps to avoid damaging the aid if your child rolls around a lot. If he insists on falling asleep with his hearing aid in, just gently take it off after he's sleeping.

* If you notice that your child always takes his hearing aids off when he's in the car or near a computer, it may be because he's bothered by the background noise they make. You should mention this to his audiologist, who may be able to change the settings to make him more comfortable.

* If your child's hearing aids don't stay in, because they fall out or he continues to take them out, you should talk to your child's audiologist and speech therapist. Perhaps the ear-molds are too old and don't fit well anymore, or too new so their shape isn't perfect, or made of a material your child is allergic to. Your child's doctor should check for an ear infection or hardened ear wax in his ear canal since either can make wearing hearing aids painful.

* To keep the hearing aids in and avoid losing them (they are expensive!), some parents have their child wear a close-fitting bonnet made of light, comfortable material that ties under the chin and keeps little fingers out. You can buy one that's specially designed for this purpose, or simply find or make a cute one yourself. You can also use clips or a security strap for hearing aids, or secure them with a special adhesive that is safe on a child's skin. Hearing aid covers and ear molds come in bright colors that are much easier to spot than beige ones when they fall out. Children love them! To buy these special products and also to find practical tips from other parents, see *Resources* on page 593.

* Check the volume setting on your child's hearing aid several times a day, and remember to have him put his aid in as soon as he wakes up. When he's old enough to understand what it does, he'll be asking for it.

It may also help you to talk to a counselor yourself to make sense of your own reactions to your child's hearing loss. You may have a hard time, especially at first, accepting the sight of your beautiful baby wearing a hearing aid (which, though not obtrusive, is not invisible) and adjusting your expectations for the future. You'll need to be very patient since it may take a long time for your child to learn to use a hearing aid and begin to talk. To succeed, he needs all the optimism, reassurance, and stimulation that you can give him. As soon as you realize that your baby is becoming day by day more responsive to the sound of your voice and engaging you with his developing communication skills, you'll know that your efforts are being well compensated.

Visual Impairment

We just found out that our child has very little sight. We're completely lost.

To be told that your child is severely visually impaired is to feel a devastating sense of loss. To help parents get through this, it's important for them to know that an infant won't have the same sense of loss of vision that an older child or adult would feel. We don't want to minimize the present and future difficulties for you and your child. But remember that few activities in life involve just one sense, and your baby will have a chance to enjoy all of the others. Bathing, for example, has the smell of soaps, the sound of running water, the feel of rough sponges or light water splashing against one's skin, and the loving touch of being cleaned and rubbed by one's parents. Even small amounts of vision, which you might consider almost useless, can be a tremendous help and source of enjoyment to your child. Even the perception of light and dark can be worthwhile, enhancing her ability to navigate and increasing her sensory enjoyment of the world.

You may hear your child described as legally blind, so you should understand what that means. The term "legal blindness" is employed for legal and educational purposes in our society—for example, to determine whether a child is eligible for certain benefits or services—but does not necessarily mean she has no useful vision. Most children who are legally blind still have some sight. A person is legally blind if, even with glasses, she can see clearly at 20 feet away an object that someone with normal vision can see at 200 feet away, or if her visual field is limited to 20 degrees or less compared with about 160 degrees provided by normal sight. In many cases a child who is legally blind can still read large symbols, see her hands, and perceive forms and light.

There are many organizations that offer programs and expert advice on how to help your child profit from whatever vision she has, and ensure that she doesn't miss valuable opportunities for intellectual, motor, and emotional development. You'll find that they can help address your many unanswered questions and fears, and also give you information on getting financial support for your child's needs. If no one has mentioned these developmental services yet, ask your eye doctor, pediatrician, or preemie follow-up clinic for a referral to the right kind of organization for your daughter. If they aren't good sources of referrals, your county's public health department or your state's division that handles services for the blind (every state has one; they go by different names) should be able to point you to both state-run and private organizations. Keep in mind that some organizations specialize in children whose only impairment is visual while others work with children who have more than one disability. If you're having trouble finding an organization, the National Association for Parents of the Visually Impaired (NAPVI) may be able to help. You can find it at www.spedex.com/napvi, or call 800-562-6265.

The sooner a specialist starts working with your baby, the better it will be for her development. The development of infants who can see is inextricably tied to their sense of vision. By noticing that people and things can move from place to place, they learn about object permanence (that objects continue to exist even when they disappear from view); by reaching out to grasp something and seeing it move, they learn about cause and effect, and so on. What is fascinating and gratifying for parents of blind babies to realize is that in the absence of other disabilities, and with people to help them learn how to interact with their environment in nonvisual ways, blind children are able to progress through the same developmental stages, along almost the same timetable, as infants who can see.

For example, by about six months of age, both blind and sighted babies can recognize their parents—who, by that time, are very ready to be recognized and appreciated for all of the nurturing they've been doing!—and tense up or cry when they're held by a stranger. (To help your baby distinguish you by sight early on, try to wear clothing of the same bright color whenever you are with her. If she cannot see much at all, you can enhance her ability to recognize you with her other senses by always wearing the same fragrance or by softly talking or singing to her as you approach. You'll also protect her from being startled if you use your voice to let her know you are near, rather than touching her or picking her up unexpectedly.) Blind and sighted babies are able to sit up at about the same age. If someone is teaching them how to explore their environment, they develop comparable language skills. (An exception is that blind children often have temporary confusion with personal pronouns like "I" and "you" between the ages of two and three.)

There are a few, significant differences in the typical development of a blind child that are important for you to be aware of, so they won't worry you. Early on, many parents worry about their baby's often-blank facial expression and rare smiles, wondering if this is a sign of either unhappiness or lack of intelligence. Most often it is neither, and simply results from not having the opportunity to imitate other people's varied expressions. You can help your baby by allowing her to feel your face with her hands and by looking out for other signs, such as body movements, of her emotions.

For a blind infant, some motor milestones also come later. Sighted infants start reaching out for things they see, almost automatically, at about four to five months of age. Blind infants have to wait until they have learned a lot about objects through sounds, and are then motivated to reach out and grasp things, at around nine months. Similarly, independent walking often comes later, typically at around one-and-a-half to two years of age. You can help your baby by playing games involving the way that sounds, the feel of things, and their position in space relate. For example, you can shake your key ring in front of her, then to one side and the other. Have her grab your jangling keys to see where they are and to help her realize that hard metal things clink when they hit each other and are silent when their movement is stopped.

Most commercial toys are fine for visually impaired babies, especially those that do more than one thing, play music, or have various textures. You can also look at the American Foundation for the Blind's catalog of recommended toys for blind children or contact specialized companies, such as Dragonfly Toys, that sell toys especially for children with disabilities. You'll find both in the resources in the appendix.

Despite many parents' instincts to the contrary, you won't be helping your daughter by exposing her for long periods to the sounds of TV or radio dialogue. This kind of auditory stimulation—words that just go on, without being tied to any apparent cause and effect—can actually hurt rather than help by teaching your child that words are meaningless and irrelevant to communication. Music is great, though, and children's songs can be a good way to teach your child some language and early concepts (that animals make sounds, wheels on a bus go around, and so on).

Similarly, you can use light productively in your home to encourage the use of whatever vision your baby has. It's better for her not to spend most of her time looking up into ceiling lights; instead, shine light on objects you would like her to see.

If you notice that your child has certain repetitive mannerisms, such as rocking her body, rubbing her eyes, or swinging her head back and forth, don't worry: Experts believe that blind children may resort to this kind of self-stimulation at times when there isn't enough external stimula-

Does Your Child Have Cortical Visual Impairment?

Some preemies have trouble seeing, temporarily or permanently, due to a disruption of the visual pathways of their brain. Even though their eyes may send good pictures to their brain, their brain isn't able to process or understand them well. Most commonly, so-called cortical visual impairment results from a serious intraventricular hemorrhage or some other injury to the brain.

You can ask your pediatrician or ophthalmologist whether your baby's vision problems appear to be due partly to cortical visual impairment, which is present in some preemies who also had ROP. Children who have it often love looking at lights and prefer to use their peripheral vision; you may notice them trying to look at objects out of the corners of their eyes. Their vision may seem variable over time; they may seem to see better one day, or hour, than the next.

If your baby's main problem seems to be cortical visual impairment rather than damage to the eye itself, there's reason to be hopeful: this condition might improve gradually over months or years. No one can predict how much sight an individual child will recover. The resulting vision may not be good, but it may be much, much better than before. Special therapy to improve a child's vision as much as possible is often recommended, so make sure to ask your eye doctor, pediatrician, or preemie follow-up clinic whether your child might benefit, and for a referral in your area.

tion to be satisfying. You can try to distract your child by encouraging her to focus on people or objects around her. Even if that doesn't always work now, be reassured that these mannerisms usually go away as a child grows up. (The more disabilities a child has in addition to visual impairment, the longer they may last.)

As she grows, your child will be able to lead a rich life, to enjoy books (which she can read in Braille), become adept on computers (there is an extensive library of software for the visually impaired), and even play some sports (especially swimming, dance, and tumbling), depending on her abilities and interests. You'll weigh the pros and cons of regular, neighborhood schools, where she'll be in the "mainstream," versus specialized schools for blind children, which are tailored to her needs, but more insular. Many professions will be open to her because of great advances in technology for the blind and the willingness of more companies to provide it.

Experts suggest that, ideally, a blind child have both a certified teacher of the visually impaired (who specializes in helping her use her remaining vision and other senses to optimize all areas of development) and a certified orientation and mobility specialist (who specializes in helping her understand and safely move through spaces). They might teach your child directly or be consultants to the early intervention specialist who works with her. These specialists will be useful to your child throughout her early childhood and adolescent years. Early on, for example, the orientation and mobility specialist might help your toddler move from her room to the kitchen, where she'll play with your pots and pans, and at the start of high school might teach her how to take public transportation, or become familiar with the layout of her new school.

One piece of advice that is most stressed by experts is that you shouldn't give in to your normal, parental instinct to be overprotective of your young child who is visually impaired. Yes, she will bump into things and fall more often than many other children. It's not easy to sit back and let this happen! But it's important to start looking at gentle knocks and bruises as good things, not bad. They're a sign that your child is getting around and exploring her environment rather than suffering from the much worse consequences of passivity and under stimulation—and that through your loving efforts, you're giving her the confidence, desire, and trust to do so.

Sensory Processing Problems

Our daughter, who was a preemie born at 32 weeks, hates the noise of the vacuum cleaner and the touch of wool or fur. I was told she could have a sensory processing disorder. What is that?

The term "sensory processing" refers to one of the jobs performed by everybody's brain: organizing and interpreting noises, sights, smells, tastes, body movements, textures and temperatures—in other words, all of the signals from our senses—so that we can respond to them appropriately. A person who doesn't process sensory signals in quite the right way might not tolerate some kinds of touch or sound well, as you've noticed in your daughter, or alternatively might be unusually oblivious to them. This is what is meant by a sensory processing disorder (also called "sensory integration dysfunction" or "sen-

sory modulation" problems), which some experts believe can lead to unusual behavior and sometimes social and emotional difficulties.

Of course, all of us find some sensations disturbing (you may be bothered by a scratchy wool sweater, the squeaking of a knife against a plate, or lumps in your mashed potatoes), and different people are disturbed by things to different degrees. But while a lot of people, like your daughter, hate the noise of the vacuum cleaner, most know how to defend themselves against it by simply moving to another room or shutting it out by concentrating on something else. The theory is that some former preemies don't learn to do that as well, or as early, as their peers. Your daughter, for example, may not know how to modulate—in this case dampen—the signal coming through her ears and her negative responses to it. Overwhelmed by the noise, she flies off the handle. The same thing could be happening when she touches a fabric that gives her an unpleasant sensation.

Sensory processing problems can take two forms, and both can be present in the same child:

* **Over-responsiveness to stimulation.** Some children with sensory processing problems find many more sensations, and milder ones, grating and often react inappropriately. They may be unable to tolerate certain noises (such as the sound of air conditioners or people singing), smells (like perfumes or detergents), movements (like swinging or rocking), textures (very soft ones like a stuffed animal's fur, or very coarse ones like hairbrushes), sights (like rapidly changing facial expressions), or foods that feel mushy, squishy, or lumpy. Babies who are hypersensitive may cry a lot and be difficult to soothe, or may simply "shut down," reacting less and less to their increasingly frustrated parents. A baby who is over-

responsive may not be able to tolerate several different kinds of sensation at the same time. (This is typical of very young preemies, but they've usually outgrown it by the time they go home from the NICU.) For instance, an infant may feed well only if his mother is not looking at him or not holding him, accepting a bottle only when it is propped up in his crib. Older children with hypersensitivity may respond with crying, terror, gagging, lashing out, or avoidance and withdrawal. Some toilet training problems can be linked to sensory issues; for example, a child may not like the feel of the toilet seat, or the cool air on his undiapered skin and insist on continuing to use his diaper. (A quick tip: try cutting a hole in the diaper, so your child can keep it on but still use the toilet. This will introduce him gradually to the different sensations.)

* **Under-responsiveness to stimulation.** Other children may be unusually under-responsive or unaware of sensations. For instance, a baby may not suck readily because she's less aware of a nipple being put in her mouth. Under-responsiveness can lead to a craving for especially intense stimulation like deep touch, fast swinging, or spinning. A toddler may even make himself fall on purpose, or frequently lift and throw heavy objects. It is thought that the need for strong physical stimulation may arise from a dampened sense of proprioception (meaning that signals about the body's position, balance, and motion are dulled).

According to one theory, preemies may be more prone to sensory processing problems because of the overstimulation they were exposed to in the NICU. Invasive medical therapies, a noisy, bright environment, and overfrequent contact, all at a gestational age when a baby is supposed to be getting only dampened sensory signals in the womb, may lead to a subtle brain imbalance that forms the root of sensory processing problems. But no one knows if this is really what happens.

You should know that many physicians and educators still consider sensory processing disorder to be a controversial concept. Doubters say that the problems it describes are too varied and vague to be a distinct diagnosis, that they overlap with learning and behavior problems such as attention deficit disorder, hyperactivity, or autism, or even with perfectly normal differences in temperament. Moreover, researchers have not done large studies to support it.

Other professionals—occupational therapists, in particular—have found that sensory processing problems make sense as a way to understand difficult or fragile children who are fussy and easily stressed by too much stimulation. But even they tell parents that sensory processing problems are not so much a medical diagnosis as a description of a more sensitive personality, or a more immature stage of development that can make it harder for a child to handle certain aspects of the world around her. It doesn't mean she's "sick," although living with her can sometimes be difficult.

Believe us, you're not alone if you feel like you're tearing out your hair, or stuck for ideas on how to deal with your overly sensitive child. Fortunately, occupational therapists have developed some useful strategies for dealing with sensory processing issues. They often work with a child in an OT gym, a special environment in a private office or clinic that offers a lot of different sensory stimulation. Your child can have fun trying out new sensory experiences in a controlled, gradual, and nonchallenging way, encouraged by the therapist. This can be very effective in helping a child learn new ways to process and tolerate the normal, common sensations she experiences during her daily activities, from playing to feeding to sleeping.

(Continued on page 510)

Tips for Feeding Hypersensitive Preemies

It's not surprising: when children are hypersensitive to touch in their mouth or on their face, they can develop feeding problems.

They may refuse to eat any foods with a certain taste, temperature, or texture (for instance, all soft foods like pasta or gelatin, or all crunchy foods like pretzels or crackers)—or absolutely insist on eating only them. Some babies refuse all finger foods or anything with chunks, taking only smooth processed food for a long time. Others reject smooth foods and will accept only finger foods. Frequent gagging or vomiting, when not caused by a condition like reflux, may be due to hypersensitivity, or to one step beyond it: what is called "oral aversion," a tactile defensiveness in the mouth and throat accompanied by strong negative emotions, such as fear and disgust.

Preemies who were on a ventilator for a long time in the NICU or had a lot of medical intervention involving their mouth and throat are more likely to react negatively to feeding, possibly because they were tube-fed for so long that they didn't get a chance to experience the pleasure of sucking and the taste of sweet, satisfying milk early enough in their lives. Imagine, if you were used to nothing but plastic in your mouth, how strange and unsettling it would be to feel liquid spurting from a nipple into the back of your throat!

Feeding specialists have come up with some amazingly creative ways to reduce a child's oral hypersensitivity (you'll find even more in *Resources* listed on page 592).

* Touch her body playfully while slowly working your way toward her face and mouth. A firm touch usually works better than a light or ticklish one, which can be irritating. Eventually, see if you can get your child to handle kissing games (for instance, take turns kissing a stuffed animal).

* Brush her teeth with a regular or electric toothbrush to "wake up" her tongue and mouth with sensations and movements that don't involve eating.

* Separate food play from mealtime, so she can explore and experience the sensory aspects of food (its different colors and smells, its wetness or roughness, its crackling or smushing sounds) without being under pressure to ingest it. This way, too, she won't feel like food games are just tricks to get her to eat.

* Distract her during feeding with games or songs so she's less aware of what she's actually doing.

* Let your child take control, teasing her with the spoon instead of pushing it into her mouth. Reverse psychology might lead her to lean forward and decide she wants to "catch" the food.

* Put the spoon away if just the sight of it upsets your child, and let her taste food on a toy or on your finger. Try dipping a lollipop in crumbs.

* Try desensitizing your child's gag reflex by swabbing her tongue with lemon ice.

Fruit-flavored lollipops, which also are acidic, may work, too.

* Rub deeply on her hands and cheeks with a washcloth before presenting food to her, to stimulate the body parts involved in feeding.

* Blend food more thoroughly to make it absolutely chunk-free, or disguise lumps by thickening the blended food with dehydrated baby food, instant potatoes, instant pudding, or ground graham cracker crumbs.

* Very gradually add textures (perhaps with Cheerios) or tastes (with cinnamon, spicy sauces, or pickles) to make food more intensely flavored and interesting.

* Start by serving your child's favorite foods at room temperature or at the temperature she likes best, and very slowly increase or decrease how hot or cold they are.

* Follow the principle of "see it; touch it; taste it," taking these steps one at a time. First, just put food on your child's plate and let her get used to seeing it there. Then let her play with the food or put it in her mouth without eating it. Suggest blowing bubbles with straws, spitting out colors (give her red, yellow, and green foods), maybe making a picture with her food, smelling it, mashing it. When the time comes, you can ask her, "Can you make this crunch?"

Try to keep calm and cool even if your child vomits, cleaning up without too much fuss. This can be hard! But it is essential for you to learn how to control your own stress, or mealtime will become an even more unpleasant experience that she won't want to repeat—or will use vomiting to bring to a quick end. In general, you should try as hard as you can not to focus on the amount of food your child takes in, but on having fun at mealtime.

Above all, don't ever hesitate to ask for help from an occupational therapist, a feeding specialist, or your baby's doctor. You'll end up feeling more empowered—and your child will respond positively, too.

(Interestingly, if your child has difficulty with language, too, she may get an added boost. Some therapists have noticed that when sensory issues get addressed, language delays often improve as well, possibly because the brain becomes more organized and efficient.)

You, too, will learn from the occupational therapist ways to soothe your baby, calm her, and help her cope. For example, if she becomes easily agitated when she's stimulated in more than one way at once, you might be advised that when you are feeding or dressing her, you should keep the lights low, cut out as much noise as possible or try a gentle, constant humming to neutralize background noise, and maintain a stable facial expression (what therapists call a "still face"). Some preemies respond well to strong, rhythmic touch, or the repetitive, intense movements of a rocking chair or swing, to calm them. The American Occupational Therapy Association (AOTA)—on the web at www.aota.org or by phone at 800-377-8555 or 301-652-2682—can give you a list of occupational therapists in your region.

Just one or a few OT sessions might be all you and your child need. Experts believe that in most cases these sorts of problems can be solved within the family, without a lot of outside help. Remember that your daughter, through her sometimes exaggerated or unusual responses, is sending you clues. By picking up on them, you'll help her avoid the things that disturb her; then, little by little, with time and patience and by gently and gradually challenging her, you'll help her become accustomed to them.

Long-Term Feeding Problems

The doctor says that if my eight-month-old daughter's eating and weight gain don't get better, she will need a feeding tube.

It's a test of emotional strength when your child has difficulty eating and you're racked by feelings of frustration, anxiety, and guilt at every meal. For many families, a feeding tube (called a gastrostomy tube, or g-tube) turns out to be a much better alternative—for the child's growth and for the parents' peace of mind.

But the decision to have a g-tube placed in your child's stomach, so that you can supplement the amount of food she eats by mouth, is a painful and difficult one you usually don't need to rush into. Most doctors won't bring up the option of gastrostomy as long as there's still a good chance that a child's eating and growth will improve soon. Luckily, even if a g-tube is needed for a while, most feeding difficulties are eventually overcome, but it takes time, patience, and often expert advice and guidance. The earlier you get help, the better. So, the first thing to understand is why your child is having feeding problems, and who can offer you the best advice on how to deal with them.

Certain preemies tend to develop feeding problems, in particular, those who have severe chronic lung disease, a tracheostomy, severe reflux, or cerebral palsy. These children make very slow progress—and sometimes even backtrack—in their ability to eat by mouth. It's important for you to realize that the way your child eats is affected by her medical problems and her physical and neurological development, not just by her temperament or personal tastes. For instance, a baby with BPD may have trouble breathing while she eats, and may not be able to eat successfully until her lungs have more fully recovered. Eating may cause pain in a preemie who suffers from reflux. Preemies with cerebral palsy may have difficulty coordinating the many complicated movements of the tongue, lips, jaw, and neck that are needed for sucking, chewing, and swallowing. And some preemies who have temporary developmental delays may simply reach their feeding milestones later than other babies do.

Preemies who were on a ventilator for months and had a lot of medical procedures around their mouths (such as intubations, suctioning, and taping) may also develop a reaction that doctors call oral aversion. Instead of associating eating with pleasure, they associate it with medical treatment and discomfort. Babies with oral aversion may refuse to suck on a nipple (so they need to be fed by tube temporarily) but they are often willing to eat from a spoon and cup when they're older. Some experts believe that preemies who had very long hospitalizations are especially prone to have problems processing the sensations related to feeding such as the feel of a nipple in their mouth or the taste and smell of milk or formula. When a child has sensory processing problems (see page 507), she may intensely dislike certain food textures, tastes, or temperatures.

You should certainly have your baby seen by experts who can diagnose her specific feeding problems and may be able to boost her eating and weight gain. Your doctor may already have arranged for this. If not, here are some specialists who might help:

* **A pediatric nutritionist or dietician** can calculate your baby's daily calories and estimate how much more she needs to eat to meet her nutritional needs. He can also help you enrich your child's current diet to get the most out of every mouthful.

* **A pediatric gastroenterologist** can assess whether your baby has reflux, isn't absorbing

nutrients adequately, or whether any other medical condition might be contributing to her feeding problems.

✳ **An occupational therapist** can determine whether the muscles your child needs for eating are working properly and how to help them become better coordinated. An occupational therapist can also address any sensory processing problems that may be interfering with your child's eating.

✳ **A speech-language therapist** can diagnose and treat problems with oral movements and coordination (the same movements needed for speech are needed for sucking, chewing, and swallowing), and can perform special diagnostic tests to see how food is moving inside your child's mouth and throat while she's eating. You can read more about these tests on pages 315–318. (By the way, a baby doesn't have to be talking yet to be seen by a speech-language therapist.)

✳ **Other families whose children have problems similar to yours** are specialists in their own right. You can join a support group or find an on-line community of parents who share your experiences and concerns. Families who have children with sensory processing problems or who are getting tube feedings at home are especially likely to have a wealth of tips for you—as well as generous doses of empathy, compassion, and much-needed humor.

To help you with the decision about whether to get a g-tube, have a look at the information on pages 365 and 366 and in the Getting Acquainted with: G-tube Feedings at Home box on pages 513–517. Some of the reassuring things you will find out are that a g-tube is usually only a temporary measure, that most children continue eating by mouth after getting one—using the tube only for extra feedings, often during the night while she

and the rest of the family are sleeping—and that many parents who fought for a long time against a g-tube afterward changed their minds about it when mealtimes became more peaceful and they finally saw their child's growth blossom.

Weaning a Child from Tube Feedings

Now that my baby has a g-tube, he's growing well. The doctor says not to be discouraged, but I'm afraid he'll never come off tube feeds.

If your baby's doctor tells you that she doesn't think your child will need tube feedings forever, you can believe her. It may seem impossible now, but so much can change in the next weeks, months, or years. Your baby will grow bigger and stronger—making it more likely that his feeding ability and endurance will improve—as you, his doctor, and feeding therapist work on any other issues that are impeding his progress. You just need to practice faithfully the therapies and techniques you're taught, and give them time to work. Patience is the virtue that parents of tube fed children need the most!

Weaning a child from tube feedings is usually a slow, gradual process, and its pace will depend on your child's health, physical abilities, and willingness to eat. There are some major landmarks you can watch for, to know where you are on the road.

First, before asking a baby who's being tube fed to begin eating by mouth, the doctor will want to be sure he's growing well and able to eat safely without breathing trouble or possible aspiration. Your baby will need to be a willing partner, so he should be showing some enjoyment when he's touched around his mouth or given tastes.

The next milestone is moving from simply tasting food to actually eating mouthfuls.

(Continued on page 517)

Getting Acquainted with: G-Tube Feedings at Home

When a child gets a g-tube or a convenient skin-level "button" to which the tube is attached just for feedings, her parents receive a full training course on it. The doctors and nurses will make sure you're comfortable using the g-tube or button for feedings and are ready to deal with its daily care before you take your child home from the hospital.

Most likely, the relief you feel that surgery is behind you is tempered with a lot of anxiety about the effect tube feedings will have on your child's and family's lives. You may be asking yourself: Will our child look awful? Will she be able to play with other kids and have fun? How will we fit these unnatural, complicated feedings into our busy schedule? Will we ever be able to go out and leave her with a babysitter? (The answers to all of these questions are reassuring, as you will soon discover.) To top it off, the fear of possible complications or of pulling the tube out accidentally can be almost unbearable.

First, be assured that it is totally normal to have these feelings. Adapting to and accepting your child's tube-feeding is a process like, some mothers say, learning a new job. You might make mistakes, but that's OK. With the help of doctors, nurses, and other parents, you'll gradually find yourself becoming more comfortable. Remember that the love and care you'll put into tube feeding your baby are the same you would give no matter how she was fed.

Most preemies will continue to work on eating by mouth after getting a g-tube and eventually outgrow their need for one. When the time comes for surgery to remove their child's tube and close the gastrostomy, many parents find they look back with relief and gratitude at the time

their child had it—a change of life that was not only for the better, but even a blessing.

The following information is not meant to cover all of the detailed instructions you'll get from your baby's medical specialists on how to feed her. It is just a reminder of the basics, with some added tips from feeding therapists and other parents who have "been there." Be sure to check the *Resources* section (page 592) for web sites and books that other parents have found valuable, including *Feeding and Nutrition for the Child with Special Needs* by Martha Dunn Klein and Tracy Delaney, from which we have drawn considerable wisdom.

The basics: How and what to tube feed your child

When you give your child tube feedings at home, you have to learn a new vocabulary—on top of everything else! You'll hear medical folks talk about a "stoma," the opening in your child's skin leading to her stomach. You'll also hear them refer to "bolus" feeds (meaning the whole quantity is given at once) versus "continuous" feeds (in which formula is dripped into your child's stomach continuously).

Bolus feedings are given by pouring breast milk, formula, or blended foods into a large syringe, connecting it to the top of the g-tube, and letting the liquid flow into your child's stomach by gravity. It usually takes about 15 minutes for the syringe to empty. Continuous feedings are dripped into the g-tube automatically from a bag connected to an electric pump. The pump can also be programmed to deliver a bolus feeding over a longer period than it would take to flow in by gravity alone (over an hour, for example).

The kind of formula you give your child, and how much, will change over time as she grows and her nutritional needs change. She may start out with preemie formula, then switch to regular infant formula (perhaps with prune juice added for constipation), then possibly graduate to pureed foods. You'll want to introduce new formulas or foods gradually, to give your child time to adjust to them.

You'll see that in many ways, a feeding is a feeding! Like any parent, you'll be watching for your child's cues when she's being tube fed, just as you would do if she were eating by mouth. For example, widening eyes and squirming can be signs that she's becoming uncomfortably full. You may need to stop her feeding for a few minutes, burp her, or give her a smaller amount next time. Be sure to tell your child's doctor and feeding therapist what you notice, so you can troubleshoot together.

Her doctor will check on her growth and diet every few months, often with the help of a nutritionist and feeding therapist. He'll also evaluate the progress she's making toward eating by mouth, and the day when she'll finally leave tube feedings behind.

What are the best times, positions, and places for tube feedings?

In principle, it's simple: Your goal is to make your child's mealtimes as close to "normal" as possible, so the best time and place for tube feedings is where and when your child would be eating if she didn't have a tube. If your baby would be nursing at your breast, then hold her in your lap. If she would be eating in a high chair, give her tube feedings there. But don't feel bad if you don't achieve this at first, while you're still overwhelmed with mastering the logistics of tube feeding, or your baby still has medical conditions that take

priority. Just work toward it, and you will get there!

Most tube-fed children get bolus feedings during the day and continuous feedings at night. Like babies who are breastfed or bottle fed, they usually eat every 3 to 4 hours throughout the day. Older kids may get their tube feedings on a schedule designed to mimic normal mealtimes and snack times (bigger boluses for meals, smaller boluses for snacks). Continuous feeding at night allows you and your child to sleep undisturbed: you replenish your energy, while she gets the nourishment she needs.

Tube feedings go best—as do mealtimes for any of us—when a child is relaxed and still. Not only does this help digestion, but if her stomach muscles are clenched tight, it may impede the flow of fluid through the tube. So, settle into a comfortable chair for a nice stretch of calm time with your baby or toddler. Try to keep her back straight when she eats (a rounded back kinks the stomach and makes reflux more likely), supporting it with your hand or arm if you're holding her, or with straps and bolsters if she's in a chair. If you feel like you just don't have enough hands to hold her, the syringe full of formula, and perhaps a pacifier, too, try wrapping some tape around the syringe and taping or pinning it to your shirt, the crib rail, or the back of a chair.

For an older child, whenever you can, feed her at the dining room table with the rest of the family. Even if she's not eating anything by mouth yet, she'll learn that mealtimes and the feeling of being satisfied go along with companionship and sociability.

Extra tips from experts

Here are some pointers from tube feeding experts for parents who are just getting started:

* **To help prevent infections,** always wash your hands before preparing and giving a feeding, and make sure the equipment is clean.
* **If your child has a balloon-type g-tube** (the doctor will have told you this), gently pull on the tube (never yank it) at the start of each feeding to make sure the balloon is resting snug against the wall of your baby's stomach. You'll feel resistance if the balloon is where it should be.
* **If you want to slow down the flow,** just lower the syringe. Remember that the higher you hold the syringe, the faster the formula flows into your baby's stomach.
* **Babies who have a small stomach or reflux** may do better when their feedings flow in especially slowly, giving their stomachs more time to empty. You might consider using a pump to extend the feeding time.
* **If your child spits up during her tube feedings**, try burping her more, slowing down her feeding, or taking a little break in the middle of a feeding to give her stomach more time to empty. To help avoid reflux, be sure to keep her head higher than her stomach, her back straight, and don't bounce her around. Also, check the temperature of the formula, since formula that is too cold makes some babies vomit.
* **When you need to give your child medication,** use a liquid form whenever possible. If you have to use tablets, crush them to a fine powder and let them dissolve in about a tablespoon (15 cc) of warm water or formula. It's usually fine to open capsules and dissolve the granules inside, but always check with your pharmacist first to be sure.
* **If your child has a fever or has been sweating** outside in the hot sun, she may need more fluid than usual but be unable to drink more on her own. Ask your doctor what to do in these situations. You may need to give her a few extra ounces of water, formula, or juice.
* **Some feeding specialists recommend making blended formulas yourself** for older children to expose them to more diverse and complex tastes and digestion. (Your child can smell the formula in her stomach as it wafts up into her nose and mouth, and when she burps—in addition to any tastes you give her by mouth, of course.) If you're interested in trying this, be sure to get the OK from your child's doctor first. Blend the foods you choose very thoroughly so they don't clog the tube, perhaps even buying a special blender. (Vita-Mix gives discounts to parents with tube-fed children.) You'll need to work with a dietician to be sure you're giving your child appropriate calories and nutrition, not introducing new foods too fast, and preparing and storing the food safely (for example, never use raw eggs, which can house bacteria that cause food poisoning).
* **For older kids who are on continuous feedings during the day,** you can get something really convenient: a small, portable pump that fits into a backpack.
* **To prevent clogs in the g-tube,** flush the tube with water after every feeding and medication dose.

Dealing with problems

G-tube problems aren't always avoidable, but there are lots of things you can do to make them less likely, or to manage them when they occur:

* **Make sure the g-tube or button isn't rubbing** against your child's skin. It can be painful and cause granulation tissue to build up; and if the tube pulls on the edges of the stoma, the stoma can stretch and widen, causing leaks. So whenever you think of it, check that the

g-tube or button can rotate freely, with ⅛" of room above your child's skin. If not, it may be time to replace it with a bigger size.

* **To keep the g-tube from pulling against the stoma,** place several gauze pads around the stoma and tape the tube to them, then tape or pin the tube higher up, too—to your baby's diaper or the back of her shirt (be careful not to stick the pin into the tube itself!). Or if she keeps pulling on it herself, tuck the tube inside a "onesie" where she can't reach it.

* **If fluid is leaking around the g-tube,** first make sure the tube isn't clogged and that it flushes easily. If you have a tube with a balloon, gently pull on the tube to make sure the balloon is in the correct position, snug up against the wall of your child's stomach under her stoma. If the leak is bad, ask the doctor whether you should readjust the amount of water inside the balloon, or whether the tube or button needs to be replaced. Occasionally, leaks occur because the valve of a button-type tube gets stuck in the open position.

* **To protect your child's skin around a leaky gastrostomy,** sprinkle a special stoma powder (such as Stomahesive or Stoma-ease) on the area, then cover it thickly with a zinc-oxide cream. (Many parents recommend Calmoseptine, which also contains menthol oil.) Always keep gauze pads or a foam dressing, such as Hydrasorb, around the tube to absorb possible leaks and replace them when they get wet. A few drops of Maalox on the gauze can help neutralize irritating stomach acid.

* **You may see some pink, raised tissue around your child's stoma** called granulation tissue. This is the body's normal way to heal a wound, but it's not what you want in this case! Not only does your child's stoma need to stay open, but granulation tissue is tender and bleeds easily. The best way to prevent it is to keep her skin from getting irritated by leaks or rubbing by the tube. If too much granulation tissue builds up, your baby's doctor will treat it, usually by numbing it with a little Xilocaine gel, then cauterizing it by touching the tissue with a silver nitrate stick. You may be instructed to repeat this procedure for a few days at home until the granulation tissue is gone. Putting some Vaseline on the normal skin around the stoma will help protect it and avoid burns. An alternative treatment is Triamcinolone cream applied three times a day.

Some parents prefer to use other remedies to treat granulation tissue, which you might try with your doctor's permission. One is diluted eucalyptus oil (available at health stores or on the Internet): two drops of oil to about a tablespoon of water. First test it on a less sensitive area, such as your baby's arm or leg, to make sure she doesn't get an allergic reaction, then dab the solution on the granulation tissue with a cotton swab.

* **What if the g-tube becomes clogged** by food or medications? Diet soda, cranberry juice, or a quarter of a teaspoon of meat tenderizer in two teaspoons of water can be more effective than warm water alone in dissolving the clog. Gently inject 10 cc of the liquid into the tube and slowly let it flow back out until the blockage is cleared. Never use a lot of pressure (even though you may want to blow the tube to smithereens!) or you could damage it. But you can gently squeeze the tube along its length, milking it to help push clogs through.

* **Babies with sensitive skin may develop a rash** or irritation from tape. You might be able to avoid tape altogether by pinning the tube to your baby's clothes. Or try sticking the tape to her shirt, pants, or diapers instead of her skin. You can also experiment with different kinds of tape, such as cloth or paper tape instead of plastic. (Hospitals carry a wide range of tapes, so next time you're there,

ask your baby's nurse if she'll give you some samples to try. Most drugstores carry different kinds, too.)

* **Infections around the stoma** are rare. But if you notice redness and swelling that extends an inch around the button or tube, smells bad, or just won't go away, have your child seen by his pediatric surgeon. Most likely it will turn out to be just irritation and not an infection, but you want to be sure so that your child will get the right treatment and you can relax.

* **If your baby's button or g-tube comes out,** the first rule is: Don't panic! Cover the opening with a clean gauze pad or cloth to catch leaks. Then, if your child is crying, take a few minutes to calm her down. (You may need to calm yourself first. A few deep breaths and a silent pep talk—"I can handle this; it will be fine"—does wonders.) It's crucial to replace a tube as soon as possible, ideally within two hours, because after about four to six hours the opening from her skin to her stomach will start to close. Follow your doctors' and nurses' instructions about what to do in this situation. They may have taught you to replace or change the tube or button yourself, or to temporarily insert a catheter you'll have among your home tube-care supplies, or to go to the nearest hospital emergency room for expert help. Don't ever hesitate to call your support team at the hospital. Someone will take you step by step through the procedure and reassure you that you're doing the right thing. After the tube is replaced, it may need to be X-rayed to make sure it's in the right position. Until you're sure the tube is correctly placed in your child's stomach, you shouldn't use it for feeding.

* **Be sure to carry a replacement tube or button** with you when you go out, in case the tube accidentally comes out.

Moving from tube feedings to eating by mouth

For most preemies, tube feedings are just a bump on the road; eventually, they're able to eat everything they need by mouth. But there are some things you can do to move more quickly toward that longed-for destination. The feeding plan that you and the therapist develop will take your child—usually with baby steps—from one feeding milestone to another, based on her own particular problems and needs, likes and dislikes, and the cues she gives that she's ready to move forward. You'll find a fuller description of this process on page 512.

As you go through the often frustrating, but ultimately rewarding, process of weaning your child off g-tube feeds, above all remember that you are not alone. Don't ever hesitate to reach out to the many other parents who have children with g-tubes, too. You can find them online, and your child's feeding therapist and doctor can put you in touch with families who live near you.

The experience you're embarking on will almost certainly feel hard at times, especially at first. But you'll be surprised at how quickly you become an expert tube feeder. Believe it or not, the anxiety you feel now will soon start to fade away, and one day you'll marvel at how normal your child's feedings have come to seem.

A feeding therapist can be immensely helpful in making this transition—a huge one for some kids!—with as little stress and discomfort and as much pleasure and fun as possible.

In the final phase, those mouthfuls expand into meals, which your child eats with eagerness and enjoyment.

But how do you move from here to there?

There are many small steps along the way. You've probably started already by giving your baby a pacifier with his tube feedings. The doctor or feeding therapist will tell you when your child is ready to take a few mouthfuls of food before each tube feeding, and when it's time to motivate him to eat by reducing the calories you're giving him by tube and letting him get hungry.

Hunger is important, because it sets the stage for a child to understand that sucking, chewing, and swallowing can ease his hunger pangs. If he's on continuous drip feedings now, first he'll be transitioned to bolus feedings, so he can feel what it's like to have an empty stomach and to make sure he can tolerate—and enjoy—a full one. (The feeling of fullness is distressing to some kids who've had serious breathing problems or severe reflux. An important step in the g-tube weaning process can be simply getting a child to accept having a full stomach.)

There are other strategies to stimulate hunger: for instance, you might be told to switch from giving your child the same amount of formula at regular intervals to a meal-snack-meal-snack-meal schedule (like a typical young child's), or you might be instructed to postpone a tube feeding here and there, or to dilute your child's tube feeding with water. The last step, usually, is to stop all tube feeding during the day, allowing your child to eat all he can and to make up at night, while he sleeps, any nutrient deficits he isn't quite covering on his own. So drip feedings at night are usually the last to go. Since most parents and kids mind this kind of tube feeding the least, even this not-quite-ultimate step is a very exciting one!

Although the g-tube weaning process sounds complicated—and indeed, you shouldn't make any of these changes on your own—don't worry. Your child's doctor and feeding therapist will be guiding you as you go along.

You can find more information on pages 458, 507, 511, and 513, about eating problems and tube feeding. Here are some useful reminders and tips to try as your child makes the gradual transition from tube feedings to eating everything by mouth:

* **Encourage your child to use his mouth to explore the world**. Let him lick and chew his toys, his toes, even the furniture. You don't need to be afraid of a few germs. He'll be exposed to new textures and tastes, and all that mouthing sets the groundwork for taking in food, while also strengthening his immune system.
* **Encourage your baby to make sounds.** Babbling, speaking, singing, and making nonsense noises all help with eating because of the various, controlled movements his mouth has to make for each.
* **At the beginning of a feeding**, gently massage your child's gums and teeth with a soft toothbrush or a wet washcloth wrapped around the tip of your finger. Like an athlete's warm-up exercises, this helps keep your child's mouth active and alert to stimulation, setting the stage for better eating.
* **Once your child is taking some food by mouth**, feed him first from the breast, bottle, or spoon to take advantage of his hunger and attention, then immediately follow with a tube feeding of any extra nutrition he needs. Even if he eats very little, he'll still learn to associate sensations in his mouth with satisfying his hunger.
* **Set a time limit of 15 to 30 minutes for mouth feedings.** This will keep them fun and reduce the pressure.
* **Music can bring playfulness, rhythm, and flow to mealtimes,** which will actually make eating easier—as well as calming tension and helping you and your child focus better. You can try singing, or just playing music in the

background. Experiment with kiddie music, folk songs, jazz, classical, even rock-and-roll.

* **If your child is older than six months and isn't eating anything by mouth yet,** consider asking his doctor or dietician whether you may give him homemade pureed foods as part of his tube diet. These taste different from the commercial formulas he's used to and may help him accept and enjoy the juices, cereals, fruits, and vegetables he'll be asked to eat later on. Be sure to ask the dietician how to complement your homemade foods so that your child receives the same complete nutrition he would get from commercial formulas.

* **Another way to give your child tastes of milk,** juice, baby food or, if he's older, of whatever the family is eating, is by spilling some on his high-chair tray. When he plays with it and then puts his fingers to his lips, he'll get the flavor.

* **Be sure you've addressed any issues your child has with reflux and constipation.** These can make *anyone* loath to eat. Reflux can be treated by slowing down or thickening the feedings, positioning your child with his head higher than his stomach and his back sraight, and giving him prescription medications. For constipation, the doctor may instruct you to give your child a little prune juice every day, or to increase the fiber or water in his diet.

* **Don't rush—let your child set the pace—and avoid pushing excessive quantities of food.** Your well-meant eagerness could make your child feel anxious and out of control—recipes for a setback.

* **Expect that there will be plateaus,** where the gains your child has made are consolidated, before new progress is made. Periods of time when it seems that nothing is happening are a normal, essential part of the process.

* **Take some deep breaths and pauses to calm yourself,** because you can pass your moods on to your child. In particular, if you fear that progress isn't happening and tube feedings may become permanent, you might make changes too rapidly, or do the opposite and become passive and hopeless. Keep in mind that your child has fears as well—that pain and harm can come from eating—and overcoming them is a gradual process, with fits and starts.

* **Acknowledge what all parents in this situation know**—that this is a *really* frustrating process—and don't feel bad about asking for help from your partner, other family members, or friends. It can be especially hard on mothers, who are usually the primary caregivers and feeders, and whose identity and sense of competence are often wrapped up in how well their baby eats and grows.

* **No matter how eager you are to get rid of the tube, you shouldn't press to have it removed** until you and the doctor are sure that your child can take in enough food and water to be safe, even when he's sick. Taking the tube out too soon may lead to overlong and pressured mealtimes, and possibly failure to grow and thrive.

* **Remember that time and maturation are on your side.** Improvement in breathing, growth in the size of a child's jaw and throat, and the natural development of all of the muscles and nerves that control eating help to promote a child's feeding ability as he grows. (This doesn't mean, however, that early treatment is unnecessary. You want to nip problem behaviors in the bud, before they become habits that are extremely hard to break.)

The most important thing you can do is to make eating fun and enjoyable, rather than another unpleasant "procedure" or a battleground for control. Your child must come to trust the adult who's feeding him, and his own abilities.

(*Continued on page 525*)

In Plain Language: What Is Cerebral Palsy?

Although their child's diagnosis of cerebral palsy initially brings pain and anguish to a family, it's wrong to be overly pessimistic. Many people imagine someone with CP as intellectually impaired, tied to a wheelchair, and unable to live an independent life. But in fact, most people with CP have normal (and sometimes even very high) intelligence, and the severity of their physical problems can vary greatly, making a world of difference for a child's future. CP can be so mild that it is barely noticeable, apparent only when someone is doing certain, specific tasks, like brushing her long hair or pouring from a heavy coffeepot. While a child with mild CP can't be expected to be a professional football player or pianist, she is likely to lead a virtually normal life—going to school, playing recreational sports and games, getting married, having children, and working, like all of her peers. At the other end of the spectrum, CP can be so severe that it leads to poor control of most movements, including speaking and eating. In between are many people who use a wheelchair, or need ongoing physical therapy and medical treatment but still lead fulfilling lives.

Your own child's situation will become clearer over the next few years, as it becomes apparent what she can and cannot do. Much will depend on whether she suffers only from this disability, or from other disabilities and problems, as well. If a larger area of her brain was injured, she might be mildly or severely intellectually impaired (having learning disabilities or mental retardation). Children with CP are also more likely than other kids to suffer from hearing or visual impairments, seizures, sleep disorders, reflux, or behavior problems. Remember that CP is not something you grow out of, but it is also not progressive, meaning it doesn't get worse. If your child has mild

CP, she is not at risk of having more severe CP later on.

You'll learn that cerebral palsy is classified into different types, depending on what part of the child's body it affects most, and what kind of muscle tone or movement problems it causes.

✳ **Spastic diplegia:** This is the most common type of CP among preemies. *Spastic* refers to stiff muscle tone, and *diplegia* to the fact that the legs and feet are mainly affected. (Preemies with spastic diplegia can have some trouble with hand movements, but to a much lesser extent.) This means that walking and running might be hard for them—they may, for example, not walk independently until the age of two or three, perhaps with the help of braces on their lower legs—but they'll probably be able to use their upper body well, holding themselves upright, and using their hands and arms for everything from eating to writing. Many preemies with spastic diplegia can speak well, and, fortunately, are spared many of the other medical problems that often go along with CP.

It's also possible to have spastic hemiplegia (stiff tone affecting the arm and leg on one side of the body, but not the other) or spastic quadriplegia (affecting all limbs, and often the head and trunk, as well). Quadriplegia can often be diagnosed within the first six months of life.

✳ **Athetoid CP:** Preemies who do not have spastic cerebral palsy may have what is called athetoid CP, in which muscle tone is changeable, and varies between too low and too high. Children with athetoid CP, who are often very bright intellectually, may have trouble holding themselves in an upright posture while walking or sitting, getting their hands to the right spot to grasp something, or holding on to things. They often make involuntary movements of the face and upper body.

* **Ataxic CP:** A few preemies have ataxic CP, which is characterized by clumsy, uncoordinated movements, and poor balance. Children with ataxic CP, whose intelligence is usually not affected, may walk unsteadily and with a wide gait, placing their feet far apart to compensate for their uncertain balance. Movements that are quick or require precision, such as writing or buttoning a jacket, are hard for them, and they may have a tremor when making voluntary movements, such as reaching for a cup of juice.

One thing many parents worry about is their future feelings for their child with cerebral palsy. As with any special needs child, you may wonder: Will I love her? Will I ever be able to accept what has happened to her, and to me? These are normal fears, and we can assure you: you almost certainly will. Parents who have children both with and without CP say their feelings for them are not that different. In both cases, they range across the typical parental spectrum from anxiety, frustration, and fatigue to delight and pride. Just as their love for their children who don't have CP is not related to their IQ scores or athletic victories, their love for their child who does have CP is not related to the results of her developmental evaluations.

Treatment of cerebral palsy focuses not on curing it—it is a life-long condition—but on helping a child achieve her maximum potential. (As you can read below, researchers are hoping that if new, experimental therapies continue to show promise, in years to come it may be possible to repair some of the damage to the brain in some children.) Experts believe that the earlier treatment begins, the more chance there is of improving abnormal movements and developing normal

abilities. If your child has been diagnosed with CP, she should be referred by her pediatrician or preemie follow-up clinic to your state's early intervention program, whose job it is to do a complete, developmental evaluation, and arrange for the appropriate, specialized interventions for your child. Therapy for a child with cerebral palsy may include:

* **Physical therapy:** to help with gross motor skills, such as standing, walking, running, and sports, and to recommend any special equipment, such as shoe inserts or braces (to keep the foot and ankle in normal positions);

* **Occupational therapy:** to help with fine motor and self-help skills, such as eating, dressing, toileting, writing, and drawing, and to recommend any special equipment, such as adapted silverware or pencils. Occupational therapy can also help with any sensory issues, such as aversion to certain textures (in clothing or food, for example) or kinds of touch, which some preemies with CP will have (see page 507);

* **Speech and language therapy:** because CP sometimes affects the way a child moves her lips, jaw, tongue, and respiratory muscles, all of which are necessary for speaking;

* **Medical treatments:** including medications or procedures to reduce high muscle tone, and treatments for joint problems that can result from abnormal tone or movements;

* **Family support:** to help parents or siblings cope with the emotional and practical challenges of caring for a child with CP.

Fees for physical therapy and medical treatments are often covered, fully or partially, by private insurance plans or Medicaid. Other kinds of therapy are less often covered, but if your child's doctor provides good documentation of medical necessity, you may have a better chance of being reimbursed. Many therapists also help by adjusting their fees based on a family's ability to pay.

One of the advantages of starting therapy early is that therapists can help parents learn how to understand and relate to their child better. This can be tremendously valuable, since muscle tone problems can interfere not only with the way a child does various tasks, but also with the way she responds to and communicates with her parents. A child with CP may have trouble giving nonverbal cues about her wants and needs. For example, she may not be able to turn away from her parents when she needs a rest from stimulation, and instead, may be frequently irritable, making her parents feel rejected. A therapist can help parents by teaching them that some of their child's responses and symptoms are due to her cerebral palsy, not to lack of love for her parents.

As time goes on, and if the need arises, your child's doctor will tell you about medical treatments that are used to help children with spastic CP. Most involve attempts to loosen stiff joints and muscles, which can be uncomfortable or even painful (like an intermittent or sometimes a constant cramp) as well as interfere with movement. The first line of treatment is usually medication that a child can take orally, such as diazepam (Valium) or baclofen. Oral medications are most effective in children who need just a mild decrease in muscle tone, or who have widespread spasticity.

When it's important to target certain, specific muscles, there are other options. One is Botox—yes, that trendy medication used to erase facial wrinkles is also a widely used treatment for cerebral palsy. This medication is injected into tight muscles to reduce the high tone and make them more pliant. It is effective in many cases of mild or moderate CP, helping a child improve her leg positioning and walk better. The effects are temporary—from three to six months—and provide a good opportunity for physical therapy or casts that aim to correct positioning problems.

Some children get Botox every three or four months on an on-going basis.

Another treatment for spastic CP is a baclofen pump, a small pump that is surgically inserted under the skin of the abdomen and releases doses of the medication baclofen, a muscle relaxer, into the spinal fluid every few hours. This treatment has the advantage of relaxing a broad area of the body's muscles, rather than just a few specific ones, and is often extremely effective. It is generally used in children after the age of three.

A surgical procedure called selective dorsal rhizotomy can be used to reduce high tone in the legs. In the lower back area, nerves that lead to the legs and are functioning abnormally are identified and cut. The benefits—reduced pain, greater muscle strength and balance, and an improved ability to walk, either independently or with more ease using a walker or crutches—are permanent, but weeks or months of intensive physical therapy are needed after the procedure to strengthen the legs that have been weakened and to train them to make new movements. You can ask your child's doctor about the newer, minimally invasive approach to rhizotomy that is offered by a few hospitals; recovery time is far faster, so a child can start physical therapy within a few days after surgery.

All of these treatments have pros and cons that you should discuss in detail, along with other treatment options, with your child's doctor and therapists before making any decisions. When the time comes, keep in mind that high muscle tone is not the only thing that prevents good motor function in children with cerebral palsy. (Abnormal balance and weakness of muscles can, also.) Thus, reducing spasticity will improve some children's function more than others.

The mainstay of non-medical treatment for CP is physical therapy. While the effectiveness of physical therapy is hard to prove in research (one problem is that it's difficult to do controlled studies, in which some children are denied physical therapy for the experiment's sake), it is generally believed to improve quality of movement, to reduce the eventual occurrence of muscle contractures that might require orthopedic surgery, and to give parents a better understanding of how best to help their children. Some experts, though not all, believe that motor skills, like cognitive skills, can be enhanced by enriching stimulation, thus compensating for some biological deficits. Occupational therapy and speech and language therapy also are long-standing, widely used therapies to help children who have CP with the skills of daily life.

You're likely to hear about a myriad of newer therapies, but be sure to ask your child's doctor before trying one, since some make claims they can't live up to. Among those enthusiastically recommended by parents is hippotherapy (horseback riding with a specially trained therapist). Parents say it helps their children who can't walk get a sense of what movement feels like, stretches their legs, arms, and back, helps their balance and the strength of their muscles, allows them to bond with an animal—and is just plain fun. For exercise, swimming with a recreational therapist is highly recommended, since movements in the water work muscles more strenuously, and the buoyancy offers your child a chance to experience the thrill of independent mobility.

For the future, medical researchers are working on two experimental therapies that hold a great deal of promise. While up to now it has been thought that the damage to the brain that caused cerebral palsy was permanent and physical therapists aimed to minimize the stiffness or abnormal movements that resulted, these therapies have raised hopes that it may be possible to actually heal damaged parts of the brain. For instance, constraint-induced therapy, which has been used with adult stroke survivors for over a decade, has been more recently tried with children whose CP affects just one side of their body. In constraint-induced therapy, a child's good arm is restrained, and the child works intensively—at least six hours a day for three weeks—with a physical therapist to practice repetitive movements with the other. A recent study found enormous improvement in children that lasted even after the therapy stopped; for example, one four-year old boy who had never been able to use his affected arm began to play ball and later joined a Little League team, using a specially adapted glove as an aid.

A similar principle is behind robotic therapy, also used initially in stroke patients and in the testing phase for children with cerebral palsy. Placing his arm in the arm of a robot connected to a computer screen, for example, a child might try to move the cursor on the screen for many, exact repetitions—hundreds in an hour long session—with the computer gently assisting him if he doesn't move or moves in the wrong direction. Early findings seem to indicate significant, lasting improvements in the children's movements. If you're interested in finding out whether it's possible for your child to participate in a clinical trial, ask for more information from United Cerebral Palsy (at www.ucp.org or 800-872-5827) or the National Institute of Neurological Disorders and Stroke (at www.ninds.nih.gov/disorders/cerebral_palsy/detail_cerebral palsy.htm or 800-352-9424).

Most people with cerebral palsy and normal intelligence reach high levels of function and independence. Children with disabilities have a legal right to public education through high school, and a significant number go on to study at colleges and universities, including some of the nation's best. An adult with moderate CP should be able to do almost any job that involves intellectual more than manual dexterity; you'll find lawyers, doctors, and teachers, among others. An adult with severe CP is more likely to live at home longer, or in an apartment with a personal aide or a group home set up for people with disabilities, but may be able to work, utilizing new breakthroughs in assisted technology such as voice-activated computers.

In most cases, children with CP outlive their parents, although the survival rate to adulthood is lowest, about 70 percent, for children with quadriplegic cerebral palsy and severe intellectual impairment.

According to experts, there are periods of particular stress in the life of a family with a child with cerebral palsy. The first, of course, is at the time of diagnosis and for a while afterward, when parents are dealing with their own grief while having to meet the practical and emotional demands of starting various kinds of treatment. The second period of particular stress comes when the child enters school. Next are the adolescent years, when children with CP, even if it is mild, struggle with particularly tough social and self-esteem issues. Finally, there's the advent of adulthood, when parents have to figure out living arrangements, how to get any needed special services (which were previously available through the school system or pediatric clinics), and how their child will cope, in general, in the less protective adult world.

As you make your way through the first period, we suggest that you take a few minutes to read *In Depth: Parenting a Child with Special Needs* on page 537, where you may find some answers to questions you have about the journey you are facing. One question shared by many parents is: Will our lives ever be the same again? The answer is no, as it would be for any parents with a new baby. What is hard to realize now, but what most parents gradually do, is that the change won't necessarily be for the worse. Just as childless couples have never experienced the joys of children, and don't realize how worthwhile it is, on balance, to be awakened at dawn every morning or to lose the opportunity for nightly romantic dinners, couples without disabled children can't possibly understand the joys and profound meaning that they bring to their parents.

A study of the impact of cerebral palsy on families was revealing. Asked about the negatives, about 65 percent of the parents interviewed said they lived on a "roller coaster," about 40 percent said they had trouble finding good childcare, and about 35 percent said they had had to quit a job at some point. Asked about the positives, about 90 percent of the parents said that the experience had increased their self-esteem and brought the family closer together. "Again, we learn that having a child with a disability means hard work for parents, but it is rewarding work," concluded United Cerebral Palsy, the study's sponsors.

Don't ever doubt the power that your love and care have to make your child's life rich and rewarding. A recent small study looked at whether parenting style has a major effect on the quality of life of children with CP. Researchers rated each set of parents in two ways: whether they were more controlling and protective or gave more freedom to their child, and whether they were more critical and emotionally distant or more accepting and warm. They concluded that parenting style had a far greater influence on the children's psychological and social quality of life than any other factor—including how severe the cerebral palsy was. The children of parents who gave more independence, and were accepting and warm, had higher self-esteem, better behavior, and fewer social or emotional limitations.

As your child grows, experts advise that you allow her to do everything she's capable of, avoid overindulging her, listen to her opinions and feelings, and above all, recognize and value her efforts and achievements. Keep in mind that the most valuable thing you can give your child is not a new developmental skill, but an environment of unconditional love and a strong foundation of self-esteem.

And you must come to trust your child's inner timetable and ultimate development. Later, you'll find that the lessons in faith and acceptance you gain now will serve you and your child well, long after you reach the end of this huge journey you're taking together.

Predicting Intelligence

My one-year-old son is doing some things later than his twin sister, and at preemie clinic they told us his mental development is slower than it should be. Does this mean he's mentally retarded?

Of course you're anxious. But don't necessarily come to that conclusion yet. First of all, keep in mind that some of the differences you are noticing in your twins may be due to the fact that one is a boy and one is a girl. Because of differences in brain development, baby girls tend to acquire language more quickly than boys do and are usually more interested in social interactions. (Boys tend to have a better sense of spatial relations and mechanics, but those skills emerge later, when toddlers begin to play with puzzles and blocks.) Also, although severe intellectual disability can usually be diagnosed in early infancy, experts often can't tell which infant preemies will end up with milder problems, and which will be normal. Minor developmental delays often come and go. It's hard to predict whether a young child will end up being a quick or slow learner, with a higher or lower IQ, before he reaches school age.

Overall, former preemies do have somewhat lower IQ scores on average and a higher rate of mental retardation than children born at term (see page 527). But averages don't tell you anything about your individual child.

Parents whose children have mild cognitive delays in the first couple of years have many good reasons to be optimistic. Here's why:

* **The younger a child is, the less likely it is that his score on a developmental test will persist over time.** The most commonly used developmental assessment tool for babies and toddlers is the Bayley Scales of Infant Development, which has a mental and a motor component. The Bayley evaluates the development of a child up to about two years of age—but cannot measure his IQ. It is useful because it allows delays to be picked up early, and helps identify infants and toddlers who can benefit from early intervention services.

But a Bayley score doesn't reliably predict how a child will develop in later years. First of all, normal development can proceed in different children at very different rates. Also, infants have only a small repertoire of behaviors and skills that can be assessed. For instance, a baby can reach for things he wants, and find sights or sounds amusing, but no baby can build a model airplane or write a funny story. As a child gets older, there are more skills and abilities that should emerge and can be measured. Finally, the family environment of a child, and the experiences he's exposed to as he grows, are going to play a major role in his learning.

When a Bayley is given at six months of age, only one in four scores corresponds to a child's IQ at three years of age. When a Bayley is given at two years, its predictive value increases: Three in four scores are confirmed by an IQ test a year later. But studies show that even IQ scores can change and improve over time, thanks to a child's family's and teachers' efforts.

* **When an infant or toddler has Bayley scores that are only slightly lower than average, his delays may be only a temporary consequence of his prematurity.** Preemies can develop more slowly than full-term babies in their first 18 months because long hospital-

izations and medical treatments can interfere with normal stimulation and learning, and some may still be recovering from the effects of illnesses, and some may have transient problems with muscle tone (see page 469). Children who are found to have mild cognitive delays in the first couple of years are also the most responsive to early intervention. With appropriate education and stimulation, by the time they are four or five years old and ready to enter preschool, quite a few of these slow developers have caught up and have IQ scores in the normal, or even high range.

* **The predictive value of a Bayley assessment is greater for extremely low scores,** which are more likely to stay low over time and to be confirmed later by IQ testing indicating mental retardation. Severe cognitive impairments can usually be diagnosed before 18 to 24 months of age. If this happens with your child, it's important to know that the vast majority of children who are mentally retarded can still learn a lot—much more than you probably think they can—and steadily progress over the years.

What neurologists and baby specialists are looking for when they assess an infant's development are certain well-defined milestones—mental, physical, and social—that reflect his ability to explore the world and to learn. For example, some of the milestones an infant normally achieves by 12 months of age or earlier are:

* Good head control (he can lift and hold his head steady and look where he wants);
* A pincer grasp (he can pick up small objects between his thumb and forefinger);
* He can bring his hands together, hold two objects at once, and transfer objects from hand to hand;
* He tracks moving objects with his eyes;

* He orients his attention toward a sound;
* He can move his arms and legs in a coordinated, alternating motion (important for later taking his first steps);
* He babbles (a prelude to speech);
* He can imitate behaviors and actions, such as a smile or a sound (important for sociability and learning);
* He recognizes the permanence of objects, as shown by looking for a hidden object that he remembers having seen (evidence of his developing attention, memory, and knowledge about the world);
* He is wary of strangers, and gets upset at separation from a loved one (a sign of a secure emotional attachment to parents and caregivers, which is a strong predictor of a baby's cognitive development and future academic success).

After a child turns three, there are several tests that can measure his IQ. Developmental psychologists often use more than one tool to assess a wide range of cognitive abilities that normally develop before a child enters preschool. Their goal is also to determine a child's strong and weak points in particular areas of learning, so that specific educational techniques can be used to help him. Families should take each result as a piece of information that may be useful, but also be aware of these tests' limitations, such as:

* **The presence of a motor or sensory impairment (like cerebral palsy or a hearing loss)** can make a child perform at a level lower than his intellectual capabilities. An IQ score can also be biased by the behavior of a child during testing (if he doesn't pay attention, for example), his language and culture (if his first language isn't English or he's not a white American), and the skills of the examiner.

(Continued on page 528)

Prematurity and IQ

The normal range for IQ scores is from 85 to 115. About three in four preemies have scores in this range, indicating that they have normal intelligence.

Of course, just like for term babies, there's a wide distribution, and some preemies have above normal—or even way above normal—intelligence, while others have below normal intelligence. For preemies as a whole, the average IQ tends to be about 10 points below the average for children born at term—a mean score of 93 compared to 103, according to recent studies. It is believed that loss of cognitive faculties in preemies may result from numerous factors that can interfere with a developing brain, such as medical complications that cause a lack of blood flow or oxygen, poor nutrition over long periods of time, infection, inflammation, or exposure to drugs or stimulation that adversely affect the brain.

Smaller and younger preemies score lower than older and bigger preemies in general, but recent studies point out that family factors, and in particular the parents' level of education, predict a child's later intelligence even better than weight and gestational age at birth. This is reassuring news, indicating that the stimulating environment, loving support and learning opportunities you give your child—as well as the genes you pass down—can balance or even outweigh the risks of a premature birth.

This doesn't mean you need to teach your child aggressively, with flash cards or other rote learning. That might even be counterproductive. Rather, if you spend time with him for many hours a day, playing attentively, reading books,

talking, and telling him what you're doing as he accompanies you in your daily routine, you'll increase his cognitive capacity and flexibility—the roots of intelligence. Child development specialists also believe that creating a strong emotional attachment with your baby is crucial for his intellectual development. This will give him confidence in the responsiveness of people around him, which will support his ability to explore, learn, interact with other adults and children, adjust to school, develop a positive sense of self, and recover from upsets and failures.

Different degrees of intellectual disability lead to dramatically different developmental outcomes. About 10 percent to 15 percent of the total population have IQ scores between 70 and 80, indicating borderline intelligence, or slow learning abilities; in preemies born at less than 1,000 grams, the prevalence is somewhat higher, about 15 percent to 30 percent. Borderline intelligence is not mental retardation, and can go unrecognized if a child is enrolled in a class in which the mean IQ of the other students is in the low average range. But if a child who is a slow learner is in a more demanding school environment, he may fail, or may be wrongly reproached for laziness. When given adequate early intervention and educational support, children with borderline intelligence can learn and progress in mainstream schools at an almost normal rate.

An IQ score below 70 is classified as mental retardation. About 5 percent of preemies with birth weights greater than 1,000 grams, and 10 percent to 15 percent of preemies with birth weights less than 1,000 grams, have IQs in this range, compared to 2 percent to 3 percent of the total population. Mental retardation in former preemies frequently goes along with other disabilities, like cerebral palsy or loss of vision, and most children who are affected do best with multidisciplinary interventions, as well as special education.

Most former preemies diagnosed with mental retardation will have a mild (IQ score of 55 to 70) or moderate (IQ score of 40 to 55) degree of cognitive impairment, and will be able to dress and feed themselves, use the bathroom, talk, learn, make friends, find work, and carry on a productive life. Family environment and participation, together with special education, can have a great impact on the cognitive abilities of children with mild or moderate mental retardation. Those who are mildly retarded can usually reach a sixth-grade academic level, and develop enough social and vocational skills to live semi-independently. Those with moderate retardation can usually be educated to a second-grade level, and function independently in environments that are orderly and familiar, such as their home or a sheltered workshop.

Children with severe mental retardation (an IQ score of 20 to 40) can develop language, but usually not until after age five, and can think very simply. Those with profound mental retardation (an IQ score of below 20) usually need constant aid and supervision.

Hearing that your child may have an intellectual disability can be extremely painful. But parents should keep in mind that there's a lot they can do, with their active and loving involvement at home and the quality of the early intervention and education they provide, to support a child's cognitive development and everyday functioning. There is also a blessing you will discover over time. Children with mild or moderate mental retardation may be slow to learn, but their emotional responsiveness is usually normal or better, bringing deep joy to their families, friends, and, not least of all, themselves.

* **IQ scores can change over time,** depending on the support and stimulation a child gets. The IQs of many children who come from disadvantaged families, for instance, rise once they're enrolled in a good quality preschool program. (The reverse is unfortunately true, too. Children who are not appropriately stimulated can lose IQ points over time.) To promote a child's intellectual ability, research shows that you should play with him, read to him, talk to him, and turn off the TV.

* **True, a high IQ is usually a good indication of a child's future academic success.** IQ tests measure aptitudes like memory, language comprehension, and the ability to discern patterns, which are important in school work. But human intelligence is too complex to be described by one number, and a high IQ doesn't necessarily predict how successful a person will be in life. Some of the many meaningful abilities an IQ *cannot* measure are social skills, creativity, athleticism, musicality, artistic ability, humor, curiosity, resilience, and empathy. The concept of emotional intelligence has become widely accepted in recent years, and so-called EQ is considered even more important for success at work than the intellectual abilities measured by IQ.

There may be only one Albert Einstein (a preemie who was considered a slow student and later recognized as a genius), but there are huge numbers of children who start out as poor students and become very successful later in school and in life. In particular, IQ scores that are classified as low average, borderline, and mildly retarded should be interpreted with caution, before jumping to pessimistic conclusions.

Detecting Learning Disabilities

We think our son is really bright, yet he's slower in learning to read than his friends. Are preemies at special risk for learning disabilities?

If you asked around among a group of normal adults, you would find that some of them learned to read earlier than average and others later. You would also find that some who eventually became the most successful students were late readers. Some kids just aren't neurologically ready or interested in reading as soon as others. It could be that your son is more focused on mastering jungle gyms, or exploring the world of dinosaurs or action toys, than on sitting down to read at this point in his life, and that he'll catch up as soon as he gets around to it.

Nevertheless, since your child was a preemie, it's important not to just wait and see. Former preemies are at greater risk for learning disabilities than other children, and if your son does have one, an early diagnosis (ideally, before he's in third grade) could help him a lot. The academic problems caused by learning disabilities can be a source of great frustration to a child, particularly if they're mistaken for lack of intelligence, talent, effort, or interest in school. So, talk to your pediatrician and your child's teacher about your concerns. If either agrees that it's warranted, or you remain concerned, ask for a referral to a professional who specializes in learning disabilities, and arrange to have your son evaluated.

Learning disabilities are quite common in the general population, affecting more than one in ten children. When preterm and term children with normal IQs are compared, though, learning disabilities occur approximately twice as frequently in preemies—mostly in those with smaller birth weights and gestational ages, more medical complications, and more social stresses (like poverty, low parental education, and unstimulating or chaotic home environments). They're also more common in preemies with a family history of learning disabilities.

Although a few kinds of problems that affect learning, such as hyperactive behavior, short attention span, and problems with fine motor coordination (which can later affect a child's penmanship) are sometimes evident earlier, most learning disabilities aren't picked up until elementary school, when children are challenged with the demanding tasks of reading, spelling, writing, and arithmetic. A learning disability is diagnosed when there's a significant gap between a child's intelligence and the skills he's achieved in one or more academic areas. Children with learning disabilities may have more difficulty than other kids their age with spoken or written language, math, memory, reasoning, or attention and self-control. Besides delaying academic achievement in one or more areas, learning disabilities can also be a cause of social problems.

Even if he does turn out to have a learning disability, your child's long-term prospects may be very good. Because these deficits affect only specific aspects of development, they usually don't limit a child's general potential to learn. Special education programs, tutoring, counseling, or medication can often help a lot. Young people with learning disabilities can aim to achieve a college education or higher, and to find professions in which they make the best use of their gifts, becoming successful, fulfilled, and well-adjusted adults.

Preemies and Learning Disabilities

What is a learning disability? This broad term covers many kinds of problems in the key areas of learning:

* **Reading disorders.** Difficulty with reading is called dyslexia. Dyslexia can refer to problems with any of the steps involved in reading, such as being able to recognize letters as symbols rather than as meaningless shapes, perceive the different sounds that make up words, or remember words that one has read before. Other reading disabilities, involving difficulty with comprehension of concepts rather than identification of single words, may be found in later grades. These might arise if a child has difficulty forming mental images from a written sentence, or relating a concept she's reading about to one stored in her memory.
* **Writing disorders.** If a child has difficulty reproducing the shapes and symbols of letters, words, and numbers in writing, dyslexia may be to blame. She may have trouble recognizing or remembering them, or she may have a problem with "visual-motor coordination": linking what she sees to the appropriate movements of her fingers and hands. Delayed fine motor skills—for instance, holding and controlling a pencil with precision—may also contribute to this difficulty. Children with disorders of visual-motor coordination often produce less in writing than their peers, because they can't write as fast or as well.
* **Arithmetic disorders.** Problems with math can arise from difficulty distinguishing numbers and symbols, memorizing facts like the multiplication table, aligning numbers (a task requiring visual-motor coordination), or understanding abstract concepts.

Some learning disabilities, because they're so broad, hinder performance in more than one subject, and can also affect a child's social interactions:

* **Difficulty understanding speech, despite normal hearing (central auditory processing or receptive language disorder).** These children may be unable to distinguish one sound from another, or to understand a complex sentence they hear, making it difficult for them to follow instructions.
* **Difficulty articulating sounds (articulation disorder), using words (expressive language disability), pronouncing words, or stuttering.** These children may lack fluency in expressing themselves and what they've learned, orally and in writing. Many have difficulty retrieving words they know from their memory.
* **Difficulty focusing and concentrating (attention deficit disorder, or ADD).** ADD can show up, especially in preemies, as excessive daydreaming, easy distractibility, and a tendency to mentally drift off. Or it can be accompanied by the fidgety, hyperactive, and impulsive behavior more commonly associated with ADD, in which case it's called attention deficit/hyperactivity disorder, or ADHD. Not surprisingly, any difficulty paying attention can make the consequences of other learning disabilities worse. Boys are more frequently diagnosed with ADD or ADHD than girls.
* **Difficulty with cognitive functioning.** This includes problems with logic, abstract thinking, or memory. It also can include problems

with so-called executive functions: planning, problem solving, and being able to work independently. A child may have difficulty handling new information, remembering assignments, or planning a course of action. She may show poor judgment, lack common sense, or have problems with decision making. Delays often appear in the later grades, as more activities that involve abstract reasoning are required. Young people with this kind of cognitive learning problem may show normal or even higher than normal intelligence in other areas.

* **Non-verbal learning disabilities.** These children have difficulty with space and time. They may have trouble understanding how much space things—including their own bodies—take up, which can result in clumsiness, or in telling time and planning within a time frame, which can lead to problems doing homework. They often have trouble with the big picture: they know a lot, but struggle to write an essay with a beginning, middle, and end; or learn rote arithmetic skills well, but struggle with math problems. They are at risk for social problems, also, since they don't perceive or use facial expressions as skillfully as other kids do.

* **Autism-spectrum disorders.** Some recent studies suggest that former preemies may have a higher risk of autism than children born at term. Autism is associated with a variety of learning disabilities, such as attention deficit/hyperactivity disorder, gross and fine motor problems, difficulty imitating gestures and movements (which can interfere, for example, with writing and drawing), and problems with reading comprehension. (Children with autism may have an outstanding ability to read words but still not fully grasp the meaning of what they read.) Speech and language disorders are also common. As a result, most children with autism, even if they have very high

IQs, need special education. Keep in mind, though, that this diagnosis is a wide umbrella including very mild forms of autism and other related disorders—like Asperger's syndrome—which don't preclude mainstream schooling and happy, normal lives (people with Asperger's may be socially awkward but are highly intelligent, and can achieve extremely successful careers in fields like science and mathematics).

Mostly because of learning disabilities, up to half of preemies with a birth weight less than 1,000 grams, and one-third of those with a birth weight less than 1,500 grams, will need some kind of special tutoring or educational services.

The sooner a learning disability is detected and a child receives special support, the better he'll do. Most elementary schools will have a child evaluated if he has a two-year or greater delay in some area (for instance, if a fourth grader is writing at only a second-grade level), but his parents and teachers can raise a red flag sooner than that and request an earlier evaluation. Don't berate yourself too hard if you miss the signs, though; they can be subtle. Especially if a child is very smart, he may have figured out how to compensate for a mild learning disability and still do well in school. On the other hand, not all children with normal intelligence who fail in school have a learning disability. Some of them may just be slower to develop a skill (normal development encompasses a wide range of different abilities that mature at different times), have emotional disturbances, have previously unrecognized visual or hearing losses, or simply lack motivation.

Diagnosing and identifying learning disabilities is done after an extensive evaluation by a psychologist who specializes in learning disabilities. You can make an appointment yourself, or get a referral from your child's teacher or pediatrician. Sometimes a psychologist will suggest that your child also be seen by another specialist, such as an audiologist, speech-language pathologist, occupational therapist, or special educator, to confirm the diagnosis.

The origin of learning disabilities lies in problems in the way that different areas of the brain are linked together; the result is difficulty interpreting and using information that comes through the senses or from another part of the brain. Scientists have shown that some brain regions in children with dyslexia are smaller and function differently from those of children who are good readers, and that educational intervention can change some of their brain patterns to make them more efficient.

Preemies may be at higher risk for learning disabilities because a premature birth, and the unusual experiences that follow it, may interfere with the way brain cell networks normally would have formed in late pregnancy and early infancy. The cause of a premature birth (for instance, an infection or other medical complication) might also cause a learning disability, perhaps because of damage to nerve cells as their connections were developing. In addition, disorders like dyslexia tend to run in families, and scientists have found a genetic link to some subtle brain dysfunctions.

You should realize that children with learning disabilities are often bright and, with help, can succeed academically—even excel. Public schools are required by federal law to provide special programs for learning disabled children, either in separate, all-day classrooms or in extra classes that a child attends in addition to his regular ones. Some parents hire a private tutor to help their child. If you decide to do that, wait until after he's been evaluated, when you'll have specific recommendations about your child's needs and strengths. A good tutor doesn't have a "one size fits all" approach, but will tell you whether she has the skills to help your child. If not, she can refer you to someone who does. (See pages 594–595 for a list of resources on learning disabilities, including organizations that can provide references for private special educators.) Although learning disabilities are life-long conditions, by giving a child individual attention and focusing on ways to overcome or work around his particular deficits, and by keeping learning fun, special education can have remarkable success.

Specialists other than teachers may also be called on to help:

* **Audiologists** can help children develop better strategies for listening to and understanding what they hear, sometimes by using technologies like hearing aids or amplification, even for children who aren't hard of hearing, or computer programs that slow down words, making it easier to understand their sounds.
* **Speech Therapists** can work with children who don't articulate well, practicing specific sounds through imitation, play, and exercise.
* **Occupational therapists** can help with fine motor delays, improving hand movements for writing and drawing, and coordinating them with visual attention.
* **Doctors** can treat attention and hyperactivity disorders with medications.
* **Psychotherapists,** usually using a combination of behavioral therapy and family therapy, can help to decrease a child's restlessness and improve his concentration and ability to learn.

No matter what kind of learning disability your child has, the therapists following him should also teach you the best strategies for interacting with him, stimulating his interest with activities and toys, and encouraging appropriate behavior and skills. Since some kids with learning disabilities can't read facial expressions well, they may do or say the wrong thing to other children and turn them off. So parents should also try to help their child learn how to make friends by teaching him how to understand people's attitudes and feelings.

If your former preemie is diagnosed with a learning disability, remember that he's not alone.

They are found in millions of school-age children, often relieving them from the pressure and stigma of being considered lazy, difficult, or unintelligent. A parent's unconditional support and optimism is crucial to help a child take a positive attitude toward his problems at school and lessen their possible psychological consequences, which may include withdrawal, anger, depression, and loss of self-esteem.

It takes great patience to sustain a child who has a learning disability, and many parents find comfort in talking to a counselor when they're still searching for solutions. Support groups, books, and Internet resources can also help parents better understand and face their child's learning disability, connecting them to the many other families who are dealing with a similar problem.

MULTIPLES

One Twin with Disabilities

What can I do to help my twin who has a disability? She'll feel so bad when she compares herself to her sister.

For a parent, nothing is more difficult than seeing a child of yours in pain, physical or emotional. You would take it onto yourself, if you could. But pain is a part of every person's life, whether she has a disability or not. All parents learn that the most valuable thing they can offer is to help their children develop the emotional strength and inner resources to deal with whatever hurdles they face—and perhaps even to be strengthened rather than weakened by them.

Although it's natural to be most concerned about your daughter with a disability, you should also make sure not to overlook your other twin's needs. It's difficult, and occasionally painful, growing up with a sibling who has a chronic illness or disability. But try not to get discouraged or depressed about her situation. There is a hidden—and profound—positive impact of these problems. In many growing children, they give rise to unusual amounts of self-confidence, compassion, and responsibility. In fact, biographers have noticed that a disproportionate number of the prominent, historically important people in our century faced adversity—of this kind and many others—in their childhoods, rather than having the idyllic childhood that we all strive to give our children and assume is best for them. Strong children who are fighters can overcome a lot, and benefit in unique ways from doing so.

What's most important is for you to check in often with your children about their feelings. This is true for both of your daughters, the one who has a disability and the one who does not. Ideally, you'll develop the kind of relationships that make them feel they can confide in you, telling you their feelings, and counting on you for support.

Still, it's sometimes a challenge to know how to help your children, each with her own difficulties. First some advice from experts to help your daughter who has a disability:

* **Affirm her feelings.** As your daughter gets older and has a growing awareness of being different, she will often feel sad, embarrassed, angry, lonely, fragile, or discouraged. When she does, acknowledge her feelings and let her cry about them, holding her and letting her know that you realize things are hard for her. Don't say things like "Buck up" or "Other children have even worse problems." No matter how well-meaning you are, you'll give her the

impression that you find her feelings unacceptable, or just don't want to hear about them.

* **Don't pity her.** Even though you are empathizing, don't convey pity. Once you've let her know that you understand her feelings, you can teach her that everyone feels pain and has struggles—and that her disability neither defines her nor limits her future. It's important for you to believe this, too.

* **Be open and honest about her disability.** Openly discuss your daughter's disability with her: what it is, how it happened, and whether it is likely to get better or worse in the future. Use clear, simple, age-appropriate explanations rather than telling her more details than she really wants to know at one time. Also practice with her some answers she can give to kids at school if they ask questions or make comments. You'll find good suggestions in the books and web sites listed in *Resources* on pages 594 and 597–598.

* **Be a model of acceptance.** Model for her, through your daily actions, that you accept all aspects of every child, and admire every child for who he is. When you meet new children (say, in a social setting or at the doctor's office), comment on their strong points, not their weak ones. If they have disabilities, don't treat them differently from other children—be just as open and engaged. If you think they have beautiful eyes, say so. If they're really good at something, or have accomplished something that required effort, mention your admiration.

* **Respect her by being firm and demanding of her.** Whenever possible, apply to her the same rules, discipline, and expectations for being a responsible member of the household that you apply to her sister. At times this may seem overly demanding (to you or to her), as she will have to struggle and find alternative ways of doing things. But over time, it

will build her self-respect. Overprotecting and indulging her will diminish her sense of competence. However, it's also important to let her know often that you're aware of the extra effort she has to expend and that you treasure it.

* **Show clearly that it's the amount of effort that you value in your children, rather than the extent of their specific achievements.** It's important that your daughter who has a disability realize that you would not admire or love her more if she were free of it. Keep in mind that all of the therapy and medical treatments can send the wrong signal: that you are desperately trying to make her normal and will be disappointed with anything less.

* **Go out of your way to find an activity at which your daughter can excel.** Everyone needs to feel successful and to have pride of accomplishment. It may be anything from horseback riding to swimming, using computers or reading. Pay attention when your daughter tells you she particularly enjoys something, and get tips from her therapists or special education teachers about things she may be able to excel in. Do whatever is needed to facilitate her involvement, and share her pleasure!

* **Don't discourage her from mixing with other children who have disabilities.** While you may want to give your daughter a mainstream education and as normal a life as possible, find some arena in which she can interact with others who have disabilities. It will help her social self-confidence to meet other children with disabilities, and give her direction and ambition to meet adults who can become mentors and role models.

What about your other daughter? Most studies show that children who have siblings with a disability or chronic illness are well-adjusted, on average, and some indicate that they are more likely to develop positive qualities like strong social skills, sensitivity, and compassion for others. But that doesn't mean things are easy for them. Their lives are different from most other children's and frequently more challenging. You can expect a number of normal reactions.

Your daughter who does not have a disability will feel understandably jealous of all the attention her twin is getting from you and other caregivers. As she gets older, it will dawn on her that you may repeatedly have to cancel your plans to attend her events, or anticipated family events, to cater to her twin's needs. Also, she may have to cope with an unusual amount of early separation from you, because of hospital visits and doctors and therapists appointments.

It's common for children with siblings who have a disability to feel anger, blaming their sibling or parents for the fact that they don't get enough attention, or even for somehow causing their sibling's condition (before they are old enough to understand it). When they're young, it's typical for them to fear that they may get the condition, too, or that they did something to cause it. When they're a little older, they often feel embarrassed about having a sibling who is different, and may want to hide her from schoolmates, only to be hit by another negative feeling, shame, for doing that. And some feel guilty just for being healthy themselves.

Some ways to help your child who does not have a disability:

* **Be open and honest about her sibling's disability and ongoing problems.** Give her as much information as she wants, but communicate it in age-appropriate ways. For example, a young child whose sibling has cerebral palsy and wears braces might be told, "It's hard for her to keep her legs in the right position for walking the way we do. The doctor gave her these to help her." When she's older, it may help to give her an update after each of her sibling's visits to the doctor, especially if there's more family stress. Be sure to explain to your young child that her twin's condition is not contagious and that she didn't cause it. These are common misconceptions that you may not even realize your child has.

* **Spend time alone with her.** Set aside some time each day, even if it's just at bedtime, and a longer period of a few hours each week. Siblings of children with disabilities often get very little time alone with their parents—when it's easiest for you to show her, and for her to realize, how much you love her.

* **Focus your attention entirely on her from time to time when her sibling is present, too.** It can be difficult not to be completely absorbed by your child with a disability if she has lots of needs or her behavior is a problem. But you have to learn how to let go of your protectiveness and sometimes give your other daughter undivided attention. For instance, when you're shopping or in a crowded waiting room, even if her twin with a disability is making too much noise and you fear she's bothering other people, try to answer your daughter's questions and meet her expectations. Be particularly sure not to ignore her just because she's well-behaved.

* **Take the time to listen to her feelings.** Acknowledge that you understand that her life is different, and more stressful, than that of other kids, and encourage her to share her feelings with you. Don't criticize them as selfish or mean. When it's appropriate, let her take part in family decision making and take her feelings into account.

* **Make sure to treat her like a child, not like a helping hand.** Involving your child in her sister's care can be a very positive thing—she may feel extremely proud of being able to help her disabled twin and the family—but

only to the extent that she likes it. When she's young, simple tasks like handing you diapers, singing, and playing with her sister may be appropriate. Above all, follow her cues. The aim is to make her feel included and helpful, but never burdened. Also beware of putting pressure on her to behave much more responsibly than a child of her age normally would. Some children feel that they have to overachieve to compensate for their parents' grief, or act more mature or understanding just because it's so hard to take care of their sibling, and end up missing out on the parental support that is appropriate and important for them.

∗ **Teach her how to respond to comments about her sister.** As she gets older, unfortunately, she's going to get both questions and barbs from her peers, and she'll be at an age when they will hurt. Coach her on exactly what to say, and role-play with her so that she becomes comfortable saying the words herself. Explain to her that sometimes people say hurtful things simply because they don't understand disability.

∗ **Clearly demonstrate that you accept and admire both of your children exactly as they are.** Researchers have found that when parents appear to be unaccepting of their child who has a disability, siblings are more likely to have problems adjusting.

∗ **Consider a sibling support group.** There are many support groups for siblings of children with disabilities where they can freely voice their feelings and see that others have them, too. If you think your daughter would benefit, you can call the organization listed on page 597 to see if they know of a group that is convenient for you.

Try to remember that every single sibling relationship is different, and being a twin is always complex, whether or not a disability is involved. There are siblings who are close from childhood through adulthood, some who never are, and some who start out close and grow apart as they grow up and vice versa. Even if you do all you can, your children may fall into any of these categories—just like everyone else's.

IN DEPTH

Parenting a Child with Special Needs

A Trip You Never Planned

Emily Perl Kingsley, a writer for *Sesame Street* and the mother of a child with special needs, once compared her parenting experience to being forced to take a trip to a place you never planned to visit. Parents who are going to have a baby feel like they are planning a fabulous vacation to a dreamland like Italy, she says. But if their child has a disability, they find out that their plane has landed in Holland instead.

> *. . . So you must go out and buy new guidebooks. And you must learn a whole new language. And you will meet a whole new group of people you would never have met. It's just a different place. It's slower-paced than Italy, less flashy than Italy. But after you've been there for a while and you catch your breath, you look around and you begin to notice that Holland has windmills . . . and Holland has tulips. Holland even has Rembrandts. But everyone you know is busy coming and going from Italy . . . and they're all bragging about what a wonderful time they had there. And for the rest of your life, you will say, "Yes, that's where I was supposed to go. That's what I had planned." And the pain of that will never, ever, ever, ever go away . . . because the loss of that dream is a very, very significant loss. But if you spend your life mourning the fact that you didn't get to Italy, you may never be free to enjoy the very special, the very lovely things about Holland.*

How Families React to the Birth of a Child with Special Needs

Many parents of children with disabilities have responded to Kingsley's words, not denying that their paths have been difficult, but affirming that over time, they also have found the "very lovely things about Holland."

The sociologist Rosalyn Benjamin Darling, co-author of *Ordinary Families, Special Children*, points out that although personal details may differ, most parents in this situation follow similar paths before being able to bring their lives back to normal. The steps along the way include:

* **Anomie, or disorientation.** When a baby's disability is diagnosed and for some time afterward, his parents may be disoriented, confused, and uprooted from their normal habits and frame of mind since so many of their plans and expectations have been shattered. Anomie is a mainly passive stage. Psychologists suggest that during this period, parents experience the normal process of grief for the loss of a healthy baby. First comes the initial shock, accompanied by numbness, and sometimes denial or disbelief. It may be too overwhelming at first to deal with the truth. For some parents, offers of information or emotional support can set off waves of panic, anger, and despair. Even those parents who want more information on their child's disability in order to help him may not know where to find it

and, as a result, feel powerless. Self-pity may alternate with guilt, and parents may feel lost, not knowing what to think or where to turn to get their bearings again.

* **Seekership.** Seeking answers to make sense of one's experience is a natural human reaction to the stage of anomie. To reestablish order and find meaning and solutions, most parents begin searching for resources to help them with their child. They may look for medical treatments, intervention programs, or educational and social support. They may also begin to ask openly for their child to be loved by family members, respected by friends, and accepted socially. By focusing their energies on meaningful tasks, most parents gradually begin to modify their expectations and come to accept their situation.

  The stage of seekership may never end completely, as new problems or obstacles can arise at any time, particularly when a child with a disability has a health or developmental setback, or when new challenges arise in adolescence and adulthood. Psychologists and parents report that flashbacks of the negative, passive feelings from the stage of anomie can periodically reappear (in a process that some experts have called chronic sorrow, see page 483), but they become easier to deal with, through experience.

* **Normalization.** Once they've discovered or created solutions to their problems, and if they receive good medical, social, and educational support, most families of children with disabilities succeed in reorganizing and normalizing their lives. In most cases, their lifestyle is not very different from that of families with normal children, although their expectations have been modified. Most parents still worry about their child's future, and many cope by adopting the philosophy of taking one day at a time. At the same time, most also feel hope.

Although given the choice many families would not bring a baby with a disability into the world again, they all say that they deeply love their child and that their parenting experiences have been fulfilling.

A Longer Phase of Anomie, for Parents of Preemies

A permanent disability in a premature baby is often diagnosed only after months have gone by, prolonging for his parents the initial stage of anomie. Their "plane" doesn't land in Holland right at birth, but is forced to make an emergency landing in an unexplored place.

For these families, the first reason for grieving is the loss of a normal pregnancy and a full-term baby to take home right away. In addition, if their preemie is very small and fragile, or very sick, the fear that he might not survive causes them to experience anticipatory grief over the possibility of losing him. Worries about a future disability may only lurk in the background, during the hospitalization. Even when a premature baby is finally ready to go home, his future development may still be uncertain, and doctors only able to tell his family about an increased risk of a future disability. Some parents deal better with this uncertainty than others; some can maintain an optimistic outlook, while for others, having to wait and see is torture.

When a definite diagnosis of disability is finally reached, it's a hard blow. Painful questions are faced: "Will my child ever walk, or will he always use a wheelchair?" "Is my baby ever going to see my face?" "Why did this have to happen to us? What did we do to deserve it?" Mothers and fathers who already felt guilty about their child's early birth, blaming themselves or their doctors for not preventing it, may find their remorse growing to unbearable heights. Parents who are unprepared, because their preemie had an easy hospital course and seemed to be OK, may feel acutely betrayed. Other families, who suspected all along that something was wrong with their child, may actually feel relieved that their suspicions are confirmed at last.

If you have just discovered that your premature baby has a disability, you're probably still disoriented and in the stage of anomie. Be reassured that your feelings, even if they're extremely negative, are normal: You need to feel them deeply in order to move on. But try not to despair. Ask for help from your partner, a close friend, or relative. Even if your friends are worried about you, they may need a word or sign from you to feel entitled to reach out and talk about the painful things that are happening to you. If you're afraid you're sinking into a depression, you should talk to a therapist (you can ask your child's pediatrician or your own doctor for advice on finding one) or a religious adviser. With some support you'll find yourself learning day by day what can help you cope, slowly leaving the climax of your crisis behind.

Moving on: The Role of Social Relationships

Before and shortly after their child's birth, many parents may share some of the negative or ambivalent societal attitudes toward children with special needs. People often consider having a child with a disability to be one of the worst tragedies that can happen to a family. When first hit by the harsh reality of their baby's condition, a mother and father have to review their ideas from a personal perspective they never imagined they'd have, and really think: "Exactly how bad is this? What specifically is no longer possible for us, and what is?" Bonding with a baby who has a disability is sometimes more difficult and can

take longer because the infant may not respond to his parents' attention and loving gestures with predictable and rewarding behavior, such as smiling, cuddling, or becoming soothed. (Many preemies, with or without disabilities, can be fussier and more difficult to handle than term infants, because of their still immature senses and neurological responses.)

Fortunately, barriers and obstacles are usually swept away by the strong bond that develops between parents and their baby, no matter how he looks or behaves. "As time goes by, you fall in love. You think, this kid's mine and nobody's gonna take her away from me," said one mother interviewed by the sociologist Darling. Like any parent, you notice and relish your baby's unique beauties. You feel the urge to hold and protect him. Your love, nourished by the love you'll get in return, will steadily grow. It will be your primary source of strength, helping you to abandon most of your initially negative feelings.

Especially at first, some parents may not talk openly to relatives and friends about their child's disability, out of shame, self-protection, or fear of causing pain or worry to people they love. But later, when they fully understand the nature of their baby's problem, parents begin to ask for attention and consideration for their child, first from significant others and then from the rest of the world. In Darling's interviews, most parents described their close relatives, friends, and work colleagues as generally sympathetic and a great source of both emotional and practical help. Only in a few cases did some relatives or friends react negatively, not wanting to get involved with a child who is disabled, or treating him differently from his siblings or cousins (sometimes in an overly affectionate, but not genuine, fashion).

If this happens to you, don't be too surprised. People who react oddly out of self-defense or ignorance often change their behavior over time.

But even if some relationships become impossible for you to carry on, you won't be abandoned. Your loyal friends will be supplemented by families of other children with disabilities, whom you'll meet through your child, and who will become meaningful friends and soulmates for you, like a second family.

Initially, facing strangers or acquaintances with a child who has a disability can be hard. If a baby doesn't look different, his parents may choose not to mention his condition, or tell a white lie about his age, to make it match his behavior or size. Don't feel bad about doing that—you have no obligation to open yourself up to everyone you meet. Questions can make a mother or father feel uncomfortable, and lead them to isolate themselves to avoid conflicts or embarrassment. That's also an understandable reaction. But after awhile, most parents begin to feel stronger and more secure when they take their child out in public. They find the right answers to give even to indelicate questions, and find that explaining their situation to others helps them put it in perspective themselves. Slowly, families resume old habits, like going to restaurants or shopping malls with their child without feeling that people's eyes are pointed at them. If somebody stares, they eventually learn not to be hurt by it or to lash out in anger, but simply to ignore it.

Sometimes a family risks isolation because of their child's restrictions: He has to avoid infections, it's difficult to move him around with his equipment, or he just can't enjoy certain activities. Parents may not get out much because they can't find competent babysitters and are scared that their child will get sick while they're gone, or are simply too tired to want to leave home. In time, you'll feel more comfortable getting your child out and about or going out without him. In the meantime, it can help to hire nurses as babysitters, or to form a babysitting co-op with other parents of children with disabilities. (Try contacting local early intervention and disability agencies, or advertising in the local paper.) You can also train several willing relatives and friends to take care of your child. And be sure to explore your options to receive respite care services. Respite care—advocates call it "the gift of time"—is short-term temporary care for people with disabilities, provided in your home or elsewhere. You get a precious break from your daily caregiving responsibilities, perhaps for a night or a few hours each week or month on a regular basis, or for an even longer time so that you can take a well-deserved vacation, all the while knowing that your child is in the good hands of a well-trained caregiver. Respite care services are usually payable on a sliding scale based on your family's income. (Check page 594 for ways to find out what is available in your area. Your child's service coordinator or hospital social worker can also help you find respite care and financial resources to help pay for it.)

A significant interaction is the one with doctors. Many parents in Darling's studies say their doctors were tactful and supportive, pointing out positive aspects of their child's condition without minimizing their concerns, and helping them to overcome their initial grief and immobilization. But many parents say they've also dealt with medical professionals who were lacking compassion and concern. If a doctor uses the wrong words or tone in communicating a child's risk for a disability, confirming a diagnosis, or even recommending institutionalization to parents who would never consider it, he can deeply hurt them, leaving an open wound that won't heal for a long time. If you're not happy with your baby's doctors and therapists, you should find the courage to leave them and look for other medical professionals who make you feel good about your child. All parents eventually find them and cherish those relationships.

How Parents Become Researchers and Experts

A powerful way for parents to move out of anomie and on to normalization is to seek answers to their questions and become well-informed about their child's disability. Mothers or fathers can feel particularly isolated because nobody around them is concerned about their issues or is available to answer their questions. Supportive relatives and friends simply can't provide a lot of practical advice about a child with a disability. Pediatricians and general practitioners may be good doctors, but may not know much about a child's particular disability and the latest treatments or possible interventions. A few parents have the shocking revelation that their pediatrician can't (or worse, doesn't want to) manage their child's condition or one of its complications. As a result, many families decide to look for medical information on their own, and for a doctor who specializes in their child's condition.

There are some very good books on children with disabilities, which you should read and keep handy as reliable references (some are listed on page 597). Also, a mine of information is readily available for you on the web. A quick search of "special needs" will lead you to dozens of web sites, some of them carefully designed and updated by national nonprofit organizations or medical professionals, some leading you to online parent support groups, others telling you personal stories. Even if you're a seasoned web surfer, you'll be surprised by the vast and rich human network that thrives online.

Parents of children with special needs have claimed for themselves a big chunk of the Internet, and rightfully so, because it's a fantastic way to break out of isolation. Chat groups and e-mail discussion lists allow you to listen to parents like you freely describing their daily joys and battles to each other. You can participate in discussions by sending your own messages, or just be a silent reader. Many families and children have created personal web sites where they post pictures and notes to share their experiences with anybody who's interested. Emotional support, guidance, and valuable information are only a few seconds away from you. Just be aware that when it comes to claims of miracle cures and therapies, or to medical information, what you read on the web isn't always reliable. Remember to check the source before building up false hopes, and ask your doctor before trying anything—a medication, a therapy—that might not only be a waste of time, money, and energy, but perhaps even harmful to your child.

If you don't yet feel a drive for knowledge, or can't take the initiative to reach out because you feel empty or overwhelmed, take your time. But be assured that when the right moment comes, you won't have to do everything alone. You can think of it as embarking on a new career—a venture that isn't easily undertaken without the help of others in the field who can educate and guide you and share their accumulated wisdom. In this case, the other "professionals" are parents of disabled children who have gone through the experience before you. Besides joining online support groups and chat rooms, you should also forge personal relationships with people who live nearby. You can meet them in a support group or parents' association that you may find through your child's school or early intervention program, or one of the many national or local organizations on disabilities (see page 597).

The sense of empowerment and of deep mutual understanding that another parent can offer you is unequaled. It's one thing to get advice from a counselor or developmental expert: it's another to see how someone has put it into practice. You'll be able to ask or answer questions, share experiences, agree or disagree as a peer. Through other parents' eyes, you'll also learn how to better appreciate your child with his special needs and special gifts. (He certainly has many!) And by breaking your isolation, you'll be able to make a normal life for yourself more quickly.

From Seekership to Normalization

Many parents become excellent advocates for their children, thanks to other families' support and suggestions, and their own efforts. Your goal should be to learn as much as possible about your child's condition, finding out about existing medical treatments, the effectiveness of interventions and therapies, and any available educational and financial help.

Today, thanks to early intervention programs, developmental support for infants and young children is usually readily available immediately after, or even before, they are diagnosed with a disability. (You can read more about early intervention on page 492.) But despite the fact that legislation has also aimed to secure free and appropriate public education for older children with disabilities, parents may still face some difficulties during the preschool and school years. Inappropriate settings, a lack of qualified staff for special education and health services, inadequate transportation, and financial barriers can still create challenges for families, especially if they live in an underserved or rural area. As a result, it is extremely important for parents to be well-informed and persistent in claiming their child's right to get help to grow to his maximum potential.

In other words, you should be a squeaky wheel, and never take no for an answer if it means getting your child the help he needs. That doesn't mean you should become unnecessarily confrontational or aggressive, since the school and public health officials you'll have to deal with are not your enemies, and are often the route to what you want. But since some of them may not be as forthcoming as they should be, you had better be prepared to find a way around them, talking to their supervisors and making your voice clearly heard.

Many parents and experts offer advice on establishing fulfilling lives for you and your child, and a normal routine for your family. Try to switch off your worries about your child's delays or limitations when you're with him and really play or relax together. Learn how to praise him frequently, but without exaggerating, as you would any other child. As much as possible, apply the same rules and discipline to him that you expect from your other children. Set challenging goals for him and avoid overprotectiveness and overindulgence so that he can truly do his best.

Keep in mind that kids with disabilities, like all children, don't have fixed skills, but need to be exposed to activities and helped to master them in order to move forward. Much of what any child can accomplish will depend on his education, the expectations he's trying to live up to, and the resources at his disposal. No one is born knowing how to swim, or read, or use the toilet, or behave politely. These come with education and a lot of hard work and practice. So you should nurture and educate your child as you would any child (although sometimes with different techniques) so that you can recognize his potential and help him reach it.

Talk to your child openly about his condition as soon as he can understand it so he can accept himself without embarrassment. Let him mingle with other children, with and without disabilities, to help him be comfortable in both spheres and to get the best educational opportunities—

without denying the limitations that go along with his disability, or implying that other children with disabilities are less desirable friends. Thanks to your efforts, along with early intervention and special education, you should see your baby progress and develop into a happy, well-adjusted child. That will give you an incredible sense of accomplishment, the most significant reward you could ever get. You'll soon realize that you too can be a proud and happy parent—and that your family's life can be wonderful.

Darling's studies indicate that the vast majority of families who have a child with a disability adapt well to the demands of their situation, and some even seem to function better in some ways than before. Most parents say they feel that their other children have not been negatively affected by a sibling with special needs; on the contrary, many say that their children became more responsible, aware, and compassionate, often assuming the role of protectors and defenders of their special brother or sister and taking over caregiving tasks without complaining. Parents often find that they have become better people and achieved a sense of growth and mastery through their experience. Many couples are rewarded with a deeper, more fulfilling relationship after going through this experience together.

But in some situations, a mother and father can get entangled in their different emotional reactions, particularly in the stage of anomie, or become so busy dealing with seekership that they grow apart. Some siblings of children with special needs feel neglected, or that their childhoods were hijacked by their family situation. (You can find advice on how to meet the needs of your children in *One Twin with Disabilities*, page 533; it applies just as much to nontwin siblings.) Most important is to be aware of possible marital and family problems, make extra efforts to keep communication alive, and, if needed, seek marital or family counseling promptly, to help you address difficulties at the first sign, overcome them when possible, and make your bonds stronger.

How Former Preemies with Disabilities View Their Lives

When parents of a child with special needs realize they have overcome their acute sense of loss and are enjoying life again, they often still have wrenching doubts about their child's future. "The world can be cruel." "How will she feel when her friends begin to date?" "Will he be miserable that he can't play sports?" In early childhood, parents can provide reassurance, encouragement, protection. But what about later, in adolescence, when peers become so important in shaping a child's self-image?

Encouraging answers come from several studies looking at how preemies judge their quality of life at adolescence and beyond. In one study, 141 former preemies—83 percent of all surviving premature babies with a birth weight less than 1,000 grams who were born between 1977 and 1982 in central-west Ontario, Canada—were interviewed when they were 12 to 16 years old. In addition, parents of nine severely impaired teenagers gave responses for them. Due to their extreme prematurity, more than a quarter of the adolescents had some serious impairment, such as cerebral palsy, mental retardation, blindness, or deafness. Yet, to the surprise of the researchers and the public, the vast majority of these young people, including those with disabilities, thought their lives were very good and certainly well worth living. As a matter of fact, their ratings of their quality of life were similar to those of a group of term-born adolescents of comparable age and socioeconomic background, none of whom had disabilities.

In another study, the same adolescents were interviewed about their self-esteem in various areas—scholastic, social, athletic, job-related—

and also about their physical appearance, romantic appeal, behavior, and ability to make friends. Experts point out that how teenagers rate themselves on these abilities, and their overall sense of self-worth, greatly influences the choices they make in their lives. Again, the researchers found encouraging results. The former preemies had levels of self-esteem similar to those of adolescents who were born at term, except with regard to athletic competence.

Yet other research studies followed a large group of preemies with a birth weight under 1,500 grams, born in the late 1970s in Ohio, from infancy to young adulthood, and compared them to a similar group of children who were born at term. At age 20, the former preemies reported that they were as satisfied with their emotional and physical health, academic achievements, and work performance as their full-term peers, and had similar levels of self-esteem. The only area in which they felt they lagged was physical resilience, which limited activities like sports and family outings. Not surprisingly, such self-perceived limitations were higher in those with neurosensory disabilities.

These research studies are particularly meaningful because they give former preemies the chance to speak for themselves. How heartening and encouraging it is to learn that they have a much more positive perspective on their lives than society, health professionals, and even some of their parents may have. Maybe they won't choose to become professional athletes, but many will still play sports for fun, and a world of opportunities is open to anyone who feels competent in school, in work, and with friends. Indeed, when reporting on some of these findings, one newspaper told the story of a former preemie who was in the Canadian study, a 16-year-old girl who weighed 640 grams at birth. She is blind, but she could play the flute (and hoped to be a professional musician), was a downhill skier, and rode a tandem bicycle. The portrait was of a vibrant, spirited, proud young woman in love with life.

Of course, we must ask: Is it possible that some of the children with disabilities in these studies were hiding their true feelings out of defensiveness, or were in denial about their limitations? While that cannot be completely ruled out, the evidence points more to a positive process of adaptation, self-acceptance, and affirmation. Other research on adolescents with disabilities (not former preemies) have found their self-worth and quality of life ratings to be high, too. The authors of the Canadian study point out that these children and their parents should get credit for how well they learned to cope with their disabilities. That may be the most important message coming from this research.

You are a mirror for your child. The way you see him will mightily shape his body image and sense of self. That is why you shouldn't deny his disability, try to change it, or hide it, but make an effort to accept it, work with it, and even love it as a part of your child's whole identity. Listen carefully to what so many others like him have to say about their lives—those who know first hand what it's like to live with a disability. They say their lives are full and good. So convince yourself that he can be happy and that he will be able to fulfill his dreams. That, after all, is what really matters.

Part IV

OTHER CONSIDERATIONS

CHAPTER 10
LOSING A BABY

. . . .

Helping you deal with a profound grief and guiding you through the necessary arrangements.

. . . .

INTRODUCTION: LOSING A BABY

Of all of the issues we cover in this book, this is the one for which words are most inadequate. Facing the loss of a child shatters all of a parent's expectations of how birth and life are supposed to go. You may feel shaken to your core right now, struggling to get your emotional bearings and keep going.

In this chapter, you can find the answers and guidance to help you deal with some of the questions, feelings, and choices you are now confronting, many of which you may never have thought about before. Some parts of this chapter may be useful to you now; others you may want to come back to as time passes and you find that new feelings and questions come to the surface.

While everyone must make his or her own way through this intensely personal experience, we hope that reading this will help you feel a little less lost, and a little less alone.

When You Lose Your Baby:
The Complicated Feelings of Grief

Nothing hurts like the loss of a child. Maybe the observation that comes closest to expressing what it means to a parent is that when your child dies, part of you dies also. You can never get over it, or go back to what you were. To be sure, you will eventually recover from the grief, in the sense that you will become happy and work and play normally again. But you will never forget the part of you, your child, who should have been with you.

Infants die so infrequently in our society that

most parents have no models for what they are expected to feel or do. Many wonder whether since they knew their child so briefly the excruciating pain they are feeling is abnormal. Because people who haven't lost a baby cannot truly imagine what you are feeling, friends and family don't know how to react and may say the wrong things. Another reason a parent's grieving over a newborn child is lonely is that hardly anybody knew and loved your baby but you. While others may soon forget his importance to you, you will still be aching to hold him in your arms.

How You May Feel in the Initial, Acute Phase of Grief

Grieving for your baby may involve more intense and long-lasting feelings than you expected. Try to remember that while grief is painful to live through, psychologists say it is healthy and necessary; only by facing your feelings, and expressing them will you be able to heal your wound and adjust to your loss.

Grieving is as individual as people are. Much has been written on the typical stages and nature of grief, but remember that nobody's feelings follow a fixed formula or neat progression. More likely you will have good days and bad days, good moments and bad moments—and you may feel a vast range of emotions at the same time.

Many bereaved parents have both emotional and physical symptoms. Physical symptoms often occur in waves, and may include extreme fatigue, dizziness, pain, nausea or a feeling of emptiness in your stomach, loss of appetite, headaches, heaviness in your chest with rapid or deep breathing, difficulty sleeping, and sleeping all day or not wanting to get out of bed. Some mothers even say their arms ache, as though they are aching for the baby they want to hold. You may cry a lot, or you may cry a little. This doesn't indicate how much you're suffering inside, but only how much you're openly releasing your pain.

Emotionally, you may feel depression, numbness, helplessness or fear, anger (at yourself, your doctors, or even your baby), emptiness and longing, disbelief that this really happened, and guilt. Be assured that almost all grieving parents feel guilty—for things they did or didn't do during the pregnancy or their baby's life that might have made him healthier or happier. The instinctive drive to protect one's child is so strong that many bereaved parents feel an underlying sense that they failed their child, even if saving him would have required miracles. Always remember that no parent is perfect, and whether our children live a short time or a long time, we all do some things we're proud of and some things we aren't. Try to ban yourself from thinking the inevitable "if only" thoughts, because they are unfair and harmful.

You may find that you can't concentrate, and are uninterested in things you used to enjoy before. You may spend tremendous amounts of time replaying every detail of your baby's life in your mind. You may feel like you are in a trance, invisible to the people around you because they cannot see your pain. You may wonder how the world around you can be going on as if everything were normal.

With all of these disturbing reactions, it's common for mothers and fathers who have lost a child to wonder, at some point, whether they might be going crazy. You aren't. You are experiencing one of the greatest losses anyone can, and grief is a lot more complicated than mere sadness.

Even if what you are going through is normal, however, you may find it a comfort to get professional counseling. Your obstetrician or hospital's social worker may be able to recommend a psychologist or family counselor who specializes in grief. There are also support groups especially for parents who have lost babies (some are listed on page 595), where it can be a relief to talk to people who really understand what you are going through. Some hold meetings, while others bring parents together by telephone or online.

You should definitely seek professional help if serious marital strains arise, you have persistent thoughts about committing suicide, you are doing things that are harmful to yourself (including over-using alcohol or drugs), or, if after several weeks, you are still having trouble sleeping, aren't eating much, or can't carry out normal daily activities.

As Time Passes

When can you expect to start feeling better? Thankfully, as with a physical injury, the most acute, searing pain may ease fairly soon. But most people find that the gradual process of healing, and making peace with the loss, takes longer than they expected. Researchers who looked at how bereaved parents were doing in the months after their infant had died found that by eight months, mothers' symptoms of depression and anxiety had eased a lot, but not completely. Although be-reaved fathers, like mothers, were significantly de-pressed and anxious two months after the death, by eight months they had largely recovered. (It's possible that these fathers still had some other grief symptoms; anxiety and depression were the only ones measured in this study.)

Most parents find that there are ups and downs over the months, when their pain seems to worsen or ease for a while, for no obvious reason. But at some point, whether it's seven months, or one year, or two years, you will adjust to the loss and realize that it doesn't hurt as much as it did before. Some psychologists say the goal of mourning is to allow you to get to the point when you can remember everything about your baby, from conception through his brief lifetime, without acute suffering.

Later on in the years to come, you may find that the weeks leading up to your baby's birthday or the anniversary of his death are hard again. Like some parents, you may want to start a tradition of doing something special on these occasions, such as lighting candles, or giving a children's book to your library in your baby's name, or hav-ing everyone in the family write a note to your baby.

Because you will be your baby's parent for-ever, a portion of your grief may reappear at other times, too, for the rest of your life, when something provokes a memory. But this "shadow grief" won't be debilitating. Indeed, many parents feel that far from being diminished by their loss, they've become better people—more sensitive to both the riches of life and the suffering of others—and stronger than they ever expected.

The Impact on a Marriage

It's important for you to be aware that the death of a baby can be very tough on a marriage. In fact, more than half of all couples who lose a child get divorced within a few years. Under-standing why some couples develop problems may help you become aware of any in your own marriage before they become serious.

One reason that grieving doesn't always draw partners closer together is that there is something inherently lonely about it. Even when you are mourning the same person, your suffering can't really be shared. Each partner has to deal with his own acutely personal feelings. Each is unable to alleviate the other's pain. Another reason is that a couple may be so weary from grief that they forget to nurture each other.

Men and women also tend to grieve differ-ently, often without awareness or respect for the differences. It goes without saying that no two men or women are the same. But in general, it has been observed that fathers tend to cope with grief by keeping busy. They may throw them-selves into physical activities, work, or hobbies that distract them from the pain. Mothers are more likely to want to process the loss—to cope by talking about it, reading books about grief, seeking out support groups, and going back over every memory and question about what their baby went through in their mind. Fathers tend to be more logical, mothers more intuitive and emotional, though sometimes just the opposite is true. This can easily result in doubting your partner's love for your child, or feeling like your partner is bullying you to get over the loss. Or you may hear your partner complaining that you are running away from life. Sexual tensions can also arise if one partner wants the comfort and closeness of making love while the other feels guilty about seeking pleasure at a time of sadness or associates it with memories of creating the baby who died. Sometimes strains deepen if one partner recovers more fully than the other after a few months, as fathers often do.

Just by keeping these things in mind, you'll have a better chance of avoiding the strains that build up and divide some couples. Try to respect differences as just differences, not as right or wrong ways of feeling or acting. Try to understand that they don't reflect how much love each of you had for your child. Be patient with each other. Above all, when tensions do arise, talk them through openly and as soon as possible so that they don't build up over time.

QUESTIONS AND ANSWERS

Dying at Home or in the Hospital

We've been told that our baby does not have long to live and that he can stay in the hospital or come home with us until then. We're afraid we couldn't bear watching him die at home.

When you can no longer hope that your beloved baby will live, being afraid is one of the most natural emotions. Afraid of feeling too much like a mother or father to your baby, and loving him too much when he is going to be stolen away from you. Afraid of not being able to alleviate his suffering. Afraid of your own pain, which is nearly unbearable already, and will become even worse.

If you also feel afraid when the doctor says that you can take your baby home with you, don't think that your initial reaction is strange or coldhearted; instead, it probably reflects the vulnerability that you feel. The important thing is to think this decision over carefully so you don't look back on this time with regret, feeling that you lost precious opportunities in your fleeting time with your child.

Not many premature babies who are dying can go home with their parents. It is possible only for a baby who has an illness or condition that is incurable but who can survive for a while, usually several days or more, independent of a ventilator or other intensive-care technology. Most often these are preemies who have genetic or other congenital problems, such as severe heart or kidney disease or brain abnormalities. It may also be possible, for instance, for a premature baby with short gut syndrome (an intestinal condition), who can live for a week or two on regular feedings at home. If you feel that your baby fits this description and his doctor hasn't asked whether you would like to take him home, make sure to ask whether it is an option. Some hospitals don't think to offer this choice to parents, but may be willing to consider it.

You may fear that caring for your dying baby at home would open the door to more suffering and pain that you simply couldn't handle. You know yourself and your family best. For some parents, it may truly be the best decision to have their baby cared for in the hospital, with them coming to visit as they have been.

We want to be sure you know, though, that many parents with the same initial concern end up caring for their baby at home with much more confidence than they expected and are very glad they did. Most parents find that they treasure the moments of being a mother or father to their baby in the traditional ways, holding him when he cries, wiping his mouth or nose when he needs it, diapering and feeding him, and putting him to sleep in his crib or beside them in their bed as they always had planned. Later, these are memories they cherish forever.

Some parents who have older children worry that it would be harmful to them to have the baby at home, to see him so sick and witness his death. Research has shown, however, that it may actually help children to spend time with their sick sibling. In one study of terminally ill children with cancer, children whose siblings died at home seemed to show less fear and to adjust better to the loss than those whose siblings spent their last days in the hospital, out of view.

Your baby's doctor and nurses will teach you how to care for your baby and what to do as his health worsens. Ask whether your baby is likely to be in any pain or discomfort, and what you should do to keep him as comfortable as he would be in the hospital. Many babies won't suffer, but if there is a chance that your baby will, you may be taught to give him drops of oral morphine when he needs it. The NICU may also arrange for a hospice nurse, whose expertise is in pain control and other comfort measures for dying patients, to come to your home and help you. Of course, if you are ever concerned that your baby is suffering, or feel you can't care for him adequately, you can always bring him back to the hospital. And you will be told whom to call if you have questions, day or night. (If the doctor or nurses don't mention this, don't hesitate to ask.)

If you are specifically worried about the last moments, and afraid for your baby to die at home alone with you, you can arrange with your family doctor or a hospice nurse to come to your house and be with you at the end (ask your hospital's social worker or your neonatologist to help you with these arrangements), or you can take him back to the hospital when the time comes. (You shouldn't call 911, though, because the emergency medical team may try to resuscitate him, even though you don't want them to.) If you take him to the emergency room, tell the staff right away that your baby is there for comfort care, not to be resuscitated. Your neonatologist or family doctor can call your local emergency room in advance so they'll know to expect you.

No matter which choice you make, whether your baby stays in the hospital or comes home with you, nothing can take away how difficult this is for you. The question to ask yourself is whether one way will bring you more peace.

Naming and Birth Announcements

We don't know what to do about naming our daughter, who lived so briefly. Should we give her our favorite girl's name, as we had planned? Should we send out birth announcements?

True, your daughter lived only briefly. But in your memory, she will be alive for as long as you are, always your child. A decade from now, if you have two other children and someone asks you how many children you have, you will find that you think, "I have three children. One died ten years ago."

For that reason, it is very important to name

your baby, and to consider giving her the name that you always intended. You will think of her by her name, you will use her name when you talk to friends about her life and death, and you will use her name when you talk with your partner or other children about her place in your family. You will want it to be a beautiful name, to represent the profound feelings you have for her.

While there is no set tradition or right or wrong answer on whether to send out announcements of your baby's birth and brief life, from personal experience we can say that you'll be happy if you give your cherished baby this recognition, also. Experts on grieving say that parents of babies who die often feel extremely lonely in their grief since there are so few people who knew and remember their child. An announcement is one way of including other people in your baby's life and death—and of asking them to support you in your grief. It can be very simple, giving your baby's name, birth date, death date, and some expression of your feelings. Your friends and family will probably be deeply moved by your open demonstration of love and loyalty to your child.

A name and a birth announcement are among the few things you had time to give to your baby. If you had only had the chance, you would have given her so much more.

Funeral

Our baby was so young, and our friends and family never even got to meet her. Is a funeral really appropriate?

When you lose a baby, you learn that there is no greater trauma than the loss of a child, no matter how big, no matter how old. Love can't be calculated on the basis of ounces or years.

For a long time it was thought that parents would recover fastest if all signs and memories of

their infant were erased as quickly as possible. But now it's understood that parents don't forget their baby, and never put the loss behind them. Experts recommend strongly that parents attend to their grief and express it. In the long run, it will be important for you to feel satisfied with the way your baby's death was recognized, and the way you said goodbye.

In the initial devastation or numbness of your grief, it is easy to decide that it is too difficult or too costly to make funeral arrangements and that a formal service isn't necessary because there are many other ways to say goodbye. While that may be true, many parents do feel later that a funeral or memorial service was an important element. It doesn't have to be big; it can be as intimate and private as you wish. You can introduce your baby to your family and friends, or just have your immediate family send off your darling child with love. If you start by talking to your clergy or the hospital's social worker, you'll discover that it isn't so hard to arrange and can be done inexpensively. If you're a member of a religious congregation, many of the arrangements may be made for you.

To help you decide whether you prefer to have a funeral and burial, a funeral and cremation, or only a memorial service, here are some things to consider:

✻ **Burial**. Think about where you want to bury your baby. Remember that if you bury her where you live now and move away later, it may be very hard to leave her. You can choose a cemetery for its location, or beauty, or because some of your family members are buried there. If cost is a concern, know that there is a wide price range among cemeteries, and many religious denominations have low-cost or free cemeteries. Your nursery's social worker may have a list of options in your region or be able to help you locate them. Be sure to ask whether your baby will be buried in a common or an individual grave, and whether you'll be able to visit her and put a marker where she is buried.

Unless the hospital is handling the burial, you will need a funeral home. If you don't know of one, you can ask the social worker or your clergy to suggest one, or you can find one online. Many funeral directors go out of their way to be considerate of parents who have lost babies. Some even provide funeral services for babies free of charge, or for much less than their normal fees. If you find a funeral director unpleasant or he is quoting prices that are high for you, don't hesitate to call another one.

One possibility is to ask the funeral home to handle everything for you: They will pick your baby's body up at the hospital, take it to the funeral home, prepare her body and lay her in the casket you choose, and manage the burial. But if that is too expensive, or you simply want to be more involved, you can take over some of these tasks. Some parents choose to take their baby's body from the hospital to the funeral home in their own car. If you want to do that, ask the social worker whether you need to take along a special permit or certificate of death. Some parents even build their own little casket or ask a woodworking friend to do it for them.

* **Cremation.** Some parents are drawn to cremation's sense of finality, and it is generally much less expensive than burial. Usually, all of the arrangements and the cremation are handled by a funeral home. (Just as with burial, you can be the ones to take your baby's body to the funeral home if you prefer.) Think about where you would like to place the ashes afterwards. You may want to buy a special urn or choose a pretty container you already own. Some parents decide to keep the urn at the funeral home, bury it in a special place, or take it home. Or you may prefer to scatter the ashes in a place that is meaningful to you, and beautiful and peaceful for your baby.

Some hospitals offer cremation at no charge to parents, but you should find out beforehand whether you will be given your baby's ashes. If not, take into consideration that many parents say they're sorry if they don't have a specific place to go to visit their deceased baby on her birthday, holidays, or whenever they feel the need.

* **The service.** A service can be a funeral, which is performed with the burial or cremation, usually at the funeral home or gravesite, or it can simply be a memorial service, separate from the arrangements you make for your baby's body. Your baby's funeral or memorial service can take any form you wish: It can follow religious traditions or it can be one that you adapt or create yourself, to be led by a religious leader, a friend or family member, or you and your partner.

Don't feel inhibited about incorporating some loving parental touches. This is your baby, and you have the same need that any mother or father has to take care of your child. Some parents bury their baby with a blankie, a family photograph, a stuffed animal, or a toy. Some drape a soft quilt over the coffin. You could dress your baby in a special outfit that you had waiting for her, but that she never got the chance to wear. Instead of flowers, you can ask you family and friends to bring stuffed animals, toys, or balloons that your baby would have loved.

All of these are personal decisions, a matter of what feels right to you. If at all possible, both you and your partner should be involved in planning your baby's goodbye so that neither of you later regrets the choices that were made.

Blessings and Benedictions

For some parents, it is important to bless or baptize their baby before she dies. NICUs are used to doing this, and you shouldn't hesitate to ask. A small service can be held right in the nursery led by the hospital chaplain or someone from your home congregation. In most nurseries, parents are able to bring some close friends and family members for the service, as long as the nursery doesn't become too crowded. Often, a screen or curtain can be put up so you can have some privacy during the service. This expression of spirituality and love can be very meaningful for a family whose child is dying and, if you want to include them, for the doctors and nurses taking care of her. Just talk to your baby's nurse or the NICU's social worker or chaplain to make the arrangements.

Donating Organs and Breast Milk

We want to give something of our baby so that she will live on in some way and do some good. What can we do?

Nothing can make up for the loss of your beloved baby, but some parents hope that their child can leave a legacy that lives on, or gives some other sick child a better chance in life.

If you are thinking about donating your baby's organs, you should know that unfortunately, this is seldom an option for parents of premature babies. Organ donation, which is subject to strict guidelines, usually requires that the donor die in a way that is rare for preemies: brain death occurs while the body's other organs are still functioning well. Occasionally, a baby who is ineligible to donate organs but had no possibility of an infection or genetic problem is able to donate corneas, heart valves, or other tissues. But there are age and weight requirements, which rule out most premature babies who die soon after birth. However, if you are interested in making this ex-traordinarily generous gift, ask your baby's doctor about it. You should know that every hospital in the United States is required to report all deaths to its local organ procurement organization, which reviews the medical facts and determines whether organ or tissue donation is possible. A coordinator will let your baby's doctor know and come talk to you if your baby is eligible.

There is another valuable donation you may be able to make: the breast milk that your body made for your baby. All preemies receive unparalleled health benefits from being fed breast milk. For some, whose health is particularly fragile, it can be an especially important advantage. But not all mothers of premature babies are able to provide it for their own children, so there are human milk banks that collect breast milk from the mothers of preemies who can spare it, and send it to premature babies who need it. (As you can read on page 139, milk produced by mothers of preemies is different from milk produced by mothers of full-term babies.)

If you have already been pumping, the easiest thing to do is to tell your nurse not to throw away the breast milk that you had stored for your baby. Then, you or someone from the NICU staff can contact the closest breast milk bank and make arrangements to send them your milk. If your nursery staff does not know which one is closest, you can find out by contacting the Human Milk Banking Association of North America at 919-861-4530 or www.hmbana.org. Some mothers whose babies have died continue to pump their breasts for several days or weeks longer, to send as much milk as possible to the breast milk bank. They say this helps them as they grieve and assures them that something good is coming out of their tragedy. Since breast milk banks usually run short of preterm milk for preemies who need it, your milk will be a very precious gift.

Autopsy

Our baby just died, and we've been asked whether we want to have an autopsy. Why would we do that?

The last thing you're ready for now is decisions, yet a few of them have to be made. Whether to have an autopsy needs to be decided quickly because it must be performed within a day or two of your baby's death in order to provide the fullest answers.

Usually, parents are asked whether they want an autopsy if there is uncertainty about the cause of their baby's death. Some hospitals have a policy that parents are always asked. In a few situations, an autopsy may even be legally required, such as when there was no doctor or nurse attending to the baby, and her death was sudden and unexpected. (This might arise, for example, if your baby died unexpectedly at home.) Even if the doctor doesn't mention it, parents always have the right to request an autopsy.

You may have been told that one reason for an autopsy is to help medical science and other preemies by clarifying the exact cause of your baby's death and helping doctors learn more about how to prevent it in the future. That's true. But what matters more at this terribly painful time is whether an autopsy would be emotionally helpful or hurtful to you. Some doctors recommend autopsies because they find that for many parents, questions tend to surface weeks, months, or even years after their infant's death. If there are questions in your mind as to why your baby died, whether it was preventable by the doctors, or whether anything you did or didn't do was to blame, information from an autopsy might provide you with reassurance and peace of mind. While the answers won't alleviate your grief, because nothing can, they may allow you to grieve without unnecessary doubts or guilt. You should also consider, with your doctor's help, whether you might want the information for future pregnancies, to know whether the problem your baby had might happen again.

On the other hand, you may find the idea of subjecting your innocent baby to an internal examination to be disturbing or even inconceivable. You may not be able to bear the idea of putting her through something more, when she's been through so much already. Just remember, before dismissing the idea out of hand, that your baby is at peace now and nothing can change that. But it is a personal decision whether the additional information is worth it. In fact, an autopsy doesn't always provide all the answers, so you're not guaranteed to learn what was wrong. Be assured that many parents skip an autopsy and never regret it.

Autopsies are usually performed at the hospital by a staff pathologist. If your hospital doesn't have one who does autopsies, it will be performed elsewhere. (Ask about this, since you'll want to know exactly where your baby is.) Incisions are required, so the pathologist can carefully examine the internal organs and tissues, but they can be completely covered by your baby's clothing or a blanket later. If you want to impose some limits on the autopsy, you may be able to. For example, some parents request that only their baby's lungs be examined or that no incisions be made in his head. If you decide to place limits on the autopsy, make sure they are written on the autopsy permit before you sign it.

Autopsies are usually done free of charge, but ask about your hospital's policies. Generally, preliminary results are available within a week or two. The full report, including the results of lab tests, may not be ready until a few months later. At that point, parents usually meet with their baby's doctors to discuss the findings. You may find it helpful to make a list of your unanswered questions beforehand, so you're less likely to forget them on the spot. But if more questions come to mind as you reflect on the meeting later, you can always call the doctor again.

As with many decisions surrounding your baby's death, there is often no right or wrong answer on whether to have an autopsy—just the answer with which you feel most comfortable.

How to Help Older Siblings

We can't tell how our older daughter is reacting to our baby's death. We don't know how much to involve her, or what to say to her about it.

It can be hard for parents to tell how their other children are feeling about their baby's death. Often, a young child doesn't react initially when told about a death in the family, and doesn't show obvious grief. It is widely accepted, though, that children do grieve, sometimes deeply, but in their own, childlike way—a different way than yours.

Until the age of seven or so, most children don't understand that death is permanent, and keep wondering when the baby will come back. But every child, no matter how young, can sense when something is wrong in her family, and has strong feelings—such as fear, guilt, anger, and sadness—in response. If, because of your own suffering, you are withdrawn, either physically or emotionally, your child is going to be dealing with a serious secondary loss: the temporary loss of her mother or father.

Don't expect your child to be able to verbalize her feelings. It may be too scary for her even to try. Your child's grieving will be expressed mainly through her behavior and the questions she asks. (You'll probably be struck by the directness and honesty with which your child discusses death. Parents often find it healthy and refreshing—although at first it can seem inappropriate, by adult standards.)

Every child will react to death and grief in her own, individual way, partly depending on her age and temperament, and partly on other factors, such as how much time she spent with the baby and how the rest of the family is grieving. Adults usually mourn a loved one from one to two years, with the most intense grief reactions occurring in the first two months. It hasn't been well-researched, but children who lose baby brothers or sisters are thought to grieve on a similar schedule.

Here are some typical responses that you should be prepared for:

❋ **Fear.** Probably the most frequent and powerful feeling for a child when there is a death in her family is fear. These questions loom: "Who is going to die next?" "Who will take care of me if my parents die?" "Where will I go if I die?"

You can help your child by helping her to understand why your baby died and reassuring her that you and she are not going to die for a long, long time. You can tell her that most people die when they are very old or very sick. In explaining your baby's death, use truthful language that is simple enough for her to understand. To a young child, you might say: "He was born too soon, so he was too small," or "He was born too soon, so he became very sick." A slightly older child may understand: "His lungs were not ready to breathe yet." Answer all of your child's questions honestly and directly, but with explanations that do not provide unnecessary or complex information. Be prepared for her to ask them, and for you to answer them, again and again.

As you do, don't forget that children generalize from specifics. For example, if you say that your baby died because he was sick, your child may think that people die every time they get sick. Point out the huge difference between everyday sickness and a severe illness that won't get better, and remind her of this distinction repeatedly.

Don't assume that it will be easier on your child if you resort to fairy-tale descriptions of death. On the contrary, they almost always increase a child's fear. For example, if you say, "Our baby went away on a long, long trip," your child may become afraid whenever you leave her.

* **Guilt.** Many children, unable to fully understand what happened, feel guilty when there is a death in their family. They worry: "Did I cause the death?" "Did I make him sick?" "Are my parents upset because of me?" Your child may be especially worried because of the jealousy and anger she felt when you were in the hospital visiting your baby.

Even if your child doesn't verbalize those doubts, it's safe to assume that she has them and it's important to address them. Reassure her that there was nothing she did or thought that made the baby sick and nothing that anybody could do to save the baby. Make sure you tell her that you are distraught because the baby died, not because of something she did.

* **Behavior problems.** It's common for children to have some sort of behavior problems when a sibling dies. Misbehaving may be a way of getting your attention, which they've been craving while you've been remote and distracted by your grief. Regressive behavior, such as bed-wetting, thumb-sucking, or baby talk, may be a way of asking for reassurance by having you care for them the way you did when they were smaller.

Sometimes, just giving your older child more attention can make a difference, boosting her sense of security. If you're finding it too hard to talk and play as much as usual, make a point of holding your child more and communicating through touch.

* **Taking on too much responsibility.** Some children think it's up to them to resolve this family crisis. They may think that if they're perfectly well-behaved the trouble will go away, or they may search for a way to alleviate your pain. One of our small children repeatedly suggested a plan to bring the baby back by climbing a tall ladder, then boarding a jumbo jet from its top step for a flight to heaven. She would look at her mother eagerly and say, "That's what I'll do. Then you won't be sad anymore?" If you have older children, they may even take upon themselves the responsibility for keeping the household running, or may offer their shoulder for you to lean on.

Small gestures of this kind are giving and appropriate, but they shouldn't go too far. For a child to feel that she needs to be a superachiever, or to parent her parents, is a heavy burden. Try to relieve your child of it by reassuring her that you love her whether she's naughty or nice, that she doesn't have to do anything special because she already makes you happier just by being herself, and that although you're sad now, you won't be forever.

As They Grow: A Child's Understanding of Death

Your children's ages will largely determine how they understand death, though there are variations depending on a child's experience, religious training, and family's beliefs. Here are some general guidelines.

* **Children under four.** Most children under four have no real understanding of death. They do, however, absorb the pain of others around them. Three- and four-year-olds may think of death as a temporary condition that is reversible or as a similar way of living, but in another place. They may also believe that their feelings or actions can cause death.
* **Four to six.** Many children of this age are able to understand some of the biological aspects of death: the absence of breathing, heartbeat, seeing, or thinking. They are also better able to talk about death. By six or seven years of age some understand that death is permanent, but others continue to think of it as reversible. They may also think that a death in their family is a punishment or their fault. Preschoolers often fear that death is "catching," and may

need to be reassured that no one else is going to die.
* **Seven to eleven.** Over these years, children generally make the transition to a more adult understanding of death. They become interested in what happens to the body after death and may be fascinated by mutilation, graveyards, and coffins. They are also concerned with how their world may change because their sibling died.
* **Twelve and older.** By this age, most children can think abstractly and have an adult understanding of death. However, they may be less revealing of their own feelings and reactions. During their teenage years, children are apt to start searching for meanings and to explore religious or philosophical interpretations of death.

In general, be prepared for a child's grief behavior to be different from an adult's. A child is likely to spend almost all her time acting as if nothing has changed, and then suddenly, for no apparent reason, become contemplative or sad. She may try to lose herself in noisy, active games. She may use imaginative play to work through what happened, pretending that her stuffed animals have died or playing dead herself. At moments when she can't handle your feelings or her own, she may transform the scene into something more

familiar by, say, giggling foolishly at silly things or misbehaving.

Most experts agree that parents should not try to shield children from the fact that their sibling died or from the mourning rituals and grief that follow. If there is a lot of tension and sorrow in the family that no one has explained to them, it can be a lot more frightening than if they are included.

Try to take cues from your child on how much to talk about your baby's death. Most psychologists suggest that if your child is seven years or older, you should allow and even encourage—but never force—her to go to the baby's funeral. Make sure to explain in advance what will happen so she knows what to expect. If your child is younger than that, you are the best judge. If you don't want her to be present at the funeral, partly because your own reaction may upset her, try to include her in other ways—by having her attend some other service for the baby, or devising a way for her to say her own personal goodbye. You may want her to choose a toy or draw a picture for the baby to be buried with—something that will mean a little to her now, and even more in the future.

When you lose a baby, having another child at home can be difficult for a while. You wish that you could grieve for your baby undisturbed. Try not to blame yourself if you aren't the best mother or father to your older child immediately after your baby's death. That's inevitable, given what you are going through. It can be a good idea to ask your mother or someone else close to you to come and stay with you for a little while, the way you might have planned for them to come after your baby was born. She'll help you give your older child the attention she needs—and you might benefit from the closeness, too. But as soon as possible, your older child needs your help. She'll also help you, giving you love and a sense of purpose that lift your spirits immeasurably.

MULTIPLES

Loss of One Twin

One of our twins died. I feel torn apart, grieving for her while needing to care for her brother.

Although one of your babies has died, you are and always will be the mother of twins. If you had been given the chance to raise both of your twins, you would have had to juggle the time and attention you gave to each of them. Now, you are also faced with juggling, in the deepest emotional way, as you mourn one of your twins while trying to be a happy, loving parent to the other.

There is no map to lead you through this, but some advice may help you decide how to navigate your own, personal way. Although we'll talk here about twins, for readers who are parents of triplets—or multiples of any number—and have lost a baby, what follows applies just as much to you.

✳ **Don't cut short your goodbye to your baby who is dying or has died, or feel that you need to go straightaway to taking care of your surviving twin.** Many parents feel it is important to divide their time equally among their babies, but that's not what you should be concerned about now. Thankfully, you will have plenty of time ahead of you to shower your healthier baby with undivided love, but you won't get another chance with your baby who has died. If you don't take all the time you need now to hold her, say goodbye, collect keepsakes, and grieve peacefully to the temporary exclusion of your other baby, you will probably regret it later. Some parents say they even have slight feelings of resentment that interfere with their attachment to their surviving twin. So don't feel guilty about giving your surviving twin some loving caresses and telling him that you'll be back in a day or two. If he is already home with you, ask his grandparents or someone else close to you to help by taking care of him and giving you this much-needed break. Dealing with the grief of having just lost a baby, and giving your surviving baby the happiness and attention he deserves, are conflicting demands that are just plain impossible for most people to do at the same time.

* **Make sure to collect mementos while you can.** Photos, your baby's hat, tiny socks, a lock of her hair—any mementos of your beloved child will often help you in recovering from grief and will become treasured possessions in later years. If you think a photograph of your baby would be uncomfortable for you to show friends, because of the presence of a ventilator or other apparatus, consider having a drawing made from the photograph. Some parents say that mementos representing their twins' special relationship, such as a composite drawing of the two babies together or matching teddy bears bought for their cribs, became precious both to them and to their surviving child as time went on.

* **Try not to worry if you feel some resentment or distance from your surviving twin for a little while.** At first, your surviving twin may seem like a painful reminder of your loss, or even an intruder in the world of your memories and grief. Consciously or not, you may also keep some distance from him because of the fear of losing a loved child again. Don't worry; these feelings are normal and should start to diminish soon. If you haven't taken the time you need to grieve apart from your surviving baby, consider doing it now. You'll find that even a few days away from the nursery or home will give you some valuable space. On the other hand, if you find you want much more time than that away from your surviving baby, make sure to talk to a professional counselor, who will help if you have a lingering depression that could keep your baby from getting the love and attention she needs.

    When you do start to relax and become more attached to your surviving baby, don't worry, as some people do, that you're being disloyal to your child who died. You can be sure that she will never be out of your thoughts for long. When she is, try to accept the relief that you badly need. It is said that both laughter and tears are necessary to recover from grief.

* **Be prepared for the ignorant things some people will say.** You can be sure that at least one of your relatives or friends, not knowing better, will say something foolish that may offend you, such as, "At least you have one baby left," or "Be glad you have only one baby to take care of instead of two." When parents who have lost a twin hear these kinds of statements, they feel that no one understands what they are going through. In fact, studies have consistently shown that parents who lose a twin are as intensely affected by the loss of their baby as parents who lose a singleton. However, they also show that family, friends, and hospital staff sometimes downplay the death of a twin, assuming that a parent's grief would be less. Try to forgive them and realize that they don't mean to hurt you. They probably just don't have any experience with this. If you are feeling especially alone, you will find that other bereaved parents of multiples best understand your loss and what you are going through. Among the many things they will understand is that you are grieving not only over the loss of your child, but also over the loss of your identity as a mother of twins, which had become a vital part of you. If you are interested, ask the NICU's social worker about local support groups for bereaved parents, or see page 595.

* **Beware of becoming overprotective of your surviving twin.** Many parents develop an unusually close attachment to their surviving twin. At the same time, they may find themselves terrified that he will be the next to die, and unable to shake this feeling even as their child grows older and more robust. Some parents find that it takes two or three years before

The Effect on Your Surviving Twin

Many parents wonder whether their surviving baby has a sense that he's alone now when he wasn't before, and whether the loss of his twin will have a psychological effect on him later in life. The answer is that we just don't know. No systematic research has been done on the impact of losing a twin in the womb or in infancy. There are adults whose twin died just before or after birth who say that they have lingering feelings of loneliness, sorrow, or guilt and still introduce themselves as twins. There are parents who say that their surviving twin needs an unusual amount of physical closeness, perhaps seeking something that is missing. Some grown-ups even say they have the feeling that they lost a twin but have no proof—just a lifelong sense that someone who should be there isn't. Of course, there are many perfectly happy and well-adjusted children who seem to have no memory of their early loss. Some twin researchers believe there can be a lasting impact, but they caution that at this point, there is no reliable scientific evidence to support it.

they finally believe deep down that their child is going to survive. These reactions are natural. If you feel this way, just beware of overprotecting your child and discouraging him from exploring the world. Children who are overprotected may become fearful and insecure and have difficulty with social relationships—traits that researchers have found are more common in former preemies.

* **Expect to feel uneasy for a while when people ask how many children you have.** Since you will certainly be asked, the key is to plan in advance what you want to say. At the beginning, you may feel most comfortable including your deceased baby in your count, even though the ensuing conversation may lead you to have to explain what happened. As time passes, you may prefer to avoid that subject by including only your surviving children—even though, inside, most parents never reach a point where they feel that is the accurate number.

* **If you gave birth to more than two, don't be surprised if some people refer to your two surviving triplets as twins or your surviving quadruplets as triplets.** But do feel free to correct them if this upsets you. The medical staff may unconsciously make this slip even though they know better, and it's sure to happen when people unfamiliar with your babies' history see them together after you take them home. For some parents, this terminology is OK; others, though, find it deeply hurtful and offensive. Try not to blame anyone for an understandable mistake, but since your feelings are what count, don't be shy about letting your wishes be known.

* **Think now about whether you would like to find out if your twins were identical.** Experts say it's typical for mothers not to be curious at the time of their loss but to regret later not knowing since they would like to imagine their baby and family as fully as possible as time goes by. Your babies' doctor might be able to

find out from their hospital records whether they had different blood types, which means they were not identical, or shared the same amniotic sac or placenta, which means they were. If not, a DNA test can be done to give you the answer. Just know that you'll need to decide quickly in order to use the simplest method, taking a swab from inside the cheek of each of your babies to send to a specialized laboratory for analysis, since the swab must be taken within a few hours after your baby has died. (The lab may want samples from the parents also.) Since health plans generally don't cover identical twin testing, ask your babies' doctor to find out how much the analysis will cost.

✳ **Don't feel that you need to remove all traces of your baby who has died, but don't make your surviving twin grow up in her shadow.** For some parents it feels better to remove their deceased baby's furniture and clothes right away, while for others it seems like negating their baby to do that immediately. Do what feels right to you right now. Just remember that over time you can let your deceased baby be a natural part of your family and life, one whom everyone in the family knows about and remembers, without being an inescapable presence for your surviving twin. Tell your child about her twin who died as early as possible, never making it a secret. But find a way to keep celebrations of your surviving twin's birthday joyous by separating them from your recognition of the anniversary of your baby's death. As time passes and your pain lessens, it will become easier to rejoice and mourn at the same time.

IN DEPTH

Making the Hardest Decisions

There are some decisions that no parent should ever have to make.

If your baby's outlook is very poor, the time may come when his doctors ask you, or you ask yourself, whether you want to limit or stop his medical treatment: whether it is better and kinder to allow him to die, rather than using all measures to try to keep him alive for as long as possible.

Any parent faced with this question knows the deep, searing pain it causes. You search for the "right" answer, but unfortunately, there isn't one. The doctors may be telling you that your baby's outlook is not absolutely certain, and even if it were, no doctor or expert could answer the paramount question: whether living the life your child is expected to have—maybe a short one, or a long one with medical struggles and disabilities—will be a good thing for your child or not.

It is amazing to think that not long ago you and your partner were discussing the color of sheets for the crib or debating when a child should start daycare. Now those concerns seem like part of a fairytale world that you no longer inhabit.

It's common for parents to feel overwhelming guilt or shame when they even begin to think about a decision like this. That's because parents have an instinct, virtually hard-wired into them, to save their children's lives. Certainly, in most situations, this is a wonderful, protective reaction. But when one's baby is severely ill, things are more complicated. If all medical technology can do is uncomfortably postpone an infant's inevitable death, or enable a premature baby to survive but with debilitating physical or mental disabili-

ties, parents may offer greater protection to their child by not using it. For the deepest emotional reasons, the guilt you feel is understandable, but try to remember it doesn't mean you are doing something wrong.

What Ethics and Religion Say

Doctors, judges, and specialists in medical ethics agree that in this technological era, just because something *can* be done to prolong an infant's life doesn't mean that it *should* be done. The decision to use life-sustaining treatment or not is an intensely personal one that is based on one's values about what makes life worth living and how much suffering is bearable. Because a baby cannot speak for himself, his parents have to decide for him.

If you are confronting this decision, you will find that you need to examine your most fundamental values. Very few people believe that life is good no matter what and that death is always the worst possible outcome. Think of an elderly person who is terminally ill and suffering from unremitting pain; a person with severe brain damage who is permanently unconscious; history's patriots and saints who chose to die rather than live in intolerable circumstances. Most people believe that life is precious because it enables us to live out the things we really value: interacting with other people and the world around us through language and our senses, being able to make plans and work toward our goals, feeling more pleasure than pain, and loving and being loved.

If you, too, believe that there are situations in which life is not better than death, considering whether to limit medical treatment for your baby is a matter of assessing whether that tragic point has been reached for him. Where the turning point lies will be different for different parents. You may believe it has been reached if your baby has little chance of surviving. Or you may feel it has been reached if in surviving, he will probably be physically or mentally unable to do most of the things that children or adults do, or will have to endure repeated pain and medical problems with little chance of ever leaving the hospital and coming home. Of course, babies don't always take the course that doctors predict, and a child with a high likelihood of dying or having long-term disabilities still has a chance, even if it's small, of beating the odds. So, some parents may feel that life is worth battling for at all costs, until they are told that their baby has absolutely no hope of surviving and that medical care can no longer help him.

Determining where the turning point lies for you is going to take tremendous strength on your part, no matter what your values and choices. You may have to be strong enough to recognize that it has not yet been reached for you, even if it has been for your baby's doctors. Or vice versa: that it has been reached for you, even though the doctors would rather do everything possible to keep your baby alive. And if you do feel that that point has been reached for you, you will need to be strong enough to act on your intuition and conviction, and let go of the person you least want to let go of, your child.

If parents decide not to prolong their baby's life with aggressive medical treatment, they can authorize what is called a do not resuscitate order (you may hear it referred to as a DNR). A DNR order means that you do not want cardiopulmonary resuscitation given to your baby if he stops breathing or his heart stops. For a baby who is just being delivered, the doctors will do everything they can to make your baby comfortable, including drying him off, gently wrapping him in warm blankets, and giving him to you to hold close. But they won't put him on a ventilator, take blood, or put in IV lines. For a baby who is already in the intensive care nursery, a DNR order can mean withdrawing the medical support your baby is on (for example, taking him off a ventilator) or taking the smaller step of withholding any further life-sustaining treatment (for example, if his breathing weakens, not putting him on a ventilator if he isn't on one, and not giving CPR). Your baby's doctor may suggest limiting other kinds of medical treatment as well, such as procedures that hurt or blood transfusions, if your priority is making your baby's life as peaceful and comfortable as possible rather than extending it as long as possible.

Some parents, and some doctors too, instinctively believe that withdrawing treatment a baby is already receiving that may be keeping him alive, such as a ventilator, is very different from withholding new, additional treatment. They think that not adding treatment is morally justified when a baby is too sick for it to do much good, but that stopping treatment a baby is already receiving is actively killing him. It is important for you to know that most experts in medical ethics do not view these options as morally different. First of all, it is your baby's disease, arising from his prematurity, that will be the cause of his death—not you, no matter what medical treatments you authorize or stop. Second, although parents and doctors have special roles and relationships that obligate them to help their babies and patients when they're in trouble, helping can mean different things. Sometimes, stopping medical treatment is the most helpful, and continuing it is harmful. Your obligation, and your baby's doctor's, is to figure out what you believe will most help your baby and to do that.

What are the laws that guide you and your baby's doctor? Although they vary from state to state, the vast weight of federal and state law supports a patient's right to refuse or consent to medical treatment, and parents are given that right for their children, who can't decide for themselves. But there are limits. Some states restrict a parent's ability to withhold life-sustaining care unless it is clear that the child is terminally ill. And every state requires parents to make choices that can reasonably be viewed as in their child's best interests. Especially since hospitals and neonatologists can interpret the laws and their moral obligations differently—and sometimes fervently disagree—if you want to know about your rights and constraints, you can ask to talk to the ethics consultant at your hospital, if it has one (most hospitals have ethics committees or consultants who have experience making difficult ethical decisions about medical treatment and know the laws involved), or get a second opinion from a neonatologist at a different hospital.

If there is a lot of tension between you and the medical staff, you may wonder whether it would be helpful to hire a lawyer. In general, though, this should be a last resort. Private lawyers usually aren't well versed in these kinds of situations, unlike the professionals who face them frequently. They may approach the issues less delicately or in a distant and adversarial fashion, making it harder for parents and the medical staff to do what is most needed—understand each other's deeply held feelings and work closely together.

Some parents who are religious express concern about whether making life and death decisions is taking over God's role. You should talk to your clergy or the hospital chaplain if this is a concern for you, but we can assure you that there are many different ways, even within the same faith, that devoutly religious people perceive God's will and how medicine fits into God's plan. Some people believe that since God gave us medical technology, it is God's plan for us to use it. Others believe that since God gave us not just medical technology but also the knowledge and judgment to recognize when it will work and when it won't, it is God's plan for us to use medicine wisely. One belief is that we should treat premature babies to the very end because God will take the baby when God is ready. Others think that God's plan will be revealed after a baby is taken off man-made technological support by whether the baby then lives or dies.

Many religious and nonreligious people alike find comfort and peace in letting nature take its course, rather than fighting something so essential.

One worry of many parents is whether it is selfish or inappropriate to consider their family as a whole when making their decision. Raising a child with chronic health problems or disabilities will change parents' and siblings' lives, and involve physical, emotional, and financial burdens. It's possible to imagine these kinds of considerations being selfishly motivated in some cases. But it's also possible to imagine that they could arise from parents' deep sense of responsibility to all of their children, including their sick one, and a realistic view of the care they are capable of providing. According to many theologians, Christian moral tradition, for one, requires weighing everyone's needs and taking the common good, as well as the benefit for any one individual, into account.

Time and Information to Help You Make a Good Decision

If it isn't absolutely necessary for you to make a decision immediately, take your time, and make it only when you are ready. Psychologists have noted that parents are less likely to feel regret or guilt about their decision later if they had good information and time to reflect on their alternatives beforehand.

For many reasons, doctors and nurses are often several steps ahead of parents in believing that the time has come to limit medical treatment. Parents who just gave birth to a premature baby may still be in shock, or filled with an understandable, stubborn hope that they aren't ready to abandon yet. Also, experienced doctors and nurses know many things about a preemie's condition and prospects that are not obvious to parents who have never been in this situation before. They know, for instance, that a newborn who weighs only 500 grams and needs 100 percent oxygen has little chance of surviving for long, whereas parents have to listen to the unfamiliar information the doctors give them, digest it, and then accept it or not. And, of course, time passes very differently when you are contemplating the death of someone you love than when you are a medical professional with more distance.

Unfortunately, bad feelings can arise between parents and the NICU staff when parents are slower to decide to limit treatment. (The reverse situation sometimes happens, too—a baby's parents feel it's time to let go, while the staff believes medical therapy should continue longer.) While conflict is the last thing you need right now, be assured that whether you agree with the doctors and nurses or not, both you and they have your baby's best interests at heart.

Above all, before making a decision, make sure you have a clear understanding of what is wrong with your child, what his medical treatment might entail, and what his prospects are with and without treatment, both now and in the future. Many parents find that they're in such a state of shock that they can't absorb or remember much. Don't be embarrassed: the doctors understand this, and it is their role to answer as many questions as you

have, as many times as you need to ask them, until you have all the information you need.

You may discover that different doctors and nurses have varying opinions on your baby's condition and future quality of life. Different opinions can be terribly confusing when you are making life and death decisions, but try to listen to them and to understand that they reflect uncertainty about your baby's future and the right path to take. Of course, some doctors and nurses will have more experience and knowledge than others, and you should weigh their judgments more heavily. Still, getting a better sense of the uncertainties will help you make a better decision.

If you and your partner are in conflict about the decision, it may be helpful to talk together to the nursery's social worker or the hospital chaplain. Talk to other people you trust, also. Then, weigh all of the information and views you hear, listening to your own, internal voice.

Feel free to ask the chaplain, social worker, or your baby's doctor to set up a meeting for you with the ethics committee at any time if you think it might help you make your decision. A hospital ethics committee usually offers only advice, not binding decisions, and can be a good resource for you as well as for the medical staff.

How to Spend the Remaining Time

If you do decide to limit medical treatment, think about what you want for your baby's precious remaining minutes, hours, or days. There are still a lot of things to hope for, even if a long life isn't one of them. One thing to hope for is that your baby feels love. Many parents treasure the memories of the time they had together at the end when they could finally envelop their baby in their arms, free of wires and tubes and beeping monitors, whispering and singing to him, and giving him the blissful feeling of being loved.

You can also hope that your baby feels at peace. Ask whether he has been given medicine to eliminate any pain or discomfort. The medications that most intensive care nurseries use will make him feel comfortable and serene.

The doctors and nurses will want to help with any other requests you have, so be sure to tell them. If you want privacy with your baby, they may have a separate room where the two of you can sit alone together, or they may put up a curtain or screen within the nursery. You can tell the nurses whether you feel most comfortable if they check on your baby frequently or you prefer to have longer periods of time with him alone. Also tell them whether you want your baby to remain on a monitor (the alarms can be turned off so you'll have peace and quiet but you will be able to see on the screen exactly when his heart stops beating). If you cannot leave your hospital room and your baby is to be brought to you, you may want to ask that he be given breathing assistance until he gets to your room, so he will be sure to feel your arms around him in his last moments.

Both before and after your baby dies, you can hold him, cuddle him, kiss him, rock him, and tell him some of the things you want him to know—about you, his siblings, cousins, or grandparents; the places you would have taken him; and, of course, your everlasting feelings for him. You can ask the nursery staff if there is someone who can take photographs; whether you look at them often or not, you will treasure them as keepsakes of your baby later. You will especially love having a picture of him without a ventilator so that you can see his beautiful face, so try to get one during his last hours or moments, even if your heart and mind are elsewhere. If you prefer and have the time, there are organizations you can find on-line that specialize in bereavement photography, which bring parents together with photographers who can produce lovely photographs, or DVDs combining images and music, often at no charge for their services.

Don't be ashamed if you feel afraid to hold your baby while he dies, or afraid to see him afterward, thinking that you would rather remember him alive. There are no rules for what you should do, and many other parents have the same feelings. We want you to know, though, that parents who do hold their baby in his last moments are usually relieved to find that it is like holding your baby close to you as he falls asleep. The moments together feel peaceful, intimate, and far more natural then you may imagine. And they provide a valuable sense of finality and closure. Some parents spend a few minutes with their baby after he dies, while others want to spend hours. There's almost no limit—just tell your doctor what you want to do, and he'll let you know whether it's possible within your hospital's guidelines.

Some hospitals will put together a collection of mementos for you, but if yours doesn't or there are more things you'd like, don't be embarrassed to ask. In addition to photographs, among the things that parents often want are: their baby's blanket, T-shirt, and hat; a lock of hair; a set of footprints and handprints; their baby's ID bracelet; the name card from his bed or isolette; a record of his weight and measurements; and any presents or personal items that decorated his bed. Some hospitals give all parents copies of their child's birth certificate or certificate of death, but others don't. Your hospital's social worker can tell you how to get these if you want them.

Always remember that if you feel guilty or have doubts about your decision later, it doesn't mean you made the wrong one. Parents who decide to stop medical treatment can't help but wonder whether their baby might have beaten the odds and recovered. Parents whose children died after long hospitalizations or who lived on but with serious problems after they continued treatment can't help but wonder whether they did the right thing for their child or family.

As a parent, you try to make the right decision out of love, and then you revisit it out of love. If you can say that after much soul-searching you made the best choice you could, you should try to accept your decision and live with it in peace.

CHAPTER 11

I WAS A PREEMIE, TOO

. . . .

Famous people who were born premature and thrived,

even before the recent advances in neonatal medicine.

. . . .

Despite the hurdles that premature babies have to face, there's never been a better time than today to be born before term. Still, prematurity has always been a part of the human experience, and some babies who were born early have always been able to survive and thrive. We can find traces of illustrious preemies in historical sources and biographies—some whose prematurity is considered certain, thanks to precise records, and others for whom it can only be inferred, because an infant was very small, or had some typical complication of prematurity. (Sometimes, a premature birth was used as a convenient excuse to obscure the real reason—a premarital dalliance—that a baby arrived sooner than expected after the parents' wedding.) The list of former preemies includes some of the most famous names imaginable—scientific and artistic geniuses, great athletes, entertainers, statesmen, and even one of the most towering figures of the Old Testament—all of whom attest to the vastness of a preemie's potential, despite, and sometimes because of, his shortened gestation.

Take a look at the amazingly big footsteps that our children are following in:

Moses (lived sometime between 14th and 13th century BCE): Old Testament prophet, lawgiver, and leader who delivered his people from slavery in Egypt. If Moses was a preemie, he was surely one of the first on record and one of the most influential in human history. According to the Bible, the Pharaoh of Egypt ordered the killing of all Jewish male children, but Moses escaped because his mother was able to keep him hidden for three months and then famously placed him in a basket among the reeds of the Nile River. Many ancient biblical commentators explained that because Moses was born at six months gestation, the Egyptian spies didn't come looking for him until three months later, and because he was unusually quiet (typical for a preemie), he didn't give himself away. Other scholars have said that his mother gave birth earlier than expected because she was pregnant before she wed. One thing everyone agrees on is that Moses' greatness could already be detected in his infancy, in part by the extraordinary circumstances surrounding his birth.

Johannes Kepler (1571–1630): One of the fathers of modern astronomy, Kepler discovered the three laws of planetary motion that are still taught to physics students today, and paved the way for acceptance of the sun-centered planetary system. Obsessed with precision, he developed the most exact astronomical charts of his time, and even calculated his own gestational period: 224 days, 9 hours, 53 minutes (or seven months, to the rest of us). A frail child who suffered from numerous ailments, he sought refuge in education, becoming one of the most influential minds in scientific history and shaping the world's understanding of the heavens.

Isaac Newton (1642–1727): English natural philosopher and creator of modern physics. According to tradition, a ripe apple falling in Newton's garden led him to discover the law of gravity. He himself fell out of his mother's womb too green, small enough, he later said, to fit into a quart mug and to raise considerable worry for his survival.

Jean-Jacques Rousseau (1712–1778) and **Voltaire**, pseudonym of François Marie Arouet (1694–1778): Two of the most famous French writers and philosophers, they lived at the same time and had extremely influential but opposing ideas. Voltaire believed that education and reason were what elevated humankind above beasts. The egalitarian Rousseau thought that education was corrupting, separating humans from nature. Both tough characters, they despised each other. Yet they had something in common: Each came into the world as a tiny preemie. Rousseau was born

almost dead; Voltaire so sick that he received last rites and was christened only when he was nine months old.

Johann Wolfgang von Goethe (1749–1832): German poet, dramatist, and novelist, and one of the greatest figures in world literature, Goethe was born prematurely, "a puny waif whose life was despaired of." His birth became the catalyst for instituting better training for midwives in the city of Frankfurt, thanks to Goethe's powerful grandfather, who was mayor at the time.

John Keats (1795–1821): An English Romantic poet, widely celebrated for his poetry despite dying young, at the age of 26, of tuberculosis. A premature birth, a short life truncated by a very premature death, Keats was truly a "fair creature of an hour," who nonetheless left a lasting mark with his poems.

Mark Twain, pseudonym of Samuel Clemens (1835–1910): American author and humorist, Twain wrote two masterpieces of American literature, *The Adventures of Tom Sawyer* and *The Adventures of Huckleberry Finn*. Born two months premature, he didn't appear fit to grow up. "A lady came in one day," his mother wrote later, "and said, 'You don't expect to raise that babe do you.' I said I would try. But he was a poor looking object to raise." Still, the night of his birth, Halley's Comet had been seen in the sky, and his family rightly thought it was a good omen.

Winston Churchill (1874–1965): Born of a British lord and an American heiress, Churchill was Great Britain's prime minister during World War II. He secured an alliance with the United States and Russia and helped mastermind the strategy that led to Hitler's defeat. Churchill was born seven and a half months after his parents' hastily arranged wedding, at their country home far from London's excellent doctors. His father wrote to his mother-in-law, "The boy is wonderfully pretty . . . very healthy considering his prematurity." (Churchill liked to tease skeptics who questioned whether he was really premature: "Although present on the occasion, I have no clear recollection of the events leading up to it.") A born fighter, impetuous and courageous, in his first statement as prime minister, Churchill would say, "I have nothing to offer but blood, toil, tears, and sweat."

Albert Einstein (1879–1955): Discoverer of the theory of relativity, Einstein revolutionized contemporary physics and became a synonym for human genius. He was a lonely and shy child who hardly spoke until age three, and was never successful in school. He said: "I sometimes ask myself how it came about that I was the one to develop the theory of relativity. The reason, I think, is that a normal adult never stops to think about problems of space and time. These are things which he has thought about as a child. But my intellectual development was retarded, as a result of which I began to wonder about space and time only when I had already grown up."

Anna Pavlova (1881–1931): Beautiful Russian ballerina Pavlova was the most celebrated dancer of her time, who became famous as the dying swan in a solo that was choreographed for her in the ballet *Swan Lake*. She never became physically strong, despite the wrenching practice required by ballet. "You must realize that your daintiness and fragility are your greatest assets," young Pavlova was admonished by a teacher. And she did, developing rare qualities of expressiveness, delicacy, and fluidity of movement that enchanted audiences.

Willie Shoemaker (1931–2003): Legendary American jockey Shoemaker was born too early and too small, and didn't grow much afterward, either. At 4-feet-11 inches and 96 pounds, he used his small size, smarts, and strength to great advantage. In an amazing career of forty-two years, Shoemaker won 11 Triple Crown horse races and earned more than $123 million in prize money. It is said that his grandmother put him in a shoebox next to an oven to keep him alive the night he was born.

Stevie Wonder, pseudonym of Steveland Morris (1950–): Hugely successful American soul singer and songwriter, a natural talent and child prodigy who sang and mastered the piano, harmonica, and drums before the age of ten. Wonder was one of the thousands of preemies who, in the 1940s and early 1950s, were blinded by ROP (retinopathy of prematurity). Blindness didn't prevent Wonder from doing what all the kids his age were doing, he once said, and it perhaps enhanced his exceptional musical gift. He celebrated life, freedom, love, and his newborn baby, Aisha, with the song "Isn't She Lovely?"

Patrick Bouvier Kennedy (1963): Third child of Jacqueline Bouvier Kennedy and John Fitzgerald Kennedy, 35th President of the United States. Patrick was born prematurely at 34 weeks of gestation and died only two days later of RDS (respiratory distress syndrome), one of the most common complications of prematurity. Patrick's brief life had a tremendous impact. The loss of a First Family's baby deeply moved the nation and led to an outpouring of public and private resources for medical research and special newborn care units. Thanks to that support and to the many new medical treatments that followed, the lives of today's 34-weekers are not at risk from RDS. Patrick rests in Arlington National Cemetery, beside his parents.

The list of alleged premature babies goes on. It includes an emperor, **Napoleon Bonaparte,** and a king, **Farouk** of Egypt; the father of evolution and natural selection, **Charles Darwin;** the French writer **Victor Hugo;** the Impressionist painter **Pierre-August Renoir;** and the philosopher **Thomas Hobbes.** Some contemporary preemies are the actors **Colin Farrell, Michael J. Fox,** and **Sidney Poitier;** the singer **Suzanne Vega,** and the twin pro football players **Tiki** and **Ronde Barber.**

Who knows how many towering figures are being born among our preemies of today?

APPENDICES

APPENDIX 1

RISK FACTORS
FOR PREMATURITY:
WHO'S AT RISK?*

While you're going to read here about some of the things that increase the odds of giving birth early, try not to use them to draw firm conclusions about your pregnancy or the pregnancy of anyone else you love. That would be a mistake, because in any pregnancy the medical issues may be more complex than can be described here. Risk factors for prematurity may be weak or strong, and they often interact. Also, many women who have one or more of them still give birth at or near term. Remember that only your doctor can adequately evaluate your individual case and make an accurate prognosis for your pregnancy and your baby.

Obstetric History

* **Previous premature delivery.** This is one of the most significant risks for a premature birth. If you have already had a premature baby, you have a 20 percent to 50 percent chance of seeing it happen again. But don't lose heart; it may be possible to correct something that caused you to deliver early before. Getting progesterone shots during your pregnancy might also significantly lower your risk (see page 18).

* **Previous second trimester abortion.** This surgical procedure requires a wide dilation of the cervix, which can damage it and lead to cervical insufficiency. The risk of preterm birth also increases—but only slightly—with the number of first trimester abortions a woman has had, from about 1 percent for a single abortion to 2 percent to 3 percent for more than one.

* **Becoming pregnant less than six months after a previous delivery.** Your body may not be fully recovered and prepared to handle another pregnancy so soon.

* **Infertility.** Women who have had a lot of trouble conceiving, including those who become pregnant while receiving treatment for infertility, have a higher incidence of preterm delivery. It is still not certain whether this is due solely to whatever caused the infertility in the first place or whether some side effects of assisted reproduction therapies contribute to the risk (see page 37).

* Most of these risk factors for prematurity are explained in greater detail in the first chapter. Look for the cross-referenced pages if you want to read more about them.

Problems with the Reproductive Organs

✴ **Malformation of the uterus.** If a woman's uterus has fibroids or an abnormal shape, it might not be able to stretch enough to accommodate a full-term baby, so she is more likely to have a smaller than normal baby and for delivering prematurely. But many uterine malformations can be corrected with surgery, after which there's a much better chance of carrying a pregnancy to term.

✴ **Cervical insufficiency.** Some women have what's called an insufficient or incompetent cervix: Their cervix (the opening of the womb) tends to open too early in pregnancy, causing a premature birth. You can have cervical insufficiency because you were born with it, as a result of previous gynecologic or obstetric procedures, or for unknown reasons. Having it in one pregnancy doesn't necessarily mean it will occur in subsequent ones, but the risk is higher. You can read more on page 23 about cervical insufficiency and a simple surgical procedure called a cerclage, which can be done during pregnancy to keep your cervix closed until term.

Obstetric Complications During the Pregnancy

✴ **Multiple gestation.** Twins have a 25 percent to 50 percent chance of being born before term, and that rate rises with each additional fetus. The main reason is purely mechanical: The uterus gets distended by all of the babies inside, and distention is a signal for it to contract. But some multiples are born prematurely for other reasons, such as high blood pressure in the mother, because the fetuses aren't growing well in the womb, or because of twin-twin transfusion syndrome, a serious problem that identical twins can develop (see page 37).

✴ **Bleeding during pregnancy.** While most episodes of vaginal bleeding during pregnancy turn out to be nothing to worry about, your doctor will want to check for two conditions of the placenta—placental abruption and placenta previa—that can harm a mother and baby and are common causes of elective preterm delivery. A placental abruption is when part of the placenta tears away from the wall of the uterus so it can no longer do its work of passing nutrients and oxygen from mother to baby. A placenta previa is when the placenta covers the cervix, where it is prone to tear and bleed when the cervix dilates or the baby pushes against it during labor. You can read more about vaginal bleeding, placental abruption, and placenta previa on page 26.

✴ **Polyhydramnios or oligohydramnios.** Polyhydramnios means there's too much amniotic fluid around the fetus. The extra fluid stretches the uterus, sometimes leading to early contractions and preterm delivery. Since the fetus normally swallows large amounts of amniotic fluid, anything that impairs his ability to swallow can cause too much fluid to build up. This could be due to problems with his mouth, neck, or stomach, or to neurological conditions, but often the cause is unknown. Oligohydramnios—meaning too little amniotic fluid—can be due to a leak from premature rupture of the membranes, not enough blood flow through the placenta, or abnormalities of the fetus's urinary system (because the amniotic fluid consists mostly of fetal urine). When blood flow through the placenta is inadequate, it can lead to poor growth and fetal distress, and prompt an elective preterm delivery. You can read more about conditions affecting the amount of amniotic fluid and ways to treat them on pages 44–45.

* **Preeclampsia.** Preeclampsia is a disease that occurs only during pregnancy. If you have preeclampsia, your blood pressure will be high and you'll have protein in your urine. Preeclampsia causes blood vessels to tighten, including those going to the placenta, so it can reduce the amount of blood that goes to the fetus, which can impede his growth and development. If it's severe, preeclampsia can also cause life-threatening complications for the mother. Preeclampsia is the most common reason for an elective preterm delivery. Fortunately, it always goes away after delivery, usually in just a few days (you can read more about preeclampsia on page 14).

* **Fetal growth restriction.** If a baby is growing poorly in the womb, it usually means that he isn't getting enough nutrients and oxygen. If the problem is severe, it can cause damage to him, or even lead to stillbirth. Your obstetrician may opt for an elective delivery to prevent these risks, or preterm labor and delivery may occur spontaneously.

Infection

Almost any severe infection in a pregnant woman can be a threat to both mother and fetus, and can lead to a preterm delivery. If you develop an infection, the odds are that you will still carry your pregnancy to term. However, there are some hidden infections that are believed to be responsible for a large number of preterm births. For example, research has linked bacteria that normally live in a woman's genitourinary tract to low-grade infections of the fetal membranes, placenta, and uterus. These cause inflammation, which over several weeks or months can lead to preterm labor or premature rupture of the membranes (see page 27).

Chronic Disease in the Mother

If you have a chronic illness, you should discuss with your doctor how it might affect your pregnancy. Many illnesses, if not severe, don't cause substantial problems. But some chronic maternal diseases can disrupt the growth and development of the fetus or can get worse in the mother during pregnancy because of the bodily changes that occur. Sometimes a mother needs a medication that she stops taking while she's pregnant because it is dangerous to the developing baby. Her pregnancy may then be electively cut short so she can safely take her medicine again. Probably the two most common chronic diseases that lead to premature birth are diabetes and high blood pressure.

* **Diabetes.** If you have diabetes (type 1, type 2, or gestational diabetes, which is diagnosed during pregnancy), you're more likely to develop high blood pressure or preeclampsia, either of which can cause dangerous complications in you or your baby that prompt an elective preterm delivery. Diabetes itself can affect a baby's growth in the womb: Most commonly, it makes him grow too fast because of the excessive sugar in his mother's blood, but occasionally, if the diabetes is long-standing and severe, blood flow to the placenta can be inadequate and a fetus's growth can be slowed. You will be closely monitored throughout pregnancy and counseled about how you should change your diet, exercise, and insulin injections, if needed. The good news is that women with diabetes can usually control their blood sugar enough so that no harm comes to them or their baby. Sometimes an elective preterm delivery is done a few weeks before term to avoid a difficult delivery (if the baby has grown too big from all that sugar) or to

protect a mother and baby from serious health problems. You can read more about diabetes on page 15.

* **High blood pressure.** High blood pressure can be an isolated problem, or it can accompany heart disease, kidney disease, or other medical complications. High blood pressure can lead to prematurity because it can damage the placenta, or because continuing the pregnancy in the face of a severe underlying disease is harmful to the mother or to the fetus. Women who already have high blood pressure are at greater risk of developing preeclampsia, which often necessitates a premature delivery.

Abnormalities of the Fetus

Approximately two or three babies in a hundred are born with a major birth defect. Premature labor and delivery is common, often because these congenital conditions are associated with other risk factors, such as too much or too little amniotic fluid, poor fetal growth, a chronic maternal disease, or infection. Sometimes, though, the reason for preterm delivery is unknown. If you find out that your baby has a serious abnormality, you and your doctor will make plans for the best possible treatment for both you and your baby before, during, and after delivery.

Lifestyle choices

You can read more about the following lifestyle choices and others that have been linked to prematurity on page 11.

* **Smoking.** Smoking reduces blood flow to the placenta and thus oxygen to the fetus, causing poor fetal growth. It is directly linked to preterm rupture of membranes and premature birth. Cigarette smoke and nicotine also increase the chance of placental abruption and

placenta previa. Keep in mind that it's never too late for quitting to make a difference: Cutting back on the number of cigarettes you smoke, even in the second half of your pregnancy, can reduce your risk.

* **Drinking alcohol.** Women who have more than seven drinks a week during pregnancy have a higher risk of preterm deliveries than those who completely abstain. Alcohol in the first trimester is also linked to birth defects and later on can cause poor fetal growth, although an occasional small glass of wine at dinner or at a social gathering isn't going to harm your baby.

* **Recreational drug use.** Cocaine and amphetamines can cause preterm birth as well as poor fetal growth and birth defects. Cocaine also raises the risk of placental abruption. Other kinds of illicit drugs, including marijuana and heroin, don't increase the chance of a premature delivery, but if they're used regularly they can stunt a baby's growth in the womb or cause withdrawal symptoms after birth, so they're best avoided during pregnancy.

* **Sexual activity.** In general, sex during pregnancy isn't associated with a higher risk for prematurity. Still, most obstetricians will advise you to avoid sexual intercourse if you've had episodes of premature labor, rupture of membranes, or bleeding. That's because an orgasm can stimulate uterine contractions, and sex can cause some minor injury to your cervix or spread infection into your uterus, and the resulting inflammation could contribute to a preterm birth.

Ethnicity and Social Factors

* **Ethnicity.** Black women in the United States have a higher rate of preterm birth than Hispanic and Caucasian women of the same socioeconomic level. The reasons aren't well understood and are being actively investigated, but

probably involve a mixture of physical (including genetic), social, and other environmental factors (you can read more on page 10).

* **Little or no prenatal care.** Overall, women who are poorer and have less education are more likely to have premature babies. Because many social and behavioral risk factors go together, it's hard to evaluate the role of each one separately, but receiving little or no prenatal care by an obstetrician or midwife during pregnancy does raise the risk of a preterm delivery. However, attempts to make prenatal care more available have not been successful in reducing rates of prematurity.

Maternal Weight and Age

* **Low maternal weight.** Women who weigh less than 100 pounds at the start of pregnancy or who gain too little weight during pregnancy have an increased chance of delivering prematurely. Maternal malnutrition can also impair the fetus's growth. Your obstetrician will check on your weight gain throughout pregnancy, and if it isn't sufficient, he will counsel you to eat more or better. Never take the initiative of adding vitamins, minerals, or supplements to your diet without your doctor's permission, though, because some supplements, especially in large quantities, can harm your baby.

* **Overweight.** If you're overweight but don't have one of the other risk factors for prematurity, you're most likely going to deliver a healthy baby at term. But overweight women are at higher risk for diabetes and high blood pressure, both of which increase the chances of a premature birth.

* **Age younger than 18 or older than 40 years.** If you're in one of these age groups but don't have other risk factors for prematurity, your chance of having a premature baby is increased but by only a small amount.

APPENDIX 2

CONVERSION CHARTS FOR WEIGHT AND TEMPERATURE

How Many Pounds? How Many Grams?

Weight Conversion from Pounds to Grams

Ounces	0	1	2	3	4	5	6	7	8	9	10	11	12	13	14	15
Lbs. 0	—	28	57	85	113	142	170	198	227	255	283	312	340	369	397	425
1	454	482	510	539	567	595	624	652	680	709	737	765	794	822	850	879
2	907	936	964	992	1021	1049	1077	1106	1134	1162	1191	1219	1247	1276	1304	1332
3	1361	1389	1417	1446	1474	1502	1531	1559	1588	1616	1644	1673	1701	1729	1758	1786
4	1814	1843	1871	1899	1928	1956	1984	2013	2041	2070	2098	2126	2155	2183	2211	2240
5	2268	2296	2325	2353	2381	2410	2438	2466	2495	2523	2551	2580	2608	2637	2665	2693
6	2722	2750	2778	2807	2835	2863	2892	2920	2948	2977	3005	3033	3062	3090	3118	3147
7	3175	3203	3232	3260	3289	3317	3345	3374	3402	3430	3459	3487	3515	3544	3572	3600
8	3629	3657	3685	3714	3742	3770	3799	3827	3856	3884	3912	3941	3969	3997	4026	4054
9	4082	4111	4139	4167	4196	4224	4252	4281	4309	4337	4366	4394	4423	4451	4479	4508
10	4536	4564	4593	4621	4649	4678	4706	4734	4763	4791	4819	4848	4876	4904	4933	4961
11	4990	5018	5046	5075	5103	5131	5160	5188	5216	5245	5273	5301	5330	5358	5386	5415
12	5443	5471	5500	5528	5557	5585	5613	5642	5670	5698	5727	5755	5783	5812	5840	5868
13	5897	5925	5953	5982	6010	6038	6067	6095	6123	6152	6180	6209	6237	6265	6294	6322
14	6350	6379	6407	6435	6464	6492	6520	6549	6577	6605	6634	6662	6690	6719	6747	6776
15	6804	6832	6860	6889	6917	6945	6973	7002	7030	7059	7087	7115	7144	7172	7201	7228

How Many Degrees Fahrenheit? How Many Degrees Celsius?

Temperature Conversion from Fahrenheit to Celsius

To convert from °F to °C: (°F – 32) ÷ 1.8 = °C		To convert from °C to °F: (°C × 1.8) + 32 = °F	
Degrees Fahrenheit	**Degrees Celsius**	**Degrees Fahrenheit**	**Degrees Celsius**
93.2	34.0	101.5	38.6
93.6	34.2	101.8	38.8
93.9	34.4	102.2	39.0
94.3	34.6	102.6	39.2
94.6	34.8	102.9	39.4
95.0	35.0	103.3	39.6
95.4	35.2	103.6	39.8
95.7	35.4	104.0	40.0
96.1	35.6	104.4	40.2
96.4	35.8	104.7	40.4
96.8	36.0	105.2	40.6
97.2	36.2	105.4	40.8
97.5	36.4	105.9	41.0
97.9	36.6	106.1	41.2
98.2	36.8	106.5	41.4
98.6	37.0	106.8	41.6
99.0	37.2	107.2	41.8
99.3	37.4	107.6	42.0
99.7	37.6	108.0	42.2
100.0	37.8	108.3	42.4
100.4	38.0	108.7	42.6
100.8	38.2	109.0	42.8
101.1	38.4	109.4	43.0

APPENDIX 3

GROWTH CHARTS

Weight and Gestational Age at Birth

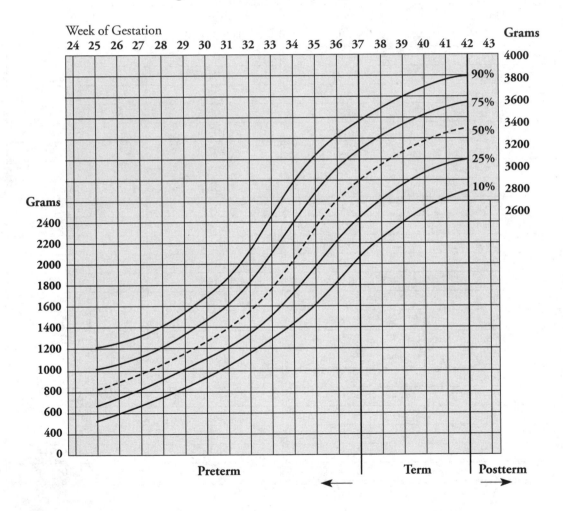

Adapted with permission from Lubchenco LO, Hansman C, and Boyd E: *Pediatrics* 37:403, © American Academy of Pediatrics 1966, and from Battaglia FC and Lubchenco LO: *Journal of Pediatrics* 71:159, © Mosby 1967

Growth in the Womb

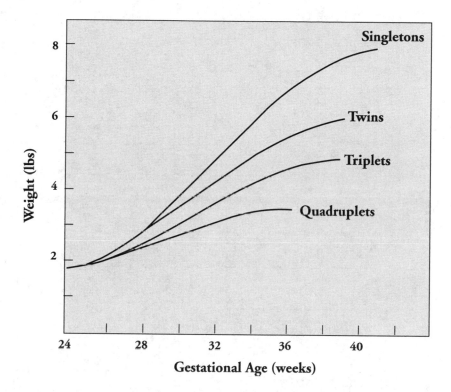

Adapted with permission from McKeown T, Record RG: Observation on foetal growth in multiple pregnancy in man, *Journal of Endo-crinology* 8:386, 1952

Growth from Birth to Age 3 for Premature Girls Who Weighed Less than 1,500 Grams at Birth

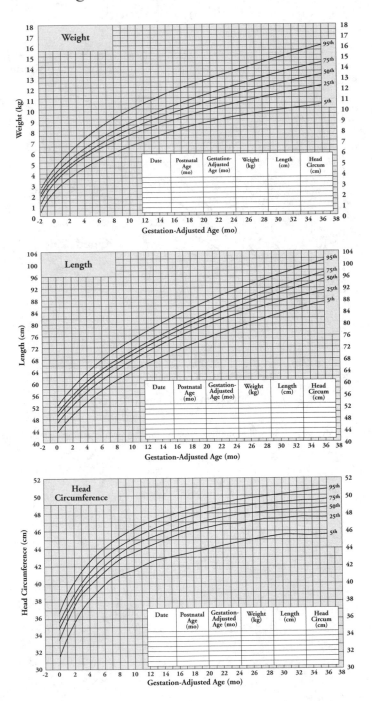

Chart provided by Ross Products Division, Abbott Laboratories, Columbus, OH

Growth from Birth to Age 3 for Premature Girls Who Weighed 1,500–2,500 Grams at Birth

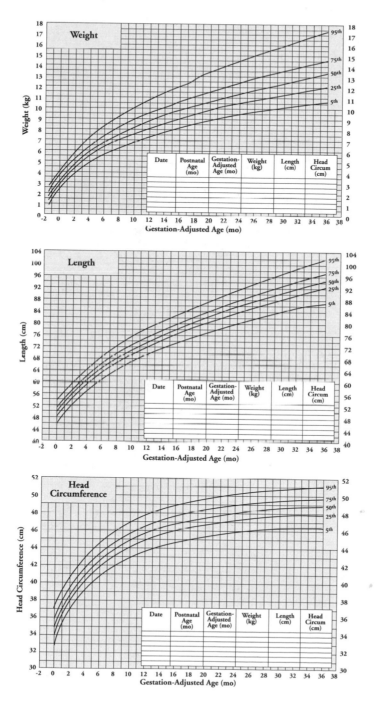

Chart provided by Ross Products Division, Abbott Laboratories, Columbus, OH

Growth from Birth to Age 3 for Premature Boys Who Weighed Less than 1,500 Grams at Birth

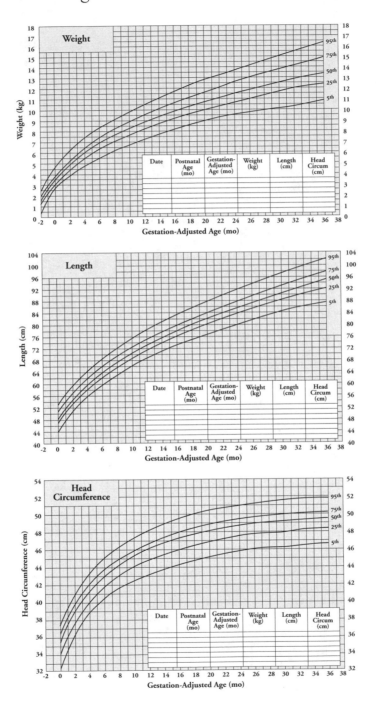

Chart provided by Ross Products Division, Abbott Laboratories, Columbus, OH

Growth from Birth to Age 3 for Premature Boys Who Weighed 1,500–2,500 Grams at Birth

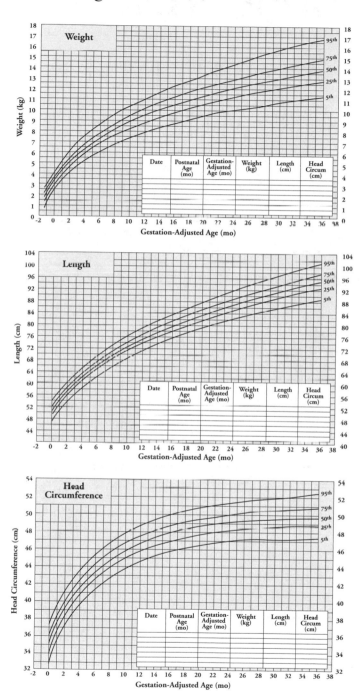

Chart provided by Ross Products Division, Abbott Laboratories, Columbus, OH

APPENDIX 4

A SCHEDULE FOR MULTIPLES

Date _____

Triplet A

Time	Feeding			Diaper	
	Nurse	Food	Formula	Urine	Bowel
12:00					
1:00					
2:00					
3:00					
4:00					
5:00					
6:00					
7:00					
8:00					
9:00					
10:00					
11:00					
12:00					
1:00					
2:00					
3:00					
4:00					
5:00					
6:00					
7:00					
8:00					
9:00					
10:00					
11:00					

Triplet B

Time	Feeding			Diaper	
	Nurse	Food	Formula	Urine	Bowel
12:00					
1:00					
2:00					
3:00					
4:00					
5:00					
6:00					
7:00					
8:00					
9:00					
10:00					
11:00					
12:00					
1:00					
2:00					
3:00					
4:00					
5:00					
6:00					
7:00					
8:00					
9:00					
10:00					
11:00					

Triplet C

Time	Feeding			Diaper	
	Nurse	Food	Formula	Urine	Bowel
12:00					
1:00					
2:00					
3:00					
4:00					
5:00					
6:00					
7:00					
8:00					
9:00					
10:00					
11:00					
12:00					
1:00					
2:00					
3:00					
4:00					
5:00					
6:00					
7:00					
8:00					
9:00					
10:00					
11:00					

Reprinted with permission of MOST (Mothers of Supertwins), Inc., Brentwood, NY

APPENDIX 5

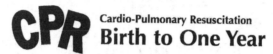 **Cardio-Pulmonary Resuscitation**
Birth to One Year

If not alone, send someone to **call 911**

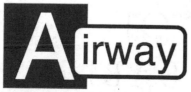**irway**

(1) Position Head - Open Airway
(2) Look - Listen - Feel for Breathing

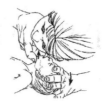

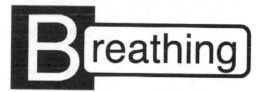**reathing**

(1) Cover nose and mouth
(2) Give 2 slow breaths
(3) Watch for chest to rise

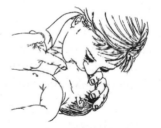

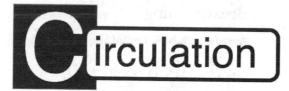**irculation**

(1) Check for signs of circulation

(2) If circulation is present, give 1 breath every
3 seconds (20 breaths / minute)

(3) If no circulation, start 30 chest compressions to
2 breaths (100 times / minute)

If alone, after 5 cycles of 30 compressions to
2 breaths (about 2 minutes) **call 911**

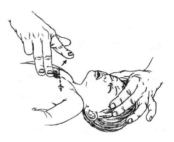

APPENDIX 6

RESOURCES FOR PARENTS OF PREMATURE BABIES

These are some organizations, web sites, and books that may be helpful to you. We do not endorse these listings, and the views expressed in them are not necessarily our own; we merely offer them to give you some leads to the many resources that are available. The phone numbers and web site addresses are correct at the time we are writing this book, but may change over time.

Allergy Products

Allergy Control Products (sells facemasks and other products for children and adults with allergies)
Danbury, CT
(800) ALL-ERGY (255-3749)
www.allergycontrol.com

Allergy Free Shop (sells facemasks and other products for children and adults with allergies)
Miami, FL
(877) 212-2828 or (305) 254-2828
www.allergyfreeshop.com

Breastfeeding

Ameda (sells breast pumps)
Lincolnshire, IL
(866) 99-AMEDA (866-992-6332)
www.ameda.com

Human Milk Banking Association of North America (provides information about milk banking and how milk is processed, how to order milk, and how to become a donor)
Raleigh, NC
(919) 861-4560
www.hmbana.org

International Lactation Consultant Association (to locate a breastfeeding consultant)
Morrisville, NC
(919) 861-5577
www.ilca.org

La Leche League (provides information and support for mothers who are breastfeeding, and helps to locate a breastfeeding consultant)
(877) 4-LALECHE (877-452-5324)
www.lllusa.org

Medela Inc. (sells breast pumps)
McHenry, IL
(800) 435-8316
www.medelabreastfeedingus.com

Cerebral Palsy

Finnie's Handling the Young Child with Cerebral Palsy at Home by **Eva Bower** (ed.), **Butterworth-Heinemann, 2008** (a book that addresses common, everyday situations and emotions to help parents manage them)

National Institute of Neurological Disorders and Stroke (provides information on cerebral palsy, including available treatments and research)
Bethesda, MD
(800) 352-9424 or (301) 496-5751
www.ninds.nih.gov/disorders/cerebral_palsy/detail_cerebral_palsy.htm

United Cerebral Palsy (offers broad information and support for people with CP and other disabilities)
Washington, D.C.
(800) 872-5827 or (202) 776-0406
www.ucp.org

Child Care

Child Care Aware (helps families locate child care programs in their communities and provides information on options, financing, and more)
Arlington, VA
(800) 424-2246
www.childcareaware.org

Clothes and Supplies

Amazon.com (sells a wide range of clothing and supplies for preemies—you can search for "preemies," "preemie clothes," "preemie diapers," "infant car bed," and more)
www.amazon.com

Children's Medical Ventures (sells products designed to enhance the development of premature babies, such as special pacifiers, positioning aids, isolette covers, and diapers)
Monroeville, PA
(888) 766-8443
www.childmed.com

Earlybirds (sells organic and cotton clothing designed for preemies)
New Brighton, MN
www.earlybirdsbabywear.com

Jacqui's Preemie Pride (sells cotton clothing designed for preemies)
Smithsburg, MD
(888) 245-1715
www.jacquispreemiepride.com

The Preemie Store . . . and more (sells a wide range of preemie clothes and other products from numerous suppliers)
www.preemie.com

Zutano (sells hip, colorful clothing designed for preemies)
www.zutano.com

Early Intervention

Early Intervention Support (offers information on early intervention and parenting tips for behavior and developmental challenges; sells products for parents raising special needs children)
www.earlyinterventionsupport.com

First Signs (helps educate parents and professionals about the early warning signs of autism and related disorders)
Merrimac, MA
(978) 346-4380
www.firstsigns.org

NECTAC (National Early Childhood Technical Assistance Center) (offers information on federally supported early intervention services for infants and toddlers, and on preschool special education; provides contact information for your state's programs)
Chapel Hill, NC
(919) 962-2001
www.nectac.org

Feeding Issues and Tube Feeding

Child of Mine: Feeding with Love and Good Sense (2nd ed) by Ellyn Satter, Bull Publishing, 2000 (a book that covers nutrition, feeding issues, and the feeding relationship from pregnancy through childhood)

Deceptively Delicious: Simple Secrets to Get Your Kids Eating Good Food by Jessica Seinfeld, William Morrow, 2007 (a cookbook that provides recipes stealthily packed with vegetables)

Feeding and Nutrition for the Child with Special Needs by Marsha Dunn Klein and Tracy Delaney, Pro-Ed, 2006 (a collection of information sheets that explain the major medical issues and feeding equipment, and offer guidance on dealing with children with feeding challenges)

How to Get Your Kid to Eat . . . But Not too Much by Ellyn Satter, Bull Publishing, 1987 (a book that provides information and guidance on how to handle children with feeding problems)

Mealtime Notions LLC (offers advice and resources for families whose children have special feeding issues and mealtime challenges, and provides recipes for homemade food for tube feeding)
Tucson, AZ
(520) 829-9635
www.mealtimenotions.com

New Visions (offers information, equipment, and educational workshops for parents and professionals dealing with children with feeding problems)
Faber, VA 22938
(800) 606-7112 or (434) 361-2285
www.new-vis.com

Parenting Tips: How to Sneak Vegetables into Your Child's Diet (a web site that provides recipes with hidden vegetables)
http://www.essortment.com/family/parentingtipsh_sasb.htm

The Sneaky Chef: Simple Strategies for Hiding Healthy Food in Kids' Favorite Meals by Missy Chase Lapine, Running Press, 2007 (a cookbook that provides recipes with disguised healthy ingredients)

Financial Assistance

Benefits for Children with Disabilities (a federal web site that offers information and links to many kinds of assistance for families who have a child with a disability)
www.disability.gov/benefits/social_security_cash
_benefit_programs/benefits_for_children_with
_disabilities

Insure Kids Now (a federal web site and hotline that provides information on government health insurance programs for children, Medicaid, and Children's Health Insurance Program [CHIP]; your baby may be eligible if you cannot afford private health insurance)
(877) KIDSNOW (877-543-7669)
www.insurekidsnow.gov

Social Security Online (a federal web site that provides the information needed to apply for SSI, or Supplementary Security Income, for which you may be eligible based on your baby's birth weight or medical history and your financial resources)
(800) 772-1213
www.ssa.gov/pubs/10026.html

For other information on financial assistance, including Katie Beckett funds (making Medicaid available to children with disabilities who are cared for at home) and any public or private sources within your state for which you might be eligible, the best approach is to contact your hospital's social worker, even after your baby has left the NICU.

GE Reflux

PAGER, or Pediatric/Adolescent Gastroesophageal Reflux Association (offers information and support on reflux)
Silver Spring, MD
(301) 601-9541
www.reflux.org

Hearing Impairments

Alexander Graham Bell Association for the Deaf and Hard of Hearing (provides broad information on hearing loss, financial aid resources, and support for parents of children who are deaf or hard of hearing)
Washington, DC
(202) 337-5220
www.agbell.org

American Speech-Language-Hearing Association (offers information on services, health insurance benefits, and how to locate an ASHA-certified pediatric audiologist or speech-language pathologist in your area)
Rockville, MD
(800) 638-8255
www.asha.org/public/

The Children's Hearing Institute (offers support and educational programs for infants and children with hearing loss or profound deafness, focusing on those who can be helped with cochlear implant technology)
New York, NY
(646) 438-7819
www.childrenshearing.org

Gallaudet University (a university and research center for the deaf and hard of hearing; its web site provides broad information on hearing loss)
Washington, DC
(202) 651-5000
www.gallaudet.edu

The Listen Up Web (provides information, educational programs, resources, and support for parents with hearing impaired children)
www.listen-up.org

SilkaWear (sells bonnets specially designed to keep hearing aids in place)
Perth Road Village, Ontario
(866) 211-3107
www.silkawear.com

High-Risk Pregnancy

High-Risk Pregnancy (information provided by the U.S. National Library of Medicine and the National Institutes of Health)
www.nlm.nih.gov/medlineplus/
highriskpregnancy.html

Sidelines (offers information and support for women going through a complicated pregnancy or on bed rest)
Laguna Beach, CA
(888) HI-RISK4 (888-447-4754)
www.sidelines.org

Home Health Care

Aaron's Tracheostomy Page (provides information on home care and support for parents who have a child with a tracheostomy)
www.tracheostomy.com

Access to Respite Care Help (ARCH) (provides information on respite care and helps parents locate respite services in their area)
Chapel Hill, NC
(919) 490-5577
http://chtop.org/ARCH.html

United Ostomy Associations of America (offers information, teaching material, and support for parents whose child has an enterostomy)
Fairview, TN
(800) 826-0826
http://www.uoa.org

Hydrocephalus

Hydrocephalus Association (provides information, parent support, and resources on hydrocephalus)
San Francisco, CA
(888) 598-3789 or (415) 732-7040
www.hydroassoc.org

Learning Disabilities

International Dyslexia Association (provides information, services, and support for families dealing with dyslexia and related difficulties in learning to read and write)
Baltimore, MD
(410) 296-0232
www.interdys.org

Learning Disabilities Association of America (provides information and support on learning disabilities, negotiating the special education process, and helping your child and yourself)
Pittsburgh, PA
(412) 341-1515
www.ldanatl.org

Attention Deficit Disorder Association (offers information and support on attention deficit disorders)
Wilmington, DE
(800) 939-1019
www.add.org

National Center for Learning Disabilities (provides information, support, and resources on learning disabilities)
New York, NY
(888) 575-7373 or (212) 545-7510
www.ncld.org

Loss and Grief

Center for Loss in Multiple Birth, or CLIMB (offers support for parents who have lost one of their twins, triplets, or higher-order multiples)
Anchorage, AK
(907) 222-5321
www.climb-support.org

The Compassionate Friends (offers support for parents who have lost a child of any age)
Oak Brook, IL
(877) 969-0010 or (630) 990 0010
www.compassionatefriends.org

Hygeia Foundation (offers support and numerous projects, including shared poetry, for parents who have lost a baby during pregnancy or after birth)
Woodbridge, CT
(800) 893-9198
www.hygeiafoundation.org

Now I Lay Me Down to Sleep (a national network of photographers who donate their services to preserve photographic memories of babies who die in the hospital)
www.nowilaymedowntosleep.org

Share (offers support for parents who have lost a baby during pregnancy or after birth)
St. Charles, MO
(800) 821-6819 or (636) 947-6164
www.nationalshare.org

When Bad Things Happen to Good People by Harold S. Kushner, Anchor, 2004 (a book by a theologian and father who faced his own son's fatal illness, and addressed the question so many parents ask: "Why us?")

Massage

International Loving Touch Foundation (offers training and information on infant and preemie massage)
Portland, OR
(800) 929-7492 or (503) 253-8482
www.lovingtouch.com

Touch Research Institute (conducts research on preemie massage and offers books and workshops on how to massage preemies)
Miami, FL
(305) 243-6781
www.miami.edu/touch-research

Preemie Issues (Various)

Dear Zoe: Letters to my Miracle Grandchild by Max De Pree, HarperCollins, 1999 (a book of letters from the author to his premature granddaughter, exploring issues of love, perfection, and faith)

March of Dimes (offers extensive information and support for parents during the NICU days and afterwards, funds research, and conducts national advocacy on prematurity)
White Plains, NY
(914) 997-4488
www.marchofdimes.com/prematurity

March of Dimes Share Your Story (an online community and discussion forum for parents of premature babies)
www.shareyourstory.org

Outcome data for extremely premature babies, offered by National Institute of Child Health and Human Development (a web site that provides statistics predicting outcomes for babies born from 22 weeks through 25 weeks of gestation who do not have genetic disorders or major birth defects. You'll need to know your baby's gestational age, weight, sex, whether she is a singleton or multiple, and whether you received steroid shots to boost her maturity while she was still in the womb. Be sure to get your doctor's help in interpreting the statistics you receive, and keep in mind that any predictions about a preemie's long-term outcome are only estimates.)
www.nichd.nih.gov/about/org/cdbpm/pp/prog
_epbo/epbo_case.cfm

Premature: **poems by Scott Landsbaum** (a collection of poems written while the author's premature niece and nephew were hospitalized in a neonatal intensive care unit; expresses emotions and reactions to medical technology, resilience, and the power of life)
www.prematurepoems.com

Speeches by Michael T. Hynan (a psychologist and father of a preemie offers insights into how parents cope emotionally with a high-risk birth)
https://pantherfile.uwm.edu/hynan/www/LIFER
.html
https://pantherfile.uwm.edu/hynan/www/MIN
NAEP.html

Treasured Memories, **by Rebecca A. Niestrath** (a comprehensive baby journal for parents of premature and sick babies)
www.amazon.com/Treasured-Memories-Rebecca
-Niestrath/dp/0967474000/ref=cm_lmf_tit_7
_rsrsrs0

Sensory Processing

Sensory Processing Disorder Foundation (offers information, educational programs, and support for parents of children with sensory processing disorder, including a guide to services in your area)
Greenwich Village, CO
(303) 794-1182
www.spdfoundation.net/

Sibling Issues

No Bigger than My Teddy Bear, **by Valerie Pankow, Family Books, 2004** (a picture book that introduces the intensive care nursery to young children)

Rosie and Tortoise, **by Margaret Wild and Ron Brooks, DK Children, 1999** (a picture book that features Rosie the hare, who is afraid to hold her premature baby brother)

Sibling Support Project (a national program that offers information, resources, and support groups for siblings of children with special needs)
Seattle, WA
(206) 297-6368
www.siblingsupport.org

Special Needs

Achievement Products (sells exercise tools and other products for children with special needs)
Carol Stream, IL
(800) 373-4699
www.specialkidszone.com

Breakthrough Parenting for Children with Special Needs: Raising the Bar of Expectations by Judy Winter, Jossey-Bass, 2006 (a book that guides parents on how to work with professionals, understand the law, plan for the future, and help their children with special needs reach their full potential)

Child Development Media (sells videos, books, and instruction material on child development and children with special needs)
Van Nuys, CA
(800) 405-8942 or (818) 989-7221
www.childdevelopmentmedia.com

The Child with Special Needs: Encouraging Intellectual and Emotional Growth by Stanley I. Greenspan, Serena Wieder, and Robin Simons, Perseus Books, 1998 (a book that provides guidance on how to identify a child's capacities and challenges, and encourage emotional and intellectual development)

Dragonfly Toys Co. (sells toys for children with special play needs, and aids for daily living)
www.dragonflytoys.com/

Family Village (an online directory of resources for children with special needs and their families, with topics from assistive technology, legal rights and legislation, to special education, recreational opportunities, helpful products, and medical information)
www.familyvillage.wisc.edu

Internet Resources for Special Children (a web site that provides links to sites for numerous disabilities)
www.irsc.org/disability.htm

More than a Mom: Living a Full and Balanced Life When Your Child Has Special Needs by **Heather Fawcett and Amy Baskin, Woodbine House, 2006** (a guide to carving out a fulfilling life while coping with the challenges of mothering a child with developmental disabilities, based on mothers' experiences)

National Dissemination Center for Children with Disabilities (a national source of information on disabilities in children of all ages, including special education and legal rights, in English and Spanish)
Washington, DC
(800) 695-0285 or (202) 884-8200
www.nichcy.org

Nobody's Perfect—Living and Growing with Children Who Have Special Needs by Nancy B. Miller with "The Moms": Susie Burmester, Diane G. Callahan, Janet Dieterle, and Stephanie Niedermeyer, Brookes Publishing, 1994 (a guide through the process of adapting to having a child with special needs, including personal reflections from four mothers)

The Special Child: A Source Book for Parents of Children with Developmental Disabilities by Siegfried M. Pueschel, Patricia S. Scola, Leslie E. Weidenman, and James C. Bernier, Brookes Publishing, 1994 (a home reference book on detection, prognosis, and treatment of children's disabilities, also providing information on education, intervention, and advocacy)

Special Kids Need Special Parents: A Resource for Parents of Children with Special Needs by Judith Loseff Lavin, Berkley Publishing, 2001 (an informational and inspirational manual based on interviews with healthcare professionals, therapists, educators, celebrities, parents, and special children)

Uncommon Fathers: Reflections on Raising a Child with a Disability by Donald J. Mayer (ed.), Woodbine House, 1995 (a collection of essays by fathers about the life-altering experience of having a child with a disability, helpful to fathers but also to their partners and families)

When Your Child Has a Disability: The Complete Sourcebook of Daily and Medical Care, Revised Edition by Mark L. Batshaw (ed.), Brookes Publishing, 2001 (a book that offers information and advice on the daily and long-term care issues of parenting a child with special needs)

You Will Dream New Dreams: Inspiring Personal Stories by Parents of Children with Disabilities by Stanley D. Klein and Kim Schive (eds.), Kensington Books, 2001 (a collection of real-life stories on healing, coping, surviving, and being happy again told by parents of children with disabilities)

Twins and Other Multiples

Mothers of Supertwins, or MOST (offers support, advice, and resources for parents of triplets, quadruplets, and more)
East Islip, NY
(631) 859-1110
www.mostonline.org

National Organization of Mothers of Twins Clubs (can connect you to a local multiples club, and offers information and advice regarding multiples)
Franklin, TN
(248) 231-4480
www.nomotc.org

Triplet Connection (offers advice and support, and sells practical information packets for expectant and new parents of triplets, quadruplets, and more)
Spring City, UT
(435) 851-1105
www.tripletconnection.org

Twins Magazine (a national magazine that focuses on topics relating to multiples)
Fort Collins, CO
(888) 55-TWINS (888-558-9467) or
(970) 377-1392
www.twinsmagazine.com

Twin-Twin Transfusion Syndrome

Twin to Twin Transfusion Syndrome Foundation (offers information and emotional and financial support to families dealing with twin-twin transfusion syndrome)
Bay Village, OH
(800) 815-9211 or (440) 899-8887
www.tttsfoundation.org

Visual Impairments

American Foundation for the Blind (provides information and resources for families and professionals, relating to visual impairment)
New York, NY
(800) AFB-LINE (800-232-5463) or
(212) 502-7600
www.afb.org

American Printing House for the Blind (offers books, games, toys, and aids for daily living for the visually impaired)
Louisville, KY
(800) 223-1839 or (502) 895-2405
www.aph.org

Family Connect (a joint web site by American Foundation for the Blind and National Association for Parents of Children with Visual Impairments that offers support, advice, a toy guide, and other resources for parents)
www.familyconnect.org

Hadley School for the Blind (offers free, distance courses for families on raising and educating children who are visually impaired)
Winnetka, IL
(800) 323-4238 or (847) 446-8111
www.hadley.edu

National Association for Parents of Children with Visual Impairments (offers information, support, and a phone referral service to more specialized information or services needed by parents for their children with visual impairment)
Watertown, MA
(800) 562-6265 or (617) 972-7441
www.spedex.com/napvi

National Library Service for the Blind and Physically Handicapped (offers a lending library of children's Braille and audio books circulated throughout the U.S. by postage-free mail)
Washington, DC
(888) NLS-READ (888-657-7323) or (202) 707-5100
www.loc.gov/nls/children/index.html

Seedlings Braille Books for Children (offers a large selection of Braille books to purchase, for children ranging from pre-readers through age 14)
Livonia, MI
(800) 777-8552 or (734) 427-8552
www.seedlings.org

INDEX

Page numbers in italics refer to illustrations.

ABOUT THE AUTHORS

DANA WECHSLER LINDEN, a journalist, was a senior editor at *Forbes* magazine when she gave birth to premature twins. She lives in New York City with her husband and two daughters.

EMMA TRENTI PAROLI, a medical news writer, has authored cover stories for *L'Espresso* and other leading publications. She and Dana met when their children shared the same room in the neonatal intensive care unit. Emma lives in New York City with her husband and son.

MIA WECHSLER DORON, M.D., a neonatalogist at the Newborn Critical Care Center at the University of North Carolina at Chapel Hill, is Dana's sister. In addition to caring for patients, she conducts clinical research, teaches, and writes on ethics and medical decision making. Mia lives in North Carolina with her husband and daughter.